# TARGETS AND EMERGING THERAPIES FOR SCHIZOPHRENIA

# TARGETS AND EMERGING THERAPIES FOR SCHIZOPHRENIA

Edited by

**JEFFREY S. ALBERT**
**MICHAEL W. WOOD**

WILEY

**A JOHN WILEY & SONS, INC., PUBLICATION**

Published by John Wiley & Sons, Inc., Hoboken, New Jersey
Published simultaneously in Canada



***Library of Congress Cataloging-in-Publication Data:***

Targets and emerging therapies for schizophrenia / edited by Jeffrey S. Albert, Michael W. Wood.
p. ; cm.
Includes bibliographical references and index.
ISBN 978-0-470-32282-6 (cloth)
I. Albert, Jeffrey S. II. Wood, Michael W. (Michael William), 1961-
[DNLM: 1. Schizophrenia–drug therapy. WM 203]

616.89'8061–dc23

2011051091

Printed in the United States of America

10 9 8 7 6 5 4 3 2 1

# CONTENTS

# PREFACE

When we began this project several years ago, we envisioned a collection of chapters that represented a summary view of a highly dynamic field and a body of work that would serve as a transient snapshot of the current state of research into new therapies for schizophrenia. The search for new treatments for schizophrenia was being robustly pursued by many pharmaceutical and biotechnology companies. New hypotheses in disease biology were being generated from the insights of gifted academic researchers. Substantial investments were being made toward the identification and validation of emerging drug targets arising from those insights. The field of schizophrenia research was teeming with opportunity and the clinical validation of promising treatment hypotheses seemed imminent. Since that time, the aura surrounding the research of emerging therapies for schizophrenia has changed considerably.

Expenditures in schizophrenia-focused drug discovery from larger pharmaceutical and biotechnology companies have been scaled back substantially. The combination of rising research and development costs, more challenging payer environments, and increasingly stringent regulatory hurdles has pushed schizophrenia-focused drug discovery toward the bottom of the risk/reward prioritization analysis advanced by industry consultants. In fact, investments in psychiatric drug discovery overall have suffered major cutbacks within industry. Moreover, the liquidity crisis in the global financial markets negatively impacted the funding of the smaller biotechnology firms, the sector that has traditionally driven the higher risk research investments exploring new therapies.

The liquidity crisis and the austere reaction to that crisis decreased the pool of money available to government granting agencies as well. Academic research in the area of schizophrenia continues, but funding is under constant threat. In addition, the funding of basic science research in many countries is confronted by public attitudes that do not appreciate the impact that these expenditures have on advancing the human condition, increasing the quality of life, and stimulating economic expansion. Moreover, in the particular case of spending on mental health research, there still exists an unwillingness to accept mental illness as a bona fide condition and a discipline worthy of research support.

The wholesale reduction in support for schizophrenia research does not stem from a lack of need for improved treatments for schizophrenia. Although the current treatment options are a major advancement over the primitive approaches to mental illness before pharmacotherapies, there remains ample opportunity for improvement. Many current therapies engender profound side effects and none treat all facets of the disease. The scientific understanding of schizophrenia will continue to evolve, and new hypotheses and novel targets will undoubtedly emerge from those findings. The need to translate these basic science findings into potential therapies in future looks to be addressed through creative, public–private partnerships, and philanthropic foundations. It remains to be seen whether these enterprises will be able to span the translation gap and fill the current void to effectively bring new therapies to patients. As new scientific frontiers are pushed back, there is some cause for hope that the basic understanding of the underlying biological mechanisms and the advance of new translational methodologies will reinvigorate investment into new, more effective therapies

Against a backdrop of diminishing investment in research and development for new therapies for schizophrenia, there is cause to consider what has been captured inside this collection of chapters. The organizing principle for the book was straightforward. We reasoned that since most drug discovery programs are traditionally focused on selectively modulating individual neurotransmitter systems, the book chapters could be arranged according to neurotransmitter systems. The collection begins by establishing the historical framework for neurotransmitter-based drug discovery in schizophrenia by examining the dopamine system. From there, individual dopamine receptors and an intracellular signaling method to modulate dopaminergic pathways are examined. The chapters that follow explore the predominant modern hypothesis of neurotransmitter-based deficits, the role of glutamatergic dysfunction. The progress on individual glutamate-based approaches is then reviewed. Finally, the chapters progress through several other important neurotransmitter systems being investigated as potential therapeutic targets; current serotoninergic, cholinergic, peptidergic, and γ-aminobutyric (GABA)ergic approaches are all discussed.

The authors that agreed to contribute their time and expertise to carefully construct and contribute their reviews were both diligent in their efforts and patient in their demeanor. In the end, they have effectively captured the state of affairs during a major paradigm shift in the field of schizophrenia research treatment. We hope that this book will be used as a starting point for future investigators. To that end, it is our sincere desire that readers will find this book both useful and inspiring. Most importantly, we hope that this snapshot will serve as a foundation for a field reinvigorated in the coming years and that future research built on this foundation will deliver new, more effective treatments for the serious and devastating illness schizophrenia.

JEFFREY S. ALBERT
MICHAEL W. WOOD

# CONTRIBUTORS

**Jeffrey S. Albert, PhD,** Department of Chemistry, CNS & Pain Innovative Medicines, AstraZeneca, Wilmington, DE, USA

**Alo Basu, PhD,** Department of Psychology, College of the Holy Cross, Worcester, MA, USA

**Michael Benneyworth, PhD,** Department of Pharmacology, University of Minnesota School of Medicine, Minneapolis, MN, USA

**Kevin N. Boyd, PhD,** Department of Pharmacology, Penn State Univerity College of Medicine, Hershey, PA, USA

**Thomas A. Comery, PhD,** Pfizer Worldwide Research & Development, Pfizer Inc., Groton, CT, USA

**Joseph T. Coyle, MD,** Department of Psychiatry, Harvard Medical School, The Laboratory of Molecular Psychiatry and Neuroscience, McLean Hospital, Belmont, MA, USA

**Alan J. Cross, PhD,** CNS & Pain Innovative Medicines Unit, AstraZeneca, Wilmington, DE, USA

**Lee A. Dawson, PhD,** Neurosciences PCU, Eisai Ltd, European Knowldege Centre, Hatfield, Herts, UK

**John Dunlop, PhD,** Pfizer Worldwide Research & Development, Pfizer Inc., Groton, CT, USA

**Roelof W. Feenstra,** Solvay Pharmaceuticals Research Laboratories, The Netherlands

**Christian C. Felder, PhD,** Neuroscience Discovery, Eli Lilly and Company, Lilly Corporate Center, Indianapolis, IN, USA

**Joseph I. Friedman, MD,** Department of Psychiatry, Mount Sinai School of Medicine, New York, NY, USA

**Jonathan Gross, PhD,** Cranbury, NJ, USA

**Mihály Hajós,** Yale University School of Medicine, New Haven, CT, USA

**Craig Jamieson, PhD,** Department of Medicinal Chemistry, Schering-Plough Corporation, Newhouse, Motherwell, UK

**Caitlin A. Jones, PhD,** Solvay Pharmaceuticals Research Laboratories, The Netherlands

**Aurelija Jucaite, MD, PhD,** CNS & Pain Innovative Medicines Unit, AstraZeneca, Södertälje, Sweden

**Isabella Kanellopoulou, MD,** Pilgrim Psychiatric Center, Clinical Neuroscience Center, W. Brentwood, NY and Manhattan Psychiatric Center, New York, NY, USA

**John H. Kehne,** Translational Neuropharmacology Consulting, LLC, Potomac, MD, USA

**Bruce J. Kinon,** Eli Lilly and Company, Lilly Corporate Center, Indianapolis, IN, USA

**Bin Liu, PhD,** Division of Chemistry and Research Technologies, Eli Lilly and Company, Lilly Corporate Center, Indianapolis, IN, USA

**Andrew C. McCreary, PhD,** Solvay Pharmaceuticals Research Laboratories, the Netherlands. Present Address: Brains On-Line, Groningen, the Netherlands

**David L. McKinzie, PhD,** Neuroscience Discovery, Eli Lilly and Company, Lilly Corporate Center, Indianapolis, IN, USA

**John K.F. Maclean, PhD,** Department of Medicinal Chemistry, Schering-Plough Corporation, Newhouse, Motherwell, UK

**Richard B. Mailman, PhD,** Departments of Pharmacology, Penn State University College of Medicine and Milton S. Hershey Medical Center, Hershey, PA, USA

**Gerard J. Marek, MD, PhD,** Abbott Laboratories, Abbott Park, IL, USA

**Karen L. Marquis,** Yardley, PA, USA

**George D. Maynard,** Axerion Therapeutics, New Haven, CT, USA

**James A. Monn, PhD,** Eli Lilly and Company, Lilly Corporate Center, Indianapolis, IN, USA

**John A. Morrow, PhD,** Department of Molecular Pharmacology, Schering-Plough Corporation, Newhouse, Motherwell, UK

**Vladan Novakovic, MD,** Pilgrim Psychiatric Center, Clinical Neuroscience Center, W. Brentwood, NY, and Manhattan Psychiatric Center, New York, NY, USA

**Svante Nyberg, MD, PhD,** CNS & Pain Innovative Medicines Unit, AstraZeneca, Södertälje, Sweden

**William J. Pitts, PhD,** Inflammation Chemistry, Bristol-Myers Squibb Co., Princeton, NJ, USA

**Bruce N. Rogers,** Pfizer Global Research & Development, Pfizer Inc., Groton, CT, USA

**Sharon Rosenzweig-Lipson, PhD,** IVS Pharma Consulting, LLC, East Brunswick, NJ, USA

**Lee E. Schechter,** Pfizer Worldwide Research & Development, Pfizer Inc., Groton, CT, USA

**Jeffrey M. Schkeryantz, PhD,** Eli Lilly and Company, Lilly Corporate Center, Indianapolis, IN, USA

**Judith A. Siuciak, PhD,** The Biomarkers Consortium, Foundation for the National Institutes of Health, Bethesda, MD, USA

**Richard C. Thompson, PhD,** Department of Chemistry, Tusculum College, Greeneville, TN, USA

**Paul W. Smith, PhD,** Novartis Institute for Tropical Diseases, Singapore

**Philip G. Strange, PhD,** Emeritus Professor of Pharmacology, University of Reading School of Pharmacy, Reading, UK

**Jeannette M. Watson, PhD,** Immune Targeting Systems Ltd, London, UK

**Michael W. Wood, PhD,** CNS & Pain Innovative Medicines Unit, AstraZeneca, Wilmington, DE, USA

# INTRODUCTION

ALAN J. CROSS

Schizophrenia is a severe and debilitating illness that is generally recognized as starting with a first diagnosis in young adulthood and lasts throughout the patient's lifetime, often with chronic progression. The incidence of schizophrenia in the general population is around 1%, and according to the World Health Organization [1], schizophrenia accounts for a significant proportion of the global burden of illness in terms of disability and mortality. The nature of schizophrenia, including fragmentation of personality, cognitive impairment, and inability to function, makes it a particularly damaging illness for patients, families, and the community.

For more than 50 years, pharmacotherapy of schizophrenia has relied on a single concept, the dopamine hypothesis [2, 3], based on the pioneering work of Carlsson and Linquist [4]. The so-called first- and second-generation antipsychotic drugs all incorporate an interaction with the dopamine $D_2$ receptor in their pharmacological properties, with differences in the degree of selectivity and the more recent introduction of partial agonism as variations on the theme. These drugs have well-defined antipsychotic properties and as such have had a tremendous impact on the treatment of schizophrenia. Despite this, it is equally well understood that antipsychotic drugs do not treat the entire spectrum of the illness, nor do all patients respond to these drugs. There thus remains a considerable unmet patient need, and novel approaches for the

*Targets and Emerging Therapies for Schizophrenia*, First Edition.
Edited by Jeffrey S. Albert and Michael W. Wood.

treatment of schizophrenia must address key areas such as cognitive deficits, negative symptoms, and poor response to current antipsychotics. Our understanding of the underlying neurobiology of schizophrenia is improving considerably, driven by the impact of genetics and neuroimaging studies. Genetic studies have identified a growing list of rare, highly penetrant structural variants many of which implicate genes involved in the development of the central nervous system (CNS) and in maintaining synaptic integrity and function [5]. Neuroimaging studies have provided the substrate for understanding abnormalities in neural circuitry and how these might underlie certain neuropsychological features of illness. These advances in our understanding of the disease biology offer hope that in the longer term, treatments may be devised which address the underlying neuropathological processes leading to the development and chronicity of illness, as well as addressing the heterogeneity of disease.

It is always tempting to speculate that disease-modifying treatments are on the horizon, but it is worth remembering that even in such well-defined neuropsychiatric illnesses as Huntington's disease, such breakthroughs have proven to be enigmatic. In the case of schizophrenia, it is clear that a great deal has to be done to fill the gap between understanding of genetic risk and identification of viable drug targets. Thus, emerging approaches to pharmacotherapy of schizophrenia rely less on an understanding of disease etiology and more on understanding changes in neurophysiology and neuropharmacology associated with the illness.

Although the dopamine hypothesis has been the cornerstone of therapeutics, our understanding of the neurobiology of dopaminergic systems and the relation to schizophrenia continues to advance, and there is scope remaining to produce improved treatments based on novel pharmacology relating to dopamine. It is clear, however, that dopamine-based approaches do not treat all features of the illness and many patients fail to respond to current antipsychotics, suggesting that alternative approaches are required. Some of the most promising approaches relate to the glutamate hypothesis, which, despite being formulated over 25 years ago, arguably has not been adequately tested in the clinic. It is to be hoped that novel glutamatergic pharmacological agents will provide the tools for adequately testing this very attractive hypothesis. Beyond this, a number of neurotransmitters systems clearly modulate the effects of dopamine. On listing these approaches one may comment that little has changed over the last few decades and indeed many of these neurotransmitters systems have been extensively reviewed in the context of involvement in schizophrenia. There are, however, several key changes worth noting, most importantly that the field has moved from formulating hypotheses to testing hypotheses using drug candidates with the appropriate pharmacology and drug-like properties to enable definitive clinical studies. Moreover, clinical and preclinical studies can be designed from a background of improved disease understanding, leading to the use of more relevant intermediate phenotypes, translational tools, and endpoints. It is encouraging that several of these emerging treatments are delivering positive signals in the clinic. Although much work still has to be done to understand how these therapies should be used optimally, it is clear that meaningful and novel pharmacological treatments for schizophrenia are moving closer to reality.

## REFERENCES


1. World Health Organization (2001) The World Health Report 2011: Mental Health: New Understanding, New Hope. World Health Organization: Geneva.
2. Crow, T.J. (1980). Positive and negative schizophrenic symptoms and the role of dopamine. *British Journal of Psychiatry*, *137*, 383–386.
3. Carlsson, A. (2002). The dopamine hypothesis of schizophrenia: new aspects. *Advances in Behavioral Biology*, *53*, 417–422.
4. Carlsson, A., Lindqvist, M. (1963). Effect of chlorpromazine or haloperidol on formation of 3-methoxytyramine and normetanephrine in mouse brain. *Acta Pharmacologica et Toxicologica*, *20*, 140–144.
5. Tam, G.W.C., Redon, R., Carter, N.P., Grant, S.G.N. (2009). The Role of DNA Copy Number Variation in Schizophrenia. *Biological Psychiatry*, *66*, 1005–1012.

# 1

# DOPAMINERGIC HYPOTHESIS OF SCHIZOPHRENIA: A HISTORICAL PERSPECTIVE

AURELIJA JUCAITE AND SVANTE NYBERG

In search of evidence for the dopamine hypothesis of schizophrenia, this review focuses on studies of patients with schizophrenia. The review is composed of two parts: the first serves as a short reminder of the anatomy and function of the dopamine system, and the second guides the reader through the history of scientific discoveries and paradigms used to investigate the role of dopamine in the pathophysiology of schizophrenia.

## 1.1 DOPAMINE SYSTEM: NEUROANATOMY AND MODE OF ACTIVITY

Dopamine is a phylogenetically old neurotransmitter intrinsic to brain function and behavior. It is of central importance in movement, reward-associated behavior, and emotions. Abnormal patterns of dopamine neurotransmission have been suggested to underlie several neurological and psychiatric disorders, for example, Parkinson's and Huntington's diseases, schizophrenia, drug abuse, and attention-deficit/hyperactivity disorder (ADHD).

*Targets and Emerging Therapies for Schizophrenia*, First Edition.
Edited by Jeffrey S. Albert and Michael W. Wood.

### 1.1.1 Macroanatomy

Dopamine is synthesized in dopaminergic neurons from the amino acid tyrosine by the enzymes tyrosine hydroxylase (forming L-3,4-dihydroxylphenylalanine [L-DOPA]) and L-amino acid decarboxylase (AACD). Tyrosine hydroxylase is a rate-limiting enzyme in the synthesis of dopamine, and its mRNA expression is abundant in human mesencephalon.

Dopaminergic neurons showing the highest expression of tyrosine hydroxylase mRNA are aggregated in distinct clusters: the ventral midbrain (A8-9-10), diencephalon (A11-15), and telencephalon (A16-olfactory bulb, A17, and the retina). Dopaminergic neurons cluster into the three major nuclei in the brain that contain cell bodies: (1) the substantia nigra pars compacta (SN, A9), located in the ventral midbrain; (2) the ventral tegmental area (VTA) or A10, lying medial to SN; and (3) the arcuate nucleus of the hypothalamus, throughout the posterior and dorsomedial nuclei of hypothalamus (A11–15, in the diencephalon) [1, 2]. Smaller groups of dopaminergic neurons are located in the retina and the olfactory bulb, in the human cerebral cortex [3, 4], in the subcortical white matter, and in the striatum [5, 6].

The dopaminergic projections from these neurons are distributed throughout the anatomically segregated neuronal systems that control motor, limbic, and cognitive aspects of behavior (Fig. 1.1). The dopaminergic projections form three major long pathways:

1. The nigrostriatal pathway contains over 80% of all dopaminergic innervation, primarily targeting the striatal medium spiny projection neurons. Dopamine modulates cortical innervation to the striatum and is involved in the control of movement.

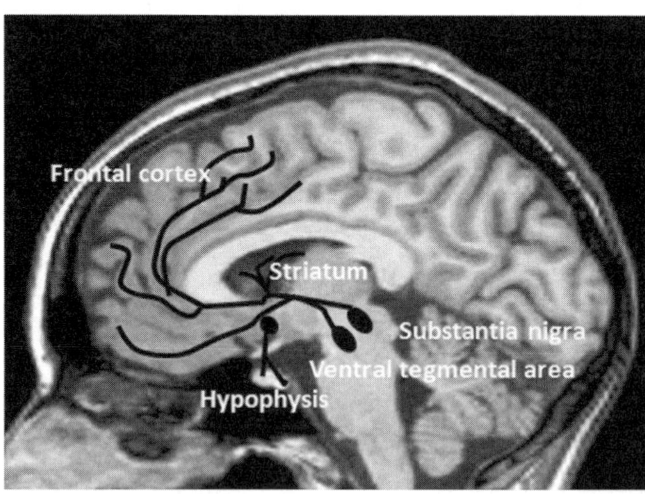


**FIGURE 1.1** Dopamine projections in the human brain. A schema of the major dopamine projection systems is superimposed on an MR image of a human brain.

2. The mesolimbic pathway, with neurons from VTA synapsing in the nucleus accumbens and amygdala, is engaged in emotions, motivation, goal-directed behavior, pleasurable sensations, the euphoria of drug abuse, and the delusions and hallucinations of psychosis [7].
3. The mesocortical pathway originates in the VTA and terminates in the forebrain with its most abundant innervation in the prefrontal cortex, anterior cingulate, insula, entorhinal cortices. The majority of target neurons are excitatory pyramidal cells and minor target group are dendrites of local inhibitory neurons [8, 9] largely involved in cognitive functions.

There is a topographic organization of the SN/VTA innervation to the cortical regions (e.g., dorsal prefrontal and anterior cingulate cortices receive innervation from the dorsal group of cells of the SN and the retrobulbar area), while ventromedial limbic cortices receive input from the VTA [10]. In addition, several shorter pathways distinct from the major projections have been identified: the tubero-infundibular pathway, which projects from the hypothalamic nucleus to the anterior pituitary and contributes to the neurohumoral regulation of lactation; the mesohippocampal tract, which originates in the SN/VTA and terminates at the hippocampus and is involved in memory formation; and the mesofrontal tract, which traverses from the SN to the prefrontal cortex and is active in reward mechanisms. Ultrashort dopaminergic pathways connecting inner and outer layers of the retina (interplexiform amacrine-like neurons) and cells in the olfactory bulb (periglomerular dopamine cells) have also been reported [11], although their function is less well understood.

### 1.1.2 Microanatomy

Neurotransmission, including the synthesis–storage–release–receptor binding of the monoamine neurotransmitter as well as its uptake or degradation, is a highly controlled process. The complex balance of this cascade determines the intensity of dopaminergic signaling.

In 1979, Kebabian and Calne [12] found that dopamine exerts its effects by binding to two classes of receptors, dubbed as the dopamine $D_1$ and $D_2$ receptors (D1R and D2R). These receptors could be differentiated pharmacologically, biologically, physiologically, and by their anatomical distribution. All dopamine receptors are G-protein-coupled receptors (GPCRs). Heteromeric guanine nucleotide-binding proteins (G-proteins) are made up of alpha ($\alpha$), beta ($\beta$), and gamma ($\gamma$) subunits, binding to which will influence effector recognition and can activate different signaling cascades. Therefore, based on the receptor coupling to GPCRs, activated subunits of G-proteins and further effects on second messengers, dopamine receptors are presently subdivided into the Gs-, Gq-, or Golf-coupled $D_1$ receptor family and Gi/o $D_2$ receptor family [13]. By their different G-protein coupling, $D_1$-family and $D_2$-family receptors have opposing effects on adenylyl cyclase activity (i.e., stimulatory vs. inhibitory effect, respectively), on cyclic adenosine monophosphate (cAMP) concentration, as well as on phosphorylation processes [14]. Gene cloning revealed that DR2 family is further subdivided into dopamine $D_2$, $D_3$, and $D_4$ receptors (D2R, D3R, D4R) and their splice forms. A short splice version of $D_2$ ($D_2$Sh) and a long splice version of $D_2$ ($D_2$Lh) coexist in the brain as the most characterized dopamine receptor splice variants. The $D_2$Sh are predominantly presynaptic receptors (autoreceptors) and participate in the feedback mechanisms, or, when situated on the terminals, affect synthesis, storage, and release of dopamine into the synaptic cleft. The $D_2$Lh are viewed as the classical postsynaptic receptors. The D1R family includes dopamine $D_1$ and $D_5$ receptors (D1R, D5R).

***1.1.2.1 Dopamine $D_2$/$D_3$/$D_4$ Receptors in the Human Brain ($D_2$-like receptors)*** The precise anatomical location of the dopamine receptors in the human brain has been most fully established for the dopamine $D_2$ receptors. In the adult human brain, D2R mRNA is markedly expressed in the striatum, neocortex, hippocampus, and amygdaloid complex, and differential expression is found in the thalamus as well as in most of the hypothalamic nuclei [15, 16]. D2R expression also follows a regional density pattern; there is a density gradient of D2R in decreasing order from the striatal structures, to the thalamus, to the midbrain, and finally, to the neocortex [17–19]. The dopamine D2R distribution in the neocortex is low, uneven, and varies between higher values in the temporal lobes (including hippocampus and amygdala) to minute receptor densities in the occipital lobes [20, 21]. Very heterogeneous D2R density is also found in the thalamus and in the striatum [22]. (Fig. 1.2a shows D2/D3R distribution as measured by molecular imaging in humans *in vivo*)

The D3R has a different anatomical distribution, being absent in the dorsal striatum, but abundant in the ventral striatum, thalamus, and hypothalamic nuclei (mainly mammillary bodies) and at low levels in the striatum and throughout the cortex. This is consistent with the mRNA expression pattern [19, 23]. However, so far there are no selective agonists available for D3Rs, and they are indistinguishable from D2Rs in *in vivo* measurements.

The D4R has eight polymorphic variants in humans [24]. The receptor is found at a high density in the limbic cortex and in the hippocampus and is absent from the motor regions of the brain. mRNA for D4R has low expression in human cortex and striatum [25]. D4Rs are preferentially co-expressed with enkephalin in GABAergic neurons, thus predominantly modulating inhibitory control in the cortex and projection pathways [26]. No compounds are yet available for *in vivo* visualization of D4R, nor are there any pharmacological tools to distinguish between the physiological or functional contributions of $D_4$ and $D_2$/$D_3$ receptors.

***1.1.2.2 Dopamine $D_1$/$D_5$ Receptors in the Human Brain ($D_1$-like receptors)*** The cells expressing D1R mRNA are localized in the striatum, cerebral cortex, and bed nucleus of stria terminalis [16]. Dopamine D1R mRNA expression in

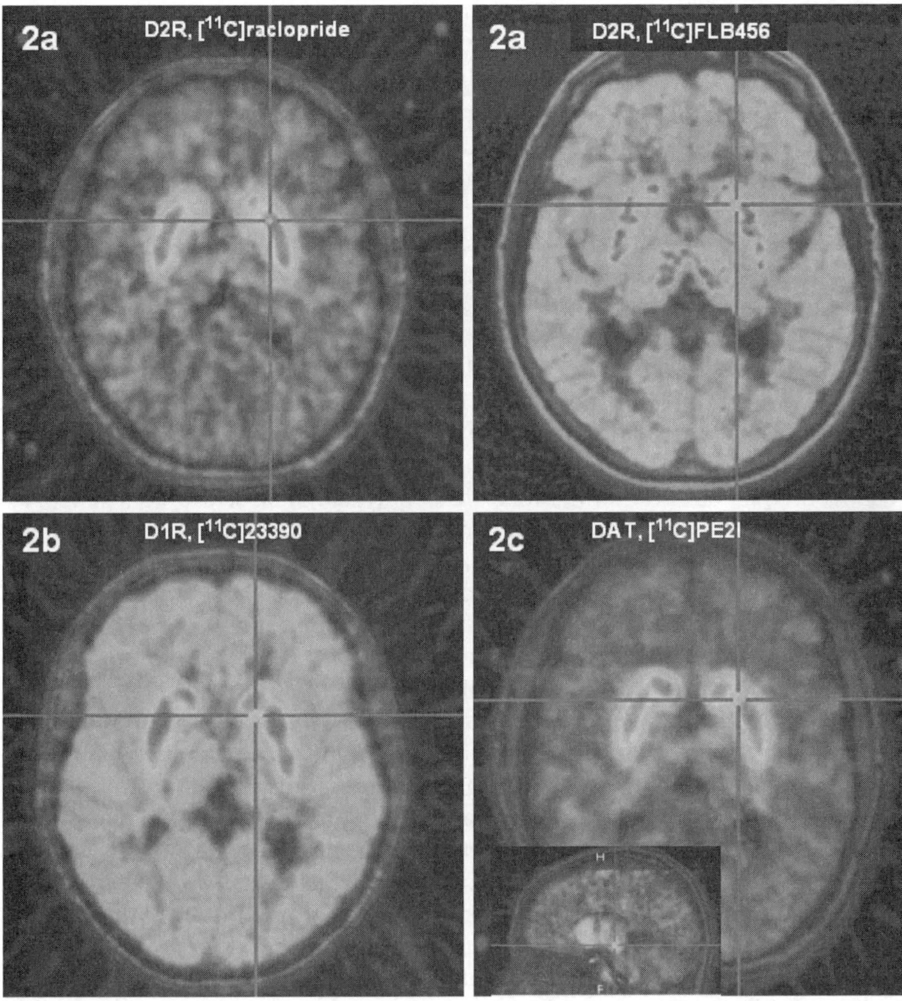


**FIGURE 1.2** Dopamine receptor ($D_1$, $D_2$, $D_3$) and dopamine transporter distribution throughout the brain as measured by *in vivo* molecular imaging in humans by PET. (a) Regional radioactivity of [$^{11}$C]raclopride, representing binding to the striatal D2/D3DRs, and [$^{11}$C]FLB 456, representing binding to the extrastriatal D2/D3DRs. (b) Regional radioactivity of [$^{11}$C]SCH23390, representing binding to the D1/D5DRs. (c) Regional radioactivity of [$^{11}$C]PE2I, representing binding to the DAT. Summation PET images at transaxial and saggital planes. Substantia nigra indicated in saggital plane. (See color insert.)

the human cerebral cortex is the most abundant of all dopamine receptors. It is distributed in a laminar pattern and differs quantitatively between the cortical regions and subregions, with the highest expression in the medial orbital, insular, and parietal cortices [27]. Extremely low levels of D1R mRNA are found in the hippocampus, diencephalon, brainstem, and cerebellum, suggesting that neurons in those areas can mediate dopamine transmission via D1R, although mainly it would be mediated via D2/D3Rs. In the normal adult human brain, D1Rs show a widespread neocortical distribution, with D1R predominantly localized on spines and shafts of projection neurons [28]. D1Rs are found in high density in the basal ganglia, including regions of the caudate, putamen, globus pallidus, and SN [18, 29]. (D1R binding distribution *in vivo* is depicted in Fig. 1.2b). D1Rs in the globus pallidus and the SN are most likely localized on terminals, as there are no D1R mRNA expresssing cells in those regions. Within the basal ganglia, D1Rs are most abundant on GABAergic neurons expressing dynorphin/substance P [30].

D5R mRNA has predominant cortical expression and scattered low expression of mRNA is found in the subcortical structures, striatum, thalamus, and claustrum [31]. No radioligand selective for D5R is available. Immunochemistry studies suggest that D5Rs are concentrated in the hippocampus and entorrhinal cortex, but are also found in the thalamus and in the striatum [32].

The major functions of dopamine receptors are the recognition of the specific transmitter dopamine and the subsequent activation of effectors, leading to altered cell membrane potential and changes in the biochemical state of the postsynaptic cell. Neurotransmission via dopamine receptors is not sufficient to generate action potentials. Investigations into a possible neuromodulatory role of dopamine from the 1970s onward (i.e., electrophysiological experimental studies and microiontophoresis *in vivo*) have demonstrated that dopamine moderately depolarizes or hyperpolarizes neurons, usually by 5–7 mV [33]. Thus, dopamine acts as a neuromodulator, potentiating or attenuating cellular responses evoked by other neurotransmitters and thereby modulating neurotransmitter release, electrical excitability, and the neural firing properties of the target cell.

***1.1.2.3 Regulation of Dopamine Neurotransmission (Synthesis, Reuptake, Storage, Degradation)*** Dopamine levels in the synaptic/extrasynaptic environment are controlled by a number of molecular mechanisms: dopamine reuptake involving the presynaptic dopamine transporter, storage by vesicular monoamine transporters, and metabolic degradation by the enzymes catechol-o-methyltransferase (COMT) and monoamine oxidase (MAO).

*Dopamine Transporter (DAT)* The topology of DAT shows that it is a plasma membrane protein, with 12 transmembrane domains. It is localized only on dopaminergic neurons and is considered the phenotypic marker of dopaminergic neurons. The DAT is encoded by a single gene [34]. The highest levels of DAT expression are found in the striatum and midbrain, and significantly less is found in the frontal cortex and hypothalamus, with low levels in the olfactory bulb and the pituitary [35, 36]. The regional distribution of DAT in humans *in vivo* is shown in Figure 1.2C. Differential expression of DAT in various populations of dopamine neurons suggests regionally specific types of dopamine transmission regulation. The classical type of regulation via the uptake mechanisms exists in the striatum and the paracrine or volume transmission type of signaling is found in the midbrain and the neocortex [37]. DAT terminates neurotransmission by removing dopamine from the synaptic cleft via uptake back into presynaptic neurons. The end result of the reuptake system is maintenance of a narrow range of neurotransmitter at the synapse. Animal models have shown that genetic elimination of DAT leads to a considerably prolonged clearance time, elevated extracellular levels of dopamine, and altered neuronal firing properties [38]. Recently it has been suggested that the function of DAT may parallel the transmission type, in that it may have a reuptake function in the striatum and be involved in release in the midbrain [39].

*Vesicular Monoamine Transporter (VMAT)* VMATs transport cytoplasmic dopamine into storage vesicles and decrease levels of cytoplasmic dopamine, thereby modulating concentrations of free dopamine in the nerve terminals. Two VMATs localized to the membranes of the synaptic vesicles have been cloned, VMAT1 and VMAT2. The VMAT2 isoform is found in dopamine, norepinephrine, serotonin, and histamine releasing cells. In humans, the VMAT2 protein is encoded by the *VMAT2* gene.

*Enzymes* A major enzyme in synaptic dopamine catabolism in the cortical regions is COMT [40]. It is a relatively nonspecific enzyme, found in the cytoplasm of most tissues and in substantial amounts in the central nervous system (CNS). The precise cellular localization of COMT is not known. It is suggested that the enzyme functions extraneuronally. It plays a specific role in the regulation of synaptic dopamine levels in the cortical regions, but not in the mesolimbic or mesostriatal tracts. A functional genetic polymorphism for COMT involves a methionine-(Met)-to-valine (Val) substitution at codon 158. The Met allele has one quarter the enzyme activity of the Val allele. Therefore, the Met/Met individuals have significantly reduced enzyme activity and thereby higher dopamine levels in the prefrontal cortex [41].

Monoamine oxidase (MAO) is an enzyme that converts catecholamines to their aldehydes. It is a particle-bound protein localized in the outer membrane of mitochondria and also in the microsomes. MAO is considered an intraneuronal enzyme, but it is also found in abundance extraneuronally. It exists in two forms, MAO-A and MAO-B. The two are coded by different genes and expressed in different brain regions, MAO-A mRNA is found in noradrenergic neurons, while MAO-B is found in serotonergic and histaminergic neurons. Its presence in dopaminergic neurons is less known, however, and both MAO-B-positive dopaminergic neurons in SN and MAO-B positive glial cells near dopaminergic neurons have been documented [42].

### 1.1.3 Mechanistic Model of Activity of Dopaminergic Neuron

The firing characteristics of dopaminergic neurons have been described by electrophysiological techniques *in vitro* and *in vivo*. Spontaneously firing dopaminergic neurons have long action potential (2–5 ms) and *in vivo* display two different characteristic firing models, single spike firing, and burst firing [43, 44]. Single spike firing is a relatively regular, low frequency firing pattern, between 1 and 10 Hz. In contrast, burst firing is a transient high frequency discharge of multiple action potentials followed by an inactive period before spiking starts again. In general, it is thought that regular firing rates serve to induce tonic release of dopamine and thereby maintain a steady-state level of dopamine in the brain. Bursting neural activity gives rise to the phasic dopamine release and consequently induces high but transient increases in the dopamine levels, which convey discrete signals. Switching the firing pattern from regular to bursting and back is thought to be dependent on coinciding glutamatergic and cholinergic inputs from the subthalamic and pedunculopontine nuclei, respectively [45].

Electrophysiological activity of VTA and SN dopaminergic neurons is regulated by both autoinhibitory mechanisms and afferent inputs. The feedback regulation is largely executed by $D_2$-like autoreceptors located in the somatodendritic region of the dopaminergic neurons [43]. These receptors are activated by dopamine release from dendrites or axon collaterals. Activation of autoreceptors opens G protein-coupled inward rectifying potassium channels (GIRKs). Opening of the GIRK channels leads to increased membrane potassium conductance, which hyperpolarizes the cell membrane and consequently decreases the basal firing rate of the cell [46]. Thus, maintenance of a spontaneous, pace-maker-like firing pattern is mediated by auto-D2Rs. In addition to autoinhibitory mechanisms, the $D_2$-like autoreceptors may contribute to the regulation of dopamine transmission by modulating its synthesis and release. This function is brain region-dependent and is mediated by the autoreceptors localized on the cell terminals [47]; for example, the dopaminergic neuron terminals of mesocortical pathway have been shown to lack or have a reduced number of $D_2$ autoreceptors [48]. Autoreceptor stimulation in this pathway reduces the synthesis and release of dopamine.

Afferent inputs are of critical importance in the regulation of dopaminergic neuron firing rate. Glutamatergic innervation to the VTA, originating in the prefrontal cortex, sends an excitatory glutamatergic input to the dopaminergic neurons [49]. As a consequence, there is activation of glutamatergic N-methyl-D-aspartate (NMDA) receptors on dopaminergic cell bodies followed by a marked increase in cell burst firing [50]. The inhibitory $\gamma$-aminobutyric acid (GABA) input to dopaminergic cells in the VTA is mediated both by afferents from other brain regions and by GABAergic interneurons within the nucleus [51], which, in turn, receive glutamatergic input from the prefrontal cortex [52]. Experimental data indicate that noradrenaline also modulates dopamine neurotransmission in mesocortical dopamine systems. Activity of dopaminergic neurons decreases following selective destruction of noradrenergic fibers while direct stimulation of the locus coeruleus strongly enhances the activity of dopaminegic neurons in the VTA, and drugs that increase central noradrenergic activity may enhance dopamine turnover [53].

### 1.1.4 Dopaminergic System in Brain Circuitry

The basal ganglia-thalamo-cortical system was hypothesized to be organized into multiple segregated circuits, which subserve different functions, including motor, oculomotor, prefrontal cognitive, and limbic functions [54]. Tract-tracing and physiological experiments have indicated a general topographic organization of the cortical-basal ganglia-thalamic loops and supported a model of basal ganglia function based on parallel and segregated pathways. Recent anatomical connectivity and neuroimaging studies reveal heterogenous neural activity patterns and show that the system is more complex. Cortico-striato-thalamo-cortical loops are not completely segregated. Pathways emanating from the cortical region and entering the striatum re-enter the initial cortical area that provides input to the striatum (close loops, serving segregated processes), but will also project back to other areas of the cortex, forming open circuits and by that serving integrative processes [55]. Furthermore, neuronal projections communicating between different loops (or functional domains) have also been discovered as well as nonreciprocal connections between the thalamus and the cortex. These terminals can influence different functional cortical areas that, in turn, will project to the striatum and back to the thalamus, where they can influence other circuits. So-called hot spots of convergence between terminals from different cortical regions may occur in the thalamus and in the striatum. Interloop connections in ventral striatum have also been shown by trans-synaptic neuronal tracing studies. Nonreciprocal connections are known to occur between striatum and SN [56].

In this complex neural circuitry, the dopamine system provides a bridge by which information circulating in the ventral limbic-cortico-striatal-thalamocortical loops connects to nigrostriatal loops (see Fig. 1.3, a connectivity diagram adapted after Reference [57]). The current understanding of the cortico-basal ganglia circuitry incorporates the model of two major pathways that transmit information through the basal ganglia, via the direct and indirect pathways. The direct pathway projects from the striatum to the internal segment of the globus pallidus and SN pars reticulata (the output structures of the basal ganglia). In the indirect pathway, information leaving the striatum flows through the external segment of globus pallidus and subthalamic nucleus before proceeding to the output structures. The function of these anatomical pathways is affected by the nature of the neurotransmitters they release. The direct pathway is purely inhibitory. The indirect pathway has both excitatory and inhibitory elements. Dopaminergic inputs to the basal ganglia arising from SN/VTA cell groups modulate the relative efficacy of these two opposing

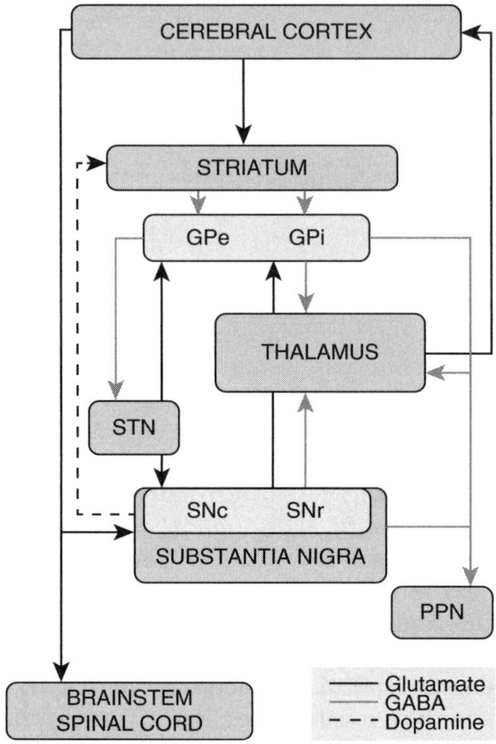


**FIGURE 1.3** A connectivity diagram of the basal ganglia thalamocortical circuitry and major neurotransmitter systems. GPi, globus pallidus internus; GPe, globus pallidus externus; SNr, substantia nigra pars reticulate; SNc, substantia nigra pars compacta; STN, subthalamic nucleus; PPN, pedunculopontine nucleus. Adapted from Reference [57].

streams of information transfer, enhancing stimulation via the direct pathway (mediated via $D_1$-like receptors) and enhancing inhibition via the indirect pathway (mediated predominantly via $D_2$-like receptors). The balance between these pathways determines whether the net relationship between the inputs and outputs of the basal ganglia will be inhibitory or excitatory. Finally, since the basal ganglia themselves inhibit the thalamus and the thalamus excites the cortex, increased outflow from the basal ganglia results in inhibition of the cortex. However, new anatomical and molecular biology studies suggest that these pathways are not so distinct. There are collaterals reaching out from the striatum to both GPe and GPi, direct striatal innervation to the cortex, without thalamic relay, direct excitatory input from the cerebral cortex to the subthalamic nucleus (hyperdirect pathway [58]), and there is evidence for co-expression of $D_1$- and $D_2$-like receptors on the same cells [59]. New models of cortico-striatal circuitry are under development.

## 1.2 DOPAMINE HYPOTHESIS OF SCHIZOPHRENIA

### 1.2.1 Emergence of the "Classical" Dopamine Hypothesis of Schizophrenia

The initial, "classical," dopamine hypothesis of schizophrenia was proposed over 50 years ago. In short, it suggested that schizophrenia may be related to an excessive activity of the dopaminergic system. Two main lines of research have contributed to the origins of this hypothesis: (1) discovery of neuroleptics and investigations of their mechanism of action and (2) investigations of the effects of psychostimulants, and observations that they may exacerbate psychosis or induce clinical symptoms mimicking positive symptoms of schizophrenia in healthy individuals.

Chlorpromazine was first synthesized in 1951 by P. Charpentier, S. Courvoisier, and colleagues at Rhône-Poulenc Laboratories (now Sanofi) [60–62]. Within half a year, chlorpromazine reached the patient clinics where it was first tested for its ability to potentiate anesthesia, as part of "lytic cocktail" [63]. Combination of contemporary clinical practice of the time (i.e., cooling of agitation with water) and the observed cooling effect of chlorpromazine led to the idea to test it in psychiatric clinics. The first administration of chlorpromazine to a patient with severe psychosis was successful [64]. Soon after, J. Delay and P. Deniker reported results of chlorpromazine application in a group of 38 manic and psychotic patients [65]. Numerous studies from all around the world facilitated the introduction of chlorpromazine into clinical practice both in Europe and the United States [66, 67]. However, side effects such as tardive dyskinesia were described from very early on. The beneficial effects of chlorpromazine (i.e., ameliorating the positive symptoms) generally occurred at doses that elicited neurologic side effects resembling Parkinson's disease. The symptoms gave rise to the term "neuroleptic" to describe these drugs (gr. *lēptos-seizing*, [68]).

Long before coming into Western medicine the sedative, calming features of the plant *Rauwolfia serpentina* had been used in India. Early scientific investigations were carried out as well. Rediscovery of *R. serpentina* and research into its sedative and antihypertensive properties at Ciba laboratories was followed by systematic clinical trials that documented the efficacy of its alkaloid, reserpine, in patients suffering from a variety of psychiatric disorders. Reserpine was introduced into clinical practice for the treatment of psychosis and research on its mechanism of action actively continued (for review, see [69]).

In parallel to the discoveries of chlorpromazine and reserpine, there were advancements in neuroscience that enabled the investigations of their mechanism of action. First, there was a shift in understanding of synaptic transmission, that is, from the idea that it is purely electrical to the concept of chemically mediated transmission. This further included the discovery of the first six neurotransmitters: acetylcholine, dopamine, GABA, norepinephrine, serotonin, and substance P [70]. Second, the introduction of the spectrophotofluorometer offered the possibility to measure drugs and endogenous substances in different tissues (review Reference [71]). Consequently, the experimental studies with reserpine led to the discovery that it was depleting serotonin from tissue storage, blood platelets [72], and neural cell terminals in the brain [73]. Furthermore, the reserpine depletion in rabbits and mice leading to the akinesia and sedation could be reversed by the administration of L-DOPA, which restored dopamine levels in the brain [74]. A series of systematic studies in the 1970s eventually led to the discovery of dopamine receptors and the finding of the primary site of action of neuroleptics (i.e., interference of neurotransmission in the mesolimbic and nigrostriatal dopaminergic subsystems) [75–77]. In summary, this series of discoveries provided evidence that (1) neurochemical alterations in the brain lie behind the clinical symptoms and (2) interference of brain neurochemistry by pharmacological means could alleviate the symptoms of neurological and psychiatric disorders. These findings suggested the role of dopamine in the pathophysiology of neuropsychiatric disorders.

Amphetamine-induced psychosis was described in the early 1940s [78]. Initially it was thought that amphetamine directly stimulated peripheral adrenergic receptors, or that it acted at norepinephrine sites in the brain. Over several years, there was increasing evidence that the psychomotor effects of stimulants were induced *via* the central dopamine system and direct action on dopamine receptors was assumed [79, 80].

Based on the findings that (1) nonreserpine neuroleptics that induced extrapyramidal rigidity were dopamine receptor antagonists, (2) that psychostimulants that could exacerbate psychotic symptoms in schizophrenia patients acted on dopamine receptors, and (3) that dopamine found in high concentrations in the striatum was lacking in Parkinson's disease, J. van Rossum suggested that alterations in the dopamine system may play a role in the etiology of schizophrenia, be it overproduction of dopamine, overstimulation of receptors, or abnormal susceptibility of receptors [80] (review Reference [81]). Thus, schizophrenia was for the first time associated with changes in brain neurochemistry. The dopamine hypothesis of schizophrenia was formulated based on the indirect evidence coming from pharmacological sciences. This hypothesis opened a new line of investigations: a search for direct evidence of changes of dopamine biomarkers in patients with schizophrenia.

### 1.2.2 In Search of Evidence for the Dopamine Hypothesis of Schizophrenia

The 1980s and 1990s were marked by an extensive search for evidence to support the dopamine hypothesis of schizophrenia. Biochemical markers, such as levels of dopamine, its precursors and its metabolites were measured in patients' cerebrospinal fluid (CSF), blood, urine samples, skin fibroblasts, and postmortem brain. Initial measurements of the levels of dopamine in postmortem brain of patients with schizophrenia showed regional changes—higher dopamine levels in caudate, nucleus accumbens, and amygdala [82, 83]. Those findings were not replicated and ultimately no clear alterations in the brain dopamine levels were confirmed. No clear changes in CSF levels of the dopamine metabolite homovanillic acid (HVA) were reported either. Thus, studies of schizophrenia patients using the peripheral biomarkers of dopamine system found no support for the hypothesis of increased dopamine metabolism [84].

Extensive development of molecular biology techniques and the cloning of five different dopamine receptors [85] stimulated the search for alterations in the dopamine receptor systems in patients with schizophrenia. Higher dopamine D2DR and D4DR binding in the striatum was found in the autoradiography studies [86, 87]. Meanwhile, developments in the area of molecular neuroimaging techniques provided new possibilities to visualize and quantify changes of dopamine receptors in the brain of living human individuals. Initial positron emission tomography (PET) studies using the nonselective radioligand [$^{11}$C]NMSP (which binds to the dopamine $D_2$, $D_4$ and 5-HT2 receptors) showed a two- to threefold elevated D2R density in the caudate nucleus of schizophrenia patients [88], a finding later attributed to the sensitizing effect of neuroleptics leading to receptor upregulation [82, 89]. No elevated D2Rs in the striatum were found in studies with drug-naïve patients and when using the more selective radioligand, [$^{11}$C]raclopride (which is selective for the D2R/D3Rs) [90–92]. High D4R density in the striatum of patients with schizophrenia seemed to suggest an explanation to the discrepant results of PET studies; however, these findings were also not replicated [93]. Thus, molecular brain imaging studies did not confirm postmortem findings of increased striatal D2Rs among patients with schizophrenia (review Reference [94]).

In summary, throughout the 1980s and 1990s, the most prevailing arguments supporting the dopamine hypothesis of schizophrenia still stemmed from an understanding of the mechanism of action of antipsychotic drugs, and in particular, the strong correlation between the antipsychotic potency of typical neuroleptics and the blockade of the D2Rs [75]. At the same time, the pharmacological evidence was questioned by the fact that clozapine, an effective atypical neuroleptic, was a weak D2R antagonist.

### 1.2.3 Dopamine Hypothesis Revisited

In the 1980s, the understanding of schizophrenia as a clinical entity was changing. Researchers began to focus attention on defining distinct dimensions of schizophrenia. Symptoms of schizophrenia were classified into separate categories such as positive (e.g., delusions, hallucinatory behavior, grandiosity) or negative (e.g., blunted affect, emotional withdrawal, motor retardation) and also the inclusion of anxiety/depression, disorganized thought, and hostility/excitement. Such questions as the change of certain symptom clusters over time, long-term outcomes, and the effect of antipsychotic treatment on different manifestations of illness were under investigation [95–97]. There was a subgroup of patients that did not respond to antipsychotics, and not all symptoms of disorder could be treated equally efficiently. Accumulating observations on the use of neuroleptics and psychostimulants indicated that drugs that ameliorate positive symptoms of schizophrenia had no effect on negative symptoms or could even worsen them (e.g., amphethamine may worsen positive, but improve negative symptoms of schizophrenia) [98].

As the clinical understanding of schizophrenia and the history of its pharmacological treatment evolved, thinking of the disorder as simply a hyperdopaminergic state was becoming insufficient. Research was directed toward the investigation of a possible primary deficit within different dopamine subsystems.

***1.2.3.1 The Theory of Regional Imbalance within Dopamine System*** In 1992, a hypothesis of "regional imbalance" in the dopamine system was suggested [99]. This hypothesis accepted dysfunction of the dopamine system in schizophrenia but did not implicate excessive dopamine transmission as the critical factor. It stated that both hypofunctional and hyperfunctional states in different brain regions may coexist in schizophrenia. Successors of this theory suggested that cognitive impairment and negative symptoms were related to the hypodopaminergic state in the cortical regions (i.e., mesocortical pathways), whereas positive symptoms of schizophrenia were associated with hyperdopaminergic activity in subcortical regions [100, 101].

Experimental studies supported the idea of regional differentiation in dopamine function. Neuroleptics were found to induce the selective effect on dopaminergic neuron firing; typical antipsychotics affected both A9 and A10 cells, while atypical antipsychotics affected only A10 cells [102]. Activation of the mesocortical dopamine system increased prefrontal glucose metabolism [103] and frontal glucose hypometabolism could be reversed by dopamine agonists [104].

In schizophrenia patients, it was the finding of reduced cerebral blood flow and glucose metabolism in the frontal cortices relative to other brain regions [105] and the "hypofrontality" concept that stimulated further search for the evidence of regional brain function differences in schizophrenia. However, a decade of neuroimaging studies yielded inconsistent results. Regional brain metabolism turned out to be dependent on a number of factors, such as medication effects, behavioral and emotional states during experiments (contextual variability), paradigms and methods of analysis used, and so on (review Reference [106]). Meta-analysis of neuroimaging studies added support for reduced frontal activation in schizophrenia, although the findings could also have been related to age or disease chronicity [107]. Studies using pharmacological functional magnetic resonance imaging (phMRI) techniques joined today in search for the link between regional brain metabolism and dopamine function in schizophrenia. It has been shown that atypical antipsychotics enhance prefrontal activity in patients with negative symptoms [101], findings that await replication.

The main controversies around this theory were and are related to the questions: (1) Are there indeed regional differences in brain activation patterns in schizophrenia? (2) Is a pattern an artifact or epiphenomenon, or it reflects true, intrinsic differences in neuronal activity specific for schizophrenia, differences in activity of the dopamine subsystems? Dysfunction of frontal cortex seen in some patients with schizophrenia that has been thought to be primary and related to a decrease in "dopamine activity" has been recently challenged by animal research. Working memory and behavioral deficits attributed to the frontal cortex have been suggested to arise secondarily to excess striatal dopamine release, implying that each exacerbation of acute psychosis with excessive dopamine turnover increases the likelihood of frontal dysfunction [108]. Thus, there is still no direct evidence that the mesocortical dopamine system is disturbed in patients with schizophrenia.

***1.2.3.2 Regional Imbalance between Dopamine and Other Neurotransmitter Systems*** What lies at the roots of the mesocortical–mesolimbic dysfunction in schizophrenia remains unknown. From the inception of the dopamine hypothesis of schizophrenia, most of the authors did not fully subscribe to it. A. Carlsson wrote in 1977: "while a primary disturbance in dopamine function in schizophrenia cannot be ruled out, the intimate relation between dopaminergic and other neuronal systems must be emphasized, the possible involvement of other amine, amino acid, or peptide transmitters in schizophrenia cannot be disregarded" [109]. Since then, several authors have proposed that dopamine levels in schizophrenia are normal but that they are elevated relative to other neurotransmitter levels. The emerging theories of schizophrenia suggest decreased levels of glutamate, NMDA receptor hypofunction [110–113], changes in serotonin system [114], and beyond (e.g., alterations among cytokines [115] or postsynaptic signal transmission system disturbances [116]). Loss of cholinergic interneurons in the striatum, hypoglutamatergia, or imbalance in glutamatergic and GABAergic projections from the prefrontal cortex have all been proposed as potential neurochemical alterations in schizophrenia. The grounds to these theories are in part built on the evidence of anatomical and functional interconnections between those neurochemical systems and dopaminergic subsystems, that is, the glutamatergic and GABAergic projections from prefrontal cortex synapse to the dopaminergic neurons of VTA and provide bidirectional control of dopaminergic neurons [100, 117].

### 1.2.4 Dopamine System in Schizophrenia: A Molecular Imaging Perspective

#### *1.2.4.1 Postsynaptic Dopamine Receptors*

*Dopamine $D_2/D_3$ Receptors* A recent meta-analysis of molecular imaging studies on striatal D2Rs in drug-naïve and drug-free patients with schizophrenia suggested that patients with schizophrenia have mildly elevated but more variable striatal D2R density compared with control subjects [118] (for a more detailed description of striatal D2R changes, see Section 1.2.2). Meanwhile, measurements of the extrastriatal dopamine system in schizophrenia are less explored. This dopamine subsystem has long been of particular interest due to the findings of altered patterns of cortical activation, which were associated with psychotic symptoms and responded to antipsychotic treatment [118, 119]. The main questions asked were: Are the extrastriatal D2Rs changed in schizophrenia and can they be the primary target of antipsychotic medications? Development of high-affinity biomarkers for extrastriatal D2R enabled researchers to look for answers to these questions ([$^{11}$C]FLB457, [$^{123}$I]epidepride, [$^{18}$F]fallypride; [120–122]).

Thus far, a few extrastriatal regions with lower D2Rs in patients with schizophrenia have been suggested—the thalamus, the anterior cingulate cortex, the amygdala, and the temporal cortices—as well as increased D2Rs in SN [123–127]. Moreover, D2R binding in the cingulate cortex and the thalamus correlated negatively with the positive symptom score [123, 128]. Meta-analysis of pharmacological studies on the effect of antipsychotics on the extrastriatal D2Rs has shown that clinically effective doses of typical and atypical antipsychotics reach high receptor occupancy in the temporal cortex [129]. Slightly higher occupancy in cortical regions compared with the striatum have been reported for aripiprazole, clozapine, quetiapine, and ziprazidone ([$^{18}$F]fallypride,[130–133]. No prefrential cortical D2R occupancy has been reported for olanzapine or haloperidol ([$^{18}$F]fallypride, [134]), for clozapine ([$^{11}$C]raclopride and [$^{11}$C]FLB457, [135]), for risperidone ([$^{11}$C]FLB457, [136]), and for sertindole ([$^{11}$C]FLB457, [137]). Importantly, there was no relation between extrastriatal D2R occupancy and drug effect on the positive symptoms [130]. The best predictor of efficacy (i.e., response in positive symptoms) and of the propensity for extrapyramidal side effects still remains striatal D2R occupancy [138].

*Dopamine $D_1$ Receptors* Within experimental studies, there is ample evidence that dopamine plays an important role in modulating neurocognitive functions. Best established is its role in working memory. Dopamine levels rise at the beginning of a working memory task and stay elevated across many trials [139]. This suggests that a dopamine signal is present during encoding and use of information processing by the prefrontal neural circuitry. Furthermore, drug applications during working memory tasks have shown that increases in dopamine levels are mediated through D1Rs [140, 141]. Given the evidence for the decrease in working memory capacity in schizophrenia, changes in the D1R system have been predicted. PET studies have examined cortical D1Rs in neuroleptic-naïve or neuroleptic-free schizophrenic patients. Decreased ([$^{11}$C]SCH23390, [142]), increased ([$^{11}$C]NNC112, [143]), or no difference in D1R binding in the prefrontal cortex ([$^{11}$C]SCH23390, [144]) in patients relative to controls was found. Higher D1R in cortical subregions (i.e., medial prefrontal cortex, superior temporal gyrus, angular gyrus) have been associated with increased genetic risk for schizophrenia, and with impairments in working memory [144, 145]. Downregulation of cortical D1Rs by clozapine, haloperidol, and remoxipride has been demonstrated in experimental studies [89] and in patients with schizophrenia using different antipsychotics [145].

In summary, blockade of the striatal D2R remains the main therapeutic target in the treatment of schizophrenia today just as it was 50 years ago. The role of the extrastriatal D2Rs in the pathophysiology of schizophrenia is still not established, although cortical D2Rs are likely to be involved in the action of antipsychotics. Experimental studies provide evidence for the role of D1Rs in cognitive functions. However, the link between cognitive dysfunctions in patients with schizophrenia and D1Rs is not yet fully understood.

***1.2.4.2 Presynaptic Dopamine System*** Investigations of presynaptic markers of the dopamine system were largely driven by the hypothesis of regional dopamine imbalance and predictions of lower dopamine synthesis rates in prefrontal cortex. Initial studies in patients with schizophrenia showed increased [$^{18}$F]fluorodopa uptake, but primarily in the ventral striatum [146], Review of cross-sectional studies on [$^{18}$F]fluorodopa uptake in schizophrenia showed that results are rather inconsistent, with elevated, reduced, or unchanged presynaptic dopamine function in patients relative to comparison subjects [147]. Interestingly, a recent follow-up study of a single patient in remission (total/positive score on a Positive and Negative Syndrome Scale (PANSS) was 55/17), and an acute severe episode of psychosis (PANSS 119/40) demonstrated that [$^{18}$F]fluorodopa influx changes little, if at all, during the development of acute psychosis [148]. This case evaluation contradicts suggested excessive presynaptic dopamine synthesis in the striatum preceding the onset of schizophrenia [149, 150]. Thus, in summary, evaluation of dopamine synthesis rate in schizophrenia showed no clear changes but has raised an interesting question for further studies: whether "state" or "trait" related changes of dopamine levels occur during psychosis.

Two other presynaptic markers, the vesicular monoamine transporter, type 2 (VMAT2), and the DAT are thought to reflect density of dopaminergic projections in the striatum. There were no changes in the striatal binding of the radioligand [$^{11}$C]dihydrotetrabenazine (DTBZ), marking VMAT2, in the schizophrenia patients on medication [151] and no changes in DAT binding in the first-episode, drug-naïve patients with schizophrenia, relative to controls ([$^{11}$C]CFT [152], [99mTc]TRODAT-1, [152]). Higher variability in DAT levels, inverse interaction between striatal DAT and D2R, loss of right–left caudate DAT asymmetry [153, 154], as well as significant negative correlation between DAT availability in the striatum and PANSS scores have been reported [155]. Thus, the hypothesis that excessive dopamine activity in schizophrenia could be explained by increased density of striatal dopamine terminals has not been confirmed.

In summary, evaluation of the presynaptic markers of dopamine system in schizophrenia suggests that changes, if any, are minor and possibly are only within a subgroup of patients with schizophrenia.

### 1.2.5 Beyond Psychopharmacology: Cognitive Models and Genetic Links

Schizophrenia involves different aspects of cognition. Early work in the field concentrated on a reduction in intelligence and a slowness in reaction time. Recently, the research focus has shifted to other cognitive domains, such as working memory, episodic memory, attention, and linguistic processing. Advanced computational network models and functional brain imaging techniques provide the possibility to look at schizophrenia at both the molecular and system levels. It has been hypothesized that the abnormal cognitive functions found in schizophrenia are a consequence of disordered anatomical connectivity, primarily dominated by a disruption in higher levels of perception and hierarchical temporal processing by the brain [156–159]. The dominant understanding today is that there might be an interplay of dysfunctional and compensatory cortical regions or networks in schizophrenia and, thus, combinations of regions with increased and decreased activation or reduced functional connectivity, which in turn is likely to be critically dependent on D1Rs and their role in enhancing NMDA receptor-mediated postsynaptic currents in prefrontal pyramidal and GABAergic neurons [141, 160]

A major enzyme in synaptic dopamine catabolism in the cortical regions is COMT. A common polymorphism in the COMT gene resulting in two valine-to-methionine Val(108/158)Met substitutions gives rise to a significant reduction in its enzymatic activity in the prefrontal cortex [41, 161]. Higher synaptic dopamine in COMT Met-homozygotes is thought to be favorable for the function of frontoparietal networks, for improved working memory after antipsychotic treatment [162, 163]. Given that COMT regulates cortical dopamine levels and that prefrontal cortical dysfunction is seen in schizophrenia, it has been predicted that the gene coding for COMT may serve as a susceptibility gene for schizophrenia (review Reference [164]). However, most recent research suggests that the relationship between COMT function and brain dopamine levels is much more complex and present knowledge is not sufficient to suggest definitive conclusions on its role in the development of schizophrenia [165, 166].

The evidence that schizophrenia can be inherited is compelling with the worldwide risk of schizophrenia of about 1%. The risk increases to about 8–10% if the patient has a first-degree relative (sibling, parents) who suffers from schizophrenia, and in monozygotic twins the risk increases to as high as 50% [167]. Despite the overwhelming evidence that schizophrenia is an inherited illness, a particular defective gene responsible for it has not been found. Genetic loci that appear to confer susceptibility for schizophrenia have been mapped to several chromosomes, including 1q21-22, 1q32-43, 6p24, 8p21, 10p14, 13q32, 18p11, and 22q11-13. Mutations in genes coding for subtypes of dopamine receptors have been explored. A network of interacting genes within the dopamine system increases the risk of schizoprenia. Suggested susceptibility genes are those encoding dystrobrevin binding protein (DTNBP1), disrupted-in-schizophrenia-1 (DISC1), neuregulin 1 (NRG1), dopamine receptors ($D_1$–$D_4$), COMT, and postsynaptic transduction mechanisms (via DARP32). There are numerous studies that support the presence of a link between gene polymorphisms and clinical symptoms, but an equal number of studies do not. Meta-analyses most often show no or only weak associations of single genes for the units of dopamine system and schizophrenia ([168]; for *D1DR* [169]; for *D2DR* [170–172] for *D3DR* [173]; for *D4DR* [174]; for *DAT* [175]; for *COMT* [176, 177]).

So far, no gene mutation that could be reliably related to schizophrenia has been found. The existence of multiple loci conferring susceptibility to schizophrenia suggests that the disease is caused by the interaction of many different genetic components. Thus, a polygene model, where multiple genes contribute to vulnerability to schizophrenia, is currently the most broadly accepted model.

## 1.3 SUMMARY AND CONCLUSIONS

Thus far, the most compelling evidence for the involvement of the dopamine system in the pathophysiology of schizophrenia remains the finding that clinical efficacy of antipsychotics is mediated via antagonism at striatal D2DRs. However, although blocking of D2DR ameliorates psychosis, this does not necessarily mean that the dopamine system is abnormal in schizophrenia. It is common in medicine that symptoms can be treated by mechanisms unrelated to disease etiopathogenesis. Vigorous search for abnormalities in the dopamine system in schizophrenia so far has yielded inconclusive results. The increasing understanding of the behavioral complexity of schizophrenia suggests that it is unlikely that a single neurotrasmitter system can explain such diverse symptoms, for example, inattention and hallucinations.

Thus, any simple, exclusive pathology of the dopamine system in schizophrenia was and is doubtful. Despite these doubts, continuing attempts to develop effective drugs for the treatment of different symptoms of schizophrenia by restoring the homeostasis of dopamine is warranted since many of the mental processes impaired in schizophrenia involve brain circuitry that is modulated by dopamine.

## ACKNOWLEDGEMENT

The authors thank the members of the PET Center at the Department of Clinical Neuroscience, Karolinska Institutet, Stockholm, Sweden, for sharing the PET images illustrating the dopamine system.

## REFERENCES

1. Dahlström, A., Fuxe, K. (1964). Localization of monoamines in the lower brain stem. *Experientia*, *20*, 398–399.

2. Lindvall, O., Björklund, A., Moore, R.Y., Stenevi, U. (1974). Mesencephalic dopamine neurons projecting to neocortex. *Brain Research*, *81*, 325–331.
3. Gaspar, P., Berger, B., Alvarez, C., Vigny, A., Henry, J.P. (1985). Catecholaminergic innervation of the septal area in man: immunocytochemical study using TH and DBH antibodies. *The Journal of Comparative Neurology*, *241*, 12–33.
4. Gaspar, P., Berger, B., Febvret, A., Vigny, A., Krieger-Poulet, M., Borri-Voltattorni, C. (1987). Tyrosine hydroxylase-immunoreactive neurons in the human cerebral cortex: a novel catecholaminergic group? *Neuroscience Letters*, *80*, 257–262.
5. Betarbet, R., Turner, R., Chockkan, V., DeLong, M.R., Allers, K.A., Walters, J., Levey, A.I., Greenamyre, J.T. (1997). Dopaminergic neurons intrinsic to the primate striatum. *The Journal of Neuroscience*, *17*, 6761–6768.
6. Prensa, L., Cossette, M., Parent, A. (2000). Dopaminergic innervation of human basal ganglia. *Journal of Chemical Neuroanatomy*, *20*, 207–213.
7. Mogenson, G.J., Yang, C.R., Yim, C.Y. (1988). Influence of dopamine on limbic inputs to the nucleus accumbens. *Annals of the New York Academy of Sciences*, *537*, 86–100.
8. Goldman-Rakic, P.S., Leranth, C., Williams, S.M., Mons, N., Geffard, M. (1989). Dopamine synaptic complex with pyramidal neurons in primate cerebral cortex. *Proceedings of the National Academy of Sciences of the United States of America*, *86*, 9015–9019.
9. Sesack, S.R., Bressler, C.N., Lewis, D.A. (1995). Ultrastructural associations between dopamine terminals and local circuit neurons in the monkey prefrontal cortex: a study of calretinin-immunoreactive cells. *Neuroscience Letters*, *200*, 9–12.
10. Williams, S.M., Goldman-Rakic, P.S. (1998). Widespread origin of the primate mesofrontal dopamine system. *Cerebral Cortex*, *8*, 321–345.
11. Dahlin, M., Bergman, U., Jansson, B., Björk, E., Brittebo, E. (2000). Transfer of dopamine in the olfactory pathway following nasal administration in mice. *Pharmaceutical Research*, *17*, 737–742.
12. Kebabian, J.W., Calne, D.B. (1979). Multiple receptors for dopamine. *Nature*, *277*(5692), 93–96.
13. Jin, L.Q., Wang, H.Y., Friedman, E. (2001). Stimulated D1 dopamine receptors couple to multiple G-alpha proteins in different brain regions. *Journal of Neurochemistry*, *78*, 981–990.
14. Nishi, A., Snyder, G.L., Greengard, P. (1997). Bidirectional regulation of DARPP-32 phosphorylation by dopamine. *The Journal of Neuroscience*, *17*, 8147–8155.
15. Gurevich, E.V., Joyce, J.N. (1999). Distribution of dopamine D3 receptor expressing neurons in the human forebrain: comparison with D2 receptor expressing neurons. *Neuropsychopharmacology*, *20*, 60–80.
16. Hurd, Y.L., Suzuki, M., Sedvall, G.C. (2001). D1 and D2 dopamine receptor mRNA expression in whole hemisphere sections of the human brain. *Journal of Chemical Neuroanatomy*, *22*, 127–137.
17. Seeman, P. (1980). Brain dopamine receptors. *Pharmacological Reviews*, *32*, 229–313.
18. Hall, H., Farde, L., Sedvall, G. (1988). Human dopamine receptor subtypes—in vitro binding analysis using 3H-SCH 23390 and 3H-raclopride. *Journal of Neural Transmission*, *73*, 7–21.

19. Hall, H., Halldin, C., Dijkstra, D., Wikström, H., Wise, L.D., Pugsley, T.A., Sokoloff, P., Pauli, S., Farde, L., Sedvall, G. (1996). Autoradiographic localisation of D3-dopamine receptors in the human brain using the selective D3-dopamine receptor agonist (+)-[3H]PD 128907. *Psychopharmacology (Berl)*, *128*, 240–247.
20. Lidow, M.S., Goldman-Rakic, P.S., Rakic, P., Innis, R.B. (1989). Dopamine D2 receptors in the cerebral cortex: distribution and pharmacological characterization with [3H]raclopride. *Proceedings of the National Academy of Sciences of the United States of America*, *86*, 6412–6416.
21. Cselényi, Z., Olsson, H., Farde, L., Gulyás, B. (2002). Wavelet-aided parametric mapping of cerebral dopamine D2 receptors using the high affinity PET radioligand [11C]FLB 457. *Neuroimage*, *32*(4), 1690–1708.
22. Gerfen, C.R. (1992). The neostriatal mosaic: multiple levels of compartmental organization. *Journal of Neural Transmission. Supplementum*, *36*, 43–59.
23. Landwehrmeyer, B., Mengod, G., Palacios, J.M. (1993). Dopamine D3 receptor mRNA and binding sites in human brain. *Brain Research. Molecular Brain Research*, *18*, 187–192.
24. Barta, C., Ronai, Z., Nemoda, Z., Szekely, A., Kovacs, E., Sasvari-Szekely, M., Guttman, A. (2001). Analysis of dopamine D4 receptor gene polymorphism using microchip electrophoresis. *Journal of Chromatography. A*, *924*(1–2), 285–290.
25. Matsumoto, M., Hidaka, K., Tada, S., Tasaki, Y., Yamaguchi, T. (1996). Low levels of mRNA for dopamine D4 receptor in human cerebral cortex and striatum. *Journal of Neurochemistry*, *66*, 915–919.
26. Meador-Woodruff, J.H., Damask, S.P., Wang, J., Haroutunian, V., Davis, K.L., Watson, S.J. (1996). Dopamine receptor mRNA expression in human striatum and neocortex. *Neuropsychopharmacology*, *15*, 17–29.
27. Mrzljak, L., Bergson, C., Pappy, M., Huff, R., Levenson, R., Goldman-Rakic, P.S. (1996). Localization of dopamine D4 receptors in GABAergic neurons of the primate brain. *Nature*, *381*, 245–248.
28. Bergson, C., Mrzljak, L., Smiley, J.F., Pappy, M., Levenson, R., Goldman-Rakic, P.S. (1995). Regional, cellular, and subcellular variations in the distribution of D1 and D5 dopamine receptors in primate brain. *The Journal of Neuroscience*, *15*, 7821–7836.
29. Thibaut, F., Hirsch, E.C., Raisman, R., Javoy-Agid, F., Agid, Y. (1990). Microtopography of D1 dopaminergic binding sites in the human substantia nigra: an autoradiographic study. *Neuroscience*, *37*, 387–398.
30. Le Moine, C., Normand, E., Bloch, B. (1991). Phenotypical characterization of the rat striatal neurons expressing the D1 dopamine receptor gene. *Proceedings of the National Academy of Sciences of the United States of America*, *88*, 4205–4209.
31. Meador-Woodruff, J.H., Grandy, D.K., Van Tol, H.H., Damask, S.P., Little, K.Y., Civelli, O., Watson, S.J. Jr (1994). Dopamine receptor gene expression in the human medial temporal lobe. *Neuropsychopharmacology*, *10*, 239–248.
32. Khan, Z.U., Gutiérrez, A., Martín, R., Peñafiel, A., Rivera, A., De La Calle, A. (2000). Dopamine D5 receptors of rat and human brain. *Neuroscience*, *100*, 689–699.
33. Herrling, P.L., Hull, C.D. (1980). Iontophoretically applied dopamine depolarizes and hyperpolarizes the membrane of cat caudate neurons. *Brain Research*, *192*, 441–462.

34. Giros, B., El Mestikawy, S., Bertrand, L., Caron, M.G. (1991). Cloning and functional characterization of a cocaine-sensitive dopamine transporter. *FEBS Letters*, *295*, 149–154.
35. Ciliax, B.J., Heilman, C., Demchyshyn, L.L., Pristupa, Z.B., Ince, E., Hersch, S.M., Niznik, H.B., Levey, A.I. (1995). The dopamine transporter: immunochemical characterization and localization in brain. *The Journal of Neuroscience*, *15*, 1714–1723.
36. Hall, H., Halldin, C., Guilloteau, D., Chalon, S., Emond, P., Besnard, J., Farde, L., Sedvall, G. (1999). Visualization of the dopamine transporter in the human brain postmortem with the new selective ligand [125I]PE2I. *Neuroimage*, *9*, 108–116.
37. Vizi, E.S. (2000). Role of high-affinity receptors and membrane transporters in nonsynaptic communication and drug action in the central nervous system. *Pharmacological Reviews*, *52*, 63–89.
38. Jaber, M., Jones, S., Giros, B., Caron, M.G. (1997). The dopamine transporter: a crucial component regulating dopamine transmission. *Movement Disorders*, *12*, 629–633.
39. Falkenburger, B.H., Barstow, K.L., Mintz, I.M. (2001). Dendrodendritic inhibition through reversal of dopamine transport. *Science*, *293*, 2465–2470.
40. Axelrod, J., Tomchick, R. (1958). Enzymatic O-methylation of epinephrine and other catechols. *The Journal of Biological Chemistry*, *233*, 702–705.
41. Chen, J., Lipska, B.K., Halim, N., Ma, Q.D., Matsumoto, M., Melhem, S., Kolachana, B.S., Hyde, T.M., Herman, M.M., Apud, J., Egan, M.F., Kleinman, J.E., Weinberger, D.R. (2004). Functional analysis of genetic variation in catechol-O-methyltransferase (COMT): effects on mRNA, protein, and enzyme activity in postmortem human brain. *American Journal of Human Genetics*, *75*, 807–821.
42. Damier, P., Kastner, A., Agid, Y., Hirsch, E.C. (1996). Does monoamine oxidase type B play a role in dopaminergic nerve cell death in Parkinson's disease? *Neurology*, *46*, 1262–1269.
43. Bunney, B.S., Walters, J.R., Roth, R.H., Aghajanian, G.K. (1973). Dopaminergic neurons: effect of antipsychotic drugs and amphetamine on single cell activity. *The Journal of Pharmacology and Experimental Therapeutics*, *185*, 560–571.
44. Grace, A.A., Bunney, B.S. (1984). The control of firing pattern in nigral dopamine neurons: burst firing. *The Journal of neuroscience*, *4*, 2877–2890.
45. Floresco, S.B., West, A.R., Ash, B., Moore, H., Grace, A.A. (2003). Afferent modulation of dopamine neuron firing differentially regulates tonic and phasic dopamine transmission. *Nature Neuroscience*, *6*, 968–973.
46. Lacey, M.G., Mercuri, N.B., North, R.A. (1987). Dopamine acts on D2 receptors to increase potassium conductance in neurones of the rat substantia nigra zona compacta. *The Journal of Physiology*, *392*, 397–416.
47. Wu, Q., Reith, M.E., Walker, Q.D., Kuhn, C.M., Carroll, F.I., Garris, P.A. (2002). Concurrent autoreceptor-mediated control of dopamine release and uptake during neurotransmission: an in vivo voltammetric study. *The Journal of Neuroscience*, *22*, 6272–6281.
48. Chiodo, L.A., Bannon, M.J., Grace, A.A., Roth, R.H., Bunney, B.S. (1984). Evidence for the absence of impulse-regulating somatodendritic and synthesis-modulating nerve terminal autoreceptors on subpopulations of mesocortical dopamine neurons. *Neuroscience*, *12*, 1–16.

49. Sesack, S.R., Pickel, V.M. (1992). Prefrontal cortical efferents in the rat synapse on unlabeled neuronal targets of catecholamine terminals in the nucleus accumbens septi and on dopamine neurons in the ventral tegmental area. *The Journal of Comparative Neurology*, *320*, 145–160.
50. Chergui, K., Charléty, P.J., Akaoka, H., Saunier, C.F., Brunet, J.L., Buda, M., Svensson, T.H., Chouvet, G. (1993). Tonic activation of NMDA receptors causes spontaneous burst discharge of rat midbrain dopamine neurons in vivo. *The European Journal of Neuroscience*, *5*, 137–144.
51. Kalivas, P.W. (1993). Neurotransmitter regulation of dopamine neurons in the ventral tegmental area. *Brain Research. Brain Research Reviews*, *18*, 75–113.
52. Carr, D.B., Sesack, S.R. (2000). Projections from the rat prefrontal cortex to the ventral tegmental area: target specificity in the synaptic associations with mesoaccumbens and mesocortical neurons. *The Journal of Neuroscience*, *20*, 3864–3873.
53. Herve, D., Blanc, G., Glowinski, J., Tassin, J.P. (1982). Reduction of dopamine utilization in the prefrontal cortex but not in the nucleus accumbens after selective destruction of noradrenergic fibers innervating the ventral tegmental area in the rat. *Brain Research*, *237*, 510–516.
54. Alexander, G.E., Crutcher, M.D., Delong, M.R. (1990). Basal ganglia thalamocortical circuits: parallel substrates for motor, oculomotor, "prefrontal" and "limbic" functions. *Progress in Brain Research*, *85*, 119–146.
55. Joel, D., Weiner, I. (1994). The organization of the basal ganglia-thalamocortical circuits: open interconnected rather than closed segregated. *Neuroscience*, *63*, 363–379.
56. Haber, S.N., Calzavara, R. (2009). The cortico-basal ganglia integrative network: the role of the thalamus. *Brain Research Bulletin*, *78*, 69–74.
57. Smith, Y., Bevan, M.D., Shink, E., Bolam, P. (1998). Microcircuitry of the direct and indirect pathways of the basal ganglia. *Neuroscience*, *86*, 353–387.
58. Nambu, A., Tokuno, H., Takada, M. (2002). Functional significance of the cortico-subthalamo-pallidal "hyperdirect" pathway. *Neuroscience Research*, *43*(2), 111–117. Review.
59. Bentevoglio, A., Morelli, M. (2005). The organization and circuits of mesencephalic dopaminergic neurons and the distribution of dopamine receptors in the brain. In: Dunnett, S.B., Bentivoglio, M., Björklund, A., Hökfelt, T., eds. *Handbook of Chemical Neuroanatomy*. Vol 21, Dopamine. Amsterdam: Elsevier, pp. 1–108.
60. Charpentier, P. (1947). The constitution of 10-(dimethylaminopropyl)phenothiazine. *Comptes Rendus*, *225*, 306–308.
61. Sneader, W. (2002). The 50th anniversary of chlorpromazine. *Drug News & Perspectives*, *15*(7), 466–471.
62. López-Muñoz, F., Alamo, C., Cuenca, E., Shen, W.W., Clervoy, P., Rubio, G. (2005). History of the discovery and clinical introduction of chlorpromazine. *Annals of Clinical Psychiatry*, *17*(3), 113–135.
63. Laborit, H., Huguenard, P., Alluaume, R. (1952). Un noveau stabilisateur végétatif (le 4560 RP). *La Presse Médicale*, *60*, 206–208.
64. Goodman, L.S., Gilman, A. (1955). *The Pharmacological Basis of Therepeutics*, 2nd ed. New York: Macmillan.

65. Delay, J., Deniker, P. (1952). 38 cas de psychoses traitèes par la cure prolongèe et continuè de 4560 RP. *Comptes rendus du Congres des Médecins, Alieniste et Neurologistes [Congr Méd Alién Neurol] (France)*, *50*, 503–513.
66. Staehelin, J.E. (1954). Einige allgemeine Bemerkungen uber die Largactil-therapie in der psychiatrischen Universitatsklinik Basel. *Schweizerische Archives für Neurologie und Psychiatrie*, *73*, 288–291.
67. Lehmann, H.E., Hanrahan, G.E. (1954). Chlorpromazine, new inhibiting agent for psychomotor excitement and manic states. *Archives of Neurology and Psychiatry (Chicago)*, *71*, 227–237.
68. Delay, J., Deniker, P. (1955). Neuroleptic effects of chlorpromazine in the therapeutics of neuropsychiatry. *International Record of Medicine and General Practice clinics*, *168*, 318–326.
69. Kapur, S., Mamo, D. (2003). Half a century of antipsychotics and still a central role for dopamine D2 receptors. *Progress in Neuro-Psychopharmacology & Biological Psychiatry*, *27*(7), 1081–1090.
70. Ban, T.A. (2001). Pharmacotherapy of mental illness. A historical analysis. *Progress in Neuro-Psychopharmacology & Biological Psychiatry*, *25*, 709–727.
71. Carlsson, A. (2001). A paradigm shift in brain research. *Science*, *294*(5544), 1021–1024.
72. Brodie, B.B., Tomich, E.G., Kuntzman, R., Shore, P.A. (1957). On the mechanism of action of reserpine: effect of reserpine on capacity of tissues to bind serotonin. *The Journal of Pharmacology and Experimental Therapeutics*, *119*(4), 461–467.
73. Pletscher, A., Shore, P.A., Brodie, B.B. (1956). Serotonin as a mediator of reserpine action in brain. *The Journal of Pharmacology and Experimental Therapeutics*, *116*, 84–89.
74. Carlsson, A., Lindquist, M., Magnusson, T. (1957). 3,4-dihydroxyphenylalanine and 5-hydroxytryptophan as reserpine antagonists. *Nature*, *180*(4596), 1200.
75. Seeman, P., Lee, T. (1975). Antipsychotic drugs: direct correlation between clinical potency and presynaptic action on dopamine neurons. *Science*, *188*(4194), 1217–1219.
76. Creese, I., Burt, D.R., Snyder, S.H. (1976). Dopamine receptor binding predicts clinical and pharmacological potencies of antischizophrenic drugs. *Science*, *192*(4238), 481–483.
77. Nagy, J.I., Lee, T., Seeman, P., Fibiger, H.C. (1978). Direct evidence for presynaptic and postsynaptic dopamine receptors in brain. *Nature*, *274*(5668), 278–281.
78. Young, D., Scoville, W.B. (1938). Paranoid psychosis in narcolepsy and the possible danger of benzedrine treatment. *The Medical Clinics of North America*, *22*, 637–646.
79. van Rossum, J.M., van der Schoot, J.B., Hurkmans, J.A. (1962). Mechanism of action of cocaine and amphetamine in the brain. *Experientia*, *18*, 229–231.
80. van Rossum, J.M. (1966). The significance of dopamine receptor blockade for the mechanisms of action of neuroleptic drugs. *Archives Internationales de Pharmacodynamie et de Therapie*, *160*(2), 492–494.
81. Baumeister, A.A., Francis, J.L. (2002). Historical development of the dopamine hypothesis of schizophrenia. *Journal of the History of the Neurosciences*, *11*(3), 265–277.

82. Mackay, A.V.P., Iversen, L.L., Rossor, M., Spokes, E., Bird, E., Arregui, A., Creese, I., Snyder, S.H. (1982). Increased brain dopamine and dopamine receptors in schizophrenia. *Archives of General Psychiatry*, *39*, 991–997.
83. Reynolds, G.P. (1983). Increased concentrations and lateral asymmetry of amygdala dopamine in schizophrenia. *Nature*, *305*, 527–529.
84. Widerlöv, E. (1988). A critical appraisal of CSF monoamine metabolite studies in schizophrenia. *Annals of the New York Academy of Sciences*, *537*, 309–323.
85. De Keyser, J. (1993). Subtypes and localization of dopamine receptors in human brain. *Neurochemistry International*, *22*(2), 83–93.
86. Seeman, P. (1981). Dopamine receptors in post-mortem schizophrenic brains. *Lancet*, *1*(8229), 1103.
87. Seeman, P., Guan, H.C., Van Tol, H.H. (1993). Dopamine D4 receptors elevated in schizophrenia. *Nature*, *365*(6445), 441–445.
88. Wong, D.F., Wagner, H.N. Jr, Tune, L.E., Dannals, R.F., Pearlson, G.D., Links, J.M., Tamminga, C.A., Broussolle, E.P., Ravert, H.T., Wilson, A.A., Toung, J.K., Malat, J., Williams, J.A., O'Tuama, L.A., Snyder, S.H., Kuhar, M.J., Gjedde, A. (1986). Positron emission tomography reveals elevated D2 dopamine receptors in drug-naive schizophrenics. *Science*, *234*(4783), 1558–1563.
89. Lidow, M.S., Goldman-Rakic, P.S. (1994). A common action of clozapine, haloperidol, and remoxipride on D1- and D2-dopaminergic receptors in the primate cerebral cortex. *Proceedings of the National Academy of Sciences of the United States of America*, *91*, 4353–4356.
90. Farde, L., Wiesel, F.A., Hall, H., Halldin, C., Stone-Elander, S., Sedvall, G. (1987). No D2 receptor increase in PET study of schizophrenia. *Archives of General Psychiatry*, *44*(7), 671–672.
91. Hietala, J., Syvälahti, E., Vuorio, K., Någren, K., Lehikoinen, P., Ruotsalainen, U., Räkköläinen, V., Lehtinen, V., Wegelius, U. (1994). Striatal D2 dopamine receptor characteristics in neuroleptic-naive schizophrenic patients studied with positron emission tomography. *Archives of General Psychiatry*, *51*(2), 116–123.
92. Nordström, A.L., Farde, L., Eriksson, L., Halldin, C. (1995). No elevated D2 dopamine receptors in neuroleptic-naive schizophrenic patients revealed by positron emission tomography and [11C]N-methylspiperone. *Psychiatry Research*, *61*(2), 67–83.
93. Reynolds, G.P., Mason, S.L. (1995). Absence of detectable striatal dopamine D4 receptors in drug-treated schizophrenia. *European Journal of Pharmacology*, *281*(2), R5–R6.
94. Farde, L. (1997). Brain imaging of schizophrenia—the dopamine hypothesis. *Schizophrenia Research*, *28*(2–3), 157–162.
95. Carpenter, W.T. Jr, Strauss, J.S., Bartko, J.J. (1981). Beyond diagnosis: the phenomenology of schizophrenia. *The American Journal of Psychiatry*, *138*(7), 948–953.
96. Andreasen, N.C. (1982). Negative symptoms in schizophrenia. Definition and reliability. *Archives of General Psychiatry*, *39*(7), 784–788.
97. Andreasen, N.C., Olsen, S. (1982). Negative v positive schizophrenia. Definition and validation. *Archives of General Psychiatry*, *39*(7), 789–794.
98. Angrist, B., Rotrosen, J., Gershon, S. (1980). Differential effects of amphetamine and neuroleptics on negative versus positive symptoms in schizophrenia. *Psychopharmacology (Berl)*, *72*(1), 17–19.

99. Davis, K.L., Kahn, R.S., Ko, G., Davidson, M. (1991). Dopamine in schizophrenia: a review and reconceptualization. *The American Journal of Psychiatry*, *148*(11), 1474–1486.
100. Sesack, S.R., Carr, D.B. (2002). Selective prefrontal cortex inputs to dopamine cells: implications for schizophrenia. *Physiology & Behavior*, *77*(4–5), 513–517.
101. Alves, F.S., Figee, M., Vamelsvoort, T., Veltman, D., de Haan, L. (2008). The revised dopamine hypothesis of schizophrenia: evidence from pharmacological MRI studies with atypical antipsychotic medication. *Psychopharmacology Bulletin*, *41*(1), 121–132.
102. Hand, T.H., Hu, X.-T., Wang, R.Y. (1987). Differential effects of acute clozapine and haloperidol on the activity of ventral tegmental (A10) and nigrostriatal (A9) dopamine neurons. *Brain Research*, *415*(2), 257–269.
103. McCulloch, J., Savaki, H.E., McCuUoch, M.C., Jehle, J., Sokoloff, L. (1982). The distribution of alterations in energy metabolism in the rat brain produced by apomorphine. *Brain Research*, *243*, 67–80.
104. Geraud, G., Arne-Bes, M.C., Guell, A., Bes, A. (1987). Reversibility of hemodynamic hypofrontality in schizophrenia. *Journal of Cerebral Blood Flow and Metabolism*, *7*, 9–12.
105. Ingvar, D.H., Franzen, G. (1974). Abnormalities of cerebral blood flow distribution in patients with chronic schizophrenia. *Acta Psychiatrica Scandinavica*, *50*, 425–462.
106. Weinberger, D.R., Berman, K.F. (1988). Speculation on the meaning of cerebral metabolic hypofrontality in schizophrenia. *Schizophrenia Bulletin*, *14*(2), 157–168.
107. Hill, K., Mann, L., Laws, K.R., Stephenson, C.M., Nimmo-Smith, I., McKenna, P.J. (2004). Hypofrontality in schizophrenia: a meta-analysis of functional imaging studies. *Acta Psychiatrica Scandinavica*, *110*(4), 243–256.
108. Kellendonk, C., Simpson, E.H., Polan, H.J., Malleret, G., Vronskaya, S., Winiger, V., Moore, H., Kandel, E.R. (2006). Transient and selective overexpression of dopamine D2 receptors in the striatum causes persistent abnormalities in prefrontal cortex functioning. *Neuron*, *49*, 603–615.
109. Carlsson, A. (1977). Does dopamine play a role in schizophrenia? *Psychological Medicine*, *7*, 583–597.
110. Kim, J.S., Kornhuber, H.H., Schmid-Burgk, W., Holzmüller, B. (1980). Low cerebrospinal fluid glutamate in schizophrenic patients and a new hypothesis on schizophrenia. *Neuroscience Letters*, *20*, 379–382.
111. Carlsson, A., Hansson, L.O., Waters, N., Carlsson, M.L. (1999). A glutamatergic deficiency model of schizophrenia. *The British Journal of Psychiatry. Supplement*, *37*, 2–6.
112. Olney, J.W., Newcomer, J.W., Farber, N.B. (1999). NMDA receptor hypofunction model of schizophrenia. *Journal of Psychiatric Research*, *33*, 523–533.
113. Pilowsky, L.S., Bressan, R.A., Stone, J.M., Erlandsson, K., Mulligan, R.S., Krystal, J.H., Ell, P.J. (2006). First in vivo evidence of an NMDA receptor deficit in medication-free schizophrenic patients. *Molecular Psychiatry*, *11*, 118–119.
114. Meltzer, H.Y. (1989). Clinical studies on the mechanism of action of clozapine: the dopamine-serotonin hypothesis of schizophrenia. *Psychopharmacology (Berl)*, *99*(Suppl S), 18–27.

115. Akira, M., Takahiro, K., Shigenobu, K. (2009). Cytokines and schizophrenia: microglia hypothesis of schizophrenia. *Psychiatry and Clinical Neurosciences*, *63*(3), 257–269.

116. Dean, B. (2000). Signal transmission, rather than reception, is the underlying neurochemical abnormality in schizophrenia. *The Australian and New Zealand Journal of Psychiatry*, *34*(4), 560–569.

117. Gao, M., Liu, C.L., Yang, S., Jin, G.Z., Bunney, B.S., Shi, W.X. (2007). Functional coupling between the prefrontal cortex and dopamine neurons in the ventral tegmental area. *The Journal of Neuroscience*, *27*(20), 5414–5421.

118. Laruelle, M., Abi-Dargham, A., Van Dyck, C.H., Gil, R., D'Souza, C.D., Erdos, J., McCance, E., Dolan, R.J., Fletcher, P., Frith, C.D., Friston, K.J., Frackowiak, R.S., Grasby, P.M. (1995). Dopaminergic modulation of impaired cognitive activation in the anterior cingulate cortex in schizophrenia. *Nature*, *378*, 180–182.

119. Winterer, G., Weinberger, D.R. (2004). Genes, dopamine and cortical signal-to-noise ratio in schizophrenia. *Trends in Neurosciences*, *27*, 683–690.

120. Halldin, C., Farde, L., Hogberg, T., Mohell, N., Hall, H., Suhara, T. et al. (1995). Carbon–11-FLB 457: a radioligand for extrastriatal D2 dopamine receptors. *Journal of Nuclear Medicine*, *36*, 1275–1281.

121. Kessler, R.M., Mason, N.S., Votaw, J.R., De Paulis, T., Clanton, J.A., Ansari, M.S., Schmidt, D.E., Manning, R.G., Bell, R.L. (1992). Visualization of extrastriatal dopamine D2 receptors in the human brain. *European Journal of Pharmacology*, *223*, 105–107.

122. Mukherjee, J., Yang, Z.Y., Das, M.K., Brown, T. (1995). Fluorinated benzamide neuroleptics—III. Development of (S)-N-[(1-allyl-2-pyrrolidinyl)methyl]-5-(3-[18F]fluoropropyl)-2, 3-dimethoxybenzamide as an improved dopamine D-2 receptor tracer. *Nuclear Medicine and Biology*, *22*, 283–296.

123. Suhara, T., Okubo, Y., Yasuno, F., Sudo, Y., Inoue, M., Ichimiya, T., et al. (2002). Decreased dopamine D2 receptor binding in the anterior cingulate cortex in schizophrenia. *Archives of General Psychiatry*, *59*, 25–30.

124. Talvik, M., Nordström, A.L., Olsson, H., Halldin, C., Farde, L. (2003). Decreased thalamic D2/D3 receptor binding in drug-naive patients with schizophrenia: a PET study with [11C]FLB457. *The International Journal of Neuropsychopharmacology*, *6*, 361–370.

125. Tuppurainen, H., Kuikka, J., Viinamaki, H., Husso-Saastamoinen, M., Bergstrom, K., Tiihonen, J. (2003). Extrastriatal dopamine D 2/3 receptor density and distribution in drug-naive schizophrenic patients. *Molecular Psychiatry*, *8*, 453–455.

126. Buchsbaum, M.S., Christian, B.T., Lehrer, D.S., Narayanan, T.K., Shi, B., Mantil, J., Kemether, E., Oakes, T.R., Mukherjee, J. (2006). D2/D3 dopamine receptor binding with [F-18]fallypride in thalamus and cortex of patients with schizophrenia. *Schizophrenia Research*, *85*, 232–244.

127. Kessler, R.M., Woodward, N.D., Riccardi, P., Li, R., Ansari, M.S., Anderson, S., Dawant, B., Zald, D., Meltzer, H.Y. (2009). Dopamine D2 receptor levels in striatum, thalamus, substantia nigra, limbic regions, and cortex in schizophrenic subjects. *Biological Psychiatry*, *65*, 1024–1031.

128. Yasuno, F., Suhara, T., Okubo, Y., Sudo, Y., Inoue, M., Ichimiya, T., et al. (2004). Low dopamine D(2) receptor binding in subregions of the thalamus in schizophrenia. *The American Journal of Psychiatry*, *161*, 1016–1022.

129. Stone, J.M., Davis, J.M., Leucht, S., Pilowsky, L.S. (2009). Cortical dopamine D2/D3 receptors are a common site of action for antipsychotic drugs—an original patient data meta-analysis of the SPECT and PET in vivo receptor imaging literature. *Schizophrenia Bulletin*, *35*, 789–797.

130. Kegeles, L.S., Slifstein, M., Frankle, W.G., Xu, X., Hackett, E., Bae, S.A., Gonzales, R., Kim, J.H., Alvarez, B., Gil, R., Laruelle, M., Abi-Dargham, A. (2008). Dose-occupancy study of striatal and extrastriatal dopamine D2 receptors by aripiprazole in schizophrenia with PET and [18F]fallypride. *Neuropsychopharmacology*, *33*, 3111–3125.

131. Kessler, R.M., Ansari, M.S., Riccardi, P., Li, R., Jayathilake, K., Dawant, B., Meltzer, H.Y. (2006). Occupancy of striatal and extrastriatal dopamine D2 receptors by clozapine and quetiapine. *Neuropsychopharmacology.*, *31*(9), 1991–2001.

132. Gründer, G., Landvogt, C., Vernaleken, I., Buchholz, H.G., Ondracek, J., Siessmeier, T., Härtter, S., Schreckenberger, M., Stoeter, P., Hiemke, C., Rösch, F., Wong, D.F., Bartenstein, P. (2006). The striatal and extrastriatal D2/D3 receptor-binding profile of clozapine in patients with schizophrenia. *Neuropsychopharmacology*, *31*, 1027–1035.

133. Vernaleken, I., Fellows, C., Janouschek, H., Bröcheler, A., Veselinovic, T., Landvogt, C., Boy, C., Buchholz, H.G., Spreckelmeyer, K., Bartenstein, P., Cumming, P., Hiemke, C., Rösch, F., Schäfer, W., Wong, D.F., Gründer, G. (2008). Striatal and extrastriatal D2/D3-receptor-binding properties of ziprasidone: a positron emission tomography study with [18F]Fallypride and [11C]raclopride (D2/D3-receptor occupancy of ziprasidone). *Journal of Clinical Psychopharmacology*, *28*, 608–617.

134. Kessler, R.M., Ansari, M.S., Riccardi, P., Li, R., Jayathilake, K., Dawant, B., Meltzer, H.Y. (2005). Occupancy of striatal and extrastriatal dopamine D2/D3 receptors by olanzapine and haloperidol. *Neuropsychopharmacology*, *30*, 2283–2289.

135. Talvik, M., Nordström, A.L., Nyberg, S., Olsson, H., Halldin, C., Farde, L. (2001). No support for regional selectivity in clozapine-treated patients: a PET study with [(11)C]raclopride and [(11)C]FLB 457. *The American Journal of Psychiatry*, *158*, 926–930.

136. Ito, H., Arakawa, R., Takahashi, H., Takano, H., Okumura, M., Otsuka, T., Ikoma, Y., Shidahara, M., Suhara, T. (2009). No regional difference in dopamine D2 receptor occupancy by the second-generation antipsychotic drug risperidone in humans: a positron emission tomography study. *The International Journal of Neuropsychopharmacology*, *12*, 667–675.

137. Nyberg, S., Olsson, H., Nilsson, U., Maehlum, E., Halldin, C., Farde, L. (2002). Low striatal and extra-striatal D2 receptor occupancy during treatment with the atypical antipsychotic sertindole. *Psychopharmacology (Berl)*, *162*, 37–41.

138. Agid, O., Mamo, D., Ginovart, N., Vitcu, I., Wilson, A.A., Zipursky, R.B., Kapur, S. (2007). Striatal versus extrastriatal dopamine D2 receptors in antipsychotic response—a double-blind PET study in schizophrenia. *Neuropsychopharmacology*, *32*, 1209–1215.

139. Watanabe, M., Kodama, T., Hikosaka, K. (1997). Increase of extracellular dopamine in primate prefrontal cortex during a working memory task. *Journal of Neurophysiology*, *78*, 2795–2798.

140. Sawaguchi, T., Goldman-Rakic, P.S. (1991). D1 dopamine receptors in prefrontal cortex: involvement in working memory. *Science*, *251*, 947–950.

141. Williams, G.V., Goldman-Rakic, P.S. (1995). Modulation of memory fields by dopamine D1 receptors in prefrontal cortex. *Nature*, *376*, 572–575.

142. Okubo, Y., Suhara, T., Suzuki, K., Kobayashi, K., Inoue, O., Terasaki, O., Someya, Y., Sassa, T., Sudo, Y., Matsushima, E., Iyo, M., Tateno, Y., Toru, M. (1997). Decreased prefrontal dopamine D1 receptors in schizophrenia revealed by PET. *Nature*, *385*, 634–636.

143. Abi-Dargham, A., Moore, H. (2003). Prefrontal DA transmission at D1 receptors and the pathology of schizophrenia. *The Neuroscientist*, *9*, 404–416.

144. Karlsson, P., Farde, L., Halldin, C., Sedvall, G. (2002). PET study of D(1) dopamine receptor binding in neuroleptic-naive patients with schizophrenia. *The American Journal of Psychiatry*, *159*(5), 761–767.

145. Hirvonen, J., van Erp, T.G., Huttunen, J., Aalto, S., Någren, K., Huttunen, M., Lönnqvist, J., Kaprio, J., Cannon, T.D., Hietala, J. (2006). Brain dopamine D1 receptors in twins discordant for schizophrenia. *The American Journal of Psychiatry*, *163*, 1747–1753.

146. McGowan, S., Lawrence, A.D., Sales, T., Quested, D., Grasby, P. (2004). Presynaptic dopaminergic dysfunction in schizophrenia: a positron emission tomographic [18F]fluorodopa study. *Archives of General Psychiatry*, *61*(2), 134–142.

147. Howes, O.D., Montgomery, A.J., Asselin, M.C., Murray, R.M., Grasby, P.M., McGuire, P.K. (2007). Molecular imaging studies of the striatal dopaminergic system in psychosis and predictions for the prodromal phase of psychosis. *The British Journal of Psychiatry*, *51*(Suppl), S13–S18.

148. Valli, I., Howes, O., Tyrer, P., McGuire, P., Grasby, P.M. (2008). Longitudinal PET imaging in a patient with schizophrenia did not show marked changes in dopaminergic function with relapse of psychosis. *The American Journal of Psychiatry*, *165*, 1613–1614.

149. Howes, O.D., Montgomery, A.J., Asselin, M.C., Murray, R.M., Valli, I., Tabraham, P., Bramon-Bosch, E., Valmaggia, L., Johns, L., Broome, M., McGuire, P.K., Grasby, P.M. (2009). Elevated striatal dopamine function linked to prodromal signs of schizophrenia. *Archives of General Psychiatry*, *66*, 13–20.

150. Kegeles, L.S., Abi-Dargham, A., Zea-Ponce, Y., Rodenhiser-Hill, J., Mann, J.J., Van Heertum, R.L., Cooper, T.B., Carlsson, A., Laruelle, M. (2000). Modulation of amphetamine-induced striatal dopamine release by ketamine in humans: implications for schizophrenia. *Biological Psychiatry*, *48*, 627–640.

151. Taylor, S.F., Koeppe, R.A., Tandon, R., Zubieta, J.K., Frey, K.A. (2000). In vivo measurement of the vesicular monoamine transporter in schizophrenia. *Neuropsychopharmacology*, *23*, 667–675.

152. Laakso, A., Vilkman, H., Alakare, B., Haaparanta, M., Bergman, J., Solin, O., Peurasaari, J., Räkköläinen, V., Syvälahti, E., Hietala, H. (2000). Striatal dopamine transporter binding in neuroleptic-naive patients with schizophrenia studied with positron emission tomography. *The American Journal of Psychiatry*, *157*, 269–271.

153. Schmitt, G.J., Meisenzahl, E.M., Frodl, T., La Fougère, C., Hahn, K., Möller, H.J., Dresel, S. (2005). The striatal dopamine transporter in first-episode, drug-naive schizophrenic patients: evaluation by the new SPECT-ligand[99mTc]TRODAT-1. *Journal of Psychopharmacology*, *19*, 488–493.

154. Laakso, A., Bergman, J., Haaparanta, M., Vilkman, H., Solin, O., Syvälahti, E., Hietala, H. (2001). Decreased striatal dopamine transporter binding in vivo in chronic schizophrenia. *Schizophrenia Research*, *52*, 115–120.

155. Schmitt, G.J., Frodl, T., Dresel, S., La Fougère, C., Bottlender, R., Koutsouleris, N., Hahn, K., Möller, H.J., Meisenzahl, E.M. (2006). Striatal dopamine transporter availability is associated with the productive psychotic state in first episode, drug-naive schizophrenic patients. *European Archives of Psychiatry and Clinical Neuroscience*, *256*, 115–121.

156. Weinberger, D.R., Berman, K.F., Suddath, R., Torrey, E.F. (1992). Evidence of dysfunction of a prefrontal-limbic network in schizophrenia: a magnetic resonance imaging and regional cerebral blood flow study of discordant monozygotic twins. *The American Journal of Psychiatry*, *149*, 890–897.

157. Bullmore, E.T., Frangou, S., Murray, R.M. (1997). The dysplastic net hypothesis: an integration of developmental and dysconnectivity theories of schizophrenia. *Schizophrenia Research*, *28*, 143–156.

158. Meyer-Lindenberg, A., Poline, J.B., Kohn, P.D., Holt, J.L., Egan, M.F., Weinberger, D.R., Berman, K.F. (2001). Evidence for abnormal cortical functional connectivity during working memory in schizophrenia. *The American Journal of Psychiatry*, *158*, 1809–1817.

159. Callicott, J.H., Mattay, V.S., Verchinski, B.A., Marenco, S., Egan, M.F., Weinberger, D.R. (2003). Complexity of prefrontal cortical dysfunction in schizophrenia: more than up or down. *The American Journal of Psychiatry*, *160*, 2209–2215.

160. Wang, J., O'Donnell, P. (2001). D1 dopamine receptors potentiate NMDA mediated excitability increase in layer v prefrontal cortical pyramidal neurons. *Cerebral Cortex*, *11*, 452–462.

161. Lachman, H.M. (2008). Does COMT val158met affect behavioral phenotypes: yes, no, maybe? *Neuropsychopharmacology*, *33*, 3027–3029.

162. Bertolino, A., Caforio, G., Blasi, G., Candia, M.D., Latorre, V., Petruzzella, V., et al. (2004). Interaction of COMT Val108/158 met genotype and olanzapine treatment on prefrontal cortical function in patients with schizophrenia. *The American Journal of Psychiatry*, *161*, 1798–1805.

163. Weickert, T.W., Goldberg, T.E., Mishara, A., Apud, J.A., Kolachana, B.S., Egan, M.F., Weinberger, D.R. (2004). Catechol-O-methyltransferase val108/158met genotype predicts working memory response to antipsychotic medications. *Biological Psychiatry*, *56*, 677.

164. Tan, H.Y., Callicott, J.H., Weinberger, D.R. (2007). Dysfunctional and compensatory prefrontal cortical systems, genes and the pathogenesis of schizophrenia. *Cerebral Cortex*, *1*(Suppl), i171–i181.

165. Williams, H.J., Owe, M.J., O'Donovan, M.C. (2007). Is COMT a susceptibility gene for schizophrenia? *Schizophrenia Bulletin*, *33*, 635–641.

166. Sand, P.G., Domani, M., Smesny, S. (2010). Critical reappraisal of a COMT transversion variant in schizophrenia. *Biological Psychiatry*, *6*, e41–e42.

167. Kendler, K.S., Diehl, S.R. (1993). The genetics of schizophrenia: a current, genetic-epidemiologic perspective. *Schizophrenia Bulletin*, *19*, 261–285.

168. Shi, J., Gershon, E.S., Liu, C. (2008). Genetic associations with schizophrenia: meta-analyses of 12 candidate genes. *Schizophrenia Research*, *104*, 96–107.

169. Cichon, S., Nöthen, M.M., Stöber, G., Schroers, R., Albus, M., Maier, W., Rietschel, M., Körner, J., Weigelt, B., Franzek, E., Wildenauer, D., Fimmers, R., Propping, P. (1996). Systematic screening for mutations in the 5′-regulatory region of the human dopamine D1 receptor (DRD1) gene in patients with schizophrenia and bipolar affective disorder. *American Journal of Medical Genetics*, *67*, 424–428.

170. Ambrósio, A.M., Kennedy, J.L., Macciardi, F., Macedo, A., Valente, J., Dourado, A., Oliveira, C.R., Pato, C. (2004). Family association study between DRD2 and DRD3 gene polymorphisms and schizophrenia in a Portuguese population. *Psychiatry Research*, *125*, 185–191.

171. Glatt, S.J., Faraone, S.V., Tsuang, M.T. (2004). DRD2-141C insertion/deletion polymorphism is not associated with schizophrenia: results of a meta-analysis. *American Journal of Medical Genetics. Part B, Neuropsychiatric Genetics*, *128B*, 21–23.

172. Glatt, S.J., Jonsson, E.G. (2006). The Cys allele of the DRD2 Ser311Cys polymorphism has a dominant effect on risk for schizophrenia: evidence from fixed- and random-effects meta-analyses. *American Journal of Medical Genetics. Part B, Neuropsychiatric Genetics*, *141*, 149–154.

173. Staddon, S., Arranz, M.J., Mancama, D., Perez-Nievas, F., Arrizabalaga, I., Anney, R., Buckland, P., Elkin, A., Osborne, S., Munro, J., Mata, I., Kerwin, R.W. (2005). Association between dopamine D3 receptor gene polymorphisms and schizophrenia in an isolate population. *Schizophrenia Research*, *73*, 49–54.

174. D'Souza, U.M., Russ, C., Tahir, E., Mill, J., McGuffin, P., Asherson, P.J., Craig, I.W. (2004). Functional effects of a tandem duplication polymorphism in the 5′flanking region of the DRD4 gene. *Biological Psychiatry*, *56*, 691–697.

175. Gamma, F., Faraone, S.V., Glatt, S.J., Yeh, Y.C., Tsuang, M.T. (2005). Meta-analysis shows schizophrenia is not associated with the 40-base-pair repeat polymorphism of the dopamine transporter gene. *Schizophrenia Research*, *73*, 55–58.

176. Egan, M.F., Goldberg, T.E., Kolachana, B.S., Callicott, J.H., Mazzanti, C.M., Straub, R.E., Goldman, D., Weinberger, D.R. (2001). Effect of COMT Val108/158 Met genotype on frontal lobe function and risk for schizophrenia. *Proceedings of the National Academy of Sciences of the United States of America*, *98*, 6917–6922.

177. Williams, H.J., Glaser, B., Williams, N.M., Norton, N., Zammit, S., MacGregor, S., Kirov, G.K., Owen, M.J., O'Donovan, M.C. (2005). No association between schizophrenia and polymorphisms in COMT in two large samples. *The American Journal of Psychiatry*, *162*, 1736–1738.

# 2

# DOPAMINE $D_2/D_3$ PARTIAL AGONISTS AS ANTIPSYCHOTICS

PHILIP G. STRANGE

## 2.1 INTRODUCTION

Schizophrenia is currently treated using antipsychotic drugs that constitute a large, chemically diverse set of compounds, all of which can be used to treat the positive (i.e., psychotic) symptoms of schizophrenia (see References [1–4] for recent reviews on the disorder and its treatment). The drugs that were introduced earlier, the typical antipsychotics such as haloperidol and chlorpromazine, have therapeutic antipsychotic effects but also cause significant motor (extrapyramidal) side effects including acute dystonia, akathisia, parkinsonism, and tardive dyskinesia. Drugs introduced more recently, the atypical antipsychotics such as clozapine, olanzapine, and quetiapine, have therapeutic antipsychotic effects but a much reduced propensity for eliciting motor side effects. These newer drugs are also reported to have some effects on the negative symptoms of the disorder. Most of the antipsychotic drugs also produce other side effects, for example, hyperprolactinemia, sedation, and weight gain.

Although the antipsychotic drugs have different affinities at a range of receptors, they all have the ability to bind with moderate to high affinity to dopamine receptors of the $D_2$-like subfamily ($D_2$, $D_3$, and $D_4$) [5]. It seems that binding to $D_4$ receptors is not a prerequisite for antipsychotic action whereas

*Targets and Emerging Therapies for Schizophrenia*, First Edition.
Edited by Jeffrey S. Albert and Michael W. Wood.

affinity at $D_2$ and $D_3$ receptors seems to be a common feature, although the relative importance of effects at $D_2$ or $D_3$ receptors is unclear. The drugs have been shown to inhibit dopamine function in a variety of tests. It has been assumed that the drugs are antagonists at $D_2/D_3$ receptors, but, in several *in vitro* assays, the drugs exhibit inverse agonism at these receptors [6]. Whether this inverse agonism is expressed *in vivo* will depend on the level of agonist-independent receptor activation. Overall, these drugs will block the effects of dopamine at $D_2/D_3$ receptors and possibly suppress basal signaling where this is present.

Because the antipsychotic drugs appear to achieve their therapeutic effects by inhibition of the effects of the neurotransmitter dopamine, theories of schizophrenia based around changes in levels of brain dopamine have been very popular. In these "dopamine theories" of schizophrenia, increased levels or activity of dopamine underlie the psychotic symptoms of the disorder. These theories are supported by the observation that dopamine release is higher in the brains (striatum) of schizophrenia patients undergoing a psychotic episode [7, 8]. It is thought that the increased dopamine release occurs in the ventral striatum (olfactory tubercle and nucleus accumbens) [9, 10]. The antipsychotic drugs then counteract the increased dopamine release in the ventral striatum. Extrapyramidal side effects are thought to result from blockade of dopamine actions in the dorsal striatum (caudate nucleus, putamen). More recently it has been proposed that dopamine release in brain regions such as the prefrontal cortex may be reduced in schizophrenia patients [9, 10]. There is less direct evidence for this proposal, although the level of dopamine in prefrontal regions may be important for cognition and reduced prefrontal dopamine could contribute to some of the negative symptoms of schizophrenia [11]. According to these ideas, schizophrenia is a disorder of dopamine imbalance with raised dopamine in the ventral striatum and reduced dopamine in the prefrontal cortex. Currently used antipsychotics will reduce the ventral striatal dopamine hyperfunction but may further inhibit dopamine function in the cortex.

It is important to realize that the currently used antipsychotics reduce ventral striatal dopamine hyperfunction but do not fully inhibit it. It can be calculated, based on dopamine release studies [7, 8], that striatal dopamine release is increased by about twofold during psychosis [5]. When olanzapine is used for therapy, the occupancy of dopamine receptors is ~55% [12], and this will restore dopamine release to normal levels [6]. If, however, too high a dose of the drug is administered, there may be too great an inhibition of ventral striatal dopamine function; the inverse agonism of these drugs may contribute here as well. This may lead to unwanted side effects such as extrapyramidal side effects.

Although the antipsychotics have been enormously helpful in treating schizophrenia, there are still problems with these drugs. This is illustrated by the recent CATIE trial where, by 18 months, 74% of the patients had discontinued drug therapy due to lack of efficacy or intolerable side effects [13]. There is still a need for new drugs that can have improved efficacy and can be tolerated better. Based on the ideas proposed above, it has been suggested that new drugs should be developed that stabilize dopamine function rather than just inhibiting it (dopamine stabilizers) [14]. Dopamine stabilizers would be drugs that decrease dopamine function where it is too high and increase dopamine function where it is too low. One class of drugs that might act as dopamine stabilizers would be dopamine $D_2/D_3$ partial agonists.

## 2.2 DOPAMINE $D_2/D_3$ PARTIAL AGONISTS

Dopamine $D_2/D_3$ partial agonists constitute another group of compounds that have been proposed as novel antipsychotic drugs. In principle, a $D_2/D_3$ dopamine receptor partial agonist should reduce ventral striatal dopamine hyperfunction while at the same time increasing dopamine function in the prefrontal cortex. Such drugs could then counteract positive and negative symptoms of schizophrenia as well as improving cognitive symptoms. Such a drug may also not elicit extrapyramidal side effects if effects of the drug on dorsal striatal dopamine function are not too high. The overall effects of the drug would depend on the intrinsic efficacy of the drug and the levels of dopamine in the various brain regions. If the intrinsic efficacy of the drug is too high, then the dopamine tone in the ventral striatum may be high enough to provoke psychosis.

It is worth considering this approach in a little more detail in order to understand the underlying ideas. Currently used drugs are all antagonists/inverse agonists at $D_2/D_3$ receptors. These compounds lie toward the negative end of the efficacy scale (Fig. 2.1) and will inhibit excess dopamine function, possibly driving it down below normal levels. Partial agonists will lie near the neutral midpoint of the efficacy scale but on the positive side and so are quite different drugs in terms of their signaling ability. These drugs are unlikely to lead to dopamine hypofunction.

There is also the question of pre- and postsynaptic dopamine receptors. Dopamine synapses possess postsynaptic receptors that are responsible for the signaling activity of the synapse (Fig. 2.2). There also exist presynaptic autoreceptors that control the release of dopamine as well as the firing rate of the

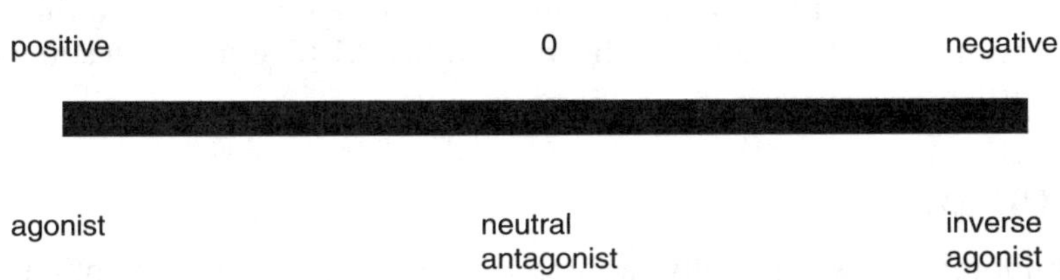


**FIGURE 2.1** Scale of efficacy. The diagram shows the relation between agonists (compounds with positive efficacy) and inverse agonists (compounds with negative efficacy) as a continuous scale.

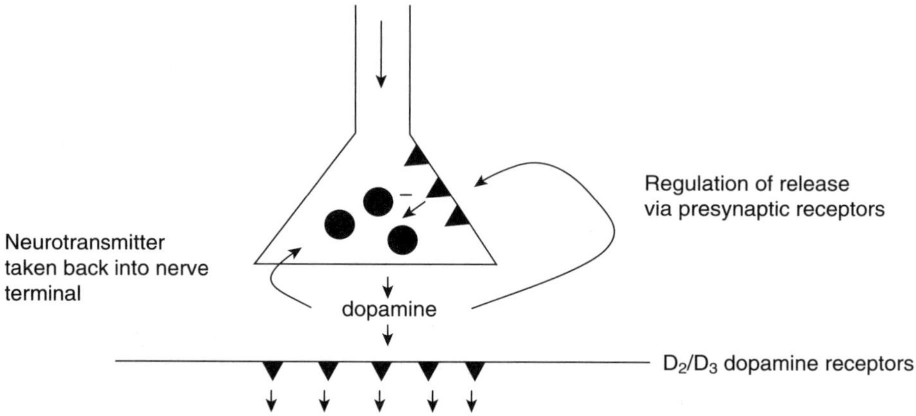


**FIGURE 2.2** Schematic of a dopamine synapse showing pre- and postsynaptic effects of dopamine.

neurons. The sensitivity of presynaptic receptors appears to be more amplified than postsynaptic receptors [15], such that a low intrinsic efficacy agonist may appear as an antagonist at postsynaptic receptors while still showing agonist activity at presynaptic receptors. The relative importance of pre- and postsynaptic effects will depend on the receptor occupancy achieved by the drugs. If receptor occupancy is high, then postsynaptic effects will dominate.

Based on these ideas, some have tried to develop dopamine stabilizers that are partial agonists, whereas others have chosen to develop presynaptic agonist/postynaptic antagonist drugs. It seems likely that these two approaches are actually equivalent when the partial agonists have low intrinsic efficacy. In that case, the drug will appear as a presynaptic agonist and postsynaptic antagonist due to the relative amplification characteristics of pre- and postsynaptic receptors.

The development of partial agonist drugs is an attractive approach to the development of new antipsychotics and has been employed by several pharmaceutical companies and academic groups, leading to the development of several new compounds and the introduction of one drug, aripiprazole. I will now consider some of the key compounds that have emerged from this work. Structures of the compounds are shown in Table 2.1 together with some comparator drugs.

### 2.2.1 UH-232

This aminotetralin was initially reported to be a selective presynaptic $D_2$-like receptor antagonist [16]. Subsequent work has shown that UH-232 is a partial agonist at $D_2$ and $D_3$ dopamine receptors but with a low intrinsic efficacy at $D_2$ receptors [17–21]. In one limited clinical trial the drug was shown to be

**TABLE 2.1 $D_2/D_3$ Dopamine Partial Agonist Drugs That Have Been Considered Potential Antipsychotics**

| Drug | Structure | Intrinsic Efficacy | Development Stage |
|---|---|---|---|
| (-)-3-PPP | 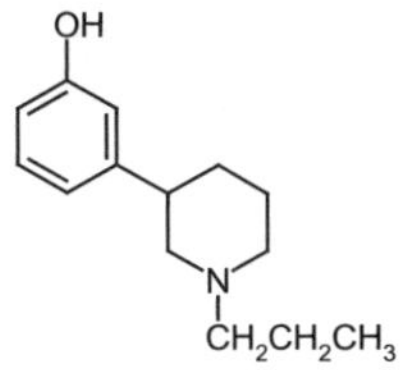 | 31.7 | Not developed |
| Aplindore | 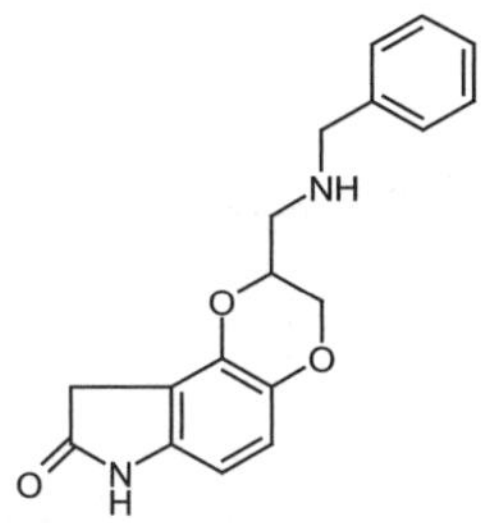 | 16.9 | Development halted |
| Bifeprunox | 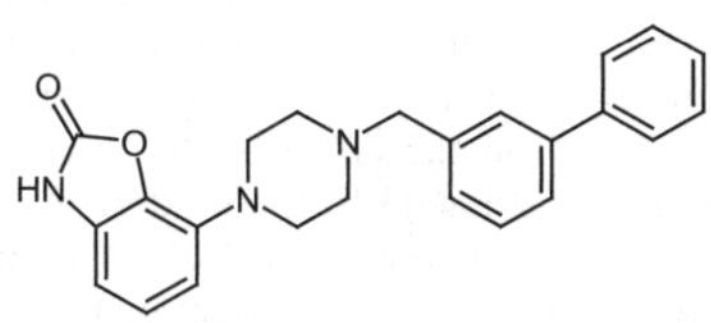 | 14.3 | Development halted |
| OPC4392 | 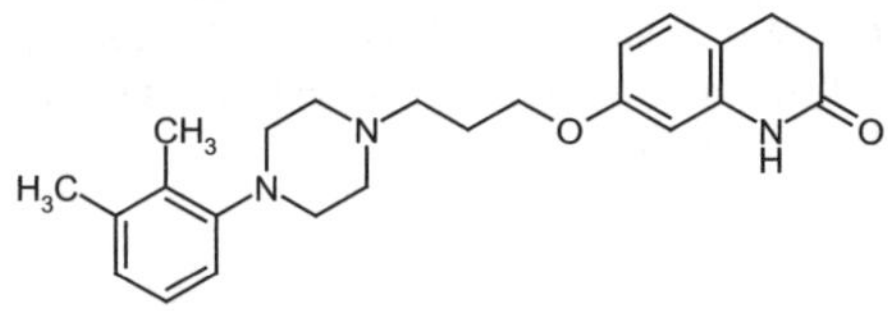 | 13.8 | Not developed |
| RGH-188 | 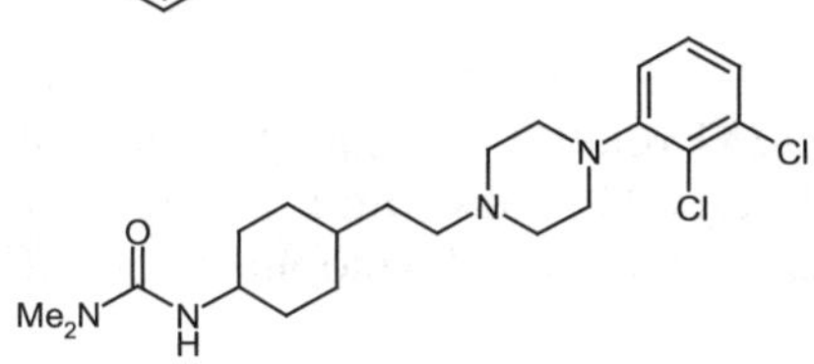 | ~6 | In Phase III trials |
| Aripiprazole | 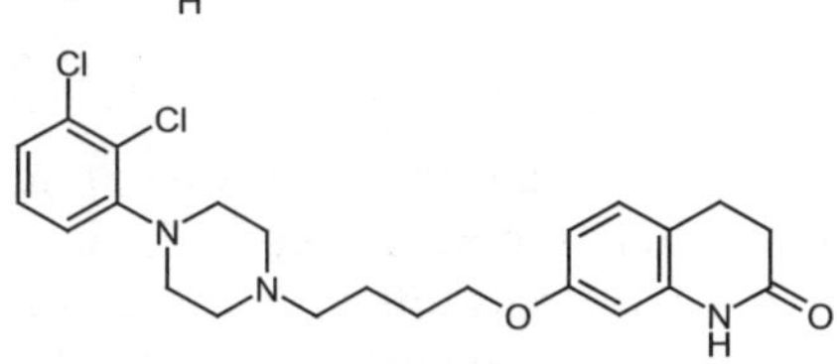 | 5.5 | Marketed |
| UH-232 | 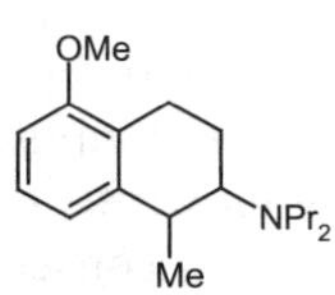 | 0.2 | Not developed |

(*Continued*)

**TABLE 2.1 (*Continued*)**

| Drug | Structure | Intrinsic Efficacy | Development Stage |
|---|---|---|---|
| Quetiapine | 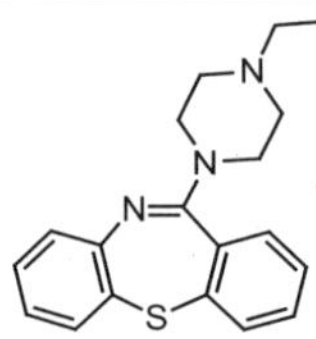  | –73 | Marketed (atypical antipsychotic) |
| Haloperidol | 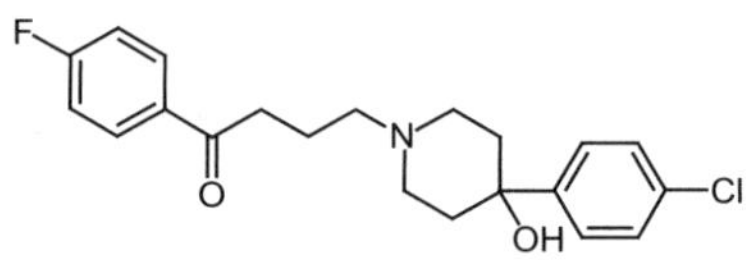  | –83 | Marketed (typical antipsychotic) |
| Risperidone | 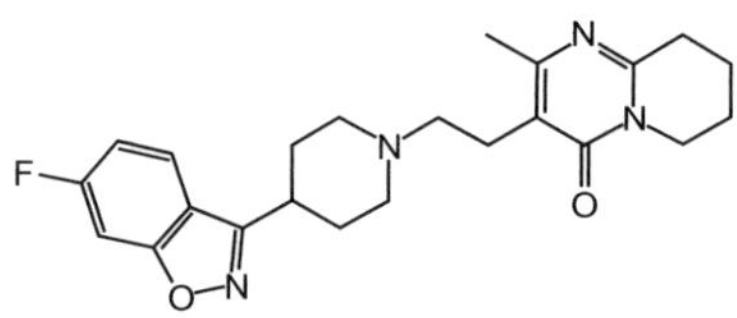  | –92 | Marketed (atypical antipsychotic) |

The structures of partial agonists that have been considered potential antipsychotics are shown together with some reference antagonist/inverse agonist antipsychotics. The development stage is shown for each compound. The intrinsic efficacy is given, mostly based on the effect of the drug to alter [$^{35}$S]GTPγS binding to membranes of cells expressing $D_2$ receptors. For (-)3-PPP, aplindore, aripiprazole, UH-232, data are from Reference [19] with the effects of dopamine taken as 100%. For haloperidol, quetiapine, and risperidone, data are from Reference [44] with the effects of (+)-butaclamol taken to represent a full inverse agonist. For bifeprunox and OPC4392, data are extrapolated from Reference [28]. For cariprazine, data are estimated from Reference [40]. It should be noted that these values are very dependent on the system for assessing such activity (see Reference [6]).

devoid of antipsychotic activity [22]. The outcome was, however, complicated by hallucinatory effects of UH-232 related to agonist effects of the drug at 5-$HT_2$ receptors. Drugs similar to UH-232 but without the serotonergic activity might therefore be good lead candidates for development of antipsychotics.

### 2.2.2 (-)-3-PPP (Preclamol)

This phenylpiperidine was reported to be a selective presynaptic agonist and postsynaptic antagonist at $D_2$-like dopamine receptors [23]. Subsequent work has shown that this compound is a moderate intrinsic efficacy agonist at $D_2$ dopamine receptors [19]. The selective presynaptic agonist actions probably reflect the greater amplification of pre- versus postsynaptic receptors, with the effects of such a compound being very dependent on the amplification state of the receptors. In one clinical trial, (-)-3-PPP was shown to have antipsychotic activity, but this waned after a week [24], possibly a consequence of its moderate intrinsic efficacy.

### 2.2.3 Aripiprazole

This substituted piperazine was developed by Otsuka in Japan. Their strategy was based on the idea that a presynaptic dopamine receptor agonist would reduce dopamine hyperfunction by inhibiting dopamine release via autoreceptors. It was suggested that this would be a novel way of reducing dopamine hyperfunction and might avoid the extrapyramidal side effects associated with standard antipsychotic medications. Such a compound would most likely be a postsynaptic antagonist based on consideration of the effects of preclamol but still quite different from standard antipsychotics in that the compound will have some positive intrinsic efficacy. OPC4392 was the first compound that Otsuka reported and was shown to be a presynaptic agonist and a postsynaptic antagonist [25]. Further compounds were synthesized with different length alkyl spacers, different phenyl substitution patterns, and different substitution on the quinoline ring. The compounds were tested in assays for postsynaptic antagonism (e.g., inhibition of apomorphine-induced locomotion) and presynaptic agonism (inhibition of $\gamma$-butyrolactone-induced L-3,4-dihydroxyphenylalanine [DOPA] accumulation), and OPC14597 (aripiprazole) emerged with a profile of higher potency as a postsynaptic antagonist, selective presynaptic agonist effects, and low activity at other receptors [26, 27]. Subsequent work has shown that aripiprazole has a lower intrinsic efficacy than OPC4392 at $D_2$ dopamine receptors but nevertheless still has the potential to be an agonist in a well-amplified system [19, 28]. It is also a moderate potency 5-$HT_{1A}$ agonist [29, 30],, and the importance of this will be considered later.

Aripiprazole exhibits activity in preclinical models suggestive of atypical antipsychotic action [31, 32]. Thus, it inhibits the conditioned avoidance response, a test that has good predictability for antipsychotic activity and in which other typical drugs also show inhibitory effects. It did not, however, cause catalepsy, a response thought to predict extrapyramidal side effects, whereas typical drugs such as haloperidol do cause catalepsy. Another preclinical test for side effects is the effect on prolactin release in which typical drugs such as haloperidol cause robust increases in prolactin levels. Aripiprazole causes only a small increase in prolactin release consistent with the partial agonist effects of the drug.

Aripiprazole was introduced into clinical practice as an antipsychotic in 2002 in the United States and its clinical effects have been reviewed [33, 34]. It appears to be an efficacious drug with antipsychotic effects similar to the standard drugs but also some effects on negative and cognitive symptoms. It has a low propensity to produce extrapyramidal side effects and tardive dyskinesia. Some akathisia has been reported in patients taking aripiprazole although the incidence is less than for haloperidol [35]. Aripiprazole has minimal effects on prolactin release, QTc interval prolongation, weight gain, and metabolism.

### 2.2.4 Aplindore (DAB 452)

This compound was developed by Wyeth as a dopamine stabilizer but was not developed as an antipsychotic. In *in vitro* assays for $D_2/D_3$ dopamine agonism, aplindore appears as an agonist with an intrinsic efficacy lying between full dopamine agonists and aripiprazole [19, 36]. Its moderate intrinsic efficacy may account for its failure as an antipsychotic and points to its use in disorders requiring agonist therapy such as Parkinson's disease and restless legs syndrome (see below). It also has moderate affinity at 5-$HT_{1A}$ serotonin receptors.

Aplindore exhibits agonist activity in *in vivo* behavioral models [36]. It elicits contralateral turning in rats given unilateral 6-hydroxydopamine lesions of the substantia nigra This suggests that aplindore may be useful for treating Parkinson's disease, and indeed it demonstrates favorable effects in primate models of the disease [37].

### 2.2.5 Bifeprunox

This substituted piperazine was developed by Solvay as an antipsychotic drug and in preclinical studies has been shown to be a $D_2/D_3$ receptor partial agonist and a 5-$HT_{1A}$ agonist [38]. In preclinical tests for antipsychotic activity and side effect profile, for example, inhibition of conditioned avoidance, induction of catalepsy, and effects on prolactin release, bifeprunox has similar properties to those of aripiprazole. In rats with unilateral 6-hydroxydopamine lesions of the substantia nigra, however, bifeprunox elicits contralateral turning whereas aripiprazole does not [39]. This suggests a greater intrinsic efficacy for bifeprunox compared with aripiprazole. In clinical trials, bifeprunox showed modest effects on positive symptoms of schizophrenia, but these effects were not as marked as for other atypical drugs (see work cited in References [28, 39]). This led in 2007 to the U.S. Food and Drug Administration refusing approval for the drug. In *in vitro* studies, bifeprunox has been shown to have a higher intrinsic efficacy than aripiprazole [28], in agreement with the animal tests in Section 2.2.3, and this may not be optimal for antipsychotic activity. Some *in vivo* evidence that the intrinsic efficacy of the drug may be too high comes from reports of increased nausea and vomiting with the drug during the clinical trials (see work cited in References [28, 39]). In 2009 development of bifeprunox was stopped.

### 2.2.6 RGH-188 (Cariprazine)

This piperazine was developed by Gedeon Richter as a potential antipsychotic drug. The pharmacological profile of the drug is similar to that of aripiprazole, that is, high affinity for $D_2/D_3$ dopamine receptors and 5-$HT_{1A}$ and 5-$HT_{2B}$ serotonin receptors [40]. Unlike aripiprazole, cariprazine shows about 10-fold selectivity for $D_3$ receptors ($pK_d$~10) over $D_2$ receptors ($pK_d$~9). In terms of their intrinsic efficacies at different receptors, the two drugs have very similar profiles, exhibiting partial agonism at $D_2$, $D_3$, and 5-$HT_{1A}$ receptors and antagonism at 5-$HT_{2B}$ receptors. Cariprazine has a favorable profile in preclinical tests for atypical antipsychotic activity, exhibiting inhibition of conditioned avoidance response and no induction of catalepsy in animal models. Preliminary results from a Phase IIb trial of cariprazine in schizophrenia were positive. In this trial 732 patients were randomized between five treatment groups (cariparazine: 1.5, 3.0, and 4.5 mg/day; risperidone 4 mg/day and placebo). The patients receiving cariprazine or risperidone showed symptom improvement compared with placebo. In 2010, cariprazine entered a Phase III trial for safety and efficacy against schizophrenia.

## 2.3 MECHANISMS OF ACTION OF THE DOPAMINE PARTIAL AGONIST DRUGS

Based on consideration of the properties of the compounds that have been tested as antipsychotics, some common themes emerge. All of the compounds are $D_2/D_3$ agonists of varying potency but mostly of low intrinsic efficacy. It seems that the intrinsic efficacy of the drugs must be quite low to produce an antipsychotic effect. This has mainly been assessed at $D_2$ receptors, and where compounds have failed in clinical trials this seems to be associated with relatively high intrinsic efficacy at $D_2$ receptors. For example, the intrinsic efficacies of (-)-3-PPP, aplindore, and bifeprunox are higher than for aripiprazole when measured using *in vitro* signaling assays, and it is these compounds that have either failed as antipsychotics or have not progressed quickly [19, 28].

Many of the compounds are also agonists at 5-$HT_{1A}$ serotonin receptors. A case has been made that the combination of $D_2$ partial agonism and 5-$HT_{1A}$ agonism provides a good profile for a novel antipsychotic, with the 5-$HT_{1A}$ agonist activity being beneficial for suppression of cognitive and negative symptoms while reducing extrapyramidal side effects [39]. This claim has been examined in detail, and it has been argued that for aripiprazole, the 5-$HT_{1A}$ activity is irrelevant to its clinical activity [31]. Thus, it was found that occupancy of rat brain 5-$HT_{1A}$ receptors by aripiprazole occurred at doses 10- to 20-fold higher than those required to occupy $D_2$ receptors. Also, ariprazole did not induce behaviors in rats typically associated with 5-$HT_{1A}$ agonism. These data suggest that although *in vitro* aripiprazole is a 5-$HT_{1A}$ agonist, this receptor is not activated *in vivo* at concentrations used to occupy $D_2$ receptors.

Given that the partial agonist drugs have quite different intrinsic efficacies at $D_2$ dopamine receptors compared with the standard antipsychotic drugs, it might be expected that the clinical effects of the drugs would be different. There is only one partial agonist currently in clinical practice, aripiprazole. Although this drug has fewer side effects than the standard drugs, its therapeutic antipsychotic effects are not very different [33].

This similarity in therapeutic effects between aripiprazole and the standard antipsychotic drugs may be rationalized as follows. Occupancy of $D_2$ receptors by standard antipsychotic drugs has been reported to be ~70% when being used to treat schizophrenia, but therapeutic effects may be obtained at lower occupancies. For example, for the drug olanzapine, therapeutic effects may be achieved when occupancy of $D_2$ receptors in the striatum is ~55% [12]. Under these conditions it may be calculated, assuming mutually competitive binding of dopamine and the drug, that the occupancy by dopamine is ~12%, similar to the level seen in normal patients (for calculation, see Reference [6]). In schizophrenia patients, dopamine levels are increased about twofold and the effects of the drug are to reduce this by about 50% (see above) [6]. For the dopamine partial agonist drugs, data show that receptor occupancy for aripiprazole is ~90% [41]. Under these conditions there will be little or no dopamine occupancy. Therefore, it may be that these two conditions (~55% occupancy by standard antipsychotic drug/~12% occupancy by dopamine and ~90% occupancy by the partial agonist aripiprazole) achieve similar levels of dopamine receptor stimulation, accounting for the similarity in therapeutic effects. This discussion underlines the importance of having a low but positive intrinsic efficacy in partial agonist drug candidates; it may be that aripiprazole has just the right level of intrinsic efficacy.

It has also been argued that aripiprazole has the ability to influence distinct signaling pathways differentially [42]. For example, aripiprazole has a low potency for the activation of extracellular-signal-regulated kinase (ERK) (mitogen-activated protein [MAP] kinase) compared with its effects to inhibit cyclic adenosine monophosphate (cAMP) accumulation [43]. The relevance of these observations to clinical outcomes is currently unclear.

## 2.4 CONCLUSION

Dopamine $D_2/D_3$ partial agonists potentially provide a novel means for treatment of schizophrenia. In principle, their mechanism of action, inhibition of dopamine hyperfunction and improvement of dopamine hypofunction, matches the underlying problems in schizophrenia better than existing drugs. One partial agonist drug, aripiprazole, is now marketed and other drugs are under development. Aripiprazole provides an alternative to existing atypical drugs with a similar antipsychotic profile and advantages in its side effect profile. It remains to be seen as to whether other partial agonists will improve on the profile of aripiprazole.

## REFERENCES

1. Miyamoto, S., Duncan, G.E., Marx, C.E., Lieberman, J.A. (2005). Treatments for schizophrenia: a critical review of pharmacology and mechanisms of action of antipsychotic drugs. *Mol Psychiatry*, *10*, 79–104.
2. Freedman, R. (2003). Schizophrenia. *N Engl J Med*, *349*, 1738–1749.
3. Howes, O.D., Kapur, S. (2009). The dopamine hypothesis of schizophrenia: version III—the final common pathway. *Schizophr Bull*, *35*, 549–562.
4. Grunder, G., Hippius, H., Carlsson, A. (2009). The “atypicality” of antipsychotics: a concept re-examined and re-defined. *Nat Rev Drug Discov*, *8*, 197–202.

5. Strange, P.G. (2001). Antipsychotic drugs: importance of dopamine receptors for mechanisms of therapeutic actions and side effects. *Pharmacol Rev*, *53*, 119–133.
6. Strange, P.G. (2008). Antipsychotic drug action: antagonism, inverse agonism or partial agonism. *Trends Pharmacol Sci*, *29*, 314–321.
7. Laruelle, M., Abi-Dargham, A., van Dyck, C.H., Gil, R., D'Souza, C.D., Erdos, J., et al. (1996). Single photon emission computerized tomography imaging of amphetamine-induced dopamine release in drug-free schizophrenic subjects. *Proc Natl Acad Sci U S A*, *93*, 9235–9240.
8. Abi-Dargham, A., Rodenhiser, J., Printz, D., Zea-Ponce, Y., Gil, R., Kegeles, L.S., et al. (2000). Increased baseline occupancy of D2 receptors by dopamine in schizophrenia. *Proc Natl Acad Sci U S A*, *97*, 8104–8109.
9. Abi-Dargham, A., Laruelle, M. (2005). Mechanisms of action of second generation antipsychotic drugs in schizophrenia: insights from brain imaging studies. *Eur Psychiatry*, *20*, 15–27.
10. Abi-Dargham, A., Moore, H. (2003). Prefrontal DA transmission at D1 receptors and the pathology of schizophrenia. *Neuroscientist*, *9*, 404–416.
11. Honey, G., Bullmore, E. (2004). Human pharmacological MRI. *Trends Pharmacol Sci*, *25*, 366–374.
12. Frankle, W.G., Gil, R., Hackett, E., Mawlawi, O., Zea-Ponce, Y., Zhu, Z., et al. (2004). Occupancy of dopamine D2 receptors by the atypical antipsychotic drugs risperidone and olanzapine: theoretical implications. *Psychopharmacology (Berl)*, *175*, 473–480.
13. Lieberman, J.A., Stroup, T.S., McEvoy, J.P., Swartz, M.S., Rosenheck, R.A., Perkins, D.O., et al. (2005). Effectiveness of antipsychotic drugs in patients with chronic schizophrenia. *N Engl J Med*, *353*, 1209–1223.
14. Carlsson, A., Waters, N., Holm-Waters, S., Tedroff, J., Nilsson, M., Carlsson, M.L. (2001). Interactions between monoamines, glutamate, and GABA in schizophrenia: new evidence. *Annu Rev Pharmacol Toxicol*, *41*, 237–260.
15. Meller, E., Bohmaker, K., Namba, Y., Friedhoff, A.J., Goldstein, M. (1987). Relationship between receptor occupancy and response at striatal dopamine autoreceptors. *Mol Pharmacol*, *31*, 592–598.
16. Svensson, K., Johansson, A.M., Magnusson, T., Carlsson, A. (1986). (+)-AJ 76 and (+)-UH 232: central stimulants acting as preferential dopamine autoreceptor antagonists. *Naunyn Schmiedebergs Arch Pharmacol*, *334*, 234–245.
17. Coldwell, M.C., Boyfield, I., Brown, A.M., Stemp, G., Middlemiss, D.N. (1999). Pharmacological characterization of extracellular acidification rate responses in human D2(long), D3 and D4.4 receptors expressed in Chinese hamster ovary cells. *Br J Pharmacol*, *127*, 1135–1144.
18. Svensson, K., Carlsson, M., Carlsson, A., Hjorth, S., Johansson, A.M., Eriksson, E. (1986). The putatively selective dopamine autoreceptor antagonists (+)-AJ 76 and (+)-UH 232 stimulate prolactin release in rats. *Eur J Pharmacol*, *130*, 237–242.
19. Lin, H., Saisch, S.G., Strange, P.G. (2006). Assays for enhanced activity of low efficacy partial agonists at the D(2) dopamine receptor. *Br J Pharmacol*, *149*, 291–299.
20. Wilson, J., Lin, H., Fu, D., Javitch, J.A., Strange, P.G. (2001). Mechanisms of inverse agonism of antipsychotic drugs at the D(2) dopamine receptor: use of a mutant

D(2) dopamine receptor that adopts the activated conformation. *J Neurochem*, *77*, 493–504.

21. Griffon, N., Pilon, C., Schwartz, J.C., Sokoloff, P. (1995). The preferential dopamine D3 receptor ligand, (+)-UH232, is a partial agonist. *Eur J Pharmacol*, *282*, R3–R4.
22. Lahti, A.C., Weiler, M., Carlsson, A., Tamminga, C.A. (1998). Effects of the D3 and autoreceptor-preferring dopamine antagonist (+)-UH232 in schizophrenia. *J Neural Transm*, *105*, 719–734.
23. Hjorth, S., Carlsson, A., Clark, D., Svensson, K., Wikstrom, H., Sanchez, D., et al. (1983). Central dopamine receptor agonist and antagonist actions of the enantiomers of 3-PPP. *Psychopharmacology (Berl)*, *81*, 89–99.
24. Lahti, A.C., Weiler, M.A., Corey, P.K., Lahti, R.A., Carlsson, A., Tamminga, C.A. (1998). Antipsychotic properties of the partial dopamine agonist (-)-3-(3-hydroxyphenyl)-N-n-propylpiperidine(preclamol) in schizophrenia. *Biol Psychiatry*, *43*, 2–11.
25. Yasuda, Y., Kikuchi, T., Suzuki, S., Tsutsui, M., Yamada, K., Hiyama, T. (1988). 7-[3-(4-[2,3-Dimethylphenyl]piperazinyl)propoxy]-2(1H)-quinolinone (OPC-4392), a presynaptic dopamine autoreceptor agonist and postsynaptic D2 receptor antagonist. *Life Sci*, *42*, 1941–1954.
26. Kikuchi, T., Tottori, K., Uwahodo, Y., Hirose, T., Miwa, T., Oshiro, Y., et al. (1995). 7-(4-[4-(2,3-Dichlorophenyl)-1-piperazinyl]butyloxy)-3,4-dihydro-2(1H)-qui nolinone (OPC-14597), a new putative antipsychotic drug with both presynaptic dopamine autoreceptor agonistic activity and postsynaptic D2 receptor antagonistic activity. *J Pharmacol Exp Ther*, *274*, 329–336.
27. Oshiro, Y., Sato, S., Kurahashi, N., Tanaka, T., Kikuchi, T., Tottori, K., et al. (1998). Novel antipsychotic agents with dopamine autoreceptor agonist properties: synthesis and pharmacology of 7-[4-(4-phenyl-1-piperazinyl)butoxy]-3,4-dihydro-2(1H)-quinolinone derivatives. *J Med Chem*, *41*, 658–667.
28. Tadori, Y., Kitagawa, H., Forbes, R.A., McQuade, R.D., Stark, A., Kikuchi, T. (2007). Differences in agonist/antagonist properties at human dopamine D(2) receptors between aripiprazole, bifeprunox and SDZ 208-912. *Eur J Pharmacol*, *574*, 103–111.
29. Jordan, S., Koprivica, V., Chen, R., Tottori, K., Kikuchi, T., Altar, C.A. (2002). The antipsychotic aripiprazole is a potent, partial agonist at the human 5-HT1A receptor. *Eur J Pharmacol*, *441*, 137–140.
30. Stark, A.D., Jordan, S., Allers, K.A., Bertekap, R.L., Chen, R., Mistry Kannan, T., et al. (2007). Interaction of the novel antipsychotic aripiprazole with 5-HT1A and 5-HT 2A receptors: functional receptor-binding and in vivo electrophysiological studies. *Psychopharmacology (Berl)*, *190*, 373–382.
31. Wood, M., Reavill, C. (2007). Aripiprazole acts as a selective dopamine D2 receptor partial agonist. *Expert Opin Investig Drugs*, *16*, 771–775.
32. Natesan, S., Reckless, G.E., Nobrega, J.N., Fletcher, P.J., Kapur, S. (2006). Dissociation between in vivo occupancy and functional antagonism of dopamine D2 receptors: comparing aripiprazole to other antipsychotics in animal models. *Neuropsychopharmacology*, *31*, 1854–1863.
33. Swainston Harrison, T., Perry, C.M. (2004). Aripiprazole: a review of its use in schizophrenia and schizoaffective disorder. *Drugs*, *64*, 1715–1736.

34. Stip, E., Tourjman, V. (2010). Aripiprazole in schizophrenia and schizoaffective disorder: a review. *Clin Ther*, *32*(Suppl 1), S3–S20.

35. Kane, J.M., Barnes, T.R., Correll, C.U., Sachs, G., Buckley, P., Eudicone, J., et al. (2010). Evaluation of akathisia in patients with schizophrenia, schizoaffective disorder, or bipolar I disorder: a post hoc analysis of pooled data from short- and long-term aripiprazole trials. *J Psychopharmacol*, *24* (7), 1019–1029.

36. Heinrich, J.N., Brennan, J., Lai, M.H., Sullivan, K., Hornby, G., Popiolek, M., et al. (2006). Aplindore (DAB-452), a high affinity selective dopamine D2 receptor partial agonist. *Eur J Pharmacol*, *552*, 36–45.

37. Jackson, M.J., Andree, T.H., Hansard, M., Hoffman, D.C., Hurtt, M.R., Kehne, J.H., et al. (2010). The dopamine D(2) receptor partial agonist aplindore improves motor deficits in MPTP-treated common marmosets alone and combined with L-dopa. *J Neural Transm*, *117* (1), 55–67.

38. Cosi, C., Carilla-Durand, E., Assie, M.B., Ormiere, A.M., Maraval, M., Leduc, N., et al. (2006). Partial agonist properties of the antipsychotics SSR181507, aripiprazole and bifeprunox at dopamine D2 receptors: G protein activation and prolactin release. *Eur J Pharmacol*, *535*, 135–144.

39. Newman-Tancredi, A., Cussac, D., Depoortere, R. (2007). Neuropharmacological profile of bifeprunox: merits and limitations in comparison with other third-generation antipsychotics. *Curr Opin Investig Drugs*, *8*, 539–554.

40. Kiss, B., Horvath, A., Nemethy, Z., Schmidt, E., Laszlovszky, I., Bugovics, G., et al. (2010). Cariprazine (RGH-188), a dopamine D(3) receptor-preferring, D(3)/D(2) dopamine receptor antagonist-partial agonist antipsychotic candidate: in vitro and neurochemical profile. *J Pharmacol Exp Ther*, *333* (1), 328–340.

41. Yokoi, F., Grunder, G., Biziere, K., Stephane, M., Dogan, A.S., Dannals, R.F., et al. (2002). Dopamine D2 and D3 receptor occupancy in normal humans treated with the antipsychotic drug aripiprazole (OPC 14597): a study using positron emission tomography and [11C]raclopride. *Neuropsychopharmacology*, *27*, 248–259.

42. Mailman, R.B. (2007). GPCR functional selectivity has therapeutic impact. *Trends Pharmacol Sci*, *28*, 390–396.

43. Urban, J.D., Vargas, G.A., von Zastrow, M., Mailman, R.B. (2007). Aripiprazole has functionally selective actions at dopamine D2 receptor-mediated signaling pathways. *Neuropsychopharmacology*, *32*, 67–77.

44. Roberts, D.J., Strange, P.G. (2005). Mechanisms of inverse agonist action at D2 dopamine receptors. *Br J Pharmacol*, *145*, 34–42.

# 3

# $D_1/D_5$ DOPAMINE AGONISTS AS PHARMACOTHERAPY FOR SCHIZOPHRENIA

KEVIN N. BOYD AND RICHARD B. MAILMAN

## 3.1 HISTORY OF $D_1$-LIKE RECEPTOR LIGANDS FOR THE TREATMENT OF SCHIZOPHRENIA

### 3.1.1 Dopamine Ligands and the Treatment of Schizophrenia

Although schizophrenia is a complex disorder, the elegant work by Arvid Carlsson [1] and others laid the foundation for the prevailing hypotheses that increased dopamine signaling underlies the pathophysiology of schizophrenia. The prototypical phenothiazine antipsychotic chlorpromazine [2] is a dopamine antagonist [3], and the introduction of other phenothiazines was followed rapidly by drugs from several chemical classes (e.g., thioxanthenes) with similar action [4]. Greengard and colleagues first demonstrated that dopamine could dose-dependently stimulate the synthesis of the second messenger cyclic adenosine monophosphate (cAMP) [5] in a fashion that was antagonized by many antipsychotic drugs (APDs) [6]. Both phenothiazine and the thioxanthene class antipsychotics competitively inhibited the dopamine-stimulated activity of adenylate cyclase in proportion to their clinical potency, leading to the hypothesis that adenylate cyclase activation was the major functional mechanism of dopamine in the central nervous system (CNS) [6, 7].

Numerous drugs from other chemical classes (e.g., benzamides, butyrophenones, and dibenzodiazepines) that also had antipsychotic action were

*Targets and Emerging Therapies for Schizophrenia*, First Edition.
Edited by Jeffrey S. Albert and Michael W. Wood.

subsequently developed. Although the clinical potency of many of these early drugs was strongly correlated with their affinity for the $D_2$ receptor [8], most demonstrated little potency in inhibiting dopamine-stimulated adenylate cyclase [9]. This dichotomy led to the currently accepted nomenclature [10, 11] in which the receptors typically linked to stimulation of cAMP synthesis were termed "$D_1$," and those that inhibited cAMP synthesis and selectively bound a class of drugs called benzamides (e.g., sulpiride) were called "$D_2$." Molecular biological studies have now shown that five genes in humans code for six dopamine receptors. Both of the "$D_1$-like" receptor genes are intron-less, and include the $D_1$ and the $D_5$ [12–15]. The "$D_2$-like" receptors include two major splice variants of the $D_2$ gene, $D_{2L}$ (long), and $D_{2S}$ (short), which together are the most highly expressed of the $D_2$-like receptors [16–19]. The other $D_2$-like receptors are $D_3$ and $D_4$ types [17, 20].

### 3.1.2 Early Ideas about Role of $D_1$-like Receptors in the Treatment of Schizophrenia

Although the early data suggested that antagonism of the $D_1$ receptor might be the mechanism of antipsychotic action of the early typical drugs [6], by the late 1970s it was clear that the useful antipsychotic actions of chlorpromazine and related drugs were due to their ability to block $D_2$ receptors [8]. It was also obvious, however, that this same $D_2$ antagonism caused many of the side effects of the early drugs, including parkinsonism and other extrapyramidal effects, as well as endocrine changes. Thus, researchers began to explore other targets for schizophrenia treatment, one of which was the potential of using selective $D_1$ antagonists. Preclinical studies initially suggested that $D_1$ antagonists reduced the extrapyramidal side effects (EPS) observed with classical antipsychotics [21–23]. Other experiments suggested that the actions of $D_2$ agonists could be markedly inhibited by $D_1$ antagonists [24], raising the possibility that a $D_1$ antagonist might actually be a better APD. The latter data, however, also suggested that $D_1$ antagonists might actually have potent parkinson-like effects. Indeed, it was later demonstrated that $D_1$ agonists have profound antiparkinson effects [25, 26] and that $D_1$ antagonists can cause parkinsonism [27]. Clinical trials with the selective $D_1$ antagonists SCH39166 (ecopipam) [28–31] and NNC 01-0687 [32] confirmed that $D_1$ antagonists would not be useful in the treatment of schizophrenia.

### 3.1.3 Second- and Third-Generation APDs and Unmet Needs

The typical APDs induced a variety of neurological adverse effects seen both acutely (EPS such as parkinsonism, dystonia, akathisia, as well as neuroendocrine effects) and with long-term exposure (e.g., tardive dyskinesia [TD]) [33]. As noted earlier, many of these adverse effects are mediated by the same dopamine $D_2$ receptors that are involved in the therapeutic effects. Indeed, a majority of patients given recommended therapeutic dosages of typical antipsychotics developed acute EPS [34]. One of the most worrisome neurological side effects was TD, often irreversible and with incidence rates estimated at about 5% per year [35]. Anticholinergic drugs are effective in attenuating EPS but have their own unpleasant side effects (e.g., dry mouth, constipation, delirium, and memory deficits), further contributing to treatment noncompliance.

Making matters even worse is the fact that negative symptoms, mood symptoms, and cognitive deficits are only minimally responsive to conventional antipsychotics. The presence of negative symptoms and cognitive impairment often leads to poor social and vocational function [36, 37]. Moreover, approximately 30% of patients with acutely exacerbated psychotic symptoms have minimal response to standard antipsychotics [35, 38]. These factors spurred research for new drugs that would have equal or better efficacy, and markedly decreased side effects. For more than a decade, the side effects that were considered most critical were the neurological (EPS and TD) and neuroendocrine. The first drugs devoid of neurological side effects were originally termed "atypical" antipsychotics but are now sometimes called second generation.

For many years, there was the common view that effective antipsychotic agents would necessarily produce EPS because these actions were mediated by blockade of the same receptor (i.e., $D_2$). A great deal of research was devoted to the discovery of drugs that were "atypical"; although there was no convention about the meaning of the term "atypical," in its broadest sense it was used to refer to drugs that had at least equal antipsychotic efficacy to the "typical" drugs, without producing EPS or sustained prolactin elevation [39]. With time, and after the development of drugs that could be called "atypical," the definition was often expanded to include compounds that might have superior antipsychotic efficacy (e.g., in treatment-resistant patients) or have beneficial effects against negative symptoms and/or cognitive deficits. Some of these issues have also been discussed in Chapter 1.

## 3.2 POTENTIAL VALUE OF $D_1$-LIKE ACTIVATION IN THE TREATMENT OF SCHIZOPHRENIA

### 3.2.1 Localization of $D_1$ and $D_5$ Receptors

Neuroanatomical distribution of $D_1$ receptor ligand binding sites within the basal ganglia is remarkably similar between several species, including rodents and primates [40–46]. Since a truly selective $D_1$ radioligand does not exist, quantitative receptor autoradiography was utilized [47–50] to examine $D_1$/$D_5$ localization using radioligands (e.g., [$^3$H]-SCH39166, [$^{125}$I]-SCH23982 and [$^3$H]-SKF-83566) with high affinity and selectivity for both receptors [51, 52]. In general, patterns of [$^3$H]-SCH23390 binding parallel the distribution of dopamine terminals [48, 52], with the highest levels of binding occurring in forebrain areas including caudate putamen, nucleus accumbens, and olfactory tubercle. $D_1$ labeling is evident in structures comprising the basal ganglia outflow pathways, including the entopeduncular and subthalamic nuclei and the substantia nigra pars reticulata. $D_1$ receptors are also expressed in a number of limbic areas, notably the dentate gyrus of the hippocampus and several amygdaloid nuclei. Moderate to low densities of $D_1$ binding sites were observed in several cortical divisions, with a preferential distribution in deeper layers. The highest cortical densities occurred within the anteromedial and suprarhinal prefrontal areas. $D_1$ mRNA localization generally is consistent with the results obtained from $D_1$ receptor binding and antibody localization studies [53–58]. This correspondence suggests that $D_1$ receptors are typically expressed on cell soma and proximal dendrites rather than at distant sites. Interestingly, the substantia nigra, entopeduncular nucleus, and subthalamic nucleus regions, areas with clearly defined $D_1$ receptor binding sites, exhibit a lack of $D_1$ mRNA indicating that $D_1$ receptors are transported to axon terminals from other nuclei [59, 60].

The $D_5$ receptor has limited expression relative to that of the $D_1$ receptor. Indeed, receptor quantification in $D_1$ null mutant mice observed binding only in the hippocampus [61]. Consistent with this finding, other reports show that $D_5$ mRNA is restricted to the hippocampus, lateral mamillary nuclei, and parafasicular nucleus [62, 63]. Interestingly, other reports have suggested that $D_5$ receptors are found in other areas, including the frontal and parietal cortices and striatum [64, 65]. $D_5$ mRNA localization studies in primate brain have shown a more widespread distribution than predicted from the rodent mRNA studies [66, 67], a finding confirmed by the use of antibodies in both rodent and primate brains [64, 68, 69]. For example, using $D_5$ selective antisera, intense staining was found in frontal and parietal cortices of rat brain [64]. Significant staining was also observed in hippocampus and dentate gyrus, whereas a lower intensity signal was also observed in olfactory tubercles, dorsal aspects of the caudate putamen, and the cerebellar vermi. For the purposes of this chapter, the reference to $D_1$ agonists includes compounds that will bind to, and have functional effects at, both $D_1$ and $D_5$ receptors. Although the majority of any pharmacological consequences are likely due to the $D_1$ receptor, this cannot be proved without the successful development of an agonist or antagonist that is selective for either the $D_1$ or the $D_5$ receptor.

### 3.2.2 Cognitive and Other Potential Benefits of $D_1$-like Receptor Activation

As noted earlier, the initial hypotheses about dopamine and schizophrenia were based on the assumption that schizophrenia was the result of increased dopamine function [70, 71]. Later studies revealed a need to modify this hypothesis as negative symptoms and cognitive deficits failed to adequately respond to dopamine antagonists. These cognitive effects appeared to be resulting from a deficit in $D_1$ receptor activity in the prefrontal cortex. The fact that $D_1$ receptors are present in high concentrations in the prefrontal cortex of nonhuman primates [40] led to the finding that optimal receptor stimulation could improve working memory processes [72]. Thus, while many of the positive symptoms of schizophrenia may be mediated by hyperactivity at $D_2$ receptors in the subcortical mesolimbic region, cognitive deficits may be due to decreased activity in the mesocortical dopamine system and the subsequent hypostimulation of $D_1$ receptors. $D_1$ agonists have been shown to improve cognitive function in rodents [73, 74] and nonhuman primates [75–78], and lesions of the mesocortical dopamine projection impair working memory performance in monkeys [79] and rats [80]. In addition, local injection of a $D_1$ antagonist into the prefrontal cortex induced deficits in working memory in rhesus monkeys [81]. Thus, $D_1$ receptor activation may provide cognitive benefits and suggests a target for new therapeutic compounds to combat the working memory deficits associated with schizophrenia.

The development of dopaminergic drugs has provided examples of the significance of $D_1$ receptor stimulation for cognition. The partial agonist SKF-38393 improves the memory performance of reserpine-depleted monkeys, but not young control animals. Conversely, the full agonist dihydrexidine (DHX) improved the memory performance in young control monkeys, as well as in a subset of aged monkeys [75]. Schneider [78] also demonstrated that DHX can cause performance improvements in 1-methyl-4-phenyl-1,2,3,6-tetrahydropyridine (MPTP)-lesioned nonhuman primates. One of the most striking reports indicated that brief administration of ABT-431 can induce long-lasting reversal of antipsychotic-induced working memory deficits in monkeys [82]. Although there are overwhelming data supporting the beneficial effects of $D_1$ stimulation in cognition and memory, there is also complex dose-dependency for these effects. Paradoxically, higher doses of $D_1$ agonists have been demonstrated to impair memory performance in aged monkeys [82]. Interestingly, time is also an important factor as a dose of the $D_1$ receptor agonist SKF-81297 that disrupted working memory when administered after a 30-minute delay, improved memory retrieval when administered after a 12-hour delay [83].

The mechanism by which $D_1$ receptors affect memory and cognition is not fully understood. There is a link between acetylcholine and dopamine, as well as interactions between dopamine and glutamate. For example, the $D_1$-like agonist DHX has been shown both to increase extracellular acetylcholine levels in the rat striatum and frontal cortex, and to improve cognitive performance [73, 84]. Interestingly, $D_1$ receptors in both pyramidal and nonpyramidal neurons may interact with glutamatergic inputs, and a model of dopamine modulation of working memory posits a central role of $D_1$ receptors in enhancing glutamatergic input to such neurons [85]. Indeed, studies have suggested that the interaction between dopamine $D_1$ receptors and NMDA receptors is critical for working memory and other cognitive functions (for review, see Reference [86]). These and other mechanisms will, no doubt, be further explored, but it is clear that the $D_1$ receptor has an important role in modulating cognitive performance under the control of the prefrontal cortex. The findings support the potential use of $D_1$ agonists in the treatment of cognitive deficits and/or negative symptoms in a variety of conditions, including schizophrenia, Parkinson's disease, and age-related memory decline.

### 3.2.3 Prefrontal Cortical Circuits Involved with Working Memory

During the past decade, dopamine neurotransmission in the prefrontal cortex has become of great interest because of the critical role of the prefrontal cortex in working memory and executive function [72, 87, 88]. The localization of dopamine receptor subtypes in prefrontal pyramidal and nonpyramidal neurons, coupled with a host of pharmacological studies, has supported an essential role of $D_1$-like receptors in the elemental basis of these working memory processes [72, 75, 81, 85, 88–94]. There is a great deal of evidence for this being a highly regulated, interactive system in which $D_1$ receptors located on pyramidal cells and interneurons of several types play a major role in the physiology of working memory. There is a widely held view that this system functions at less than optimal efficiency with either too much or too little $D_1$ activation. Indeed, the full $D_1$ agonists DHX, SKF-81297, and A-77636 all affect working memory in aged monkeys in a dose-dependent manner, where low doses improve cognition and higher doses impair working memory tasks [75, 76]. Another study with nonhuman primates found morphologic changes in prefrontal cortical neurons resulting from chronic dopamine dysregulation that are similar to changes observed in patients with schizophrenia [95]. Together, these studies suggest that dopamine activity in the prefrontal cortex is critical for proper cognitive functioning. In support of these results, brain imaging studies in patients with schizophrenia have shown that impaired cognitive performance is associated with decreased $D_1$ receptor binding [96] and abnormal activation of the prefrontal cortex [97, 98]. Further imaging and postmortem studies have also suggested that decreased dopamine $D_1$ receptor activity in the dorsolateral prefrontal cortex is involved with cognitive decline, but more conclusive studies are necessary to elucidate the underlying mechanisms (for review, see Reference [99]). Interestingly, $D_1$ receptor availability was found to be upregulated in the dorsolateral prefrontal cortex of patients with schizophrenia and correlated with poor performances in working memory tasks. This deficiency, however, may be a compensatory change resulting from dopamine deficiency [100].

### 3.2.4 $D_1/D_5$ Receptors in the Hippocampus

Although $D_1$-like receptors are involved in executive functions and prefrontal cortical activity, they can also alter hippocampal memory formation. Indeed, both subtypes of $D_1$-like receptors are expressed in the hippocampus [61, 62, 101], and dopaminergic cells from the substantia nigra and the ventral tegmental area (VTA) project to the dentate gyrus and the CA1 region of the hippocampus. Interestingly, dopamine can modulate acetylcholine release as well as activation of N-methyl-D-aspartate (NMDA) receptors [102, 103], both of which are involved with learning and memory. In fact, $D_1$-like receptor agonists stimulate acetylcholine release in the hippocampus and attenuate cognitive deficits in memory-impaired aged rats [74, 104, 105]. Moreover, a study by Hersi et al. [106] suggests that these hippocampal effects are likely due to $D_5$ receptors.

Dopamine receptors in the hippocampus also modulate NMDA receptors. NMDA receptor activation is known to be crucial for the induction of long-term potentiation (LTP), the mechanism thought to underlie initial memory consolidation. Indeed, dopamine $D_1$-like agonists have been shown to potentiate late-phase LTP in the CA1 region [107, 108]. Because many memory deficits are associated with problems during late-phase LTP, $D_1/D_5$ agonists are a potential treatment for memory deficits. In fact, $D_1$-like receptor agonists, previously shown to enhance late-phase LTP, have also been reported to improve spatial memory deficits in aged mice [109]. The possibility that these agonists could treat cognitive impairments is particularly intriguing for schizophrenia as memory deficits are resistant to improvement by current antipsychotics. At present, there are no radioligands that can differentiate between the two $D_1$-like receptors ($D_1$ and $D_5$), so studies cannot determine whether specific drugs target one receptor subtype over the other. This issue will be further discussed later in the review.

### 3.2.5 Peripheral Dopamine Receptors

Although this chapter, as well as the majority of published research, focuses on dopamine receptors in the CNS, there are key functional roles for dopamine receptors in the periphery. Dopamine increases myocardial contractility and cardiac output in the heart as well as vasodilatation in the vasculature. Dopamine receptors are also present in the kidneys where they cause natriuresis and vasodilatation. A limited number of studies have examined the expression pattern and the precise role of peripheral dopamine receptors, but they likely contribute to the clinical pharmacology of dopaminergic therapies. This area has been the subject of several recent scholarly reviews [110–113].

## 3.3 MECHANISMS OF DOPAMINE AGONIST ACTION

### 3.3.1 $D_1$-like Signaling

Dopamine $D_1$-like signaling stimulates adenylate cyclase activity, subsequently activating phosphokinasc A (PKA) and a variety of other signaling cascades. These increases in adenylate cyclase activity are mediated by the heteromeric G proteins $G\alpha_s$ and $G\alpha_{olf}$. $D_1$-like receptors have been shown to activate adenylate cyclase in numerous cell lines and tissues. Indeed, $G\alpha_s$ is ubiquitously expressed and couples to both $D_1$ and $D_5$ receptors. Although $G\alpha_s$ appears to mediate $D_1$-like receptor signaling, $G\alpha_{olf}$ also stimulates adenylate cyclase activity and is highly expressed in dopaminergic regions, such as the neostriatum, where there is little $G\alpha_s$ expression [114]. Interestingly, mutant mice lacking $G\alpha_{olf}$ show no $D_1$-mediated adenylate cyclase stimulation in the striatum [115] and do not exhibit a hyperlocomotor response to $D_1$ agonists or cocaine [114]. From such data, the conclusion might be drawn that $D_1$-like receptors signal through $G\alpha_s$ and $G\alpha_{olf}$ via activation of adenylate cyclase and subsequent PKA activation. Although this seems likely, other signaling pathways have been observed for $D_1$-like receptors, including coupling to other heteromeric G proteins and signaling through $\beta\gamma$ subunits. Indeed, $\beta\gamma$ subunits can play a selective role in $D_1$-like signaling as $D_1$-, but not $D_5$-, mediated adenylate cyclase activity is attenuated by depletion of $\gamma 7$ subunit [116]. Moreover, $D_1$-like receptors can mediate signaling at a variety of voltage-gated ion channels as well as NMDA and $\gamma$-aminobutyric acid $(GABA)_A$ receptors, either directly or indirectly, through actions on DARPP-32, kinases, and phosphatases. There is also evidence that dopamine receptors (and G proteins) can have other protein–protein interactions, such as receptor oligomerization or interactions with scaffolding or other regulatory proteins, that also affect dopamine receptor signaling. There are some excellent recent reviews of this subject area [117, 118].

## 3.4 CURRENT STATUS OF $D_1$ AGONIST DEVELOPMENT

Although $D_1$ agonists may have therapeutic utility for schizophrenia, the majority of these drugs were developed to treat Parkinson's disease. Some years ago, we reviewed the status of the development of $D_1$ agonists as it applied to Parkinson's disease [119], and it is unfortunate that little has changed since that time [120, 121]. Despite the promise of $D_1$ agonists for Parkinson's disease, including both monkey [25] and human trials [26], there are currently no selective full $D_1$ agonists approved for general clinical use. Figure 3.1 shows the structure of dopamine and of some of the conceptually important $D_1$ agonists on which data are public. We have summarized our best editorial judgment of the state of the field in Table 3.1.

### 3.4.1 Status of Clinically Available Drugs

There are several drugs with $D_1$ properties that have been approved clinically. Fenoldopam [122, 123] is a phenylbenzazepine (see Table 3.1) and, like other members of that class, has a very rapid metabolism and short duration of action. In addition, unlike most of the other benzazepines, it does not cross the blood–brain barrier. Like dopamine itself, it is used in emergency medicine for its ability to decrease blood pressure and increase tissue perfusion. Apomorphine, pergolide, and bromocriptine all have been approved for treatment

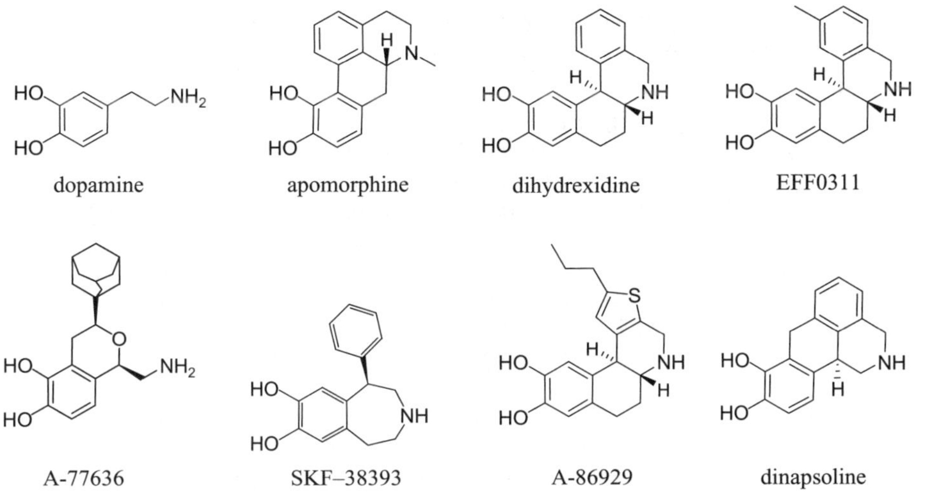


**FIGURE 3.1** Comparison of the structures of several of the experimental $D_1$ agonists that have been or are being studied.

of Parkinson's disease and all are $D_2$-preferring but have modest $D_1$ affinity. Interestingly, their relative efficacy as antiparkinson drugs in monotherapy correlates not with their $D_2$ affinity but with their intrinsic $D_1$ activity [124], with apomorphine having high, pergolide moderate [125], and bromocriptine no intrinsic activity. Unfortunately, the $D_2$ agonist effects of apomorphine and pergolide (and the $D_1$ antagonist properties of bromocriptine) make their use in the treatment of cognitive and negative symptoms more problematic as they likely could only be used in conjunction with typical antipsychotics that have high $D_2$ antagonist properties.

To our knowledge, the only relatively selective $D_1$ agonist that is currently available for human experimental studies is DHX [126, 127]. Although DHX caused profound hypotension when given intravenously in a small Phase IIa study [128], later studies demonstrated that for the lower plasma $D_1$ agonist concentration presumed to be needed to treat schizophrenia, DHX might be a useful experimental medication [129, 130]. There is at least one Phase IIa study ongoing (http://projectreporter.nih.gov/project_info_details.cfm?aid=7126751) with DHX, but it is unclear if the very short duration of action of DHX may compromise this study.

### 3.4.2 Research Status of $D_1$ Agonists

***3.4.2.1 Benzazepines*** The most widely studied class of $D_1$ agonists are based on the 3-phenylbenz[*d*]azepine backbone that we shall refer to generically as

**TABLE 3.1 Summary of Some Experimental and Clinical Ligands with $D_1$ Agonist Activity**

| | |
|---|---|
| Experimental | |
| *3-Phenylbenz[d]azepines (partial list)* | |
| SKF-38393 | First agonist with $D_1$ selectivity; modest $D_1$ IA. Short duration of action; no oral bioavailability |
| SKF-82958 | $D_1$ agonist with near-full agonist properties. Short duration of action; no oral bioavailability |
| SKF-81297 | SKF-38393 analog; $D_1$ agonist with near-full agonist properties Short duration of action; no oral bioavailability. |
| SKF-83959 | SKF-38393 analog; low $D_1$ IA at adenylate cyclase. Short duration of action; no oral bioavailability. |
| *Non-benzazepines* | |
| Dihydrexidine | First $D_1$ full agonist; high $D_1$ affinity. Injectable only and very short duration of action. Currently in National Institute of Mental Health-funded Phase IIa clinical study. |
| EFF-0311 | Dihydrexidine analog with somewhat higher $D_1$ selectivity; full $D_1$ agonist with much longer duration of action than dihydrexidine. |
| Doxanthrene | Relatively selective full $D_1$ agonist. *In vivo* characteristics unknown. |
| CY208-243 | Ergoline-like partial $D_1$ agonist; modest beneficial effects in PD. No longer in development (specifics NIPD) |
| A-68930 | High affinity $D_1$ agonist; full agonist; profound acute antiparkinson effects but caused rapid tolerance. Also caused seizures in many species. |
| A-77636 | High affinity full $D_1$ agonist (analog of A-68930). Profound acute antiparkinson effects but also caused rapid tolerance. No longer in development (specifics NIPD). |
| A-86929 (ABT-431) | $D_1$ full agonist; caused profound antiparkinson effects in humans. Modest duration of action; prodrug failed to give oral or sublingual bioavailability, hence injectable only. Development ceased (specifics NIPD). |
| Dinapsoline (DAR-0200) | Full $D_1$ agonist. Toxicity ended development (specifics NIPD). |
| Approved | |
| Fenoldopam | $D_1$ partial/high IA agonist; does not cross blood–brain barrier; approved drug for emergency medical uses. |
| Apomorphine | High affinity agonist selective for $D_2$ receptors but with high $D_1$ intrinsic activity. |
| Bromocriptine | Ergoline derivative; $D_2$ agonist with $D_1$ antagonist/low IA properties. |
| Lisuride | Serotonin agonist; ergoline derivative with activity at various serotonin receptors and $D_2$ agonist properties. Low IA $D_1$ agonist. |
| Pergolide | Ergoline derivative; $D_2/D_3$ agonist with modest $D_1$ IA. |

IA, intrinsic activity; NIPD, not in public domain.

benzazepines (see Table 3.1 for some examples). The prototype of this class is the first selective $D_1$ agonist SKF-38393 [131, 132]. Unfortunately, SKF-38393 failed to show antiparkinson actions in the bilateral MPTP primate model [133–140, 140] or in Parkinson's patients [141]. Moreover, studies have shown that SKF-38393 decreases the efficacy of levodopa and the $D_2$ agonist quinpirole [135, 136, 139] when co-administered with these latter agents to MPTP-treated monkeys. This is likely due to the fact that SKF-38393 has relatively low $D_1$ intrinsic activity [142–144] and therefore acts as a partial antagonist against levodopa. Despite relatively similar affinity to the full $D_1$ agonist DHX, in primate studies of working memory SKF-38393 was less potent and was less effective in younger animals [75].

There have since been dozens of modifications made to the benzazepine core structure [145]. Some of these have led to the standard antagonists used in the field both experimentally [21] and clinically [146]. They have also led to a variety of compounds with agonist activity at the $D_1$ receptor. As will be discussed later, it has not been possible to replace the 7- and 8-hydroxyl groups and still retain agonist activity. Thus, a common property of this class of $D_1$ agonists is rapid metabolism and little or no oral bioavailability, almost certainly due to the inherent catechol moiety. Some of these compounds include SKF-82958 [140, 144, 147, 148] and SKF-81297, both drugs having high or full $D_1$ intrinsic activity and $D_1$-like effects on motor activity [149, 150]. One of the more interesting compounds from this series is SKF-83959, which is relatively devoid of agonist activity in the commonly used adenylate cyclase assay *in vitro* but displays behavioral efficacy (at least in antiparkinson motor assays) that is similar to full agonists [151, 152]. As these examples illustrate, the benzazepines have been very useful in experimental studies in animals, but their pharmacokinetic properties have limited clinical utility.

### 3.4.3 Other Chemical Classes

The first drug purported to be a full $D_1$ agonist was SKF-89626, a thienopyridine analog of des-amino-dihydroxynomifensine first synthesized by Nichols and co-workers [153] and later studied by Andersen et al. [154]. This compound was reported to be a full agonist of adenylate cyclase with good selectivity for $D_1$ receptors. Whereas injection into the nucleus accumbens in rats gave a strong behavioral response, the compound did not cross the blood–brain barrier and its development was not extensively pursued. Later work demonstrated that although the drug has high intrinsic activity, it was not a true full agonist [144]. CY208-243 was another early $D_1$ agonist that was tested as an antiparkinson drug, but after displaying only modest efficacy [138, 147, 155–159], it appears to have been abandoned.

DHX was the first high-affinity, centrally available, full $D_1$ dopamine receptor agonist [126] that became available, and the drug appears to equal dopamine in every known functional $D_1$ system [127, 142–144, 160, 161]. This drug was used to show the importance of the $D_1$ receptor in Parkinson's disease

[25], and it also has been shown to have useful effects on working memory in young, aged [75], and MPTP-intoxicated monkeys [78]. As noted earlier, it is the only relatively selective $D_1$ agonist that is available for human experimental studies [126, 127] and, based on recent studies [129, 130], is currently being tested in schizophrenia.

The isochromans, such as A-68930 [162] and A-77636 [163], were the second class of true full $D_1$ agonists. These drugs had initial promise because they appeared to have overcome the bioavailability problems of DHX, and both compounds had antiparkinson effects [140, 164]. Unfortunately both compounds also produced rapid behavioral tolerance when administered either to animals or to patients [163, 165–167], and A-68930 also caused seizures [168]. The group at Abbott later discovered A-86929, a drug structurally similar to DHX but having a bioisosteric substitution of a thiophene for a phenyl in what is termed the accessory hydrophobic region [169]. A-86929 has similar pharmacological properties to DHX [170] and has been tested in the form of a diacetyl prodrug candidate, ABT-431 [171]. ABT-431 had dramatic antiparkinson effects in nonhuman primates [172], and the compound was also used experimentally in models of cognition [82] and drug abuse [173, 174]. Although DHX and ABT-431 have promising clinical implications, both have poor oral bioavailability. ABT-431 has been withdrawn from development for reasons that are not in the public domain. More recently, dinapsoline (DAR-0200) was reported to be a full $D_1$ agonist [175]. Although dinapsoline has little $D_1$:$D_2$ selectivity, it exhibits agonist behavioral actions that have been shown to be due predominately to $D_1$ effects [175–178]. Although dinapsoline was promising because it had some oral availability and a longer duration of action than DHX [176], it apparently also has failed in preclinical development. Finally, there were recent preliminary communications showing that a DHX analog, EFF-0311 (Fig. 3.1), was a full $D_1$ agonist with good $D_1$:$D_2$ selectivity and, most importantly, a much longer duration of action than DHX [179]. Its preclinical development status is not known.

### 3.4.4 Challenges and Opportunities for $D_1$ Discovery and Development

To date, there has been no success in attempts to develop a full $D_1$ agonist that does not contain a catechol group. Except for the isochromans that seem to "stick" to the $D_1$ receptor [180, 181], most other $D_1$ agonists have been relatively short-acting, presumably because of the requirement for the catechol moiety. It is interesting that, at least to date, the $D_1$ receptor is the only member of the Class A G protein-coupled receptors (GPCRs) in which this functionality (i.e., the catchol moiety) is essential for having a high affinity full agonist. The definition of "full agonist" that we have used to this point has been based on activity in the canonical pathway that activates adenylate cyclases. With the recognition that other signaling pathways can be critical in the action of GPCRs [182–185], it has also been suggested that such pathways may be relevant to the action of $D_1$ ligands [186–188], although this has been controversial [117, 120]. It may be possible to discover $D_1$ ligands without a catechol moiety that have high intrinsic activity for noncyclase signaling pathways (if not the cAMP system), which might still be useful in attenuating cognitive and attentional deficits.

Although the prospective clinical utility of dopamine $D_1$ agonists has been demonstrated in the laboratory, potential side effect and tolerance issues have kept current $D_1$ agonists out of the clinic. One concern has been $D_1$-induced hypotension, which led to the premature termination of the pilot human trial on intravenous DHX [128]. $D_1$-induced hypotension may be mediated by peripheral dopamine receptors in the heart and kidneys [189]. Although further studies are required to elucidate the role of $D_1$ dopamine receptors in blood pressure control before $D_1$ agonists can be safely used in humans, the lower doses of $D_1$ agonists that are presumed to be required for cognitive and memory problems may make the hypotension a null issue relative to the higher receptor occupation needed for antiparkinson effects (for comparison, see [25, 75]). Induction of seizures has been another concern with the clinical use of $D_1$ agonists. $D_2$ receptor activation can elicit anticonvulsant actions, but selective $D_1$ agonists can actually lower the seizure threshold [190]. Although selective $D_1$ agonists have been shown to be proconvulsant, these studies were conducted in animals where brain dopamine was previously lowered with reserpine or 6-hydroxydopamine (6-OHDA) [191, 192]. In normal animals, as well as humans, even full $D_1$ agonists like DHX and ABT-431 do not appear to cause seizures [193]. A-68930, however, has been reported to cause seizures [168], and its analog, A-77636, has been shown to induce seizures in nonlesioned rodents as well, but only at doses markedly greater than those that induce rotations [163]. In general, $D_1$ receptor activation alone is not sufficient to cause seizures. The mechanisms involved and the relative safety margin of $D_1$ agonists as a class are yet to be clearly determined. It is possible that seizures may be a side effect of $D_1$ agonists in Parkinson's disease where dopamine is depleted and would be less likely to occur in schizophrenia.

One final issue that may be the most important when contemplating the use of $D_1$ agonists in patients is behavioral tolerance. The daunting task is to develop a $D_1$ agonist that does not lead to rapid behavioral tolerance because to date, increasing the bioavailability and duration of action of $D_1$ agonists has resulted in rapid behavioral tolerance. For example, the selective and long-acting $D_1$ agonists, A-68930 and A-77636, produce rapid behavioral tolerance after the first day of treatment in 6-OHDA-lesioned rats, but tolerance does not develop in normal animals [165, 166]. These results suggest that tolerance may only develop under conditions of reduced dopamine levels. It is not clear if this is a property of all $D_1$ agonists, and, if so, whether it will affect the lower doses/concentrations of $D_1$ agonist that appear to be most useful in treating cognitive and negative aspects of schizophrenia. It is interesting, however, to speculate that tolerance to $D_1$ agonists may not occur in schizophrenics, where dopamine is not depleted. One must be cautious, however, because the referenced studies measured tolerance to locomotor activity. Future studies will need to examine whether tolerance to neuroprotective or cognitive enhancing effects of dopamine $D_1$ agonists occurs. More research is needed to characterize or clarify the factors mediating unwanted side effects of $D_1$ agonists. Nevertheless, development of a functionally selective $D_1$ agonist is an exciting possibility that may attenuate the negative side effects by targeting subpopulations of dopamine $D_1$ receptors.

## 3.5 FUTURE RESEARCH DIRECTIONS

### 3.5.1 Novel Approaches to Modulation of $D_1$ Function

***3.5.1.1 Functional Selectivity*** When a receptor has the ability to activate several different signaling pathways, a ligand may differentially alter these pathways through the same receptor. This concept is a modification of classical pharmacology where a full agonist would be expected to activate all of the signaling pathways linked to a receptor to the same degree as the endogenous ligand for that receptor. In addition to effects from targeting specific molecular isoforms of receptors, function may be selectively regulated by unique conformations induced by signaling complexes composed of the receptor, G proteins, and other signaling and scaffolding proteins. For example, a ligand acting at a receptor that mediates multiple functions could act as an agonist at one pathway and an antagonist at another, a process often termed functional selectivity [185]. Of critical importance is the fact that the differential activation of various signaling pathways by functionally selective compounds is not due to affinity differences at the receptor target. In fact, studies have suggested that various ligands of the same receptor can induce specific receptor conformations that regulate which signal transduction pathways are activated [194–200]. This concept becomes critical when dealing with drug design because compounds can be selected that only activate desired signaling pathways and thus have reduced unwanted effects.

***3.5.1.2 Early Evidence for Functional Selectivity of Dopaminergic Compounds*** Although research may have hinted at the idea of functional selectivity a long time ago, this concept has recently drawn much more attention as functional selectivity has been shown for a variety of Class A GPCRs of importance to schizophrenia, such as serotonin 5-$HT_{2A/C}$ and dopamine receptors. The characterization of DHX provided the first clear example of dopamine receptor functional selectivity. Although DHX was designed as a full $D_1$ agonist, it also has $D_2$ affinity [127, 161]. The functional selectivity of DHX was first shown through its variable actions at $D_2$ receptors [201]. Aripiprazole (see Chapter 2) is another example of a functionally selective dopaminergic compound. Aripiprazole is a recently approved antipsychotic drug that displays functional selectivity for various $D_2$ receptors and can range from an agonist to an antagonist. Functional selectivity has already been demonstrated for the dopamine $D_1$ receptor [180, 202], raising the possibility that functionally selective $D_1$ agonists could separate desired from undesired effects in schizophrenia treatment.

***3.5.1.3 Theoretical Basis for Use of Functional Selectivity for Next-Generation Drugs*** Prior to the development of aripiprazole, essentially all APDs were $D_2$ antagonists. One of the hypotheses of functional selectivity is that the activation of various signaling cascades may be the result of ligand-dependent receptor conformational changes. Thus, cellular functions can be modulated in a much more specific manner than what was traditionally thought. At least for the $D_1$ receptor, however, major ligand structural differences cannot explain differences in functional selectivity as structurally dissimilar $D_1$ agonists may display similar functional selectivity [202]. Thus, changes could be due to more subtle structural differences but may also be indicative of which G proteins are coupled to the receptor.

Functional selectivity paves the way for many exciting opportunities in drug discovery and development, particularly in neuropsychiatric diseases like schizophrenia. The idea of functional selectivity means that research will have to adapt the methods by which new drug compounds are screened. For example, high-throughput screening assays will look at numerous candidate drugs but typically will only measure one endpoint. Since functional selectivity suggests that drugs can signal through alternate pathways via the same receptor, this approach may overlook the potential utility of specific compounds. Furthermore, the majority of APDs currently on the market have numerous side effects that limit their use either for health reasons or for compliance. Thus, utilizing the concept of functional selectivity for design of next-generation drugs may eliminate unwanted side effects and increase their therapeutic profile.

### 3.5.2 $D_1$-$D_5$ Selective Agonists

Development of subtype-selective $D_1$-like compounds may provide a novel way to treat disease symptoms attributable to $D_1$-like receptors. Pharmacological differences between the $D_5$ and $D_1$ receptors were suggested when the $D_5$ receptor was initially cloned in 1991 [15, 62]. More than a decade later, however, a $D_1$-subtype-selective ligand has yet to be designed, and definitive physiological roles for the individual receptor subtypes are only partially understood. Several recent discoveries have demonstrated the need for a $D_5$ subtype-selective compound. Indeed, dopamine signaling through the $D_5$ receptor controls the activity of the subthalamic nucleus in a normal state [203], suggesting that a $D_5$ selective compound may provide improved therapy for select dopamine-linked disorders. In addition, the $D_1$ and $D_5$ receptors can both modulate other receptors through direct interactions. The $D_1$ receptor is able to form a functional interaction with NMDA and adenosine $A_1$ receptors [204, 205], whereas the $D_5$ receptor can complex with $GABA_A$ receptors to alter synaptic strength [206]. These issues become even more important when thinking about functionally selective drugs because in some cases it is not known which of the two dopamine $D_1$-like receptors are responsible for the effects of what are termed "$D_1$ agonists." As $D_1$ agonists emerge as potential therapeutics for schizophrenia, knowing if particular effects are due to $D_1$, and not $D_5$, receptors would be invaluable. Hypothetically, negative effects of a newly developed dopamine $D_1$-like receptor agonist could be due to activation of $D_5$ receptors. This knowledge could help in the development of enhanced drugs for schizophrenia and other diseases but requires the discovery of selective antagonists for the $D_1$ versus $D_5$ receptor.

### 3.5.3 Can Co-administration of $D_1$ Agonists Attenuate the Parkinsonism of Typical Drugs

The involvement of dopamine in the pathology of schizophrenia is influenced by both the mesocortical and the mesolimbic projections. As previously mentioned, $D_2$ receptors play a major role in the subcortical mesolimbic signals, whereas $D_1$ receptors are important for cortical dopamine transmission. Furthermore, current typical APDs are predominately antagonists of dopamine $D_2$ receptors and are not ideal therapeutics as they not only cause EPS but are also largely ineffective against negative symptoms and cognitive deficits. Because dopamine $D_1$ receptor signaling is important in regions involved with working memory, such as the prefrontal cortex, and agonists have been shown to improve cognitive functioning, co-administration of $D_1$ agonists may be an effective therapeutic strategy to alleviate the parkinsonism of typical APDs.

The balance between cortical and subcortical dopamine activity is important for proper functioning. Indeed, prefrontal dopamine activity (largely $D_1$) has been shown to inhibit subcortical dopamine activity, where the majority of $D_2$ receptors are found [207, 208]. Because schizophrenia results in hypoactive dopaminergic activity in the prefrontal cortex, this may interfere with control over mesolimbic dopamine activity [209]. Thus, a $D_1$ receptor agonist may restore the balance in dopamine function, which would lead to inhibition of subcortical dopaminergic activity and mimic the effects of a $D_2$ antagonist. Furthermore, a reduction in subcortical dopamine levels blunts motor activity, and co-administration of a $D_1$ agonist may be able to restore dopaminergic activity to a level that prevents some of the EPS seen with typical APDs without exacerbating the positive symptoms.

### 3.5.4 Other Potentially Useful Effects of $D_1$ Agonists

Dopamine $D_1$ agonists may have important secondary benefits, and one that has received attention in recent years is the potential for these agonists to be neuroprotective. Indeed, just the fact that $D_1$ agonists can reduce some of the side effects associated with APDs could classify them as neuroprotective because they help to maintain normal functioning of the CNS in response to disease. In addition, dopamine $D_1$ agonists have been shown to induce neuroprotection following CNS injury by inhibiting regulatory T cells [210]. Furthermore SKF-83959 has neuroprotective actions that are at least partially dependent on dopamine $D_1$ receptors [211], and $D_1$ receptors can interact with NMDA receptors to regulate cell death due to excitotoxicity [212]. Apomorphine, a $D_1/D_2$ agonist, increases the production of multiple growth factors, further supporting the idea that dopamine agonists can be neuroprotective [213]. Interestingly, apomorphine has been shown to be neuroprotective against MPTP-induced neurodegeneration in mice [214], although this may be due to nonreceptor actions of apomorphine, such as antioxidant or free radical scavenging properties. There are numerous targets for neuroprotective therapeutics as there are a host of factors that can influence neurodegeneration, some of which may be related to the $D_1$ agonist itself rather than receptor activation. For example, neuronal death can result from inflammation, oxidative stress, mitochondrial dysfunction, or excitotoxicity, and the precise role of dopamine $D_1$ agonists has yet to be fully explored.

Dopamine $D_1$ agonists may also be useful in attention-deficit/hyperactivity disorder (ADHD), Parkinson's disease, and substance abuse disorders, particularly cocaine. Locomotor issues observed in patients with ADHD are similar to those seen in dopamine $D_1$ receptor knockout mice [215], and studies demonstrated a relationship between the gene for the $D_1$ receptor and ADHD [216]. In addition, full $D_1$ agonists like DHX can inhibit locomotor activity in animals [217] and could have therapeutic implications for ADHD. $D_1$ agonists may also be useful in treating cocaine addicts. Dopamine is clearly important in the addictive actions of cocaine, as well as other drugs, and $D_2$ agonists are not a viable target because they increase cocaine-seeking behavior [218]. $D_1$ agonists can decrease cocaine-seeking behavior in rodents and reduce craving in humans [174]. Finally, the $D_1$ receptor has been shown to be an important target for the treatment of Parkinson's disease [119]. Although unproven, studies have suggested that $D_1$ receptors may mediate antiparkinson effects that would only be observed with activation by a full, rather than a partial, $D_1$ agonist [142]. Indeed, DHX has antiparkinson actions in MPTP-treated monkeys [25] and humans with Parkinson's disease [128], but pharmacokinetic and side effect issues have restricted its advancement into clinical trials. DHX, however, demonstrated the potential of $D_1$ agonists for treating Parkinson's disease, and ongoing studies are searching for $D_1$ agonists with increased bioavailability and reduced side effects.

### 3.5.5 Conclusions

Given the many issues associated with currently available APDs, numerous studies are investigating novel drug targets for the treatment of schizophrenia and other psychiatric disorders. Current APDs were all designed to include the property of dopamine $D_2$ receptor antagonism. The development of aripiprazole revealed the possibility of using a functionally selective $D_2$ ligand as an effective treatment for schizophrenia patients. As discussed in this review, dopamine $D_1$-like receptors are another possible therapeutic target for schizophrenia. The functional abnormalities suspected to play a role in schizophrenia have suggested a variety of novel targets reviewed elsewhere in this volume. Some of these targets (e.g., glutamate receptors) may modulate $D_1$ function, and/or be indirectly regulated by dopamine $D_1$-like agonists. The hope is that a $D_1$-like agonist would be able to treat many of the cognitive and negative symptoms of schizophrenia that are largely resistant to current antipsychotics. Furthermore, a functionally selective $D_1$-like agonist has the potential to target specific symptoms of schizophrenia while avoiding receptors that produce unwanted side effects. This potential is hopefully spurring the discovery and development of novel and improved $D_1$ agonists. Such a drug would not only be useful for schizophrenia but could also extend to the treatment of a variety of neuropsychiatric disorders.

## ACKNOWLEDGMENTS

This work was supported, in part, by Public Health Service research grants MH082441 and MH040537.

## CONFLICT OF INTEREST

Dr. Boyd reports no conflict of interest. Dr. Mailman has equity interests in Biovalve Technologies Inc. and Effipharma Inc., which have an interest in the discovery and development of drugs related to topics discussed in this chapter. The opinions expressed are solely those of the authors and do not reflect those of either of these companies or of the Pennsylvania State University.

## REFERENCES

1. Carlsson, A. (1959). The occurrence, distribution and physiological role of catecholamines in the nervous system. *Pharmacological Reviews*, *11*, 493.
2. Delay, J., Deniker, P., Harl, J.M. (1952). [Therapeutic method derived from hibernotherapy in excitation and agitation states.]. *Annales Médico-psychologiques, revue psychiatrique (Paris)*, *110*, 267–273.
3. Carlsson, A., Lindqvist, M. (1963). Effect of chlorpromazine and haloperidol on formation of 3-methoxytyramine and normetanephrine in mouse brain. *Acta Pharmacologica et Toxicologica (Copenh)*, *20*, 140–144.
4. Mailman, R.B., Murthy, V. (2010). Third generation antipsychotic drugs: partial agonism or receptor functional selectivity? *Current Pharmaceutical Design*, *16*, 488–501.
5. Kebabian, J.W., Petzold, G.L., Greengard, P. (1972). Dopamine-sensitive adenylate cyclase in caudate nucleus of rat brain, and its similarity to the "dopamine recep-

tor". *Proceedings of the National Academy of Sciences of the United States of America*, *69*, 2145–2149.

6. Clement-Cormier, Y.C., Kebabian, J.W., Petzold, G.L., Greengard, P. (1974). Dopamine-sensitive adenylate cyclase in mammalian brain: a possible site of action of antipsychotic drugs. *Proceedings of the National Academy of Sciences of the United States of America*, *71*, 1113–1117.
7. Iversen, L.L. (1975). Dopamine receptors in the brain. *Science*, *188*, 1084–1089.
8. Creese, I., Burt, D.R., Snyder, S.H. (1976). Dopamine receptor binding predicts clinical and pharmacological potencies of antischizophrenic drugs. *Science*, *192*, 481–483.
9. Trabucchi, M., Longoni, R., Fresia, P., Spano, P.F. (1975). Sulpiride: a study of the effects on dopamine receptors in rat neostriatum and limbic forebrain. *Life Sciences*, *17*, 1551–1556.
10. Garau, L., Govoni, S., Stefanini, E., Trabucchi, M., Spano, P.F. (1978). Dopamine receptors: pharmacological and anatomical evidences indicate that two distinct dopamine receptor populations are present in rat striatum. *Life Sciences*, *23*, 1745–1750.
11. Kebabian, J.W., Calne, D.B. (1979). Multiple receptors for dopamine. *Nature*, *277*, 93–96.
12. Dearry, A., Gingrich, J.A., Falardeau, P., Fremeau, R.T., Jr, Bates, M.D., Caron, M.G. (1990). Molecular cloning and expression of the gene for a human D1 dopamine receptor. *Nature*, *347*, 72–76.
13. Monsma, F.J.J., Mahan, L.C., McVittie, L.D., Gerfen, C.R., Sibley, D.R. (1990). Molecular cloning and expression of a D1 dopamine receptor linked to adenylyl cyclase activation. *Proceedings of the National Academy of Sciences of the United States of America*, *87*, 6723–6727.
14. Zhou, Q.Y., Grandy, D.K., Thambi, L., Kushner, J.A., van Tol, H.H., Cone, R., Pribnow, D., Salon, J., Bunzow, J.R., Civelli, O. (1990). Cloning and expression of human and rat $D_1$ dopamine receptors. *Nature*, *347*, 76–80.
15. Sunahara, R.K., Guan, H.C., O'Dowd, B.F., Seeman, P., Laurier, L.G., Ng, G., George, S.R., Torchia, J., van Tol, H.H., Niznik, H.B. (1991). Cloning of the gene for a human dopamine $D_5$ receptor with higher affinity for dopamine than $D_1$. *Nature*, *350*, 614–619.
16. Dal Toso, R., Sommer, B., Ewert, M., Herb, A., Pritchett, D.B., Bach, A., Shivers, B.D., Seeburg, P.H. (1989). The dopamine $D_2$ receptor: two molecular forms generated by alternative splicing. *The EMBO Journal*, *8*, 4025–4034.
17. Giros, B., Sokoloff, P., Martres, M.P., Riou, J.F., Emorine, L.J., Schwartz, J.C. (1989). Alternative splicing directs the expression of two $D_2$ dopamine receptor isoforms. *Nature*, *342*, 923–926.
18. Monsma, F.J., Jr, McVittie, L.D., Gerfen, C.R., Mahan, L.C., Sibley, D.R. (1989). Multiple D2 dopamine receptors produced by alternative RNA splicing. *Nature*, *342*, 926–929.
19. Chio, C.L., Hess, G.F., Graham, R.S., Huff, R.M. (1990). A second molecular form of $D_2$ dopamine receptor in rat and bovine caudate nucleus. *Nature*, *343*, 266–269.
20. Sokoloff, P., Giros, B., Martres, M.P., Bouthenet, M.L., Schwartz, J.C. (1990). Molecular cloning and characterization of a novel dopamine receptor ($D_3$) as a target for neuroleptics. *Nature*, *347*, 146–151.

21. Iorio, L.C., Barnett, A., Leitz, F.H., Houser, V.P., Korduba, C.A. (1983). SCH 23390, a potential benzazepine antipsychotic with unique interactions on dopaminergic systems. *The Journal of Pharmacology and Experimental Therapeutics*, *226*, 462–468.
22. Creese, I., Chen, A. (1985). Selective D-1 dopamine receptor increase following chronic treatment with SCH 23390. *European Journal of Pharmacology*, *109*, 127–128.
23. Coffin, V.L., Latranyi, M.B., Chipkin, R.E. (1989). Acute extrapyramidal syndrome in Cebus monkeys: development mediated by dopamine D2 but not D1 receptors. *The Journal of Pharmacology and Experimental Therapeutics*, *249*, 769–774.
24. Mailman, R.B., Schulz, D.W., Lewis, M.H., Staples, L., Rollema, H., DeHaven, D.L. (1984). SCH-23390: a selective D1 dopamine antagonist with potent D2 behavioral actions. *European Journal of Pharmacology*, *101*, 159–160.
25. Taylor, J.R., Lawrence, M.S., Redmond, D.E., Jr, Elsworth, J.D., Roth, R.H., Nichols, D.E., Mailman, R.B. (1991). Dihydrexidine, a full dopamine D1 agonist, reduces MPTP-induced parkinsonism in monkeys. *European Journal of Pharmacology*, *199*, 389–391.
26. Rascol, O., Blin, O., Thalamas, C., Descombes, S., Soubrouillard, C., Azulay, P., Fabre, N., Viallet, F., Lafnitzegger, K., Wright, S., Carter, J.H., Nutt, J.G. (1999). ABT-431, a D1 receptor agonist prodrug, has efficacy in Parkinson's disease. *Annals of Neurology*, *45*, 736–741.
27. Lawrence, M.S., Redmond, D.E., Jr, Elsworth, J.D., Taylor, J.R., Roth, R.H. (1991). The D1 receptor antagonist, SCH 23390, induces signs of parkinsonism in African green monkeys. *Life Sciences*, *49*, L229–L234.
28. Karlsson, P., Smith, L., Farde, L., Harnryd, C., Sedvall, G., Wiesel, F.A. (1995). Lack of apparent antipsychotic effect of the D1-dopamine receptor antagonist SCH39166 in acutely ill schizophrenic patients. *Psychopharmacology (Berl)*, *121*, 309–316.
29. Den Boer, J.A., van Megen, H.J., Fleischhacker, W.W., Louwerens, J.W., Slaap, B.R., Westenberg, H.G., Burrows, G.D., Srivastava, O.N. (1995). Differential effects of the D1-DA receptor antagonist SCH39166 on positive and negative symptoms of schizophrenia. *Psychopharmacology (Berl)*, *121*, 317–322.
30. Labelle, A., de Beaurepaire, R., Boulay, L.J., Naber, D., Jones, B.D., Barnes, T.R. (1998). A pilot study of the safety and tolerance of SCH 39166 in patients with schizophrenia. *Journal of Psychiatry & Neuroscience*, *23*, 93–94.
31. de Beaurepaire, R., Labelle, A., Naber, D., Jones, B.D., Barnes, T.R. (1995). An open trial of the D1 antagonist SCH 39166 in six cases of acute psychotic states. *Psychopharmacology (Berl)*, *121*, 323–327.
32. Karle, J., Clemmesen, L., Hansen, L., Andersen, M., Andersen, J., Fensbo, C., Sloth-Nielsen, M., Skrumsager, B.K., Lublin, H., Gerlach, J. (1995). NNC 01-0687, a selective dopamine D1 receptor antagonist, in the treatment of schizophrenia. *Psychopharmacology (Berl)*, *121*, 328–329.
33. Fleischhacker, W.W. (2003). New developments in the pharmacotherapy of schizophrenia. *Journal of Neural Transmission. Supplementum*, *64*, 105–117.
34. Barnes, T.R., McPhillips, M.A. (1999). Critical analysis and comparison of the side-effect and safety profiles of the new antipsychotics. *The British Journal of Psychiatry. Supplement*, *38*, 34–43.

35. Kane, J.M. (1999). Pharmacologic treatment of schizophrenia. *Biological Psychiatry*, *46*, 1396–1408.
36. Miyamoto, S., Duncan, G.E., Marx, C.E., Lieberman, J.A. (2005). Treatments for schizophrenia: a critical review of pharmacology and mechanisms of action of antipsychotic drugs. *Molecular Psychiatry*, *10*, 79–104.
37. Miyamoto, S., Duncan, G.E., Mailman, R.B., Lieberman, J.A. (2000). Developing novel antipsychotic drugs: strategies and goals. *Current Opinion in CPNS Investigational Drugs*, *2*, 25–39.
38. Kane, J. (1999). Olanzapine in the long-term treatment of schizophrenia. *The British Journal of Psychiatry. Supplement*, *37*, 26–29.
39. Lieberman, J.A. (1996). Atypical antipsychotic drugs as a first-line treatment of schizophrenia: a rationale and hypothesis. *The Journal of Clinical Psychiatry*, *57*(Suppl 11), 68–71.
40. Lidow, M.S., Goldman-Rakic, P.S., Gallager, D.W., Rakic, P. (1991). Distribution of dopaminergic receptors in the primate cerebral cortex: quantitative autoradiographic analysis using [3H]raclopride, [3H]spiperone and [3H]SCH23390. *Neuroscience*, *40*, 657–671.
41. Piggott, M.A., Marshall, E.F., Thomas, N., Lloyd, S., Court, J.A., Jaros, E., Costa, D., Perry, R.H., Perry, E.K. (1999). Dopaminergic activities in the human striatum: rostrocaudal gradients of uptake sites and of D1 and D2 but not of D3 receptor binding or dopamine. *Neuroscience*, *90*, 433–445.
42. Hall, H., Halldin, C., Sedvall, G. (1993). Binding of [$^{3}$H]SCH 39166 to human post mortem brain tissue. *Pharmacology & Toxicology*, *72*, 152–158.
43. Hall, H., Sedvall, G., Magnusson, O., Kopp, J., Halldin, C., Farde, L. (1994). Distribution of D1- and D2-dopamine receptors, and dopamine and its metabolites in the human brain. *Neuropsychopharmacology*, *11*, 245–256.
44. De Keyser, J., Claeys, A., De Backer, J.P., Ebinger, G., Roels, F., Vauquelin, G. (1988). Autoradiographic localization of D1 and D2 dopamine receptors in the human brain. *Neuroscience Letters*, *91*, 142–147.
45. Montague, D.M., Lawler, C.P., Mailman, R.B., Gilmore, J.H. (1999). Developmental regulation of the dopamine $D_1$ receptor in human caudate and putamen. *Neuropsychopharmacology*, *21*, 641–649.
46. Richfield, E.K., Young, A.B., Penney, J.B. (1987). Comparative distribution of dopamine D-1 and D-2 receptors in the basal ganglia of turtles, pigeons, rats, cats, and monkeys. *The Journal of Comparative Neurology*, *262*, 446–463.
47. Boyson, S.J., McGonigle, P., Molinoff, P.B. (1986). Quantitative autoradiographic localization of the D1 and D2 subtypes of dopamine receptors in rat brain. *The Journal of Neuroscience*, *6*, 3177–3188.
48. Savasta, M., Dubois, A., Scatton, B. (1986). Autoradiographic localization of D1 dopamine receptors in the rat brain with [3H]SCH 23390. *Brain Research*, *375*, 291–301.
49. Altar, C.A., Marien, M.R. (1987). Picomolar affinity of $^{125}$I-SCH 23982 for $D_1$ receptors in brain demonstrated with digital subtraction autoradiography. *The Journal of Neuroscience*, *7*, 213–222.
50. Wamsley, J.K., Hunt, M.E., McQuade, R.D., Alburges, M.E. (1991). [3H]SCH39166, a D1 dopamine receptor antagonist: binding characteristics and localization. *Experimental Neurology*, *111*, 145–151.

51. Schulz, D.W., Wyrick, S.D., Mailman, R.B. (1984). [3H]SCH23390 has the characteristics of a dopamine receptor ligand in the rat central nervous system. *European Journal of Pharmacology*, *106*, 211–212.
52. Schulz, D.W., Stanford, E.J., Wyrick, S.W., Mailman, R.B. (1985). Binding of [3H] SCH23390 in rat brain: regional distribution and effects of assay conditions and GTP suggest interactions at a D1-like dopamine receptor. *Journal of Neurochemistry*, *45*, 1601–1611.
53. Mansour, A., Meador-Woodruff, J.H., Bunzow, J.R., Civelli, O., Akil, H., Watson, S.J. (1990). Localization of dopamine $D_2$ receptor mRNA and $D_1$ and $D_2$ receptor binding in the rat brain and pituitary: an in situ hybridization-receptor autoradiographic analysis. *The Journal of Neuroscience*, *10*, 2587–2600.
54. Fremeau, R.T.J., Duncan, G.E., Fornaretto, M.G., Dearry, A., Gingrich, J.A., Breese, G.R., Caron, M.G. (1991). Localization of D1 dopamine receptor mRNA in brain supports a role in cognitive, affective, and neuroendocrine aspects of dopaminergic neurotransmission. *Proceedings of the National Academy of Sciences of the United States of America*, *88*, 3772–3776.
55. Meador-Woodruff, J.H., Mansour, A., Healy, D.J., Kuehn, R., Zhou, Q.Y., Bunzow, J.R., Akil, H., Civelli, O., Watson, S.J., Jr (1991). Comparison of the distributions of $D_1$ and $D_2$ dopamine receptor mRNAs in rat brain. *Neuropsychopharmacology*, *5*, 231–242.
56. Levey, A.I., Hersch, S.M., Rye, D.B., Sunahara, R.K., Niznik, H.B., Kitt, C.A., Price, D.L., Maggio, R., Brann, M.R., Ciliax, B.J. (1993). Localization of D1 and D2 dopamine receptors in brain with subtype-specific antibodies. *Proceedings of the National Academy of Sciences of the United States of America*, *90*, 8861–8865.
57. Ariano, M.A., Sibley, D.R. (1994). Dopamine receptor distribution in the rat CNS: elucidation using anti- peptide antisera directed against D1A and D3 subtypes. *Brain Research*, *649*, 95–110.
58. Yung, K.K., Bolam, J.P., Smith, A.D., Hersch, S.M., Ciliax, B.J., Levey, A.I. (1995). Immunocytochemical localization of D1 and D2 dopamine receptors in the basal ganglia of the rat: light and electron microscopy. *Neuroscience*, *65*, 709–730.
59. Harrison, M.B., Wiley, R.G., Wooten, G.F. (1990). Selective localization of striatal D1 receptors to striatonigral neurons. *Brain Research*, *528*, 317–322.
60. Gerfen, C.R., Engber, T.M., Mahan, L.C., Susel, Z., Chase, T.N., Monsma, F.J.J., Sibley, D.R. (1990). $D_1$ and $D_2$ dopamine receptor-regulated gene expression of striatonigral and striatopallidal neurons. *Science*, *250*, 1429–1432.
61. Montague, D.M., Striplin, C.D., Overcash, J.S., Drago, F., Lawler, C.P., Mailman, R.B. (2001). Quantification of $D_{1B}$ ($D_5$) receptors in dopamine $D_{1A}$ receptor-deficient mice. *Synapse*, *39*, 319–322.
62. Tiberi, M., Jarvie, K.R., Silvia, C., Falardeau, P., Gingrich, J.A., Godinot, N., Bertrand, L., Yang-Feng, T.L., Fremeau, R.T., Caron, M.G. (1991). Cloning, molecular characterization, and chromosomal assignment of a gene encoding a second D1 dopamine receptor subtype: differential expression pattern in rat brain compared with the D1A receptor. *Proceedings of the National Academy of Sciences of the United States of America*, *88*, 7491–7495.
63. Meador-Woodruff, J.H., Mansour, A., Grandy, D.K., Damask, S.P., Civelli, O., Watson, S.J., Jr (1992). Distribution of $D_5$ dopamine receptor mRNA in rat brain. *Neuroscience Letters*, *145*, 209–212.

64. Ariano, M.A., Wang, J., Noblett, K.L., Larson, E.R., Sibley, D.R. (1997). Cellular distribution of the rat D1B receptor in central nervous system using anti-receptor antisera. *Brain Research*, *746*, 141–150.

65. Surmeier, D.J., Song, W.J., Yan, Z. (1996). Coordinated expression of dopamine receptors in neostriatal medium spiny neurons. *The Journal of Neuroscience*, *16*, 6579–6591.

66. Rappaport, M.S., Sealfon, S.C., Prikhozhan, A., Huntley, G.W., Morrison, J.H. (1993). Heterogeneous distribution of D1, D2 and D5 receptor mRNAs in monkey striatum. *Brain Research*, *616*, 242–250.

67. Huntley, G.W., Morrison, J.H., Prikhozhan, A., Sealfon, S.C. (1992). Localization of multiple dopamine receptor subtype mRNAs in human and monkey motor cortex and striatum. *Molecular Brain Research*, *15*, 181–188.

68. Ciliax, B.J., Nash, N., Heilman, C., Sunahara, R., Hartney, A., Tiberi, M., Rye, D.B., Caron, M.G., Niznik, H.B., Levey, A.I. (2000). Dopamine D5 receptor immunolocalization in rat and monkey brain. *Synapse*, *37*, 125–145.

69. Khan, Z.U., Gutierrez, A., Martin, R., Penafiel, A., Rivera, A., De La, C.A. (2000). Dopamine $D_5$ receptors of rat and human brain. *Neuroscience*, *100*, 689–699.

70. Matthysse, S. (1974). Dopamine and the pharmacology of schizophrenia: the state of the evidence. *Journal of Psychiatric Research*, *11*, 107–113.

71. Van Rossum, J.M. (1966). The significance of dopamine-receptor blockade for the mechanism of action of neuroleptic drugs. *Archives internationales de pharmacodynamie et de therapie*, *160*, 492–494.

72. Goldman-Rakic, P.S., Castner, S.A., Svensson, T.H., Siever, L.J., Williams, G.V. (2004). Targeting the dopamine $D_1$ receptor in schizophrenia: insights for cognitive dysfunction. *Psychopharmacology (Berl)*, *174*, 3–16.

73. Steele, T.D., Hodges, D.B., Jr, Levesque, T.R., Locke, K.W. (1997). D1 agonist dihydrexidine releases acetylcholine and improves cognitive performance in rats. *Pharmacology, Biochemistry, and Behavior*, *58*, 477–483.

74. Hersi, A.I., Rowe, W., Gaudreau, P., Quirion, R. (1995). Dopamine $D_1$ receptor ligands modulate cognitive performance and hippocampal acetylcholine release in memory-impaired aged rats. *Neuroscience*, *69*, 1067–1074.

75. Arnsten, A.F., Cai, J.X., Murphy, B.L., Goldman-Rakic, P.S. (1994). Dopamine D1 receptor mechanisms in the cognitive performance of young adult and aged monkeys. *Psychopharmacology (Berl)*, *116*, 143–151.

76. Cai, J.X., Arnsten, A.F. (1997). Dose-dependent effects of the dopamine D1 receptor agonists A77636 or SKF81297 on spatial working memory in aged monkeys. *The Journal of Pharmacology and Experimental Therapeutics*, *283*, 183–189.

77. Schneider, J.S., Sun, Z.Q., Roeltgen, D.P. (1994). Effects of dopamine agonists on delayed response performance in chronic low-dose MPTP-treated monkeys. *Pharmacology, Biochemistry, and Behavior*, *48*, 235–240.

78. Schneider, J.S., Sun, Z.Q., Roeltgen, D.P. (1994). Effects of dihydrexidine, a full dopamine D-1 receptor agonist, on delayed response performance in chronic low dose MPTP-treated monkeys. *Brain Research*, *663*, 140–144.

79. Brozoski, T.J., Brown, R.M., Rosvold, H.E., Goldman, P.S. (1979). Cognitive deficit caused by regional depletion of dopamine in prefrontal cortex of rhesus monkey. *Science*, *205*, 929–932.

80. Simon, H. (1981). [Dopaminergic A10 neurons and frontal system (author's translation)]. *Journal of Physiology, Paris*, *77*, 81–95.
81. Sawaguchi, T., Goldman-Rakic, P.S. (1994). The role of $D_1$-dopamine receptor in working memory: local injections of dopamine antagonists into the prefrontal cortex of rhesus monkeys performing an oculomotor delayed-response task. *Journal of Neurophysiology*, *71*, 515–528.
82. Castner, S.A., Williams, G.V., Goldman-Rakic, P.S. (2000). Reversal of antipsychotic-induced working memory deficits by short-term dopamine D1 receptor stimulation. *Science*, *287*, 2020–2022.
83. Floresco, S.B., Phillips, A.G. (2001). Delay-dependent modulation of memory retrieval by infusion of a dopamine D1 agonist into the rat medial prefrontal cortex. *Behavioral Neuroscience*, *115*, 934–939.
84. Steele, T.D., Hodges, D.B., Jr, Levesque, T.R., Locke, K.W., Sandage, B.W., Jr (1996). The D1 agonist dihydrexidine releases acetylcholine and improves cognition in rats. *Annals of the New York Academy of Sciences*, *777*, 427–430.
85. Muly, E.C., III, Szigeti, K., Goldman-Rakic, P.S. (1998). $D_1$ receptor in interneurons of macaque prefrontal cortex: distribution and subcellular localization. *The Journal of Neuroscience*, *18*, 10553–10565.
86. Castner, S.A., Williams, G.V. (2007). Tuning the engine of cognition: a focus on NMDA/D1 receptor interactions in prefrontal cortex. *Brain and Cognition*, *63*, 94–122.
87. Goldman-Rakic, P.S., Muly, E.C., III, Williams, G.V. (2000). $D_1$ receptors in prefrontal cells and circuits. *Brain Research. Brain Research Reviews*, *31*, 295–301.
88. Castner, S.A., Goldman-Rakic, P.S. (2004). Enhancement of working memory in aged monkeys by a sensitizing regimen of dopamine D1 receptor stimulation. *The Journal of Neuroscience*, *24*, 1446–1450.
89. Murphy, B.L., Arnsten, A.F., Goldman-Rakic, P.S., Roth, R.H. (1996). Increased dopamine turnover in the prefrontal cortex impairs spatial working memory performance in rats and monkeys. *Proceedings of the National Academy of Sciences of the United States of America*, *93*, 1325–1329.
90. Zahrt, J., Taylor, J.R., Mathew, R.G., Arnsten, A.F. (1997). Supranormal stimulation of D1 dopamine receptors in the rodent prefrontal cortex impairs spatial working memory performance. *The Journal of Neuroscience*, *17*, 8528–8535.
91. Sawaguchi, T., Goldman-Rakic, P.S. (1991). D1 dopamine receptors in prefrontal cortex: involvement in working memory. *Science*, *251*, 947–950.
92. Williams, G.V., Goldman-Rakic, P.S. (1995). Modulation of memory fields by dopamine D1 receptors in prefrontal cortex. *Nature*, *376*, 572–575.
93. Castner, S.A., Goldman-Rakic, P.S., Williams, G.V. (2004). Animal models of working memory: insights for targeting cognitive dysfunction in schizophrenia. *Psychopharmacology (Berl)*, *174*, 111–125.
94. Muly, E.C., Greengard, P., Goldman-Rakic, P.S. (2001). Distribution of protein phosphatases-1 alpha and -1 gamma 1 and the $D_1$ dopamine receptor in primate prefrontal cortex: evidence for discrete populations of spines. *The Journal of Comparative Neurology*, *440*, 261–270.
95. Selemon, L.D., Begovic, A., Goldman-Rakic, P.S., Castner, S.A. (2007). Amphetamine sensitization alters dendritic morphology in prefrontal cortical pyramidal neurons in the non-human primate. *Neuropsychopharmacology*, *32*, 919–931.

96. Okubo, Y., Suhara, T., Suzuki, K., Kobayashi, K., Inoue, O., Terasaki, O., Someya, Y., Sassa, T., Sudo, Y., Matsushima, E., Iyo, M., Tateno, Y., Toru, M. (1997). Decreased prefrontal dopamine $D_1$ receptors in schizophrenia revealed by PET [see comments]. *Nature*, *385*, 634–636.

97. Barch, D.M., Sheline, Y.I., Csernansky, J.G., Snyder, A.Z. (2003). Working memory and prefrontal cortex dysfunction: specificity to schizophrenia compared with major depression. *Biological Psychiatry*, *53*, 376–384.

98. Goldberg, T.E., Patterson, K.J., Taqqu, Y., Wilder, K. (1998). Capacity limitations in short-term memory in schizophrenia: tests of competing hypotheses. *Psychological Medicine*, *28*, 665–673.

99. Toda, M., Abi-Dargham, A. (2007). Dopamine hypothesis of schizophrenia: making sense of it all. *Current Psychiatry Reports*, *9*, 329–336.

100. Abi-Dargham, A., Mawlawi, O., Lombardo, I., Gil, R., Martinez, D., Huang, Y., Hwang, D.R., Keilp, J., Kochan, L., Van Heertum, R., Gorman, J.M., Laruelle, M. (2002). Prefrontal dopamine D1 receptors and working memory in schizophrenia. *The Journal of Neuroscience*, *22*, 3708–3719.

101. Bergson, C., Mrzljak, L., Smiley, J.F., Pappy, M., Levenson, R., Goldman-Rakic, P.S. (1995). Regional, cellular, and subcellular variations in the distribution of D1 and D5 dopamine receptors in primate brain. *The Journal of Neuroscience*, *15*, 7821–7836.

102. Frey, U., Schroeder, H., Matthies, H. (1990). Dopaminergic antagonists prevent long-term maintenance of posttetanic LTP in the CA1 region of rat hippocampal slices. *Brain Research*, *522*, 69–75.

103. Frey, U., Matthies, H., Reymann, K.G., Matthies, H. (1991). The effect of dopaminergic D1 receptor blockade during tetanization on the expression of long-term potentiation in the rat CA1 region in vitro. *Neuroscience Letters*, *129*, 111–114.

104. Hersi, A.I., Richard, J.W., Gaudreau, P., Quirion, R. (1995). Local modulation of hippocampal acetylcholine release by dopamine D1 receptors: a combined receptor autoradiography and in vivo dialysis study. *The Journal of Neuroscience*, *15*, 7150–7157.

105. Mercuri, N.B., Bonci, A., Bernardi, G. (1997). Electrophysiological pharmacology of the autoreceptor-mediated responses of dopaminergic cells to antiparkinsonian drugs. *Trends in Pharmacological Sciences*, *18*, 232–235.

106. Hersi, A.I., Kitaichi, K., Srivastava, L.K., Gaudreau, P., Quirion, R. (2000). Dopamine D-5 receptor modulates hippocampal acetylcholine release. *Brain Research. Molecular Brain Research*, *76*, 336–340.

107. Huang, Y.Y., Kandel, E.R. (1995). D1/D5 receptor agonists induce a protein synthesis-dependent late potentiation in the CA1 region of the hippocampus. *Proceedings of the National Academy of Sciences of the United States of America*, *92*, 2446–2450.

108. Matthies, H., Becker, A., Schroeder, H., Kraus, J., Hollt, V., Krug, M. (1997). Dopamine $D_1$-deficient mutant mice do not express the late phase of hippocampal long-term potentiation. *NeuroReport*, *8*, 3533–3535.

109. Bach, M.E., Barad, M., Son, H., Zhuo, M., Lu, Y.F., Shih, R., Mansuy, I., Hawkins, R.D., Kandel, E.R. (1999). Age-related defects in spatial memory are correlated with defects in the late phase of hippocampal long-term potentiation in vitro and are attenuated by drugs that enhance the cAMP signaling pathway. *Proceedings*

*of the National Academy of Sciences of the United States of America*, *96*, 5280–5285.

110. Hussain, T., Lokhandwala, M.F. (2003). Renal dopamine receptors and hypertension. *Experimental Biology and Medicine (Maywood)*, *228*, 134–142.
111. Jose, P.A., Eisner, G.M., Felder, R.A. (2003). Dopamine and the kidney: a role in hypertension? *Current Opinion in Nephrology and Hypertension*, *12*, 189–194.
112. Amenta, F., Ricci, A., Rossodivita, I., Avola, R., Tayebati, S.K. (2001). The dopaminergic system in hypertension. *Clinical and Experimental Hypertension*, *23*, 15–24.
113. Velasco, M., Contreras, F., Cabezas, G.A., Bolivar, A., Fouillioux, C., Hernandez, R. (2002). Dopaminergic receptors: a new antihypertensive mechanism. *Journal of Hypertension. Supplement*, *20*, S55–S58.
114. Zhuang, X., Belluscio, L., Hen, R. (2000). G(olf)alpha mediates dopamine D1 receptor signaling. *The Journal of Neuroscience*, *20*, RC91.
115. Corvol, J.C., Studler, J.M., Schonn, J.S., Girault, J.A., Herve, D. (2001). Galpha(olf) is necessary for coupling D1 and A2a receptors to adenylyl cyclase in the striatum. *Journal of Neurochemistry*, *76*, 1585–1588.
116. Wang, Q., Jolly, J.P., Surmeier, J.D., Mullah, B.M., Lidow, M.S., Bergson, C.M., Robishaw, J.D. (2001). Differential dependence of the D1 and D5 dopamine receptors on the G protein gamma 7 subunit for activation of adenylylcyclase. *The Journal of Biological Chemistry*, *276*, 39386–39393.
117. Neve, K.A., Seamans, J.K., Trantham-Davidson, H. (2004). Dopamine receptor signaling. *Journal of Receptor and Signal Transduction Research*, *24*, 165–205.
118. Mailman, R.B. (2007). GPCR functional selectivity has therapeutic impact. *Trends in Pharmacological Sciences*, *28*, 390–396.
119. Mailman, R., Huang, X., Nichols, D.E. (2001). Parkinson's disease and D1 dopamine receptors. *Current Opinion in Investigational Drugs*, *2*, 1582–1591.
120. Mailman, R.B., Huang, X. (2007). Dopamine receptor pharmacology. In: Koller, W.C., Melamed, E., eds. *Parkinson's Disease and Related Disorders, Part 1*. Edinburgh: Elsevier, pp. 77–105.
121. Zhang, J., Xiong, B., Zhen, X., Zhang, A. (2009). Dopamine D1 receptor ligands: where are we now and where are we going. *Medicinal Research Reviews*, *29*, 272–294.
122. Tumlin, J.A., Dunbar, L.M., Oparil, S., Buckalew, V., Ram, C.V., Mathur, V., Ellis, D., McGuire, D., Fellmann, J., Luther, R.R. (2000). Fenoldopam, a dopamine agonist, for hypertensive emergency: a multicenter randomized trial. Fenoldopam Study Group. *Academic Emergency Medicine*, *7*, 653–662.
123. Oparil, S., Aronson, S., Deeb, G.M., Epstein, M., Levy, J.H., Luther, R.R., Prielipp, R., Taylor, A. (1999). Fenoldopam: a new parenteral antihypertensive: consensus roundtable on the management of perioperative hypertension and hypertensive crises. *American Journal of Hypertension*, *12*, 653–664.
124. Poewe, W., Kleedorfer, B., Gerstenbrand, F., Oertel, W. (1988). Subcutaneous apomorphine in Parkinson's disease [letter]. *Lancet*, *1*, 943.
125. Goldstein, M., Lieberman, A., Lew, J.Y., Asano, T., Rosenfeld, M.R., Makman, M.H. (1980). Interaction of pergolide with central dopaminergic receptors. *Pro-*

*ceedings of the National Academy of Sciences of the United States of America*, *77*, 3725–3728.

126. Lovenberg, T.W., Brewster, W.K., Mottola, D.M., Lee, R.C., Riggs, R.M., Nichols, D.E., Lewis, M.H., Mailman, R.B. (1989). Dihydrexidine, a novel selective high potency full dopamine D-1 receptor agonist. *European Journal of Pharmacology*, *166*, 111–113.
127. Mottola, D.M., Brewster, W.K., Cook, L.L., Nichols, D.E., Mailman, R.B. (1992). Dihydrexidine, a novel full efficacy $D_1$ dopamine receptor agonist. *The Journal of Pharmacology and Experimental Therapeutics*, *262*, 383–393.
128. Blanchet, P.J., Fang, J., Gillespie, M., Sabounjian, L., Locke, K.W., Gammans, R., Mouradian, M.M., Chase, T.N. (1998). Effects of the full dopamine D1 receptor agonist dihydrexidine in Parkinson's disease. *Clinical Neuropharmacology*, *21*, 339–343.
129. George, M.S., Molnar, C.E., Grenesko, E.L., Anderson, B., Mu, Q., Johnson, K., Nahas, Z., Knable, M., Fernandes, P., Juncos, J., Huang, X., Nichols, D.E., Mailman, R.B. (2007). A single 20 mg dose of dihydrexidine (DAR-0100), a full dopamine D(1) agonist, is safe and tolerated in patients with schizophrenia. *Schizophrenia Research*, *93*, 42–50.
130. Mu, Q., Johnson, K., Morgan, P.S., Grenesko, E.L., Molnar, C.E., Anderson, B., Nahas, Z., Kozel, F.A., Kose, S., Knable, M., Fernandes, P., Nichols, D.E., Mailman, R.B., George, M.S. (2007). A single 20 mg dose of the full D(1) dopamine agonist dihydrexidine (DAR-0100) increases prefrontal perfusion in schizophrenia. *Schizophrenia Research*, *94*, 332–341.
131. Pendleton, R.G., Samler, L., Kaiser, C., Ridley, P.T. (1978). Studies on renal dopamine receptors with a new agonist. *European Journal of Pharmacology*, *51*, 19–28.
132. Setler, P.E., Sarau, H.M., Zirkle, C.L., Saunders, H.L. (1978). The central effects of a novel dopamine agonist. *European Journal of Pharmacology*, *50*, 419–430.
133. Close, S.P., Marriott, A.S., Pay, S. (1985). Failure of SKF 38393-A to relieve parkinsonian symptoms induced by 1- methyl-4-phenyl-1,2,3,6-tetrahydropyridine in the marmoset. *British Journal of Pharmacology*, *85*, 320–322.
134. Falardeau, P., Bouchard, S., Bedard, P.J., Boucher, R., Di Paolo, T. (1988). Behavioral and biochemical effect of chronic treatment with D-1 and/or D-2 dopamine agonists in MPTP monkeys. *European Journal of Pharmacology*, *150*, 59–66.
135. Nomoto, M., Jenner, P., Marsden, C.D. (1988). The $D_1$ agonist SKF 38393 inhibits the antiparkinsonian activity of the $D_2$ agonist LY 171555 in the MPTP-treated marmoset. *Neuroscience Letters*, *93*, 275–280.
136. Bedard, P.J., Boucher, R. (1989). Effect of D1 receptor stimulation in normal and MPTP monkeys. *Neuroscience Letters*, *104*, 223–228.
137. Boyce, S., Rupniak, N.M., Steventon, M.J., Iversen, S.D. (1990). Differential effects of $D_1$ and $D_2$ agonists in MPTP-treated primates: functional implications for Parkinson's disease. *Neurology*, *40*, 927–933.
138. Gomez-Mancilla, B., Bedard, P.J. (1991). Effect of D1 and D2 agonists and antagonists on dyskinesia produced by L-dopa in 1-methyl-4-phenyl-1,2,3,6-tetrahydropyridine-treated monkeys. *The Journal of Pharmacology and Experimental Therapeutics*, *259*, 409–413.

139. Elliott, P.J., Walsh, D.M., Close, S.P. (1992). Dopamine D1 and D2 receptor interactions in the MPTP-treated marmoset. *Neuroscience Letters*, *142*, 1–4.
140. Blanchet, P., Bedard, P.J., Britton, D.R., Kebabian, J.W. (1993). Differential effect of selective D-1 and D-2 dopamine receptor agonists on levodopa-induced dyskinesia in 1-methyl-4-phenyl-1,2,3,6-tetrahydropyridine- exposed monkeys. *The Journal of Pharmacology and Experimental Therapeutics*, *267*, 275–279.
141. Braun, A., Fabbrini, G., Mouradian, M.M., Serrati, C., Barone, P., Chase, T.N. (1987). Selective D-1 dopamine receptor agonist treatment of Parkinson's disease. *Journal of Neural Transmission*, *68*, 41–50.
142. Watts, V.J., Lawler, C.P., Gilmore, J.H., Southerland, S.B., Nichols, D.E., Mailman, R.B. (1993). Dopamine D1 receptors: efficacy of full (dihydrexidine) vs. partial (SKF38393) agonists in primates vs. rodents. *European Journal of Pharmacology*, *242*, 165–172.
143. Gilmore, J.H., Watts, V.J., Lawler, C.P., Noll, E.P., Nichols, D.E., Mailman, R.B. (1995). "Full" dopamine D1 agonists in human caudate: biochemical properties and therapeutic implications. *Neuropharmacology*, *34*, 481–488.
144. Watts, V.J., Lawler, C.P., Gonzales, A.J., Zhou, Q.Y., Civelli, O., Nichols, D.E., Mailman, R.B. (1995). Spare receptors and intrinsic activity: studies with D1 dopamine receptor agonists. *Synapse*, *21*, 177–187.
145. Iorio, L.C., Barnett, A., Billard, W., Gold, E.H. (1986). Benzazepines: structure-activity relationships between D1 receptor blockade and selected pharmacological effects. *Advances in Experimental Medicine and Biology*, *204*, 1–14.
146. Chipkin, R.E., Iorio, L.C., Coffin, V.L., McQuade, R.D., Berger, J.G., Barnett, A. (1988). Pharmacological profile of SCH39166: a dopamine D1 selective benzonaphthazepine with potential antipsychotic activity. *The Journal of Pharmacology and Experimental Therapeutics*, *247*, 1093–1102.
147. Nomoto, M., Fukuda, T. (1993). The effects of D1 and D2 dopamine receptor agonist and antagonist on parkinsonism in chronic MPTP-treated monkeys. *Advances in Neurology*, *60*, 119–122.
148. Domino, E.F., Sheng, J. (1993). Relative potency and efficacy of some dopamine agonists with varying selectivities for D1 and D2 receptors in MPTP-induced hemiparkinsonian monkeys. *The Journal of Pharmacology and Experimental Therapeutics*, *265*, 1387–1391.
149. Vermeulen, R.J., Drukarch, B., Sahadat, M.C., Goosen, C., Wolters, E.C., Stoof, J.C. (1994). The dopamine D1 agonist SKF 81297 and the dopamine D2 agonist LY 171555 act synergistically to stimulate motor behavior of 1-methyl-4-phenyl-1,2,3,6-tetrahydropyridine-lesioned parkinsonian rhesus monkeys. *Movement Disorders*, *9*, 664–672.
150. Vermeulen, R.J., Jongenelen, C.A., Langeveld, C.H., Wolters, E.C., Stoof, J.C., Drukarch, B. (1994). Dopamine D1 receptor agonists display a different intrinsic activity in rat, monkey and human astrocytes. *European Journal of Pharmacology*, *269*, 121–125.
151. Downes, R.P., Waddington, J.L. (1993). Grooming and vacuous chewing induced by SK&F 83959, an agonist of dopamine "D1-like" receptors that inhibits dopamine-sensitive adenylyl cyclase. *European Journal of Pharmacology*, *234*, 135–136.

152. Gnanalingham, K.K., Hunter, A.J., Jenner, P., Marsden, C.D. (1995). The differential behavioural effects of benzazepine $D_1$ dopamine agonists with varying efficacies, co-administered with quinpirole in primate and rodent models of Parkinson's disease. *Psychopharmacology (Berl)*, *117*, 287–297.

153. Truex, L.L., Foreman, M.M., Riggs, R.M., Nichols, D.E. (1985). Effects of modifications of the 4-(3,4-dihydroxyphenyl)-1,2,3,4-tetrahydroisoquinoline structure on dopamine sensitive rat retinal adenylate cyclase activity. *Society for Neuroscience Abstracts*, *11*, 315.

154. Andersen, P.H., Nielsen, E.B., Scheel-Kruger, J., Jansen, J.A., Hohlweg, R. (1987). Thienopyridine derivatives identified as the first selective, full efficacy, dopamine D1 receptor agonists. *European Journal of Pharmacology*, *137*, 291–292.

155. Tsui, J.K., Wolters, E.C., Peppard, R.F., Calne, D.B. (1989). A double-blind, placebo-controlled, dose-ranging study to investigate the safety and efficacy of CY 208-243 in patients with Parkinson's disease. *Neurology*, *39*, 856–858.

156. Temlett, J.A., Quinn, N.P., Jenner, P.G., Marsden, C.D., Pourcher, E., Bonnet, A.M., Agid, Y., Markstein, R., Lataste, X. (1989). Antiparkinsonian activity of CY 208-243, a partial D-1 dopamine receptor agonist, in MPTP-treated marmosets and patients with Parkinson's disease. *Movement Disorders*, *4*, 261–265.

157. Emre, M., Rinne, U.K., Rascol, A., Lees, A., Agid, Y., Lataste, X. (1992). Effects of a selective partial D1 agonist, CY 208-243, in de novo patients with Parkinson disease. *Movement Disorders*, *7*, 239–243.

158. Temlett, J.A., Chong, P.N., Oertel, W.H., Jenner, P., Marsden, C.D. (1988). The D-1 dopamine receptor partial agonist, CY 208-243, exhibits antiparkinsonian activity in the MPTP-treated marmoset. *European Journal of Pharmacology*, *156*, 197–206.

159. Gomez-Mancilla, B., Boucher, R., Gagnon, C., Di Paolo, T., Markstein, R., Bedard, P.J. (1993). Effect of adding the D1 agonist CY 208-243 to chronic bromocriptine treatment. I: evaluation of motor parameters in relation to striatal catecholamine content and dopamine receptors. *Movement Disorders*, *8*, 144–150.

160. Lovenberg, T.W., Roth, R.H., Nichols, D.E., Mailman, R.B. (1991). D1 dopamine receptors of NS20Y neuroblastoma cells are functionally similar to rat striatal D1 receptors. *Journal of Neurochemistry*, *57*, 1563–1569.

161. Brewster, W.K., Nichols, D.E., Riggs, R.M., Mottola, D.M., Lovenberg, T.W., Lewis, M.H., Mailman, R.B. (1990). trans-10,11-dihydroxy-5,6,6a,7,8,12b-hexahydrobenzo[a]phenanthridine: a highly potent selective dopamine D1 full agonist. *Journal of Medicinal Chemistry*, *33*, 1756–1764.

162. Kebabian, J.W., Briggs, C., Britton, D.R., Asin, K., DeNinno, M., MacKenzie, R.G., McKelvy, J.F., Schoenleber, R. (1990). A68930: a potent and specific agonist for the D-1 dopamine receptor. *American Journal of Hypertension*, *3*, 40S–42S.

163. Kebabian, J.W., Britton, D.R., DeNinno, M.P., Perner, R., Smith, L., Jenner, P., Schoenleber, R., Williams, M. (1992). A-77636: a potent and selective dopamine D1 receptor agonist with antiparkinsonian activity in marmosets. *European Journal of Pharmacology*, *229*, 203–209.

164. Pearce, R.K., Jackson, M., Smith, L., Jenner, P., Marsden, C.D. (1995). Chronic L-DOPA administration induces dyskinesias in the 1-methyl-4- phenyl-1,2,3,6-tetrahydropyridine-treated common marmoset (*Callithrix jacchus*). *Movement Disorders*, *10*, 731–740.

165. Asin, K.E., Wirtshafter, D. (1993). Effects of repeated dopamine $D_1$ receptor stimulation on rotation and c-fos expression. *European Journal of Pharmacology*, *235*, 167–168.

166. Britton, D.R., Kebabian, J.W., Curzon, P. (1991). Rapid reversal of denervation supersensitivity of dopamine D1 receptors by l-dopa or a novel dopamine D1 receptor agonist, A68930. *European Journal of Pharmacology*, *200*, 89–93.

167. Blanchet, P.J., Grondin, R., Bedard, P.J., Shiosaki, K., Britton, D.R. (1996). Dopamine $D_1$ receptor desensitization profile in MPTP-lesioned primates. *European Journal of Pharmacology*, *309*, 13–20.

168. DeNinno, M.P., Schoenleber, R., MacKenzie, R., Britton, D.R., Asin, K.E., Briggs, C., Trugman, J.M., Ackerman, M., Artman, L., Bednarz, L. (1991). A68930: a potent agonist selective for the dopamine D1 receptor. *European Journal of Pharmacology*, *199*, 209–219.

169. Mottola, D.M., Laiter, S., Watts, V.J., Tropsha, A., Wyrick, S.D., Nichols, D.E., Mailman, R.B. (1996). Conformational analysis of D1 dopamine receptor agonists: pharmacophore assessment and receptor mapping. *Journal of Medicinal Chemistry*, *39*, 285–296.

170. Michaelides, M.R., Hong, Y., DiDomenico, S.J., Asin, K.E., Britton, D.R., Lin, C.W., Williams, M., Shiosaki, K. (1995). (5aR,11bS)-4,5,5a,6,7,11b-hexahydro-2-propyl-3-thia-5-azacyclopent-1- ena[c]-phenanthrene-9,10-diol (A-86929): a potent and selective dopamine D1 agonist that maintains behavioral efficacy following repeated administration and characterization of its diacetyl prodrug (ABT-431). *Journal of Medicinal Chemistry*, *38*, 3445–3447.

171. Shiosaki, K., Jenner, P., Asin, K.E., Britton, D.R., Lin, C.W., Michaelides, M., Smith, L., Bianchi, B., Didomenico, S., Hodges, L., Hong, Y., Mahan, L., Mikusa, J., Miller, T., Nikkel, A., Stashko, M., Witte, D., Williams, M. (1996). ABT-431: the diacetyl prodrug of A-86929, a potent and selective dopamine $D_1$ receptor agonist: in vitro characterization and effects in animal models of Parkinson's disease. *The Journal of Pharmacology and Experimental Therapeutics*, *276*, 150–160.

172. Pearce, R.K., Jackson, M., Britton, D.R., Shiosaki, K., Jenner, P., Marsden, C.D. (1999). Actions of the $D_1$ agonists A-77636 and A-86929 on locomotion and dyskinesia in MPTP-treated L-dopa-primed common marmosets. *Psychopharmacology (Berl)*, *142*, 51–60.

173. Self, D.W., Karanian, D.A., Spencer, J.J. (2000). Effects of the novel D1 dopamine receptor agonist ABT-431 on cocaine self-administration and reinstatement. *Annals of the New York Academy of Sciences*, *909*, 133–144.

174. Haney, M., Collins, E.D., Ward, A.S., Foltin, R.W., Fischman, M.W. (1999). Effect of a selective dopamine D1 agonist (ABT-431) on smoked cocaine self-administration in humans. *Psychopharmacology (Berl)*, *143*, 102–110.

175. Ghosh, D., Snyder, S.E., Watts, V.J., Mailman, R.B., Nichols, D.E. (1996). 9-Dihydroxy-2,3,7,11b-tetrahydro-1H-naph[1,2,3-de]isoquinoline: a potent full dopamine D1 agonist containing a rigid-beta-phenyldopamine pharmacophore. *Journal of Medicinal Chemistry*, *39*, 549–555.

176. Gulwadi, A.G., Korpinen, C.D., Mailman, R.B., Nichols, D.E., Sit, S.Y., Taber, M.T. (2001). Dinapsoline: characterization of a $D_1$ dopamine receptor agonist in a rat

model of Parkinson's disease. *The Journal of Pharmacology and Experimental Therapeutics*, *296*, 338–344.

177. Lewis, M.M., Watts, V.J., Lawler, C.P., Nichols, D.E., Mailman, R.B. (1998). Homologous desensitization of the D1A dopamine receptor: efficacy in causing desensitization dissociates from both receptor occupancy and functional potency. *The Journal of Pharmacology and Experimental Therapeutics*, *286*, 345–353.

178. Gay, E.A., Urban, J.D., Nichols, D.E., Oxford, G.S., Mailman, R.B. (2004). Functional selectivity of D2 receptor ligands in a Chinese hamster ovary hD2L cell line: evidence for induction of ligand-specific receptor states. *Molecular Pharmacology*, *66*, 97–105.

179. Murthy, V., Gowdahalli, K., Blake, D., Jr, Sg, A., Mailman, R.B. (2009) EFF0311, a longer-acting full $D_1$ dopamine receptor agonist with novel properties suggesting potential in vivo uses. 2009 Neuroscience Meeting Planner Online. Program No. 628.12/I38.

180. Ryman-Rasmussen, J.P., Griffith, A., Oloff, S., Vaidehi, N., Brown, J.T., Goddard, W.A., III, Mailman, R.B. (2007). Functional selectivity of dopamine D(1) receptor agonists in regulating the fate of internalized receptors. *Neuropharmacology*, *52*, 562–575.

181. Lin, C.W., Bianchi, B.R., Miller, T.R., Stashko, M.A., Wang, S.S., Curzon, P., Bednarz, L., Asin, K.E., Britton, D.R. (1996). Persistent activation of the dopamine $D_1$ receptor contributes to prolonged receptor desensitization: studies with A-77636. *The Journal of Pharmacology and Experimental Therapeutics*, *276*, 1022–1029.

182. Mailman, R.B., Murthy, V. (2010). Ligand functional selectivity advances our understanding of drug mechanisms and drug discovery. *Neuropsychopharmacology*, *35*, 345–346.

183. Mailman, R.B., Wang, Y.-M., Kant, A., Brown, J.T. (2009). Functional selectivity of dopamine receptors. In: Neve, K.A., ed. *Functional Selectivity of G Protein-Coupled Receptor Ligands*. New York: Humana, pp. 177–209.

184. Mailman, R.B., Murthy, V. (2009). Third generation antipsychotic drugs: partial agonism or receptor functional selectivity? *Current Pharmaceutical Design*, *16*, 488–501.

185. Urban, J.D., Clarke, W.P., von Zastrow, M., Nichols, D.E., Kobilka, B., Weinstein, H., Javitch, J.A., Roth, B.L., Christopoulos, A., Sexton, P.M., Miller, K.J., Spedding, M., Mailman, R.B. (2007). Functional selectivity and classical concepts of quantitative pharmacology. *The Journal of Pharmacology and Experimental Therapeutics*, *320*, 1–13.

186. Zhang, L., Bai, J., Undie, A.S., Bergson, C., Lidow, M.S. (2005). D1 dopamine receptor regulation of the levels of the cell-cycle-controlling proteins, cyclin D, P27 and Raf-1, in cerebral cortical precursor cells is mediated through cAMP-independent pathways. *Cerebral Cortex*, *15*, 74–84.

187. Panchalingam, S., Undie, A.S. (2001). SKF83959 exhibits biochemical agonism by stimulating [(35)S]GTP gamma S binding and phosphoinositide hydrolysis in rat and monkey brain. *Neuropharmacology*, *40*, 826–837.

188. Undie, A.S., Friedman, E. (1990). Stimulation of a dopamine $D_1$ receptor enhances inositol phosphates formation in rat brain. *The Journal of Pharmacology and Experimental Therapeutics*, *253*, 987–992.

189. Amenta, F., Ferrante, F., Ricci, A. (1995). Pharmacological characterisation and autoradiographic localisation of dopamine receptor subtypes in the cardiovascular system and in the kidney. *Hypertension Research*, *18*(Suppl 1), S23–S27.
190. Starr, M.S. (1996). The role of dopamine in epilepsy. *Synapse*, *22*, 159–194.
191. Johnson, K.B., Criswell, H.E., Jensen, K.F., Simson, P.E., Mueller, R.A., Breese, G.R. (1992). Comparison of the D1-dopamine agonists SKF-38393 and A-68930 in neonatal 6-hydroxydopamine-lesioned rats: behavioral effects and induction of c-fos-like immunoreactivity. *The Journal of Pharmacology and Experimental Therapeutics*, *262*, 855–865.
192. Al-Tajir, G., Chandler, C.J., Starr, B.S., Starr, M.S. (1990). Opposite effects of stimulation of D1 and D2 dopamine receptors on the expression of motor seizures in mouse and rat. *Neuropharmacology*, *29*, 657–661.
193. Darney, K.J., Jr, Lewis, M.H., Brewster, W.K., Nichols, D.E., Mailman, R.B. (1991). Behavioral effects in the rat of dihydrexidine, a high-potency, full-efficacy D1 dopamine receptor agonist. *Neuropsychopharmacology*, *5*, 187–195.
194. Roth, B.L., Chuang, D.M. (1987). Multiple mechanisms of serotonergic signal transduction. *Life Sciences*, *41*, 1051–1064.
195. Kenakin, T. (1995). Pharmacological proteus? *Trends in Pharmacological Sciences*, *16*, 256–258.
196. Mailman, R.B., Nichols, D.E., Lewis, M.M., Blake, B.L., Lawler, C.P. (1998). Functional effects of novel dopamine ligands: dihydrexidine and Parkinson's disease as a first step. In: Jenner, P., Demirdemar, R., eds. *Dopamine Receptor Subtypes: From Basic Science to Clinical Application*. Amsterdam: IOS Stockton Press, pp. 64–83.
197. Mailman, R.B., Nichols, D.E., Tropsha, A. (1997). Molecular drug design and dopamine receptors. In: Neve, K.A., Neve, R.L., eds. *The Dopamine Receptors*. Totowa, NJ: Humana Press, pp. 105–133.
198. Clarke, W.P., Bond, R.A. (1998). The elusive nature of intrinsic efficacy. *Trends in Pharmacological Sciences*, *19*, 270–276.
199. Ghanouni, P., Gryczynski, Z., Steenhuis, J.J., Lee, T.W., Farrens, D.L., Lakowicz, J.R., Kobilka, B.K. (2001). Functionally different agonists induce distinct conformations in the G protein coupling domain of the beta 2 adrenergic receptor. *The Journal of Biological Chemistry*, *276*, 24433–24436.
200. Gonzalez-Maeso, J., Yuen, T., Ebersole, B.J., Wurmbach, E., Lira, A., Zhou, M., Weisstaub, N., Hen, R., Gingrich, J.A., Sealfon, S.C. (2003). Transcriptome fingerprints distinguish hallucinogenic and nonhallucinogenic 5-hydroxytryptamine 2A receptor agonist effects in mouse somatosensory cortex. *The Journal of Neuroscience*, *23*, 8836–8843.
201. Mottola, D.M., Kilts, J.D., Lewis, M.M., Connery, H.S., Walker, Q.D., Jones, S.R., Booth, R.G., Hyslop, D.K., Piercey, M., Wightman, R.M., Lawler, C.P., Nichols, D.E., Mailman, R.B. (2002). Functional selectivity of dopamine receptor agonists. I. Selective activation of postsynaptic dopamine D2 receptors linked to adenylate cyclase. *The Journal of Pharmacology and Experimental Therapeutics*, *301*, 1166–1178.
202. Ryman-Rasmussen, J.P., Nichols, D.E., Mailman, R.B. (2005). Differential activation of adenylate cyclase and receptor internalization by novel dopamine D1 receptor agonists. *Molecular Pharmacology*, *68*, 1039–1048.

203. Baufreton, J., Garret, M., Rivera, A., De La, C.A., Gonon, F., Dufy, B., Bioulac, B., Taupignon, A. (2003). D5 (not D1) dopamine receptors potentiate burst-firing in neurons of the subthalamic nucleus by modulating an L-type calcium conductance. *The Journal of Neuroscience*, *23*, 816–825.

204. Pei, L., Lee, F.J., Moszczynska, A., Vukusic, B., Liu, F. (2004). Regulation of dopamine D1 receptor function by physical interaction with the NMDA receptors. *The Journal of Neuroscience*, *24*, 1149–1158.

205. Gines, S., Hillion, J., Torvinen, M., Le Crom, S., Casado, V., Canela, E.I., Rondin, S., Lew, J.Y., Watson, S., Zoli, M., Agnati, L.F., Verniera, P., Lluis, C., Ferre, S., Fuxe, K., Franco, R. (2000). Dopamine D1 and adenosine A1 receptors form functionally interacting heteromeric complexes. *Proceedings of the National Academy of Sciences of the United States of America*, *97*, 8606–8611.

206. Liu, F., Wan, Q., Pristupa, Z.B., Yu, X.M., Wang, Y.T., Niznik, H.B. (2000). Direct protein-protein coupling enables cross-talk between dopamine D5 and gamma-aminobutyric acid A receptors. *Nature*, *403*, 274–280.

207. Deutch, A.Y., Clark, W.A., Roth, R.H. (1990). Prefrontal cortical dopamine depletion enhances the responsiveness of mesolimbic dopamine neurons to stress. *Brain Research*, *521*, 311–315.

208. Wilkinson, L.S. (1997). The nature of interactions involving prefrontal and striatal dopamine systems. *Journal of Psychopharmacology*, *11*, 143–150.

209. Weinberger, D.R. (1987). Implications of normal brain development for the pathogenesis of schizophrenia. *Archives of General Psychiatry*, *44*, 660–669.

210. Kipnis, J., Cardon, M., Avidan, H., Lewitus, G.M., Mordechay, S., Rolls, A., Shani, Y., Schwartz, M. (2004). Dopamine, through the extracellular signal-regulated kinase pathway, downregulates CD4+CD25+ regulatory T-cell activity: implications for neurodegeneration. *The Journal of Neuroscience*, *24*, 6133–6143.

211. Yu, Y., Wang, J.R., Sun, P.H., Guo, Y., Zhang, Z.J., Jin, G.Z., Zhen, X. (2008). Neuroprotective effects of atypical D1 receptor agonist SKF83959 are mediated via D1 receptor-dependent inhibition of glycogen synthase kinase-3 beta and a receptor-independent anti-oxidative action. *Journal of Neurochemistry*, *104*, 946–956.

212. Lee, F.J., Xue, S., Pei, L., Vukusic, B., Chery, N., Wang, Y., Wang, Y.T., Niznik, H.B., Yu, X.M., Liu, F. (2002). Dual regulation of NMDA receptor functions by direct protein-protein interactions with the dopamine D1 receptor. *Cell*, *111*, 219–230.

213. Guo, H., Tang, Z., Yu, Y., Xu, L., Jin, G., Zhou, J. (2002). Apomorphine induces trophic factors that support fetal rat mesencephalic dopaminergic neurons in cultures. *The European Journal of Neuroscience*, *16*, 1861–1870.

214. Grunblatt, E., Mandel, S., Maor, G., Youdim, M.B. (2001). Effects of R- and S-apomorphine on MPTP-induced nigro-striatal dopamine neuronal loss. *Journal of Neurochemistry*, *77*, 146–156.

215. Xu, M., Moratalla, R., Gold, L.H., Hiroi, N., Koob, G.F., Graybiel, A.M., Tonegawa, S. (1994). Dopamine D1 receptor mutant mice are deficient in striatal expression of dynorphin and in dopamine-mediated behavioral responses. *Cell*, *79*, 729–742.

216. Misener, V.L., Luca, P., Azeke, O., Crosbie, J., Waldman, I., Tannock, R., Roberts, W., Malone, M., Schachar, R., Ickowicz, A., Kennedy, J.L., Barr, C.L. (2004).

Linkage of the dopamine receptor D1 gene to attention-deficit/hyperactivity disorder. *Molecular Psychiatry*, *9*, 500–509.

217. Isacson, R., Kull, B., Wahlestedt, C., Salmi, P. (2004). A 68930 and dihydrexidine inhibit locomotor activity and d-amphetamine-induced hyperactivity in rats: a role of inhibitory dopamine D(1/5) receptors in the prefrontal cortex? *Neuroscience*, *124*, 33–42.
218. Self, D.W., Barnhart, W.J., Lehman, D.A., Nestler, E.J. (1996). Opposite modulation of cocaine-seeking behavior by D1- and D2-like dopamine receptor agonists. *Science*, *271*, 1586–1589.

# 4

# PHOSPHODIESTERASE INHIBITORS AS A NOVEL THERAPEUTIC APPROACH FOR SCHIZOPHRENIA

Judith A. Siuciak and William J. Pitts

## 4.1 INTRODUCTION: THE PHOSPHODIESTERASE (PDE) FAMILY

The PDEs are enzymes that regulate intracellular signaling through the metabolic inactivation of the cyclic nucleotides cyclic adenosine monosphosphate (cAMP) and cyclic guanosine monophosphate (cGMP), a function that serves to regulate and compartmentalize the cyclic nucleotide signaling cascades. In mammals, the PDEs comprise a superfamily of enzymes composed of 21 genes, which are divided into 11 families (PDE1–PDE11). Each family has one to four subtypes, which are products of distinct genes with multiple splice variants generated from each gene. To date, over 50 unique isoforms have been described (for reviews see References [1, 2]). These family members possess characteristic enzymatic properties as well as distinct tissue, cellular, and subcellular localization throughout the organism.

A distinctive C-terminal catalytic domain with an overall amino acid sequence identity ranging from 25% to 52% and an invariant 14 amino acid signature motif is characteristic of all mammalian PDEs. In many instances, the N-terminal domain, which shows more variability among and between families, is involved in regulating enzyme activity. Importantly, it has been possible to generate inhibitors that selectively regulate cyclic nucleotide signaling through pharmacological manipulation of a specific PDE, despite the

*Targets and Emerging Therapies for Schizophrenia*, First Edition.
Edited by Jeffrey S. Albert and Michael W. Wood.

highly conserved amino acid residues within the enzyme active site. Unique therapeutic agents have been generated using this approach with considerable promise for future opportunities.

## 4.2 PDE4 FAMILY

The PDE4 family members (PDE4A, PDE4B, PDE4C, and PDE4D) are encoded by four separate genes and share a high degree of homology with the PDE encoded by the *Drosophila melanogaster* dunce gene [3, 4]. All four family members have specificity for cyclic adenosine monophosphate (cAMP) as a substrate [5, 6]. Multiple splice variants with distinct localization and functions result from alternative splicing of PDE4 [5, 6]. Thus, the expression of distinct PDE4 splice variants may play an important functional role in controlling cAMP signaling within different cell types.

There is widespread expression of PDE4A, PDE4B, and PDE4D throughout the brain although the different subtypes show distinct regional and intracellular distribution suggesting that they may subserve at least some unique functional roles. In contrast, only minimal central nervous system (CNS) expression of PDE4C is seen, particularly in the rodent [7–11]. The key brain areas of PDE4A expression are the olfactory nucleus, cerebral cortex, and corticospinal tracts [11]. PDE4B localization has been characterized in a variety of species [10, 11]. High levels of PDE4B mRNA and protein are found in rat basal ganglia and associated areas (striatum, nucleus accumbens, globus pallidus, and substantia nigra), brain areas implicated in neuropsychiatric disorders such as schizophrenia (for review see Reference [12]). PDE4D was found in the cerebellum and in multiple forebrain regions in the rat, including cerebral cortex and hippocampus [7, 11], brain regions involved in affect and cognition, and in the actions of antidepressant drugs. In the hippocampus, an area important for learning and memory, an overlapping expression of the PDE4 isozymes has been observed [10, 13]. In several species (human, monkey, and rat), PDE4B mRNA is the most abundant PDE4 subtype in the striatum [10], a site of action for both the therapeutic efficacy and side effects of antipsychotics. In contrast, moderate or minimal levels of PDE4A and PDE4D mRNA expression, respectively, are found in this area.

### 4.2.1 Medicinal Chemistry of PDE4

Medicinal chemists have focused their attention on preparing inhibitors of PDE4 for several decades (for an example of an early reference see Reference [14]). Enzyme preparations were initially obtained from brain tissue; thus, it was natural to examine CNS applications as a therapeutic focus for PDE4 inhibitors from the earliest days. One of the most widely studied PDE inhibitors [15–18] is rolipram ([±]-4-[3-cyclopentyloxy-4-methoxyphenyl]-2-pyrrolidone), which nonselectively inhibits all PDE4 subtypes (see Fig. 4.1)

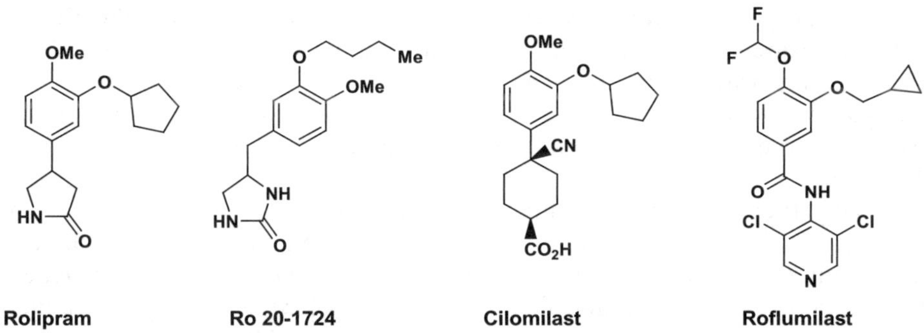


**FIGURE 4.1** Prototypical PDE4 inhibitors.

[19, 20]. Rolipram was examined clinically for the treatment of depression where it initially appeared to be similar in efficacy to the tricyclic antidepressant imipramine [21, 22]. Further progress was hampered by dose-limiting side effects including nausea and emesis [23–25]. Significant advances have been made with respect to the understanding of the structural basis of existing inhibitors; however, medicinal chemistry efforts aimed at decreasing the side effects of early inhibitors have remained a challenge to date.

### 4.2.2 PDE4 and Emesis

Nausea and emesis are complex physiologic processes with both CNS and peripheral components. There is no universally accepted and clinically validated *in vitro* assay that could guide the medicinal chemist to choose PDE4 inhibitors with significantly decreased emetic potential. However, there are several *in vitro* assays in common use.

An early hypothesis used by medicinal chemists for designing non-emetic PDE4 inhibitors was related to the discovery of a high-affinity rolipram binding site (HARBS, associated with gastric acid secretion [26]) and a low-affinity rolipram binding site (LARBS, initially associated with catalytic activity and associated with anti-inflammatory effects [27]). As a result chemists sought compounds that did not bind potently to the HARBS site. Subsequently, differential rolipram binding to PDE4 was shown to result from the presence or absence of $Mg^{2+}$ (HARBS = haloenzyme—i.e., active form with $Mg^{2+}$ bound to enzyme, and LARBS = apoenzyme, no $Mg^{2+}$ bound to enzyme) [28]. Although both forms of the enzyme are capable of binding cAMP with different affinities, it is important to note that only the haloenzyme is capable of hydrolyzing cAMP. Inhibitors that bind to both forms of the enzyme have been identified. Recent reports have linked HARBS activity to PDE4 activity in cortical neurons [29], and antidepressant activity [30]. HARBS activity has also been correlated to an animal model of emesis [31]. To date, no PDE4 inhibitors with high selectivity for LARBS have been examined in the clinic.

Another possible approach to limit emesis is to target specific PDE4 subtypes (discussed later) that might be responsible for this side effect. Experiments with PDE4D-deficient mice have suggested that this PDE4 subtype is associated with emesis [20]. As a result, significant effort is being expended to design PDE4B inhibitors with some degree of selectivity against PDE4D.

Finally, there have been a number of animal models that have been used to help delineate the emetic potential of PDE4 inhibitors prior to clinical development. These include models in dog [32], ferret [33], squirrel monkey [34] (Lamontagne et al.), and house musk shrew [35]. Rodent pica feeding has also been used as a surrogate for rodent emesis [36, 37]. These models are generally lower throughput and permit evaluation only with select compounds.

### 4.2.3 Prototypical PDE4 Inhibitors

Ro 20-1724, cilomilast, and roflumilast are second-generation PDE4 inhibitors that are structurally related to the first-generation inhibitor rolipram. Cilomilast and roflumilast have been evaluated extensively in clinical trials for the treatment of both asthma and chronic obstructive pulmonary disease (COPD) [38, 39]. Despite extensive studies, neither compound has been launched as a marketed drug, and their ultimate place in therapy remains uncertain [40]. In clinical studies, cilomilast was well tolerated at doses up to 15 mg BID (some level of efficacy observed in asthma and COPD trials) but not tolerated at a dose of 20 mg BID (nausea and emesis). The narrow therapeutic index for cilomilast has clearly hampered efforts to understand the potential benefit of PDE4 inhibition for these diseases indications, and, although to perhaps a lesser extent, a similar assessment could be extended to roflumilast and some compounds in earlier stages of development [41].

### 4.2.4 Structural Based Drug Design

The identification of subtype selective PDE4 inhibitors largely remains an unsolved problem. Comparison of the crystal structure active sites of PDE4B and PDE4D in complex with several inhibitors demonstrate a high degree of structural similarity [42] (Card et al.). This high degree of similarity between the active sites is consistent with the paucity of compounds that display a greater than 10-fold difference between reported $IC_{50}$'s for these two PDE4 subtypes. An inhibitor class that has produced examples having up to a 64-fold selectivity for PDE4D over PDE4B has been described [43]. Examination of the crystal structure of NVP (4-[8-[3-nitrophenyl]1,7-naphthryridin-6-yl] benzoic acid) co-crystallized in the active sites of PDE4B and PDE4D revealed that there is little difference between the two enzymes, with the exception of a conformational difference in a conserved methionine residue (see Fig. 4.2) [44]. It remains to be seen if these subtle structural differences between

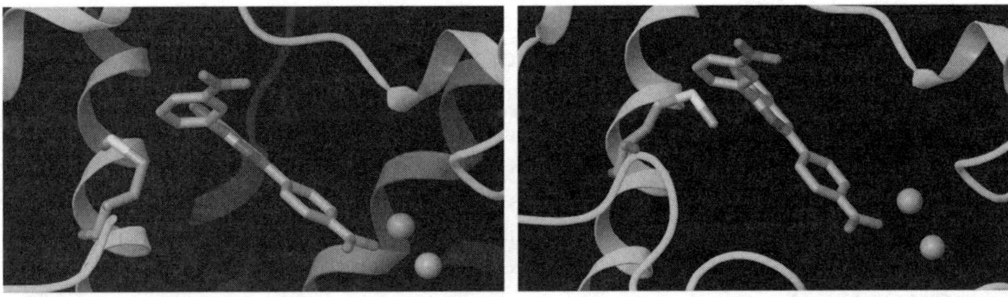

**FIGURE 4.2** NVP (4-(8-(3-nitrophenyl)1,7-naphthryridin-6-yl)benzoic acid) co-crystallized in the active site of PDE4B (left, PDB ID 2QYL) and PDE4D (right, PDB ID 2QYN). Notice the small conformational difference in the conserved methionine residue between structures. Key: carbon—gray, nitrogen—blue, oxygen—red, sulfur—yellow, zinc (left) orange, magnesium (right) orange. The protein backbone is represented by a blue ribbon. Some residues have been removed for clarity. (See color insert.)

PDE4B and PDE4D can be exploited to rationally design selective PDE4B inhibitors.

A number of groups continue to work in the area in the hopes of identifying non-emetic PDE4 inhibitors. The lack of subtype selective inhibitors has also been a major limitation within the PDE4 field. As a result, increased attention has been placed on targeting selective inhibition of PDE4 subtypes, particularly PDE4B. New models of emesis and new structural information will help medicinal chemists design the next generation of PDE4 inhibitors.

### 4.2.5 PDE4 Knockout Mice

Recently, genetically modified mice in which the genes encoding a specific PDE4 subtype have been selectively ablated have become available [45–47]. These mice provide complementary information to behavioral studies using pharmacological agents and have enabled studies exploring the central role of specific PDE4 subtypes. The various PDE4 knockout mice are constitutive knockouts and therefore the observed phenotype represents the neurodevelopmental deletion of the gene. Although little work has been done characterizing the PDE4A knockout mouse, PDE4B and PDE4D knockout mice have been studied in a variety of paradigms and show interesting CNS-related phenotypes [48–52].

PDE4B knockout mice have been characterized on two different genetic backgrounds using a battery of behavioral and neurochemical tests (see Table 4.1). PDE4B knockout mice consistently appeared to be viable, fertile, and possess no obvious impairments that might interfere with behavioral assessment. PDE4B knockout mice on the C57BL/6N background demonstrated changes in tests associated with schizophrenia (disrupted prepulse inhibition

[PPI]) and modulation of dopaminergic activity (enhanced amphetamine-induced locomotion, altered striatal dopamine levels), indicative of an pro-psychotic-like profile [48]. Interestingly, an anxiogenic-like behavioral phenotype was reported in mice on a C57/129 background [51]. Regardless of background strain, wild-type and knockout mice responded similarly in cognition models (passive avoidance, Morris water maze) [48, 51]. Since these two reports differ both with regard to genetic background and animal models used, additional studies are needed to fully understand the behavioral phenotype of the PDE4B knockout mouse.

Only limited phenotypic characterization of the PDE4D knockout mice has been performed to date (see Table 4.1). Decreased immobility in both the forced swim and tail suspension tests was indicative of an antidepressant-like phenotype in the PDE4D knockout mice [50]. In contrast, PDE4D knockout mice did not show alterations in an anxiety test as measured using the elevated plus maze [50].

### 4.2.6 PDE4 and Schizophrenia

Recent genetic studies have suggested a role for PDE4B in schizophrenia. The PDE4B gene is located at 1p31, a susceptibility region for schizophrenia [53–55]. Translocation in the PDE4B gene has been reported in two related patients with schizophrenia in Scotland [56]. Several single nucleotide polymorphisms (SNPs) in PDE4B have been recently associated with an altered genetic risk of schizophrenia in various populations [57–59]. In addition, PDE4B has been shown to bind with DISC1 (Disrupted-in-Schizophrenia 1) [56], a genetic susceptibility factor for schizophrenia (for review see [60, 61]). Two strains of DISC1 mutant mice with reduced binding to PDE4B displaying either schizophrenia-like or depression-like symptoms have been reported [62].

The behavioral profile of PDE4 inhibitors such as rolipram in preclinical animal models provides compelling data supporting the use of these compounds in schizophrenia. Rolipram demonstrated robust antipsychotic-like effects in a range of rodent animal models, in that it antagonized phencyclidine (PCP) and D-amphetamine-induced hyperactivity [49], decreased methamphetamine-induced hyperlocomotion [63], and reversed MK-801-induced deficits in latent inhibition [64].

Both rolipram and RO-20-1724 (4-[3-butoxy-4-methoxybenzyl]-2-imidazolidinone) reversed an amphetamine-disrupted auditory sensory processing [65–67]. However, inconsistent effects of these same PDE4 inhibitors have been reported in animal models of sensorimotor gating. While rolipram was reported to attenuate an amphetamine-induced deficit in PPI [66, 67], this effect was not replicated with RO-20-1724 (4-[3-butoxy-4-methoxybenzyl]-2-imidazolidinone) [65].

Rolipram suppressed conditioned avoidance responding (CAR) in rats and mice [49, 68], a model that is widely used to identify potential antipsychotic activity [69, 70]. All clinically active antipsychotic agents have shown efficacy

**TABLE 4.1 Comparison of Studies Assessing Phenotype of PDE10A Knockout Mice**

| PDE10A Knockout (KO) versus Wild-Type Mice | Siuciak et al., 2006a,b [124, 136] | Siuciak et al., 2008 [125] | Sano et al. [126] |
|---|---|---|---|
| Background strain | DBA1LacJ | C57/BL6N | C57/BL/6 |
| Gender | Male and female | Male | Not reported |
| Body weight | Decrease in female KO mice | Not reported | No change |
| Motor coordination: rotorod | ND | ND | No change |
| Baseline locomotor activity | Decrease | Decrease | Trend ($P < 0.06$) for decrease |
| Response to amphetamine/methamphetamine | No change | Increase | ND |
| Response to PCP/MK-801 | Decrease—PCP, MK-801 | Decrease—MK-801<br>No change—PCP | ND |
| CAR acquisition/response to antipsychotics | Delayed acquisition, no change in response to haloperidol or clozapine | Delayed acquisition | ND |
| Prepulse inhibition | ND | ND | ND |
| Cognition tests: Passive avoidance or Morris water maze (MWM), fear conditioning | No change—passive avoidance<br>Delayed acquisition—MWM | No change—passive avoidance | No change—fear conditioning |
| Depression tests: Forced swim test | No change | No change | No change |
| Anxiety tests: Elevated plus maze (EPM), light/dark (L/D), social interaction | No change—EPM | No change—EPM | Increased social interaction, no change—EPM and L/D |
| Analgesia tests: Hot plate | No change | No change | No change |
| Striatal cGMP, cAMP, pCREB | No change cGMP, cAMP, pCREB | No change cGMP, cAMP, pCREB | Increase in pCREB/CREB ratio and cAMP, no change—cGMP |
| Striatal turnover of dopamine, serotonin | No change | Increased—dopamine turnover | ND |

ND, not determined.

in this model, and it has been suggested that suppression of CAR is a measure of the ability of a compound to reduce stimulus salience [69]. These studies offered the first insight into the role of the various PDE4 subtypes in antipsychotic-like effects of rolipram. While rolipram administration dose-dependently suppressed CAR in wild-type mice, a decreased sensitivity was observed in PDE4B knockout mice [49]. The reduced effect of rolipram in PDE4B knockout mice was not due to a generalized impaired response to antipsychotics since the response to clozapine was not different from that of wild-type mice. In contrast, the effects of both rolipram and clozapine on CAR were not altered in PDE4D knockout mice [71]. These data suggest that the antipsychotic-like activity of rolipram in the CAR model involves, at least in part, PDE4B, but not PDE4D.

PDE4B knockout mice showed "pro-psychotic-like" phenotype (disrupted PPI, enhanced amphetamine-induced locomotion), data that appear to be at odds with the preclinical animal model data obtained using PDE4 inhibitors such as rolipram. This discrepancy may be related to several factors, as described previously [48]. First, activity at other subtypes may play a role in the actions of rolipram, as it is not selective for PDE4B. Second, relative to acute inhibition of the enzyme produced by PDE4 inhibitors, PDE4B knockout mice represent a chronic loss of the enzyme that may result in compensatory mechanisms involving genes other than the targeted one that can contribute to alterations in phenotype.

Only a single study has attempted to assess the effects of chronic antipsychotic treatment on PDE4 subtype expression [72]. In the striatum, chronic administration of clozapine, but not haloperidol, upregulated PDE4B expression, while neither treatment altered the expression of striatal PDE4A.

A therapeutic window for PDE4 inhibitors with regard to antipsychotic versus motor side effects was suggested by separation between activity in efficacy and side effect liability models such as spontaneous locomotor activity and catalepsy [49, 65]. In rats, rolipram administration produced only a modest, although statistically significant, degree of catalepsy at the highest dose tested (3.2 mg/kg, administered subcutaneously).

A core abnormality that occurs in schizophrenia is disruption of cognition [73], and the degree of cognitive impairment is the best predictor of long-term outcome [74]. Individuals with schizophrenia often experience a range of cognitive deficits including attentional and working memory impairments. Across a range of behavioral models in mice, rats, and monkeys, there is extensive evidence supporting a role for PDE4 in learning and memory (for reviews see References [75, 76]), although the PDE4 subtype mediating these effects is not yet clear. Rolipram showed pro-cognitive effects in a range of animal models including object recognition [77–80], passive avoidance [81–84], radial arm maze [81, 85, 86], Morris water maze [82, 87], contextual fear conditioning [87–89], and set-shift [90]. PDE4 inhibition has been shown to ameliorate N-methyl-D-aspartate (NMDA) antagonist-induced deficits in cognition, a finding of particular relevance to schizophrenia. Contemporary theories of schizophrenia postulate the presence of hypoactive glutamatergic pathways that may be particularly relevant to cognitive deficits and negative symptoms. Pharmacological agents that induce hypoglutamatergia, such as ketamine, MK-801, and PCP, are used as pharmacological tools to model these symptoms in animals. Rolipram reversed the MK-801-induced disruption in cognition as measured in either the radial arm maze or passive avoidance [84, 86]. Furthermore, rolipram administration attenuates the attentional set-shifting deficits induced by subchronic PCP administration [90], which produces long-lasting cognitive deficits and neurochemical changes similar to those in individuals with schizophrenia [91].

Numerous studies have evaluated the role of PDE4 in depression (for reviews see References [92, 93]). In several preclinical animal models, rolipram has an antidepressant-like profile in both mice [17, 50, 94] and rats [95–98]. Studies assessing the specific subtype involved in mediating these antidepressant-like effects have given rise to conflicting results. Repeated treatment with the antidepressants desipramine and fluoxetine increased the expression of PDE4A and PDE4B but not PDE4D subtypes in rat brain [99–101]. The results suggested that PDE4A/B subtypes are involved in signal transduction pathways in rat brain that are affected by antidepressant treatments. In contrast, chronic administration of desipramine, fluoxetine, or rolipram increased PDE4D immunoreactivity in the mouse brain, and PDE4A and PDE4B expression was regulated differently depending on drug treatment or the brain region examined [99]. Thus, additional studies are needed to clarify the reasons for these species differences in response to antidepressants.

In PDE4D knockout mice, the antidepressant effect of rolipram in the forced swim test was prevented, whereas the antidepressant effects of desipramine and fluoxetine were not altered [50]. These findings indicate that different neuronal substrates mediate the antidepressant effects of PDE4 inhibitors versus classic monoamine uptake blockers.

### 4.2.7 Clinical Studies Using PDE4 Inhibitors

Clinical evaluation of rolipram in humans has provided evidence for antidepressant activity [21, 22, 24, 25, 102, 103]. To the best of our knowledge, only a single study has reported the effects of rolipram in schizophrenia patients [104]. Although, some improvement of symptoms was observed, treatment was limited by the previously recognized side effect of emesis. Whether the problem of emesis can be overcome via subtype selective PDE4 inhibitors is not yet known, but the presence of specific PDE4 subtypes in brain areas associated with emesis (e.g., area postrema) offers some potential (see Section 4.2.2).

Currently, several PDE4 inhibitors are in development for treating the cognitive deficits associated with Alzheimer's disease. MEM1414 and MEM1917 are two development compounds listed in the pipeline of Memory

Pharmaceuticals (http://www.clinicaltrials.gov). MK-0952 (Merck) is currently being evaluated in a randomized, double-blind Phase 2 clinical trial in patients with mild to moderate Alzheimer's disease (http://clinicaltrials-nccs.nlm.nih.gov/).

## 4.3 PDE10A

PDE10A was identified in 1999 [105–107]. *In vitro*, PDE10A hydrolyzes both cAMP and cyclic guanosine monophosphate (GMP), although both $K_m$ and $V_{max}$ differ for the two substrates [107]. The PDE10 family is represented by only a single gene (PDE10A); however, multiple splice variants have been isolated [1, 92, 108, 109]. In both rodent and human brain, PDE10A2 has been identified as the major variant [108, 109]. Additional variants result from differential N-terminal splicing [1, 92, 108, 109] that does not modify either the proposed regulatory domain or the catalytic domain, and so are not expected to alter enzymatic properties of the protein. These variants may, however, account for differential expression in tissues, cells, or subcellular compartments. For example, PDE10A2 contains a unique protein kinase A (PKA)-dependent phosphorylation site that may be responsible for the membrane association of this isoform [110].

PDE10A possesses a relatively restricted distribution. While PDE10A mRNA is strongly expressed in the rodent and human brain, it is expressed minimally in peripheral tissues, with the exception of testis [108, 111, 112]. In the brain, PDE10A mRNA is predominantly expressed in the striatal complex, including caudate putamen, nucleus accumbens, and olfactory tubercule. Within these areas, intense immunostaining for PDE10A protein is reported throughout the parenchyma. PDE10A protein is found in both the cell bodies and the extensive dendritic arborizations of the medium spiny projection neurons (MSNs), which represent the majority of cells within the striatum. PDE10A mRNA is also found in MSN axonal projections, with immunostaining reported in striatopallidal and striatonigral white matter tracts as well as in the principal output targets of the medium spiny neurons (MSNs), the globus pallidus, and the substantia nigra, which themselves do not express PDE10 mRNA [112]. PDE10A protein is specifically found within striatal MSNs and was not observed in any class of striatal interneuron [113]. Striatal MSNs comprise the principal site for cortical and dopaminergic input within the basal ganglia [114]. Thus, PDE10A may play a role in regulating basal ganglia output given the high level of expression of PDE10A within this region.

PDE10A protein from rat brain, and specifically from striatal MSNs, is primarily membrane associated [110, 113] which may result from a hydrophobic interaction mediated by sequences within the unique N-terminus of PDE10A2, the primary isoform of PDE10A expressed in rat and human brain. PDE10A does not seem to be an integral part of the postsynaptic density complex, but the protein can be found within MSN spines where it may regulate postsynaptic cyclic nucleotide signaling resulting from cortical and dopaminergic inputs [113].

Lower levels of PDE10A have been reported in other brain regions, including cortex, hippocampus, dentate gyrus, cerebellum, and spinal cord [112]. Neuronal PDE10A protein distribution in these regions, however, demonstrates a pattern that is distinct from that observed in striatal MSNs. PDE10A immunoreactivity was restricted to nuclei within individual neurons in these regions with no immunostaining observed in dendritic or axonal processes within cells outside the striatum [111]. Several PDE10A RNA splice variants selectively expressed in the hippocampus have been reported [92]. These isoforms are regulated by long-term potentiation (LTP), suggesting that PDE10A may function to limit signaling associated with learning and memory. This conclusion is supported by studies in animal models of cognition using PDE10A inhibitors (see Section 4.3.3).

The overall pattern of PDE10A protein localization initially described in rat brain [112] has been confirmed and extended to mouse, dog, cynomologus monkey, and human [111]. In the periphery, consistent with the significant levels of PDE10A mRNA in testis [105, 107, 108, 112], Coskran et al. [111] have detected PDE10A immunoreactivity in dog, cynomologus monkey, and mouse testis. In contrast, PDE10A protein was below the level of detection in rat and human testis. Finally, no PDE10A immunoreactivity was seen in other peripheral tissues [111].

### 4.3.1 Medicinal Chemistry of PDE10A

Medicinal chemists have become increasingly focused on the preparation of selective PDE10A inhibitors (for reviews see [115, 116] Unfortunately, there are few detailed reports on the design of such compounds published in the primary literature at this time. Reviews of the patent literature targeting PDE10 inhibitors will provide the interested reader with an appreciation for the diversity of compounds that have been generated by medicinal chemists [117]. The alkaloid papaverine, a known inhibitor of PDE3 and PDE4, was found to also potently inhibit PDE10A (see Fig. 4.3). A medicinal chemistry approach using combinatorial and structure-based design effort based on papavarine and an internal lead produced several potent quinazoline PDE10A inhibitors [118]. One inhibitor, PQ-10 (PDE10A $IC_{50} = 4.0$ nM, PDE3A $IC_{50} = 210$ nM, PDE3B $IC_{50} = 270$ nM), was shown to elevate striatal levels of cGMP in mice similar to that observed when dosed with papaverine.

A structurally distinct series of PDE10A inhibitors typified by the examples MP-10 (subsequently designated PF-2545920) (PDE10A $IC_{50} = 0.18$) and TP-10 (PDE10A $IC_{50} = 0.3$) has been reported [119]. These compounds are highly selective (greater than 3000-fold) across the rest of the PDE family members (18 representative members PDE1 through PDE11). Both PF-2545920 and TP-10 are reported to be efficacious in a number of behavioral models in mice and rats (see Section 4.2.2).

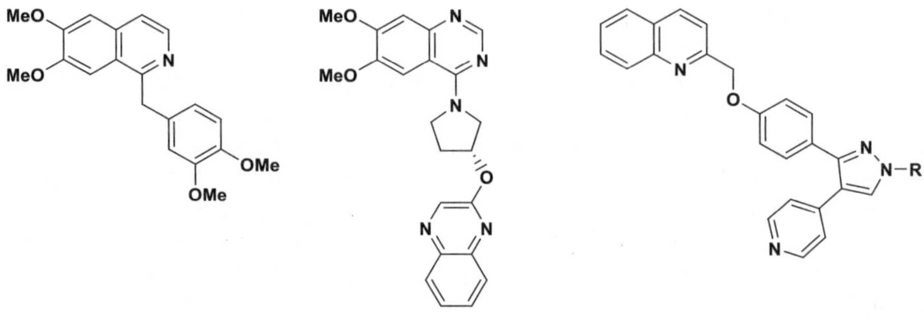

Papaverine PQ-10 PF-2545290 (MP-10), R = -$CH_3$
TP-10, R = -$CH_2CF_3$

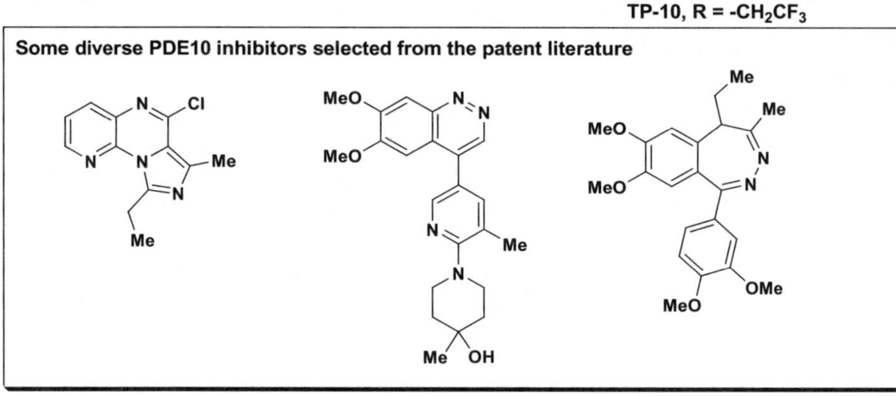


**FIGURE 4.3** Selected PDE10A inhibitors.

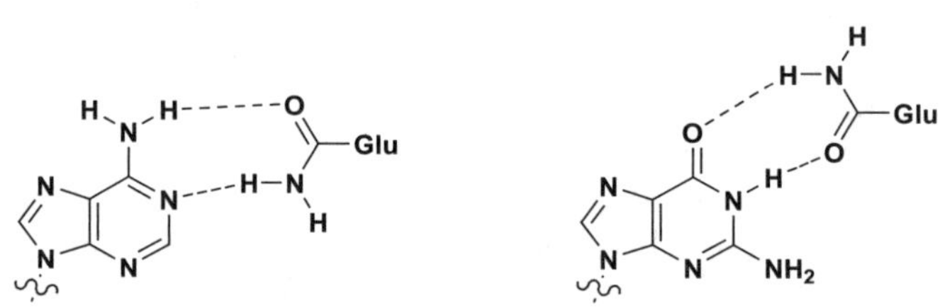

cAMP cGMP

**FIGURE 4.4** Schematic representation of "glutamine switch" substrate recognition mechanism.

PDE10A is a dual substrate PDE capable of hydrolyzing either cAMP or cGMP. Comparison of crystal structures of PDE1, PDE4, and PDE5 suggests that dual substrate PDEs may utilize a "glutamine switch" (see Fig. 4.4) in which the conserved glutamine γ-amide rotates 180° to enable complementary hydrogen binding of either cAMP or cGMP [120, 121].

A systematic evaluation of the crystal structures of cAMP and cGMP complexed with both PDE10A and a PDE10A mutant where the critical glu-

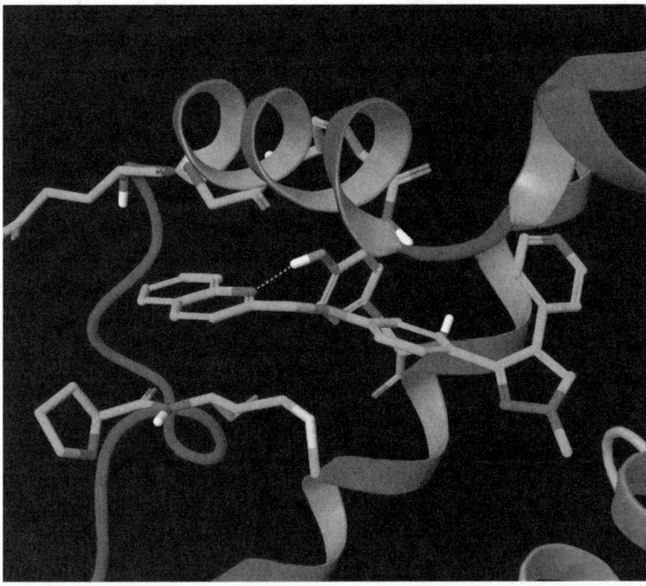

**FIGURE 4.5** PF-2454920 in complex with PDE10A (PDB ID 3HR1). Notice the hydrogen bond between the hydroxyl group on the tyrosine side chain with the quinoline nitrogen atom. Key: carbon—green, nitrogen—blue, oxygen—red, sulfur—yellow. The protein backbone is represented by a blue ribbon. Some residues have been removed for clarity. (See color insert.)

tamine has been replaced with alanine suggests that for PDE10A the glutamine switch mechanism for substrate binding may not be operative [44, 122].

PDE10A is unique in that it has a glycine residue adjacent to the conserved glutamine rather than amino acids with more sterically demanding side chains. A recent disclosure of the crystal structure of PDE10 in complex with PF-2545920 revealed that this glycine residue allows inhibitors such as PF-2545920 to access a unique lipophilic pocket in PDE10A extending beyond the conserved glutamine (see Fig. 4.5) [123]. The quinoline ring was found to effectively fill the volume of the lipophilic pocket with the nitrogen of the quinoline ring being found within hydrogen bonding distance of the hydroxyl group on a tyrosine side chain. Effective engagement of this pocket by PF-2545920 and related structures is credited with the high selectivity exhibited by this compound against other PDE family members.

The medicinal chemistry of PDE10A has advanced rapidly from discovery of lead molecules such as PQ-10, to the clinical candidate PF-2545920. The use of structure-based drug design played a critical role in the optimization of these leads. The crystal structure of PDE10A also revealed the presence of a unique lipophilic pocket in the enzyme, which provides a rationale for the high selectivity observed with PDE10A inhibitors that effectively engage this pocket. A number of pharmaceutical companies have an ongoing effort aimed at designing new PDE10A inhibitors. The future looks promising for this new class of agents.

### 4.3.2 PDE10A Knockout Mice

Constitutive knockout mice in which PDE10A activity has been genetically inactivated have been described and characterized on different genetic background strains, DBA1LacJ [124], C57Bl/6N [125], and C57BL/6 [126]. PDE10A knockout animals survived embryogenesis and were viable and fertile. Behavioral alterations such as decreased baseline locomotor activity, delayed acquisition of CAR, and a blunted locomotor response to NMDA antagonists (MK-801 and/or PCP) appeared to be core phenotypes in the PDE10A knockout (see Table 4.2), although the behavioral effects of PDE10A gene deletion vary in magnitude as a function of genetic background [124, 125]. The effects on the dopaminergic system appeared to be background-dependent as significant effects on dopamine turnover and an enhanced response to amphetamine and methamphetamine were observed only in knockout mice on the C57Bl/6N genetic background [125].

PDE10A knockout did not affect performance in other well-characterized behavioral tasks, including measures of anxiety (the elevated plus maze, light/dark test), depression (forced swim test), nociception (hot-plate test), and learning and memory (passive avoidance, fear conditioning) (see Table 4.2). However, one study did report increased social interaction [126]. In addition to differences in genetic background, these reports do vary with regard to the behavioral models utilized, making direct comparisons challenging. Additional studies in other behavioral tests or utilizing drug challenges may reveal additional phenotypes.

### 4.3.3 PDE10A and Schizophrenia

To date, there have been no reports of associations of PDE10A to schizophrenia, either through alterations in expression or activity of the protein or through SNP analysis. Limited evidence for genetic linkage is the finding that the PDE10A gene maps to human chromosome 6q26-27 [105, 106], which is close to a region identified as a schizophrenia susceptibility locus (6q25) in a large schizophrenia pedigree [127]. Additional studies are needed to explore the role of PDE10A in schizophrenia.

Given the predominant striatal localization of PDE10A, the majority of research exploring the potential therapeutic uses of PDE10A inhibitors to date has focused on preclinical models of psychosis. Papaverine had an antipsychotic-like profile in two key animal models, inhibition of PCP- and amphetamine-induced hyperactivity, as did the more selective PDE10A inhibitors, PQ-10, MP-10, and TP-10. Although PDE10A knockout mice showed a blunted response to PCP and MK-801 when compared to wild-type mice, they

**TABLE 4.2 Comparison of Studies Assessing Phenotype of PDE4B Knockout Mice**

| PDE4B Knockout versus Wild-Type Mice | Siuciak et al., 2007, 2008 [48, 52] | Zhang et al., 2008 [51] |
|---|---|---|
| Background strain | C57/Bl6N | C57/BL6 × 129/ola |
| Gender | Males | Males |
| Body weight | Decrease | Not reported |
| Baseline locomotor activity | Decrease locomotor activity | Decrease in line crossings, initial 5 minutes only |
| Response to amphetamine/ methamphetamine | Increase | ND |
| Response to PCP/MK-801 | ND | ND |
| CAR acquisition/response to antipsychotics | No change | ND |
| Prepulse inhibition | Decrease | ND |
| Cognition tests | No change—passive avoidance, Morris water maze | No change—passive avoidance, Morris water maze |
| Depression tests | Trend ($P < 0.056$) for decrease in immobility in forced swim test | Decrease in immobility in the forced swim test, no effect of desipramine<br>No change—tail suspension test |
| Anxiety tests | No change—elevated plus maze | Anxiogenic-like behavior—holeboard test, light/dark test<br>Increase—plasma corticosterone |
| Analgesia tests | No change—hot plate | No change—tail flick, acetic acid writhing |
| Striatal turnover of dopamine, serotonin | Decrease—dopamine and 5-HT turnover | ND |

ND, not determined.

responded similarly to their wild-type litter mates when challenged with dopaminergic stimulants.

PDE10A inhibition exerted an antipsychotic-like effect in both rats and mice as indicated by a suppression of CAR. The disruptive effect of papaverine on CAR was absent in the PDE10A knockout mice, confirming that the efficacy of papaverine in this assay was due to PDE10A inhibition and not some other ancillary activity. Similar results have been reported for PQ-10, MP-10, and TP-10 [119].

The CAR-suppressing effects of typical and atypical antipsychotics such as haloperidol and risperidone were not altered in PDE10A knockout mice, suggesting that these classical antipsychotics have a different locus of action relative to PDE10A inhibitors. It is important to note that PDE10A knockout mice were able to acquire the CAR task but did so at a slower rate than wild-type mice [124, 125]. One possible explanation for this finding is that the salience of the training stimuli was reduced in the knockout mice compared with wild-type mice.

Reports available on the effects of PDE10A inhibitors in models of sensorimotor gating are equivocal. Papaverine has been reported to reverse the apomorphine-induced PPI deficits in rats and the MK-801-induced deficits in rats and mice [128, 129]. In contrast, studies using the more selective and potent PDE10A inhibitor, TP-10 [119], reported that TP-10 administration did not reverse baseline PPI deficits in C57/BL-6J mice or MK-801-induced PPI deficits in rats.

Papaverine has been tested in several animal models of cognition. Papaverine has shown efficacy in the rat novel object recognition test utilizing a 48-hour delay [130]. Papaverine administration attenuated the attentional set-shifting deficits induced by subchronic PCP administration [131]. To date, there have been no published studies assessing the effects of the more selective and potent PDE10A inhibitors in cognitive assays. Curiously, chronic administration of papaverine has been reported to produce mild cognitive impairments [132], although it is unclear whether this effect is attributable to chronic PDE10A inhibition or to some other ancillary action of the compound.

In humans, papaverine has been used for decades as a muscle relaxant and vasodilator. Regarding possible cognitive enhancing effects, several studies have reported the use of cerebral vasodilators, such as papaverine, in treating geriatric dementia [133–135]. These early studies suggested some improvement in cognitive symptoms; however, no studies have to date evaluated the therapeutic utility of papaverine in cognitive impairment associated with schizophrenia. It is important to acknowledge that, while papaverine may represent a useful preclinical tool, a full understanding of the role of PDE10A in psychiatric disorders and cognitive dysfunction will necessitate the use of a more selective and potent PDE10A inhibitor.

One significant adverse effect of dopamine receptor blockade associated with current antipsychotic treatments is the occurrence of extrapyramidal symptoms. Catalepsy is used as a preclinical animal model of extrapyramidal side effects in humans. Papaverine showed efficacy in several models indicative of antipsychotic activity without inducing catalepsy, suggesting a profile of low EPS liability. However, papaverine did potentiate catalepsy induced by a low dose of the $D_2$ antagonist haloperidol [136]. Importantly, only a partial, modest induction of catalepsy in rodents has been reported in subsequent studies using more potent and selective PDE10A inhibitors [119, 136, 137] suggesting that PDE10A inhibitors may possess a pharmacological profile similar to that of the atypical antipsychotics with low extrapyramidal symptom liability.

Sedation is another common side effect associated with current antipsychotics. In animals, sedation may be measured as a reduction of spontaneous locomotor activity. Papaverine significantly reduced spontaneous locomotor activity as did all of the antipsychotic standards (haloperidol, clozapine, risperidone, and ziprasidone) tested under similar conditions [136].

An increased risk of metabolic and cardiovascular abnormalities is associated with many currently marketed antipsychotics (for review, see [138]). Results from the recent CATIE trials have provided further confirmation of the risk for obesity, impaired glucose tolerance, and hypertension in patients undergoing antipsychotic treatment [138]. The striatum may play a role in appetitive behavior [139], and given its striatal localization, the role of PDE10A in weight regulation has been assessed. PDE10A knockout mice were resistant to high fat diet-induced weight gain and increased adiposity despite equivalent daily food intake to wild-type mice. Furthermore, PDE10A knockout mice on a high-fat diet had significantly higher oxygen consumption rates, improved responses to an oral glucose tolerance test, and improved serum lipid profiles compared with the wild-type controls in indirect oxygen consumption studies [140]. These results suggest that, in contrast to many antipsychotics, inhibition of PDE10A may have an effect on metabolism to reduce body weight; however, these results are preliminary and additional studies are needed. Reduced metabolic risks that are associated with current schizophrenia therapies would be an important differentiating factor for PDE10A inhibitors.

### 4.3.4 Clinical Studies Using PDE10A Inhibitors

Currently, only Pfizer is known to be in development with a PDE10A inhibitor, MP-10 (PF-02545920), for treating schizophrenia (http://www.clinicaltrials.gov), although no results have been reported to date.

## 4.4 OTHER PDE FAMILIES

The lack of availability of tools such as selective pharmacological inhibitors and/or knockout mice has often limited the study of other PDE families. No data currently exist that suggests a role for other PDEs with regard to positive symptoms; however, it is notable that PDEs other than PDE4 and PDE10A are found within the striatum, including PDE1B [141, 142], PDE2A [143, 144], PDE7B [145–147], and PDE9A [144]. Like PDE10A, PDE1B is highly enriched in the striatal MSNs and is a dual substrate PDE. PDE1B knockout mice have been generated and profiled (see Table 4.1) in similar behavioral and neurochemical assays in several laboratories [148–151]. In contrast to the PDE10A knockouts, which are hypoactive in baseline locomotor tests, PDE1B knockout mice are hyperactive and exhibit an exaggerated locomotor response to methamphetamine and amphetamine [148–151]. PDE1B knockout mice, but not

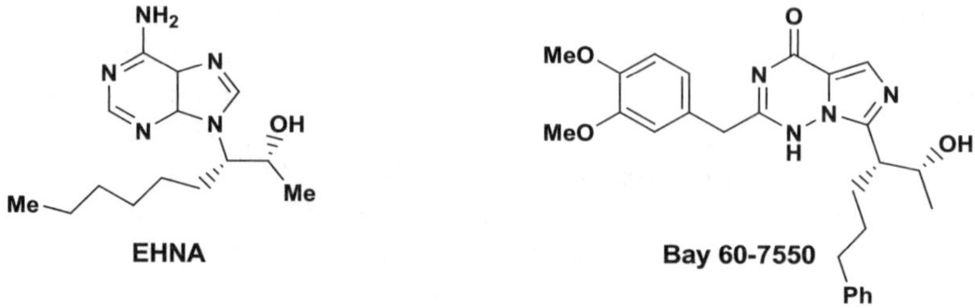


**FIGURE 4.6** Chemical structure of EHNA and Bay 60-7550.

PDE10A knockout mice, show alterations in striatal dopamine turnover [151]. The unique behavioral and neurochemical phenotypes resulting from the disruption of PDE10A, PDE4B, and PDE1B may be a reflection of differential compartmentalization within the striatum and regulation of distinct cyclic nucleotide pools. Thus, these various striatal PDEs may regulate unique signaling pathways and may work in tandem or in opposition within the same pathways. Clearly, additional study is needed to understand the interactions between different PDEs within the striatum.

The role of other PDE family members in cognition has been evaluated (see Fig. 4.6). The PDE2 inhibitor Bay 60-7550 (IC50 = 4.7 nM) (structurally related to the prototypical PDE2 inhibitor EHNA) increased cGMP levels and enhanced LTP in hippocampal slices [152]. Behaviorally, Bay 60-7550 reversed an MK-801-induced deficit in T-maze spatial alternation and was efficacious in object and social recognition assays [152, 153]. Together, these studies suggest a pro-cognitive profile accompanying PDE2 inhibition.

## 4.5 CONCLUSION

Increasing interest over the past several years has yielded intriguing data suggesting potential roles for PDEs in various aspects of schizophrenia. PDE inhibitors represent a receptor-independent mechanism of treating schizophrenia rather than direct antagonist activity at dopaminergic receptors. Although antagonism at the dopamine $D_2$ receptor remains the primary mechanism of typical antipsychotic drugs, the pharmacology of the newer atypical agents is not yet well understood and may involve other G-protein-linked receptor pathways that utilize cAMP or cGMP as a second messenger. These drugs, which work via a final common pathway to increase second messenger activity, may possess advantages over receptor selective agents, particularly for a disorder such as schizophrenia, which is known to involve multiple biochemical abnormalities. Finally, studies suggest that both PDE4 and PDE10A inhibitors may be effective in treating positive symptoms, negative symptoms, or cognitive deficits associated with schizophrenia.

## REFERENCES

1. Beavo, J., Houslay, M.D., Francis, S.H. (2007). Cyclic nucleotide phosphodiesterase superfamily. In: Beavo, J., Francis, S.H., Houslay, M.D., eds. *Cyclic Nucleotide Phosphodiesterases in Health and Disease*. Boca Raton: CRC Press, pp. 3–17.
2. Lugnier, C. (2006). Cyclic nucleotide phosphodiesterase (PDE) superfamily: a new target for the development of specific therapeutic agents. *Pharmacol Ther*, *109*, 366–398.
3. Bolger, G., Michaeli, T., Martins, T., St John, T., Steiner, B., et al. (1993). A family of human phosphodiesterases homologous to the dunce learning and memory gene product of Drosophila melanogaster are potential targets for antidepressant drugs. *Mol Cell Biol*, *13*, 6558–6571.
4. Davis, R.L., Takayasu, H., Eberwine, M., Myres, J. (1989). Cloning and characterization of mammalian homologs of the Drosophila dunce+ gene. *Proc Natl Acad Sci U S A*, *86*, 3604–3608.
5. Conti, M., Andersen, C.B., Richard, F., Mehats, C., Chun, S.Y., et al. (2002). Role of cyclic nucleotide signaling in oocyte maturation. *Mol Cell Endocrinol*, *187*, 153–159.
6. Houslay, M.D. (2005). Keynote review: phosphodiesterase-4 as a therapeutic target. *Drug Discov Today*, *10*, 1503–1519.
7. Iona, S., Cuomo, M., Bushnik, T., Naro, F., Sette, C., et al. (1998). Characterization of the rolipram-sensitive, cyclic AMP-specific phosphodiesterases: identification and differential expression of immunologically distinct forms in the rat brain. *Mol Pharmacol*, *53*, 23–32.
8. Lobban, M., Shakur, Y., Beattie, J., Houslay, M.D. (1994). Identification of two splice variant forms of type-IVB cyclic AMP phosphodiesterase, DPD (rPDE-IVB1) and PDE-4 (rPDE-IVB2) in brain: selective localization in membrane and cytosolic compartments and differential expression in various brain regions. *Biochem J*, *304*(Pt 2), 399–406.
9. McPhee, I., Pooley, L., Lobban, M., Bolger, G., Houslay, M.D. (1995). Identification, characterization and regional distribution in brain of RPDE-6 (RNPDE4A5), a novel splice variant of the PDE4A cyclic AMP phosphodiesterase family. *Biochem J*, *310*(Pt 3), 965–974.
10. Perez-Torres, S., Miro, X., Palacios, J.M., Cortes, R., Puigdomenech, P., et al. (2000). Phosphodiesterase type 4 isozymes expression in human brain examined by in situ hybridization histochemistry and[3H]rolipram binding autoradiography. Comparison with monkey and rat brain. *J Chem Neuroanat*, *20*, 349–374.
11. Cherry, J.A., Davis, R.L. (1999). Cyclic AMP phosphodiesterases are localized in regions of the mouse brain associated with reinforcement, movement, and affect. *J Comp Neurol*, *407*, 287–301.
12. Graybiel, A.M. (1995). The basal ganglia. *Trends Neurosci*, *18*, 60–62.
13. Engels, P., Abdel'Al, S., Hulley, P., Lubbert, H. (1995). Brain distribution of four rat homologues of the Drosophila dunce cAMP phosphodiesterase. *J Neurosci Res*, *41*, 169–178.
14. Goodsell, E.B., Stein, H.H., Wenzke, K.J. (1971). 8-substituted theophyllines. In vitro inhibition of 3′,5′-cyclic adenosine monophosphate phosphodiesterase and pharmacological spectrum in mice. *J Med Chem*, *14*, 1202–1205.

15. Schneider, H.H. (1984). Brain cAMP response to phosphodiesterase inhibitors in rats killed by microwave irradiation or decapitation. *Biochem Pharmacol*, *33*, 1690–1693.

16. Schwabe, U., Miyake, M., Ohga, Y., Daly, J.W. (1976). 4-(3-Cyclopentyloxy-4-methoxyphenyl)-2-pyrrolidone (ZK 62711): a potent inhibitor of adenosine cyclic 3′,5′-monophosphate phosphodiesterases in homogenates and tissue slices from rat brain. *Mol Pharmacol*, *12*, 900–910.

17. Wachtel, H. (1983). Species differences in behavioural effects of rolipram and other adenosine cyclic 3H, 5H-monophosphate phosphodiesterase inhibitors. *J Neural Transm*, *56*, 139–152.

18. Wachtel, H. (1983). Potential antidepressant activity of rolipram and other selective cyclic adenosine 3′,5′-monophosphate phosphodiesterase inhibitors. *Neuropharmacology*, *22*, 267–272.

19. MacKenzie, S.J., Houslay, M.D. (2000). Action of rolipram on specific PDE4 cAMP phosphodiesterase isoforms and on the phosphorylation of cAMP-response-element-binding protein (CREB) and p38 mitogen-activated protein (MAP) kinase in U937 monocytic cells. *Biochem J*, *347*, 571–578.

20. Robichaud, A., Stamatiou, P.B., Jin, S.L., Lachance, N., MacDonald, D., et al. (2002). Deletion of phosphodiesterase 4D in mice shortens alpha(2)-adrenoceptor-mediated anesthesia, a behavioral correlate of emesis. *J Clin Invest*, *110*, 1045–1052.

21. Bertolino, A., Crippa, D., Di Dio, S., Fichte, K., Musmeci, G., et al. (1988). Rolipram versus imipramine in inpatients with major, "minor" or atypical depressive disorder: a double-blind double-dummy study aimed at testing a novel therapeutic approach. *Int Clin Psychopharmacol*, *3*, 245–253.

22. Guiot-Goffioul, F., Gerard-Vandenhove, M.A., Troisfontaines, B., Breulet, M., von Frenckell, R., et al. (1987). [Preliminary results of a double-blind study between rolipram and desipramine in hospitalized patients with major depressive symptoms]. *Acta Psychiatr Belg*, *87*, 230–235.

23. Bobon, D., Breulet, M., Gerard-Vandenhove, M.A., Guiot-Goffioul, F., Plomteux, G., et al. (1988). Is phosphodiesterase inhibition a new mechanism of antidepressant action? A double blind double-dummy study between rolipram and desipramine in hospitalized major and/or endogenous depressives. *Eur Arch Psychiatry Neurol Sci*, *238*, 2–6.

24. Hebenstreit, G.F., Fellerer, K., Fichte, K., Fischer, G., Geyer, N., et al. (1989). Rolipram in major depressive disorder: results of a double-blind comparative study with imipramine. *Pharmacopsychiatry*, *22*, 156–160.

25. Scott, A.I., Perini, A.F., Shering, P.A., Whalley, L.J. (1991). In-patient major depression: is rolipram as effective as amitriptyline? *Eur J Clin Pharmacol*, *40*, 127–129.

26. Barnette, M.S., Grous, M., Cieslinski, L.B., Burman, M., Christensen, S.B., et al. (1995). Inhibitors of phosphodiesterase IV (PDE IV) increase acid secretion in rabbit isolated gastric glands: correlation between function and interaction with a high-affinity rolipram binding site. *J Pharmacol Exp Ther*, *273*, 1396–1402.

27. Barnette, M.S., Bartus, J.O., Burman, M., Christensen, S.B., Cieslinski, L.B., et al. (1996). Association of the anti-inflammatory activity of phosphodiesterase 4

(PDE4) inhibitors with either inhibition of PDE4 catalytic activity or competition for [3H]rolipram binding. *Biochem Pharmacol*, *51*, 949–956.
28. Liu, S., Laliberte, F., Bobechko, B., Bartlett, A., Lario, P., et al. (2001). Dissecting the cofactor-dependent and independent bindings of PDE4 inhibitors. *Biochemistry*, *40*, 10179–10186.
29. Hirose, R., Manabe, H., Yanagawa, K., Ohshima, E., Ichimura, M. (2008). Differential effects of PDE4 inhibitors on cortical neurons and T-lymphocytes. *J Pharmacol Sci*, *106*, 310–317.
30. Zhang, H.T., Zhao, Y., Huang, Y., Deng, C., Hopper, A.T., et al. (2006). Antidepressant-like effects of PDE4 inhibitors mediated by the high-affinity rolipram binding state (HARBS) of the phosphodiesterase-4 enzyme (PDE4) in rats. *Psychopharmacology (Berl)*, *186*, 209–217.
31. Hirose, R., Manabe, H., Nonaka, H., Yanagawa, K., Akuta, K., et al. (2007). Correlation between emetic effect of phosphodiesterase 4 inhibitors and their occupation of the high-affinity rolipram binding site in Suncus murinus brain. *Eur J Pharmacol*, *573*, 93–99.
32. Heaslip, R.J., Evans, D.Y. (1995). Emetic, central nervous system, and pulmonary activities of rolipram in the dog. *Eur J Pharmacol*, *286*, 281–290.
33. Robichaud, A., Savoie, C., Stamatiou, P.B., Tattersall, F.D., Chan, C.C. (2001). PDE4 inhibitors induce emesis in ferrets via a noradrenergic pathway. *Neuropharmacology*, *40*, 262–269.
34. Lamontagne, S., Meadows, E., Luk, P., Normandin, D., Muise, E., et al. (2001). Localization of phosphodiesterase-4 isoforms in the medulla and nodose ganglion of the squirrel monkey. *Brain Res*, *920*, 84–96.
35. Tashiro, N., Kataoka, M., Ozawa, K., Ikeda, T. (2007). The evaluation of whole-body plethysmography as a semiautomated method for analysis of emesis in the house musk shrew (Suncus murinus). *J Am Assoc Lab Anim Sci*, *46*, 81–85.
36. Allen, D.G., Coe, D.M., Cook, C.M., Dowle, M.D., Edline, C.D., et al. (2004). Preparation of pyrazolo[3,4-b]pyridines as phosphodiesterase inhibitors for treatment of COPD, asthma, or allergic rhinitis.
37. Takeda, N., Hasegawa, S., Morita, M., Matsunaga, T. (1993). Pica in rats is analogous to emesis: an animal model in emesis research. *Pharmacol Biochem Behav*, *45*, 817–821.
38. Field, S.K. (2008). Roflumilast: an oral, once-daily selective PDE-4 inhibitor for the management of COPD and asthma. *Expert Opin Investig Drugs*, *17*, 811–818.
39. Giembycz, M.A. (2006). An update and appraisal of the cilomilast phase III clinical development programme for chronic obstructive pulmonary disease. *Br J Clin Pharmacol*, *62*, 138–152.
40. Lipworth, B. (2006). Phosphodiesterase type 4 inhibitors for asthma: a real breakthrough or just expensive theophylline? *Ann Allergy Asthma Immunol*, *96*, 640–642.
41. Giembycz, M.A. (2005). Life after PDE4: overcoming adverse events with dual-specificity phosphodiesterase inhibitors. *Curr Opin Pharmacol*, *5*, 238–244.
42. Card, G.L., England, B.P., Suzuki, Y., Fong, D., Powell, B., et al. (2004). Structural basis for the activity of drugs that inhibit phosphodiesterases. *Structure*, *12*, 2233–2247.

43. Hersperger, R., Bray-French, K., Mazzoni, L., Muller, T. (2000). Palladium-catalyzed cross-coupling reactions for the synthesis of 6, 8-disubstituted 1,7-naphthyridines: a novel class of potent and selective phosphodiesterase type 4D inhibitors. *J Med Chem*, *43*, 675–682.

44. Wang, H., Robinson, H., Ke, H. (2007). The molecular basis for different recognition of substrates by phosphodiesterase families 4 and 10. *J Mol Biol*, *371*, 302–307.

45. Jin, S.L., Conti, M. (2002). Induction of the cyclic nucleotide phosphodiesterase PDE4B is essential for LPS-activated TNF-alpha responses. *Proc Natl Acad Sci U S A*, *99*, 7628–7633.

46. Jin, S.L., Lan, L., Zoudilova, M., Conti, M. (2005). Specific role of phosphodiesterase 4B in lipopolysaccharide-induced signaling in mouse macrophages. *J Immunol*, *175*, 1523–1531.

47. Jin, S.L., Richard, F.J., Kuo, W.P., D'Ercole, A.J., Conti, M. (1999). Impaired growth and fertility of cAMP-specific phosphodiesterase PDE4D-deficient mice. *Proc Natl Acad Sci U S A*, *96*, 11998–12003.

48. Siuciak, J.A., McCarthy, S.A., Chapin, D.S., Martin, A.N. (2008). Behavioral and neurochemical characterization of mice deficient in the phosphodiesterase-4B (PDE4B) enzyme. *Psychopharmacology (Berl)*, *197*(1), 115–126.

49. Siuciak, J.A., Chapin, D.S., McCarthy, S.A., Martin, A.N. (2007). Antipsychotic profile of rolipram: efficacy in rats and reduced sensitivity in mice deficient in the phosphodiesterase-4B (PDE4B) enzyme. *Psychopharmacology (Berl)*, *192*, 415–424.

50. Zhang, H.T., Huang, Y., Jin, S.L., Frith, S.A., Suvarna, N., et al. (2002). Antidepressant-like profile and reduced sensitivity to rolipram in mice deficient in the PDE4D phosphodiesterase enzyme. *Neuropsychopharmacology*, *27*, 587–595.

51. Zhang, H.T., Huang, Y., Masood, A., Stolinski, L.R., Li, Y., et al. (2007). Anxiogenic-like behavioral phenotype of mice deficient in phosphodiesterase 4B (PDE4B). *Neuropsychopharmacology*, *33*(7), 1611–1623.

52. Siuciak, J.A., McCarthy, S.A., Chapin, D.S., Martin, A.N. (2008). Behavioral and neurochemical characterization of mice deficient in the phosphodiesterase-4B (PDE4B) enzyme. *Psychopharmacology (Berl)*, *197*, 115–126.

53. Faraone, S.V., Hwu, H.G., Liu, C.M., Chen, W.J., Tsuang, M.M., et al. (2006). Genome scan of Han Chinese schizophrenia families from Taiwan: confirmation of linkage to 10q22.3. *Am J Psychiatry*, *163*, 1760–1766.

54. Milatovich, A., Bolger, G., Michaeli, T., Francke, U. (1994). Chromosome localizations of genes for five cAMP-specific phosphodiesterases in man and mouse. *Somat Cell Mol Genet*, *20*, 75–86.

55. Szpirer, C., Szpirer, J., Riviere, M., Swinnen, J., Vicini, E., et al. (1995). Chromosomal localization of the human and rat genes (PDE4D and PDE4B) encoding the cAMP-specific phosphodiesterases 3 and 4. *Cytogenet Cell Genet*, *69*, 11–14.

56. Millar, J.K., James, R., Christie, S., Porteous, D.J. (2005). Disrupted in schizophrenia 1 (DISC1): subcellular targeting and induction of ring mitochondria. *Mol Cell Neurosci*, *30*, 477–484.

57. Fatemi, S.H., King, D.P., Reutiman, T.J., Folsom, T.D., Laurence, J.A., et al. (2008). PDE4B polymorphisms and decreased PDE4B expression are associated with schizophrenia. *Schizophr Res*, *101*, 36–49.

58. Numata, S., Ueno, S.I., Iga, J.I., Song, H., Nakataki, M., et al. (2008). Positive association of the PDE4B (phosphodiesterase 4B) gene with schizophrenia in the Japanese population. *J Psychiatr Res*, *43*(1), 7–12.

59. Pickard, B.S., Thomson, P.A., Christoforou, A., Evans, K.L., Morris, S.W., et al. (2007). The PDE4B gene confers sex-specific protection against schizophrenia. *Psychiatr Genet*, *17*, 129–133.

60. Chubb, J.E., Bradshaw, N.J., Soares, D.C., Porteous, D.J., Millar, J.K. (2008). The DISC locus in psychiatric illness. *Mol Psychiatry*, *13*, 36–64.

61. Millar, J.K., Mackie, S., Clapcote, S.J., Murdoch, H., Pickard, B.S., et al. (2007). Disrupted in schizophrenia 1 and phosphodiesterase 4B: towards an understanding of psychiatric illness. *J Physiol*, *584*, 401–405.

62. Clapcote, S.J., Lipina, T.V., Millar, J.K., Mackie, S., Christie, S., et al. (2007). Behavioral phenotypes of Disc1 missense mutations in mice. *Neuron*, *54*, 387–402.

63. Mori, T., Baba, J., Ichimaru, Y., Suzuki, T. (2000). Effects of rolipram, a selective inhibitor of phosphodiesterase 4, on hyperlocomotion induced by several abused drugs in mice. *Jpn J Pharmacol*, *83*, 113–118.

64. Davis, J.A., Gould, T.J. (2005). Rolipram attenuates MK-801-induced deficits in latent inhibition. *Behav Neurosci*, *119*, 595–602.

65. Halene, T.B., Siegel, S.J. (2008). Antipsychotic-like properties of phosphodiesterase 4 inhibitors: evaluation of 4-(3-butoxy-4-methoxybenzyl)-2-imidazolidinone (RO-20-1724) with auditory event-related potentials and prepulse inhibition of startle. *J Pharmacol Exp Ther*, *326*, 230–239.

66. Kanes, S.J., Tokarczyk, J., Siegel, S.J., Bilker, W., Abel, T., et al. (2007). Rolipram: a specific phosphodiesterase 4 inhibitor with potential antipsychotic activity. *Neuroscience*, *144*, 239–246.

67. Maxwell, C.R., Kanes, S.J., Abel, T., Siegel, S.J. (2004). Phosphodiesterase inhibitors: a novel mechanism for receptor-independent antipsychotic medications. *Neuroscience*, *129*, 101–107.

68. Becker, A., Grecksch, G. (2008). Phosphodiesterase inhibitors—are they potential neuroleptic drugs? *Behav Brain Res*, *186*, 155–160.

69. Kapur, S. (2003). Psychosis as a state of aberrant salience: a framework linking biology, phenomenology, and pharmacology in schizophrenia. *Am J Psychiatry*, *160*, 13–23.

70. Wadenberg, M.L., Hicks, P.B. (1999). The conditioned avoidance response test reevaluated: is it a sensitive test for the detection of potentially atypical antipsychotics? *Neurosci Biobehav Rev*, *23*, 851–862.

71. Chapin, D.S., McCarthy, S.A., Martin, A.N., Siuciak, J.A. (2007). Rolipram, a PDE4 inhibitor, shows efficacy in animal models of antipsychotic-like activity: studies using PDE4B and PDE4D knockout mice. *Schizophr Bull*, *33*, 470.

72. Dlaboga, D., Hajjhussein, H., O'Donnell, J.M. (2008). Chronic haloperidol and clozapine produce different patterns of effects on phosphodiesterase-1B, -4B, and -10A expression in rat striatum. *Neuropharmacology*, *54*, 745–754.

73. Tamminga, C.A. (2006). The neurobiology of cognition in schizophrenia. *J Clin Psychiatry*, *67*, e11.
74. Fujii, D.E., Wylie, A.M. (2003). Neurocognition and community outcome in schizophrenia: long-term predictive validity. *Schizophr Res*, *59*, 219–223.
75. Blokland, A., Schreiber, R., Prickaerts, J. (2006). Improving memory: a role for phosphodiesterases. *Curr Pharm Des*, *12*, 2511–2523.
76. Rose, G.M., Hopper, A., De Vivo, M., Tehim, A. (2005). Phosphodiesterase inhibitors for cognitive enhancement. *Curr Pharm Des*, *11*, 3329–3334.
77. Bourtchouladze, R., Lidge, R., Catapano, R., Stanley, J., Gossweiler, S., et al. (2003). A mouse model of Rubinstein-Taybi syndrome: defective long-term memory is ameliorated by inhibitors of phosphodiesterase 4. *Proc Natl Acad Sci U S A*, *100*, 10518–10522.
78. Rutten, K., Lieben, C., Smits, L., Blokland, A. (2007). The PDE4 inhibitor rolipram reverses object memory impairment induced by acute tryptophan depletion in the rat. *Psychopharmacology (Berl)*, *192*, 275–282.
79. Rutten, K., Prickaerts, J., Blokland, A. (2006). Rolipram reverses scopolamine-induced and time-dependent memory deficits in object recognition by different mechanisms of action. *Neurobiol Learn Mem*, *85*, 132–138.
80. Rutten, K., Prickaerts, J., Hendrix, M., van der Staay, F.J., Sik, A., et al. (2007). Time-dependent involvement of cAMP and cGMP in consolidation of object memory: studies using selective phosphodiesterase type 2, 4 and 5 inhibitors. *Eur J Pharmacol*, *558*, 107–112.
81. Egawa, T., Mishima, K., Matsumoto, Y., Iwasaki, K., Iwasaki, K., et al. (1997). Rolipram and its optical isomers, phosphodiesterase 4 inhibitors, attenuated the scopolamine-induced impairments of learning and memory in rats. *Jpn J Pharmacol*, *75*, 275–281.
82. Ghelardini, C., Galeotti, N., Gualtieri, F., Romanelli, M.N., Bucherelli, C., et al. (2002). DM235 (sunifiram): a novel nootropic with potential as a cognitive enhancer. *Naunyn Schmiedebergs Arch Pharmacol*, *365*, 419–426.
83. Imanishi, T., Sawa, A., Ichimaru, Y., Miyashiro, M., Kato, S., et al. (1997). Ameliorating effects of rolipram on experimentally induced impairments of learning and memory in rodents. *Eur J Pharmacol*, *321*, 273–278.
84. Zhang, H.T., Huang, Y., Suvarna, N.U., Deng, C., Crissman, A.M., et al. (2005). Effects of the novel PDE4 inhibitors MEM1018 and MEM1091 on memory in the radial-arm maze and inhibitory avoidance tests in rats. *Psychopharmacology (Berl)*, *179*, 613–619.
85. Zhang, H.T., Crissman, A.M., Dorairaj, N.R., Chandler, L.J., O'Donnell, J.M. (2000). Inhibition of cyclic AMP phosphodiesterase (PDE4) reverses memory deficits associated with NMDA receptor antagonism. *Neuropsychopharmacology*, *23*, 198–204.
86. Zhang, H.T., O'Donnell, J.M. (2000). Effects of rolipram on scopolamine-induced impairment of working and reference memory in the radial-arm maze tests in rats. *Psychopharmacology (Berl)*, *150*, 311–316.
87. Gong, B., Vitolo, O.V., Trinchese, F., Liu, S., Shelanski, M., et al. (2004). Persistent improvement in synaptic and cognitive functions in an Alzheimer mouse model after rolipram treatment. *J Clin Invest*, *114*, 1624–1634.

88. Barad, M., Bourtchouladze, R., Winder, D.G., Golan, H., Kandel, E. (1998). Rolipram, a type IV-specific phosphodiesterase inhibitor, facilitates the establishment of long-lasting long-term potentiation and improves memory. *Proc Natl Acad Sci U S A*, *95*, 15020–15025.
89. Nagakura, A., Niimura, M., Takeo, S. (2002). Effects of a phosphodiesterase IV inhibitor rolipram on microsphere embolism-induced defects in memory function and cerebral cyclic AMP signal transduction system in rats. *Br J Pharmacol*, *135*, 1783–1793.
90. Nguyen, T., Lewis, S.R., Moschak, T.M., Yorek, M.S., Rodefer, J.S. (2007). Cognitive enhancing and antipsychotic effects of phosphodiesterase inhibitors. 2007 Neuroscience Meeting Planner San Diego, CA: Society for Neuroscience: Online.
91. Jentsch, J.D., Roth, R.H. (1999). The neuropsychopharmacology of phencyclidine: from NMDA receptor hypofunction to the dopamine hypothesis of schizophrenia. *Neuropsychopharmacology*, *20*, 201–225.
92. O'Connor, V., Genin, A., Davis, S., Karishma, K.K., Doyere, V., et al. (2004). Differential amplification of intron-containing transcripts reveals long term potentiation-associated up-regulation of specific Pde10A phosphodiesterase splice variants. *J Biol Chem*, *279*, 15841–15849.
93. Renau, T.E. (2004). The potential of phosphodiesterase 4 inhibitors for the treatment of depression: opportunities and challenges. *Curr Opin Investig Drugs*, *5*, 34–39.
94. Saccomano, N.A., Vinick, F.J., Koe, B.K., Nielsen, J.A., Whalen, W.M., et al. (1991). Calcium-independent phosphodiesterase inhibitors as putative antidepressants: [3-(bicycloalkyloxy)-4-methoxyphenyl]-2-imidazolidinones. *J Med Chem*, *34*, 291–298.
95. Itoh, T., Tokumura, M., Abe, K. (2004). Effects of rolipram, a phosphodiesterase 4 inhibitor, in combination with imipramine on depressive behavior, CRE-binding activity and BDNF level in learned helplessness rats. *Eur J Pharmacol*, *498*, 135–142.
96. Mizokawa, T., Kimura, K., Ikoma, Y., Hara, K., Oshino, N., et al. (1988). The effect of a selective phosphodiesterase inhibitor, rolipram, on muricide in olfactory bulbectomized rats. *Jpn J Pharmacol*, *48*, 357–364.
97. O'Donnell, J.M. (1993). Antidepressant-like effects of rolipram and other inhibitors of cyclic adenosine monophosphate phosphodiesterase on behavior maintained by differential reinforcement of low response rate. *J Pharmacol Exp Ther*, *264*, 1168–1178.
98. Overstreet, D.H., Double, K., Schiller, G.D. (1989). Antidepressant effects of rolipram in a genetic animal model of depression: cholinergic supersensitivity and weight gain. *Pharmacol Biochem Behav*, *34*, 691–696.
99. Dlaboga, D., Hajjhussein, H., O'Donnell, J.M. (2006). Regulation of phosphodiesterase-4 (PDE4) expression in mouse brain by repeated antidepressant treatment: comparison with rolipram. *Brain Res*, *1096*, 104–112.
100. Takahashi, M., Terwilliger, R., Lane, C., Mezes, P.S., Conti, M., et al. (1999). Chronic antidepressant administration increases the expression of cAMP-specific phosphodiesterase 4A and 4B isoforms. *J Neurosci*, *19*, 610–618.
101. Ye, Y., Conti, M., Houslay, M.D., Farooqui, S.M., Chen, M., et al. (1997). Noradrenergic activity differentially regulates the expression of rolipram-sensitive,

high-affinity cyclic AMP phosphodiesterase (PDE4) in rat brain. *J Neurochem*, *69*, 2397–2404.

102. Fleischhacker, W.W., Hinterhuber, H., Bauer, H., Pflug, B., Berner, P., et al. (1992). A multicenter double-blind study of three different doses of the new cAMP-phosphodiesterase inhibitor rolipram in patients with major depressive disorder. *Neuropsychobiology*, *26*, 59–64.
103. Zeller, E., Stief, H.J., Pflug, B., Sastre-Y-Hernandez, M. (1984). Results of a phase II study of the antidepressant effect of rolipram. *Pharmacopsychiatry*, *17*, 188–190.
104. Pietzcker, A., Muller-Oerlinghausen, B., Kehr, W. (1979). Antipsychotic activity of rolipram in schizophrenic patients. A pilot study. *Naunyn Schmiedebergs Arch Pharmacol*, *308*, R44.
105. Fujishige, K., Kotera, J., Michibata, H., Yuasa, K., Takebayashi, S., et al. (1999). Cloning and characterization of a novel human phosphodiesterase that hydrolyzes both cAMP and cGMP (PDE10A). *J Biol Chem*, *274*, 18438–18445.
106. Loughney, K., Snyder, P.B., Uher, L., Rosman, G.J., Ferguson, K., et al. (1999). Isolation and characterization of PDE10A, a novel human 3′,5′-cyclic nucleotide phosphodiesterase. *Gene*, *234*, 109–117.
107. Soderling, S.H., Bayuga, S.J., Beavo, J.A. (1999). Isolation and characterization of a dual-substrate phosphodiesterase gene family: PDE10A. *Proc Natl Acad Sci U S A*, *96*, 7071–7076.
108. Fujishige, K., Kotera, J., Omori, K. (1999). Striatum- and testis-specific phosphodiesterase PDE10A isolation and characterization of a rat PDE10A. *Eur J Biochem*, *266*, 1118–1127.
109. Kotera, J., Fujishige, K., Yuasa, K., Omori, K. (1999). Characterization and phosphorylation of PDE10A2, a novel alternative splice variant of human phosphodiesterase that hydrolyzes cAMP and cGMP. *Biochem Biophys Res Commun*, *261*, 551–557.
110. Kotera, J., Sasaki, T., Kobayashi, T., Fujishige, K., Yamashita, Y., et al. (2004). Subcellular localization of cyclic nucleotide phosphodiesterase type 10A variants, and alteration of the localization by cAMP-dependent protein kinase-dependent phosphorylation. *J Biol Chem*, *279*, 4366–4375.
111. Coskran, T.M., Morton, D., Menniti, F.S., Adamowicz, W.O., Kleiman, R.J., et al. (2006). Immunohistochemical localization of phosphodiesterase 10A in multiple mammalian species. *J Histochem Cytochem*, *54*, 1205–1213.
112. Seeger, T.F., Bartlett, B., Coskran, T.M., Culp, J.S., James, L.C., et al. (2003). Immunohistochemical localization of PDE10A in the rat brain. *Brain Res*, *985*, 113–126.
113. Xie, Z., Adamowicz, W.O., Eldred, W.D., Jakowski, A.B., Kleiman, R.J., et al. (2006). Cellular and subcellular localization of PDE10A, a striatum-enriched phosphodiesterase. *Neuroscience*, *139*, 597–607.
114. Ring, H.A., Serra-Mestres, J. (2002). Neuropsychiatry of the basal ganglia. *J Neurol Neurosurg Psychiatry*, *72*, 12–21.
115. Brandon, N.J., Rotella, D.P. (2007). Potential CNS applications for phosphodiesterase enzyme inhibitors. *Annu Rep Med Chem*, *42*, 3–12.

116. Chappie, T., Humphrey, J., Menniti, F., Schmidt, C. (2009). PDE10A inhibitors: an assessment of the current CNS drug discovery landscape. *Curr Opin Drug Discov Devel, 12*, 458–467.

117. Kehler, J., Kilburn, J.P. (2009). Patented PDE10A inhibitors: novel compounds since 2007. *Expert Opin Ther Pat, 19*, 1715–1725.

118. Chappie, T.A., Humphrey, J.M., Allen, M.P., Estep, K.G., Fox, C.B., et al. (2007). Discovery of a series of 6,7-dimethoxy-4-pyrrolidylquinazoline PDE10A inhibitors. *J Med Chem, 50*, 182–185.

119. Schmidt, C.J., Chapin, D.S., Cianfrogna, J., Corman, M.L., Hajos, M., et al. (2008). Preclinical characterization of selective phosphodiesterase 10A inhibitors: a new therapeutic approach to the treatment of schizophrenia. *J Pharmacol Exp Ther, 325*, 681–690.

120. Zhang, H.T., Zhao, Y., Huang, Y., Dorairaj, N.R., Chandler, L.J., et al. (2004). Inhibition of the phosphodiesterase 4 (PDE4) enzyme reverses memory deficits produced by infusion of the MEK inhibitor U0126 into the CA1 subregion of the rat hippocampus. *Neuropsychopharmacology, 29*, 1432–1439.

121. Zhang, K.Y., Card, G.L., Suzuki, Y., Artis, D.R., Fong, D., et al. (2004). A glutamine switch mechanism for nucleotide selectivity by phosphodiesterases. *Mol Cell, 15*, 279–286.

122. Wang, H., Liu, Y., Hou, J., Zheng, M., Robinson, H., et al. (2007). Structural insight into substrate specificity of phosphodiesterase 10. *Proc Natl Acad Sci U S A, 104*, 5782–5787.

123. Verhoest, P.R., Chapin, D.S., Corman, M., Fonseca, K., Harms, J.F., et al. (2009). Discovery of a novel class of phosphodiesterase 10A inhibitors and identification of clinical candidate 2-[4-(1-methyl-4-pyridin-4-yl-1H-pyrazol-3-yl)-phenoxymethyl]-quinoline (PF-2545920) for the treatment of schizophrenia. *J Med Chem, 52*, 5188–5196.

124. Siuciak, J.A., McCarthy, S.A., Chapin, D.S., Fujiwara, R.A., James, L.C., et al. (2006). Genetic deletion of the striatum-enriched phosphodiesterase PDE10A: evidence for altered striatal function. *Neuropharmacology, 51*, 374–385.

125. Siuciak, J.A., McCarthy, S.A., Chapin, D.S., Martin, A.N., Harms, J.F., et al. (2008). Behavioral characterization of mice deficient in the phosphodiesterase-10A (PDE10A) enzyme on a C57/Bl6N congenic background. *Neuropharmacology, 54*, 417–427.

126. Sano, H., Nagai, Y., Miyakawa, T., Shigemoto, R., Yokoi, M. (2008). Increased social interaction in mice deficient of the striatal medium spiny neuron-specific phosphodiesterase 10A2. *J Neurochem, 105*, 546–556.

127. Lindholm, E., Ekholm, B., Shaw, S., Jalonen, P., Johansson, G., et al. (2001). A schizophrenia-susceptibility locus at 6q25, in one of the world's largest reported pedigrees. *Am J Hum Genet, 69*, 96–105.

128. Bleickardt, C.J., Lu, S.X., Cohen-Williams, M.E., Varty, G.B., Hodgson, R.A. (2007). Effects of pde10a inhibition with papaverine in rat models of schizophrenia. 2007 Neuroscience Meeting Planner San Diego, CA: Online.

129. Lu, S.X., Del Vecchio, R.A., Kazdoba, T.M., Leach, P.T., Werner, B.J., et al. (2007). Characterization of the PDE10A inhibitor, papaverine, in mouse models of schizophrenia. 2007 Neuroscience Meeting Planner San Diego, CA: Online.

130. Liu, F., Zhang, G., Kelley, C., Day, M., Marquis, K., et al. (2006). Biochemical analysis of mechanism action of PDE10A inhibitor papaverine in pro-cognitive effects. 2006 Neuroscience Meeting Planner.

131. Rodefer, J.S., Murphy, E.R., Baxter, M.G. (2005). PDE10A inhibition reverses subchronic PCP-induced deficits in attentional set-shifting in rats. *Eur J Neurosci*, *21*, 1070–1076.

132. Hebb, A.L., Robertson, H.A. (2007). Role of phosphodiesterases in neurological and psychiatric disease. *Curr Opin Pharmacol*, *7*, 86–92.

133. Cole, J.O., Branconnier, R.J., Martin, G.F. (1975). Electroencephalographic and behavioral changes associated with papaverine administration in healthy geriatric subjects. *J Am Geriatr Soc*, *23*, 295–300.

134. Nelson, J.J. (1975). Relieving select symptoms of the elderly. *Geriatrics*, *30*, 133–139. 142.

135. Yesavage, J.A., Tinklenberg, J.R., Hollister, L.E., Berger, P.A. (1979). Vasodilators in senile dementias: a review of the literature. *Arch Gen Psychiatry*, *36*, 220–223.

136. Siuciak, J.A., Chapin, D.S., Harms, J.F., Lebel, L.A., McCarthy, S.A., et al. (2006). Inhibition of the striatum-enriched phosphodiesterase PDE10A: a novel approach to the treatment of psychosis. *Neuropharmacology*, *51*, 386–396.

137. Siuciak, J.A., Chapin, D.S., McCarthy, S.A. (2006). Novel potent and selective phosphodiesterase 10A (PDE10A) inhibitors show activity in animal models of psychosis. 2006 Neuroscience Meeting Planner, Society for Neuroscience. Online.

138. Newcomer, J.W. (2007). Metabolic considerations in the use of antipsychotic medications: a review of recent evidence. *J Clin Psychiatry*, *68*(Suppl 1), 20–27.

139. Kelley, A.E. (2004). Ventral striatal control of appetitive motivation: role in ingestive behavior and reward-related learning. *Neurosci Biobehav Rev*, *27*, 765–776.

140. Black, S.C., Gibbs, M., McNeish, J.D., Menniti, F.S., Siuciak, J.A., et al. (2006). Genetic deletion of phosphodiesterase 10A results in a phenotype of resistance to high fat diet-induced obesity, elevated circulating adiponectin and improved glucose tolerance: a new drug target. Keystone Symposium Abstracts, Adipogenesis, Obesity and Inflammation: 149.

141. Polli, J.W., Kincaid, R.L. (1992). Molecular cloning of DNA encoding a calmodulin-dependent phosphodiesterase enriched in striatum. *Proc Natl Acad Sci U S A*, *89*, 11079–11083.

142. Yan, C., Bentley, J.K., Sonnenburg, W.K., Beavo, J.A. (1994). Differential expression of the 61 kDa and 63 kDa calmodulin-dependent phosphodiesterases in the mouse brain. *J Neurosci*, *14*, 973–984.

143. Juilfs, D.M., Soderling, S., Burns, F., Beavo, J.A. (1999). Cyclic GMP as substrate and regulator of cyclic nucleotide phosphodiesterases (PDEs). *Rev Physiol Biochem Pharmacol*, *135*, 67–104.

144. Van Staveren, W.C., Steinbusch, H.W., Markerink-Van Ittersum, M., Repaske, D.R., Goy, M.F., et al. (2003). mRNA expression patterns of the cGMP-hydrolyzing phosphodiesterases types 2, 5, and 9 during development of the rat brain. *J Comp Neurol*, *467*, 566–580.

145. Cho, C.H., Cho, D.H., Seo, M.R., Juhnn, Y.S. (2000). Differential changes in the expression of cyclic nucleotide phosphodiesterase isoforms in rat brains by chronic treatment with electroconvulsive shock. *Exp Mol Med*, *32*, 110–114.

146. Reyes-Irisarri, E., Perez-Torres, S., Mengod, G. (2005). Neuronal expression of cAMP-specific phosphodiesterase 7B mRNA in the rat brain. *Neuroscience*, *132*, 1173–1185.

147. Sasaki, T., Kotera, J., Omori, K. (2002). Novel alternative splice variants of rat phosphodiesterase 7B showing unique tissue-specific expression and phosphorylation. *Biochem J*, *361*, 211–220.

148. Ehrman, L.A., Williams, M.T., Schaefer, T.L., Gudelsky, G.A., Reed, T.M., et al. (2006). Phosphodiesterase 1B differentially modulates the effects of methamphetamine on locomotor activity and spatial learning through DARPP32-dependent pathways: evidence from PDE1B-DARPP32 double-knockout mice. *Genes Brain Behav*, *5*, 540–551.

149. Reed, T.M., Browning, J.E., Blough, R.I., Vorhees, C.V., Repaske, D.R. (1998). Genomic structure and chromosome location of the murine PDE1B phosphodiesterase gene. *Mamm Genome*, *9*, 571–576.

150. Reed, T.M., Repaske, D.R., Snyder, G.L., Greengard, P., Vorhees, C.V. (2002). Phosphodiesterase 1B knock-out mice exhibit exaggerated locomotor hyperactivity and DARPP-32 phosphorylation in response to dopamine agonists and display impaired spatial learning. *J Neurosci*, *22*, 5188–5197.

151. Siuciak, J.A., McCarthy, S.A., Chapin, D.S., Reed, T.M., Vorhees, C.V., et al. (2007). Behavioral and neurochemical characterization of mice deficient in the phosphodiesterase-1B (PDE1B) enzyme. *Neuropharmacology*, *53*, 113–124.

152. Boess, F.G., Hendrix, M., van der Staay, F.J., Erb, C., Schreiber, R., et al. (2004). Inhibition of phosphodiesterase 2 increases neuronal cGMP, synaptic plasticity and memory performance. *Neuropharmacology*, *47*, 1081–1092.

153. Rutten, K., Prickaerts, J., Steinbusch, H., Blockland, A. (2007). Inhibitors of PDE2, PDE4 and PDE5 enhance spatial memory in a time-dependent manner in the object location task in rats. 2007 Neuroscience Meeting Planner San Diego, CA: Society for Neuroscience. Online.

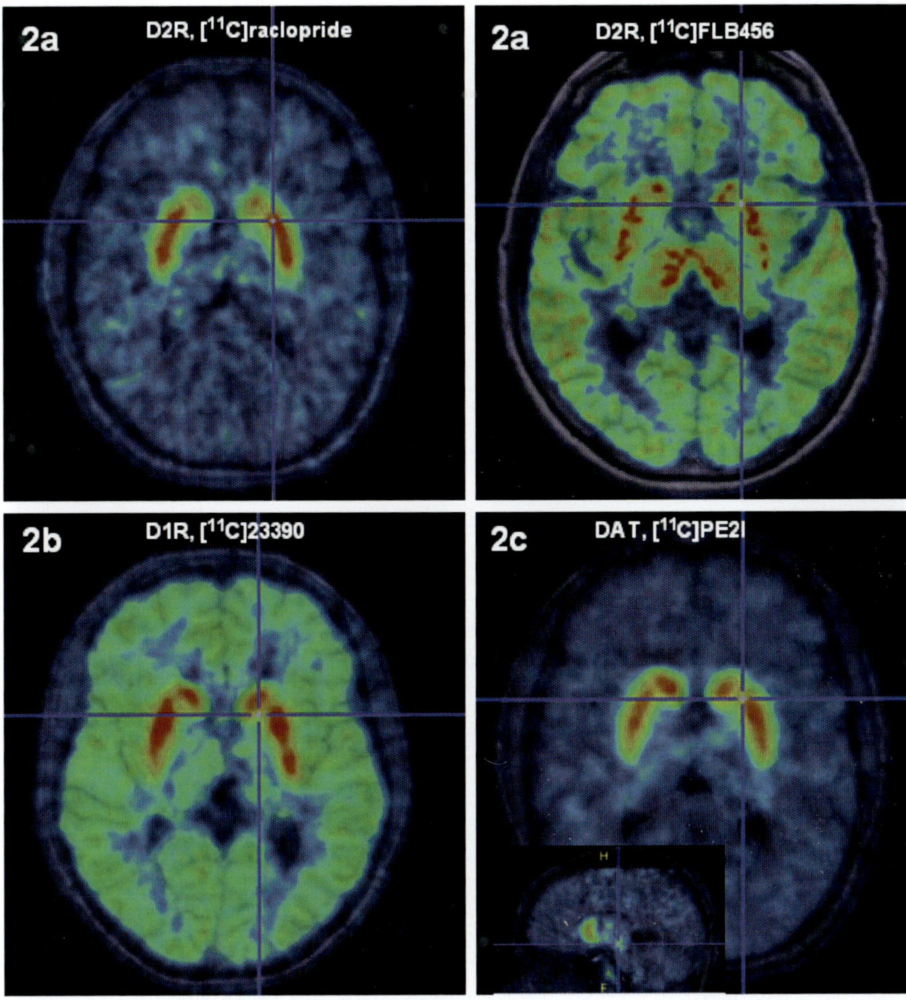


**FIGURE 1.2** Dopamine receptor ($D_1$, $D_2$, $D_3$) and dopamine transporter distribution throughout the brain as measured by *in vivo* molecular imaging in humans by PET. (a) Regional radioactivity of [$^{11}$C]raclopride, representing binding to the striatal D2/D3DRs, and [$^{11}$C]FLB 456, representing binding to the extrastriatal D2/D3DRs. (b) Regional radioactivity of [$^{11}$C]SCH23390, representing binding to the D1/D5DRs. (c) Regional radioactivity of [$^{11}$C]PE2I, representing binding to the DAT. Summation PET images at transaxial and saggital planes. Substantia nigra indicated in saggital plane.

*Targets and Emerging Therapies for Schizophrenia*, First Edition.
Edited by Jeffrey S. Albert and Michael W. Wood.

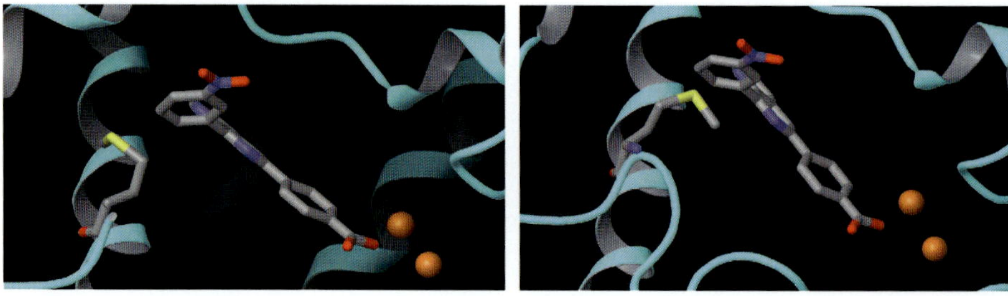

**FIGURE 4.2** NVP (4-(8-(3-nitrophenyl)1,7-naphthryridin-6-yl)benzoic acid) co-crystallized in the active site of PDE4B (left, PDB ID 2QYL) and PDE4D (right, PDB ID 2QYN). Notice the small conformational difference in the conserved methionine residue between structures. Key: carbon—gray, nitrogen—blue, oxygen—red, sulfur—yellow, zinc (left) orange, magnesium (right) orange. The protein backbone is represented by a blue ribbon. Some residues have been removed for clarity.

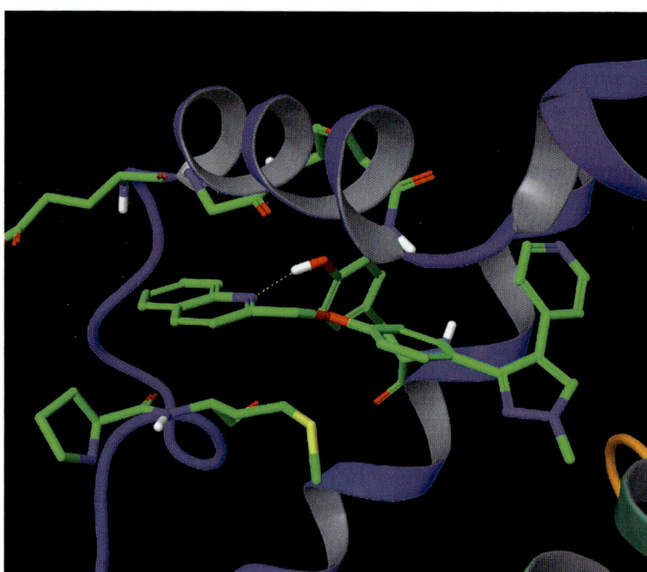

**FIGURE 4.5** PF-2454920 in complex with PDE10A (PDB ID 3HR1). Notice the hydrogen bond between the hydroxyl group on the tyrosine side chain with the quinoline nitrogen atom. Key: carbon—green, nitrogen—blue, oxygen—red, sulfur—yellow. The protein backbone is represented by a blue ribbon. Some residues have been removed for clarity.

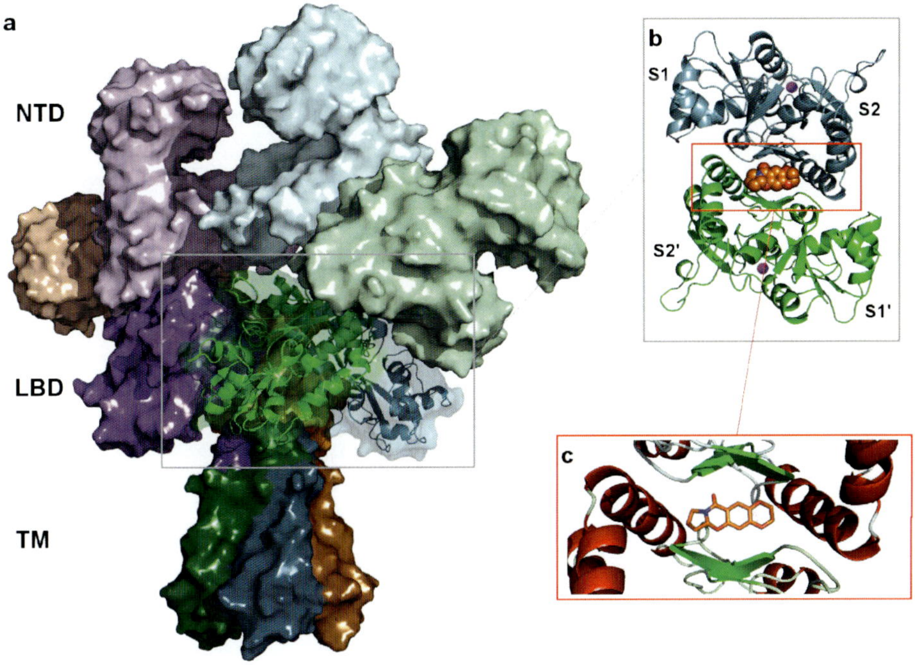


**FIGURE 7.5** Tetrameric AMPA receptor structure, modeled from PDB entry 3KG2 [8, 118]. (a) Colors discriminate individual monomers (green, cyan, purple, orange). One ligand binding domain (LBD) dimer is shown as a transparent surface. (b) Ribbon structure of the complex between the AMPA LBD dimer and the positive modulator CX614, viewed down the twofold symmetry axis relating the monomers. CX614 binds across the symmetry axis. Agonist (glutamate) binding sites are shown as magenta spheres—the agonist and allosteric binding sites are clearly distinct. (c) Close-up view of the binding site for positive allosteric modulators. As the site spans a symmetry axis, a ligand can bind in two equivalent orientations, related by rotation about the axis. A single orientation is shown here for clarity. TM, transmembrane domain; NTD, amino terminal domain.

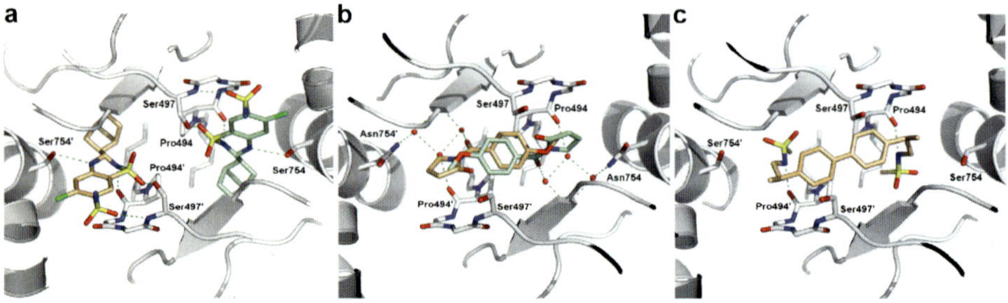


**FIGURE 7.6** Binding modes of the benzothiadiazine (a), benzamide (b), and arylsulfonamide (c) classes of AMPA modulators. Two equivalent, symmetry-related orientations are shown for (a) and (b), while only one orientation is shown for the symmetric ligand (c). **a:** Binding mode of cyclothiazide (**25**; Fig. 7.3), which forms hydrogen bonds with the side chains of Ser497 and Ser754, and with main chain atoms of Pro494 and Ser497. The norbornyl moiety is buried within a hydrophobic pocket, displacing a network of solvent molecules. **b:** Binding mode of aniracetam (**21**; Fig. 7.3), in which the two possible orientations span the symmetry axis and therefore overlap. Aniracetam makes no hydrophilic interactions with protein atoms, and forms just one hydrogen bond with a network of solvent molecules occupying the buried hydrophobic pocket. **c:** Binding mode of the aryl sulfonamide compound (**15**; Fig. 7.2). The sulphonamide occupies a hydrophobic pocket, displacing a network of solvent molecules in a similar way to cyclothiazide, while the sulphonamide NH forms a hydrogen bond with the carbonyl of Pro494.

# 5

# GLUTAMATERGIC SYNAPTIC DYSREGULATION IN SCHIZOPHRENIA

Joseph T. Coyle, Alo Basu, and Michael Benneyworth

## 5.1 INTRODUCTION

Schizophrenia affects approximately 1% of the population, and it is the seventh most costly medical disorder to society [1]. With an age of symptomatic onset in late adolescence-young adulthood, the majority of patients suffer lifelong disabling symptoms that interfere with employment and stable interpersonal relationships. The persistent disability of schizophrenia, in spite of over 50 years of innovation in antipsychotic drug development, suggests that the hypothesized abnormality in dopaminergic neurotransmission [2] does not account for the primary pathophysiolgy of the disorder. Indeed, three separate large-scale studies indicate that the second-generation or atypical antipsychotics that act at dopamine receptors are no more efficacious or tolerable than first-generation typical antipsychotics [3–5]. Both typical and atypical antipsychotics are associated with limited clinical response and poor compliance.

The dopamine hypothesis posits excessive activation of dopamine $D_2$ receptors as the primary pathophysiologic feature of schizophrenia [2]. The hypothesis is based on two critical observations: (1) the clinical potency of antipsychotics in schizophrenia correlates with their affinity for the dopamine $D_2$ receptor, and (2) high doses of stimulants, which release brain dopamine, cause psychosis [6, 7]. The major limitation of the hypothesis is that typical

*Targets and Emerging Therapies for Schizophrenia*, First Edition.
Edited by Jeffrey S. Albert and Michael W. Wood.

and atypical antipsychotics, with the possible exception of clozapine, have negligible effects on cognitive impairments and negative symptoms [8, 9]. Negative symptoms include emotional blunting, reduced motivation/drive, and asociality. Cognitive symptoms often affect executive function, attention, and working memory. It is the cognitive impairments and negative symptoms that result in persistent disability [10]. Furthermore, the severity of negative symptoms and cognitive impairments correlates with the degree of cortical atrophy and ventricular enlargement [11–15], a pathologic process that proceeds for 5 to 10 years after onset of psychosis. Interestingly, this progressive loss of cortical volume does not appear to be due to degeneration and the subsequent loss of neurons but rather to their atrophy [16, 17]. Thus, a plausible theory for the pathophysiology of schizophrenia must take into account cortical atrophy and cognitive symptoms.

## 5.2 ORIGINS OF THE GLUTAMATE HYPOTHESIS: DISSOCIATIVE ANESTHETICS AND SCHIZOPHRENIA

Since dissociative anesthetics including ketamine and phencyclidine were first introduced 40 years ago, it has been appreciated that they can produce in adults a clinical picture closely resembling, if not indistinguishable from schizophrenia, especially if they are chronically abused [18, 19]. Lodge and colleagues discovered that among the many other neuropharmacologic effects of anesthetics, the dissociative anesthetics are use-dependent, noncompetitive antagonists of the N-methyl-D-aspartic acid (NMDA)-subtype of the glutamate receptor family [20]. Ligand binding studies further clarified the NMDA receptor (NMDAR) localization of the "phencyclidine (PCP) receptor" [21]. Javitt and Zukin noted that the concentration of phencyclidine (PCP) associated with psychosis was in the same range that would bind to the NMDA receptor, and proposed that schizophrenia might result from hypofunction of NMDA receptors [22]. However, there were concerns with this causal interpretation, an alternative explanation being that individuals who abused PCP or ketamine might be at high risk for a schizophrenic-type reaction.

In a landmark study, Krystal and colleagues directly addressed this concern by demonstrating that infusion of low, subhypnotic doses of ketamine into normal volunteers in a laboratory setting produced negative symptoms including blunted affect and withdrawal and rather selective impairments in memory and cognition that are specifically associated with schizophrenia [23]. Acute administration of ketamine in normal subjects did not produce a robust recreation of positive symptoms such as hallucinations, although paranoia, thought disorder, and loose associations were evident. Nevertheless, patients with schizophrenia who were not receiving antipsychotics exhibited a significant exacerbation of positive symptoms that were unique to the given patient after administration of low dose ketamine [24]. The remarkable similarities in the subtle cognitive abnormalities observed in schizophrenia and the effects of low dose ketamine in normal volunteers were elaborated upon by others [25, 26].

Subsequent studies using the low dose ketamine paradigm in normal subjects demonstrated that it also produced physiologic abnormalities associated with schizophrenia. These abnormalities, which are not considered in the clinical diagnosis of schizophrenia, are nonetheless reflective of the underlying pathology of the disease and are therefore called "endophenotypes." Smooth pursuit and antisaccade eye tracking abnormalities are an endophenotype of schizophrenia (Holtzman et al., [27]). Low dose ketamine disrupts eye tracking in normal individuals [28]. PET imaging studies that monitor the displacement of [$^{11}$C] raclopride by endogenous dopamine demonstrated increased dopamine release in the striatum with an amphetamine challenge in schizophrenia patients as compared with controls [29]. Pretreatment with a low dose ketamine caused healthy control subjects to also exhibit increased dopamine release with amphetamine challenge as compared with placebo-treated controls. Sensory gating abnormalities are common in schizophrenia and reflect abnormal cortical and subcortical information processing. Such abnormalities can be studied noninvasively in a laboratory setting in humans as well as animals. For example, prepulse inhibition (PPI) of the acoustic startle response is observed when the response to a startling stimulus is reduced when preceded by a few milliseconds by a nonstartling tone. Individuals with schizophrenia exhibit impaired PPI [30]. Treatment of experimental animals such as rodents with ketamine causes disruption in PPI in an analogous fashion to what is observed in schizophrenia [31]. Individuals with schizophrenia exhibit behavioral evidence of temporal information processing deficits and reduced mismatch negativity (MMN) in sensory event-related brain potentials [32], which can be produced in healthy control subjects by low dose ketamine [33].

## 5.3 NEUROCHEMISTRY OF THE GLUTAMATERGIC SYNAPSE IN SCHIZOPHRENIA

Many features of the pathophysiology of schizophrenia implicate neuroanatomic, organizational, and functional features of the corticolimbic glutamatergic system. Glutamatergic pyramidal cells are the projecting neurons that interconnect prefrontal cortex, temporal cortex/hippocampus, and thalamus, regions of the brain that structural and functional brain imaging studies have demonstrated to exhibit abnormalities in schizophrenia [34]. Furthermore, the NMDA subtype of glutamate receptor plays multiple roles in brain functions that have been implicated in the cellular pathology of schizophrenia. These include regulating neuronal migration [35], neuronal differentiation [36], response to trophic factors [37], functional plasticity such as long-term potentiation (LTP) [38] of synaptic transmission, and the development of dendritic spines [39]. Abnormal migration of cortical γ-aminobutyric acid (GABA)ergic interneurons [40], neuronal atrophy [41], impaired memory, and reduced dendritic spines [42] have all been observed in schizophrenia.

Postmortem studies have provided convincing evidence that disruption in the modulation of NMDA receptors is part of the pathophysiology of schizophrenia. In addition to the glutamate recognition site on NR2 subunit, the NR1 subunit has a binding site for glycine and D-serine (also known as the glycine B receptor to distinguish it from the inhibitory glycine receptor) [43] that must be occupied in order for glutamate to open the ion channel [44, 45]. D-serine is a full agonist at the glycine B receptor on the NMDAR [46]. Tissue levels of D-serine are determined by the activity of its synthetic enzyme, serine racemase, and the activity of its catabolic enzyme D-amino acid oxidase [47–49]. Notably, serine racemase expression is high in the corticolimbic regions of the brain, whereas D-amino acid oxidase expression is quite low in these regions [47, 50]. Postmortem studies have demonstrated increased D-amino acid oxidase activity and transcript levels in subregions of the cerebral cortex in subjects with a diagnosis of schizophrenia as compared with controls or those with a diagnosis of bipolar disorder [51–53]. The increases in D-amino acid oxidase in schizophrenia vary from approximately 30% to twofold and are unrelated to neuroleptic exposure. In contrast, serine racemase activity and mRNA are relatively unaffected in schizophrenia. Measurement of the cerebral spinal fluid (CSF) of living subjects with schizophrenia has revealed reduced levels of D-serine although postmortem brain tissue levels do not appear abnormal [54, 55]. However, postmortem tissue levels of D-serine may imperfectly reflect its functional status since the regulation of its synthesis is dynamic and influenced by presynaptic glutamatergic neuronal activity [56].

Glutamate carboxypeptidase II (CGPII) hydrolyzes the neuropeptide N-acetyl-aspartyl glutamate (NAAG) [57], which is colocalized with and released by corticolimbic glutamatergic pyramidal neurons [58, 59] as well as components of other neuronal systems (noradrenergic locus coeruleus neurons, cholinergic motor neurons, limbic GABAergic neurons) [60]. NAAG selectively inhibits NMDAR currents in a glycine-reversible fashion [59]. It also is an agonist at mGluR3 receptors that downregulate glutamate release [61, 62] although recent findings in the mouse perforant pathway contradict these conclusions [63]. Five postmortem studies carried out with different patient cohorts have demonstrated reduced activity, protein, and mRNA for GCPII in corticolimbic structures in schizophrenia [64–68].

Kynurenic acid is a metabolite of tryptophan that inhibits NMDA receptors by blocking the glycine B receptor site [69, 70]. It is also an antagonist of the alpha 7-nicotinic receptor [71], which has been implicated in schizophrenia. Systemic treatment of rats with kynurenic acid, like dissociative anaesthetics, causes the ventral tegmental area (VTA) dopaminergic neurons to exhibit burst firing, which can be reversed by treatment with the partial glycine B receptor agonist, D-cycloserine (DCS) [72]. A postmortem study revealed elevated kynurenic acid levels in the prefrontal cortex of schizophrenics as compared with controls [73]. Several studies of cerebrospinal fluid (CSF) have shown elevated levels of kynurenic acid in schizophrenia [74–76].

NMDA receptors are anchored in the postsynaptic density (PSD), a protein complex with which over a hundred other proteins are associated [77]. Postmortem studies have measured subunits of the NMDA receptors as well as components of the PSD. Meador-Woodruff and colleagues described reductions in NMDA, AMPA (2-amino-3-(5-methyl-3-oxo-1,2-oxazol-4-yl)propanoic acid), and kainate receptor subunits in the thalamus (Ibrahim et al., [78]), as well as PSD-95, SAP102, and NF-L; PSD-95 and NF-L were reduced in the anterior cingulated cortex [79, 80], with the latter also affected in bipolar disorder. Toyooka et al. similarly found significant reductions in the expression of SAP97 in the prefrontal cortex and SAP102 in the hippocampus and prefrontal cortex in schizophrenia [81, 82]. The most consistent changes involved NF-L, SAP102, PSD-95, and PSD-93, which were reported to be reduced in the anterior cingulate cortex and the dorsolateral prefrontal cortex (DLPFC). An increased transcript expression was associated with decreased protein expression of PSD-95. Other synaptic components involved in glutamatergic neurotransmission are also affected in schizophrenia. The excitatory amino acid transporters (EAAT1 and EAAT2) are elevated in the thalamus [83], which should further compromise glutamatergic neurotransmission. Consistent reductions in the kainic acid receptor have been described using ligand binding [84] and *in situ* hybridization or reverse transcriptase polymerase chain reaction (RT-PCR) of mRNA encoding its subunits [85, 86] in studies of prefrontal cortex and hippocampus in schizophrenia [87, 88]. Furthermore, immunohistochemical studies revealed significant reductions in the density of GluR5, GluR6, and GluR7 immunoreactivity on the pyramidal cell dendrites found both in the stratum radiatum and in the stratum moleculare of hippocampal sectors CA1, CA2, and CA3 in patients with schizophrenia [89]. These findings are consistent with the results of several case control and association studies that implicate genes encoding the kainic acid receptor subunits and risk for schizophrenia [90, 91].

## 5.4 ARE THERE SENSITIVE DEVELOPMENTAL PERIODS FOR NMDAR HYPOFUNCTION IN SCHIZOPHRENIA RISK?

The ~50% concordance rate for schizophrenia in monozygotic twins indicates that the disease is both genetic and environmental in etiology [92]. It is therefore important to consider environmental factors and their biological substrates. In contrast to the modest amount of risk conferred by any individual putative schizophrenia gene identified to date, environmental events such as prenatal influenza infection and severe maternal stress increase schizophrenia risk ~3- to 5-fold [93]. These strong epidemiological findings point to a sensitive period in brain development during which the fetus may be more vulnerable to accumulating insults that predispose the individual to schizophrenia in adulthood. Although the specific biological mechanisms of these insults have not yet been elucidated, the multiple roles of NMDAR-mediated neurotransmission in brain development of preclinical species are widely documented [94–96].

Application of NMDAR antagonists during early postnatal development results in many phenomena related to the schizophrenia endophenotype in adulthood. Based on detailed modeling of the timing of key neurodevelopmental events, the first two postnatal weeks in the rat are considered roughly equivalent to human fetal development at the second trimester of pregnancy [97]. Perinatal blockade of NMDARs with PCP or MK-801 within this time frame has been shown to cause deficits in PPI of the acoustic startle reflex in adult rats [98, 99]. Elevated PCP- and amphetamine-induced hyperlocomotion have been observed during adolescence and adulthood in rats treated perinatally with PCP, indicating dysregulation of glutamatergic and dopaminergic neurotransmission, respectively [100, 101]. Early postnatal MK-801 treatment results in persistent cognitive deficits in set-shifting and working memory [102]. Treatment with PCP during this period has resulted in deficits in spatial reference, reversal, and spatial working memory, during adolescence and adulthood [103, 104]. Encouraging for the prospects of novel therapeutics, some adult deficits have been attenuated by treatment with D-serine or a selective inhibitor of glycine transporter-1, both of which result in increased NMDAR-mediated neurotransmission [101, 104].

Early postnatal NMDAR blockade also recapitulates a pathologic hallmark of schizophrenia, a decrease in parvalbumin (PV)-positive interneurons in the hippocampus and cortex [105–108]. Transient postnatal administration of PCP resulted in a selective decrease in PV-positive neurons in adult primary somatosensory, motor, and retrosplenial cortices [109]. Prenatal administration of MK-801 resulted in a selective decrease in PV-positive neurons in adult medial prefrontal cortex [110]. Although selective reduction in PV can be achieved by sub-acute administration of NMDAR blockers in adult rodents, the findings that this neuropathology can be induced by perinatal administration and be evident several weeks later in the mature brain demonstrate that the developing brain is vulnerable to NMDAR hypofunction and that this type of manipulation leaves a lasting lesion.

If the perinatal period is the first environmental “risk window” for schizophrenia, late adolescence/early adulthood is the next phase of the disease in which neurodevelopmental events are of acute interest, as this is the period during which psychotic symptoms typically emerge. Onset of schizophrenia corresponds to the timing of significant pruning of cortical synapses that are located on dendritic spines [111]. Postmortem studies have shown that the density of these spines on layer III frontal and temporal cortical pyramidal neurons are significantly reduced in schizophrenia [112–114]. The pruning process is regulated by neuronal activity [115], and one can hypothesize multiple ways in which the pathological and genetic findings related to NMDA-mediated neurotransmission might contribute to dysregulation at this stage.

For example, the depressed NR1 expression and elevated NR2B expression observed in schizophrenia [116] may interfere with the pruning process in a variety of ways, by resulting in hypofunction of NMDAR-mediated neurotransmission, or excitotoxicity or the potentiation of inappropriate synapses due to increased $Ca^{2+}$ influx through NMDARs.

Another major process of brain development peaking during late adolescence/early adulthood is the myelination of the brain, which supports the connectivity between different brain areas implicated in schizophrenia pathology [117]. Diffusion tensor imaging of white matter has revealed white matter abnormalities in schizophrenia, although it is difficult to distinguish between loss of coherence of white matter tracts, loss of fibers, and loss of myelination using these methods [118, 119]. Results of functional imaging studies have suggested that there is disruption of the temporal synchrony of functional neural networks in the brain in schizophrenia [120]. The oligodendroglial processes that extend to myelinate axons express NMDA receptors during development [121]. The recent finding that prenatal PCP exposure retards oligodendrocyte maturation, resulting in fewer myelin-producing cells, provides a direct link between NMDAR-mediated neurotransmission, early development, and myelination [122].

## 5.5 SCHIZOPHRENIA RISK GENES AND GLUTAMATERGIC NEUROTRANSMISSION

Currently, there is debate over the reliability of findings for risk genes identified in association studies. Some have argued that genetic evidence, unbiased with respect to candidate-gene-based hypotheses, suggests that copy number variants (CNVs) involving deletions or reduplications of stretches of DNA or new mutations are more clearly related to schizophrenia risk [123]. Nevertheless, meta-analyses of the results of whole genome-wide association (WGA) studies do point to several genes that plausibly confer risk for schizophrenia [124, 125]. The underlying assumption is that schizophrenia is a disorder of complex genetics in which multiple risk alleles of moderate effect interact with environment to produce the phenotype.

One of the first putative risk genes to emerge from an expanded association study involving 191 single nuceotide polymorphisms (SNPs ) over a 5-Mb region of 13q34was *G72* [126]. It encodes for a protein that binds to D-amino acid oxidase (DAAO), the enzyme that catabolizes D-serine and plays an important role in regulating its tissue levels. It is of relatively recent evolutionary appearance, being present only in primates. Originally, it was thought that *G72* activated DAAO, thus its designation DAO activator (DAOA). However, more recent research has shown that cultured cells, which have been transfected with *G72*, generate a protein that inhibits DAAO [127]. Thus, mutations in *G72* would likely result in disinhibition of DAAO, thereby reducing the availability of D-serine. Since *G72* was first proposed as a risk gene for schizophrenia, over a dozen studies have supported this association [128]. The impressively replicable association of *G72* with the risk for schizophrenia converges with clinical findings that serum and CSF D-serine levels are reduced in subjects with schizophrenia [54, 129]. Furthermore, placebo-controlled clinical trials have demonstrated that D-serine reduces negative symptoms, improves cognition, and reduces positive symptoms in patients with chronic schizophrenia who are receiving concurrent typical antipsychotic medications [130, 131].

Several association studies have shown that the gene encoding DAAO itself is also linked to the risk of schizophrenia [126, 132, 133]. Although the enzymatic consequences of DAAO allelic variation are not known, the fact that postmortem studies reveal elevated activity and expression levels of DAAO in the hippocampus and forebrain of patients with schizophrenia suggests that variants associated with the disorder should alter DAAO in this direction [52, 134]. Notably, one study found a robust epistatic interaction between the DAAO gene and the DAOA gene in schizophrenia with an odds ratio of 9.3 [135]. A less robust but replicated finding suggests that serine racemase itself may be a risk gene for schizophrenia [136]. A single nucleotide polymorphism is the 5′ promoter region of the gene is associated with schizophrenia and results in reduced expression of serine racemase [137]. This would result in reduced D-serine levels and consequent NMDAR hypofunction. PICK 1, a protein that interacts with serine racemase [138], has also been identified as a possible risk gene for schizophrenia in a Han Chinese population [139]. A recent meta-analytic study has implicated the gene encoding the NMDAR subunit NR2B (GRIN2B) in schizophrenia risk [140]. This subunit is associated with greater conductance of $Ca^{2+}$ than the other NR2 subunit isoforms, is highly expressed during development, and normally drops off in expression in adulthood [141].

Dysbindin (DTNP1;6p24) is another promising risk gene for schizophrenia, in that its association with schizophrenia has been replicated in several independent studies and it has strong biological plausibility (for review see Reference [142]. The dysbindin protein is concentrated in the presynaptic glutamatergic terminals where it interacts with synapsin 1 and SNAP, modulating the vesicular release of glutamate [143]. The expression of dysbindin is reduced in the prefrontal cortex and hippocampus in schizophrenia [144, 145]. Consistent with the profile of a risk gene, the dysbindin genotype associates inversely with general cognitive ability and poor premorbid function in schizophrenia [146, 147].

The association of the gene encoding neuregulin (NRG) with the risk for schizophrenia is quite robust [148]. NRG is a member of the ErbB signaling pathway that regulates neuronal development, migration, myelination, and synaptic maintenance (for review, see Reference [149]. An NRG1 hypomorph mouse displays abnormal behaviors that are reversed by the atypical antipsychotic clozapine and exhibits reduced phosphorylation of the NR2B subunit at Y1472, resulting in NMDAR hypofunction [150]. A hypomorph of the type

3 NRG1 isoform has enlarged lateral ventricles, decreased spine density, hypofunction of the prefrontal cortex and hippocampus, and deficits in PPI [151]. Thus, both mouse models share important endophenotypic features with schizophrenia. Using a postmortem tissue stimulation approach, Hahn and colleagues showed a marked increase in NRG1-induced activation of ErbB4 in the prefrontal cortex in schizophrenia although the absolute levels of NRG1 ErbB4 did not differ significantly between schizophrenia and control groups [152].

## 5.6 CORTICOLIMBIC GABAERGIC DEFICITS IN SCHIZOPHRENIA

Thirty years ago, Spokes et al. first reported reduced activity of glutamic acid decarboxylase (GAD) in cortex and GABA in the nucleus accumbens and thalamus in a postmortem study in patients with schizophrenia as compared to suitable controls [153]. However, the findings were highly variable, and other studies suggested that the loss of GAD activity may be an artifact of a slow death, to which institutionalized schizophrenic patients were particularly prone [154, 155]. Recent studies from several laboratories utilizing brain bank tissue from diverse sources have described compelling reductions of the presynaptic markers for a subpopulation of GABAergic interneurons in the frontal cortex and in the hippocampal formation (for review see Reference [156]). Two genetically distinct forms of glutamic acid decarboxylase (GAD) have been identified on the basis of molecular weight (65 and 67 kDa) [157]. GAD67 is preferentially expressed in perikarya and dendrites, whereas GAD65 is more prominently expressed in axons and terminals [158]. Several studies have described reduced numbers of GAD67 mRNA expressing neurons in the prefrontal cortex and an overall reduced expression of GAD67 as compared with GAD65 [159–162]. In a laminar analysis, Volk et al. reported that the density of neurons with detectable GAD67 mRNA was significantly decreased in the intermediate layers of the prefrontal cortex but that the level of GAD67 mRNA expression per neuron did not differ from control subjects [163].

GABAergic interneurons also express calcium-binding proteins including calretinin, calbindin, and PV [164]. The levels of expression of these proteins are modulated by afferent synaptic activity [165]. PV is expressed predominantly in chandelier and basket cells in the cortex, which receive direct input from pyramidal neurons. Their synaptic contacts are concentrated on the proximal axon in structures known as "cartridges" and the soma of the pyramidal cell, thereby exerting a major influence over pyramidal cell firing. These are fast firing interneurons that coordinate cortical excitatory output. Calbindin is localized to double bouquet cells; calretinin is found in both double bouquet and bipolar neurons. The expression of PV, but not calretinin, was reduced in the prefrontal cortex in schizophrenia [166]. In contrast to GAD67, which was associated with a significant reduction of positive neurons, the number of neurons with PV mRNA in the prefrontal cortex was unchanged in patients with schizophrenia, whereas the amount of mRNA per neuron was significantly decreased [129]. Reduced expression of GAD67 and PV in the prefrontal cortex has been replicated in studies using DNA chip array [167]. Furthermore, real-time quantitative PCR of the prefrontal cortex, anterior cingulate cortex, the primary motor cortex, and primary visual cortex has shown that there were comparable reductions in the mRNA encoding for somatostatin, PV, GAD67, the GABA membrane transporter, GAT1, and the alpha1 and delta subunits of the $GABA_A$ receptors [168]. In contrast, the expression of calretinin mRNA did not differ between schizophrenia patients and matched controls [169].

GAT1 is another specific presynaptic marker for GABAergic neurons. Initial studies describe significant reductions in GAT1 expression in the prefrontal cortex and hippocampus in schizophrenia as determined by ligand binding methods [170, 171]. Using *in situ* hybridization, Volk et al. reported that GAT1 expression was decreased below the level of detectability in a subpopulation of GABAergic interneurons in the intermediate layers of the DLPFC [163]. GAT1 immunochemistry revealed a reduced density of the cartridges of GABAergic terminal boutons innervating the pyramidal cell proximal axons [172].

Reduction in GAT1 would lead to enhanced GABAergic neurotransmission, whereas a reduction in GAD67 might be associated with reduced GABAergic neurotransmission. Studies of GABA-A receptors support the latter scenario. Early studies using ligand binding techniques revealed a 40% increase in $B_{max}$ but no change in the $k_D$ for the specific binding of $[^3H]$GABA [173]. Later studies demonstrated significant increases in $[^3H]$ muscimol binding to $GABA_A$ receptors in subfields of the hippocampal formation, the anterior cingulate cortex, and the prefrontal cortex [174]. With high resolution, the increase in $GABA_A$ receptors could be localized to pyramidal neurons in the intermediate layers of the cortex [175]. Volk et al. reported a doubling of the $GABA_A$ $\alpha$2-immunoreactive axon initial segments of the pyramidal neurons where the GABAergic chandelier cell cartridges are concentrated [176]. Alpha 1 and alpha 5 subunits of the $GABA_A$ receptor were also reported increased in the prefrontal cortex [177].

## 5.7 WHICH NMDA RECEPTORS ARE HYPOFUNCTIONAL?

NMDA receptors are ubiquitous in the brain and peripheral nervous system. The studies in which low dose ketamine was used to induce symptomatic features of schizophrenia in normal individuals, given their normal performance on the Mini Mental Status Exam, suggests that a very discrete subpopulation of NMDA receptors were being affected under these experimental conditions. The first hint of differential sensitivity of neurons to NMDAR antagonists may have been the study by Grunze et al. [178], which reported that GABAergic interneurons in the CA1 region of the hippocampus were 10-fold more sensitive to the canonical NMDAR antagonist, amino-phosphono-valeric acid (APV), and to NAAG than those on the pyramidal neurons receiving the same Schaffer collateral input. In rodents, the pyramidal neurons in the limbic cortex, especially the retrosplenial cortex, are vulnerable to the excitotoxic effects of dissociative anaesthetics with dramatic overexpression of heat shock proteins [179]. These cytopathologic effects were attenuated by muscimol, a $GABA_A$ receptor agonist [180]. On examining the electrophysiologic mechanisms responsible for these neuropathologic changes induced by dissociative anaesthetics, Li et al. found that in acute slice preparations from the rat limbic cortex, the NMDA receptors on the GABAergic interneurons were disproportionately more sensitive to the antagonist effects of MK-801 as compared with NMDA receptors on pyramidal neurons [181]. Homayoun and Moghaddam [182] reported that NMDAR inhibition in acute prefrontal slices from rat caused a reduction in GABAergic interneuron firing and a delayed disinhibition of the pyramidal neurons. Research by Jodo et al. [183] demonstrates that increased firing of prefrontal pyramidal neurons can be produced by local infusion of MK-801 in the ventral hippocampus.

Several studies now demonstrate that sub-acute or chronic treatment with dissociative anaesthetics including phencyclidine, ketamine, and MK-801 produces a downregulation of presynaptic GABAergic markers including GAD67, PV, and GAT1 in the frontal cortex of rats and mice. Pratt and colleagues have also demonstrated reduced expression of Kv3.1, hypofrontality as demonstrated by 2-deoxyglucose autoradiography, and impairments in executive functions (for review see Reference [184]). Kinney found that the changes in PV and GAD67 immunoreactivity were reversible and were fully replicated with an NR2A-selective antagonist but only partially by an NR2B-selective antagonist [185]. Behrens and colleagues further demonstrated that NMDAR blockers produce a burst of superoxide due to activation in neurons of reduced nicotinamide adenine dinucleotide phosphate (NADPH) oxidase [186]. Pharmacologic treatments that decrease superoxide production prevent the effects of ketamine on inhibitory interneurons of the prefrontal cortex. An electrophysiologic analysis of acute frontal cortical slices prepared from mice treated subchronically with ketamine indicated that the frequency and magnitude of inhibitory postsynaptic potentials (IPSPs) were significantly reduced on pyramidal neurons, and the excitability of the pyramidal neurons were significantly increased [187].

Lisman and colleagues put forward a hypothesis that the counterintuitive disinhibition of the glutamatergic pyramidal neurons after treatment with an NMDAR antagonist reflected the substantial contribution (~30%) of NMDAR channels to the excitatory postsynaptic currents (EPSCs) on GABAergic interneurons so that reduced NMDAR channel activity would have substantial impact on interneuron excitability [188]. Intracellular $Ca^{2+}$ levels could serve as a proxy for GABAergic neuronal firing. AMPA receptors, unlike NMDA receptors, generally do not conduct $Ca^{2+}$. Thus, in spite of increased glutamatergic input to these fast firing GABAergic interneurons, they "misperceive" a reduced glutamatergic tone because of blockade of their NMDA receptors by exogenous dissociative anesthetics or endogenous kynurenic acid, thereby restricting $Ca^{2+}$ influx. To correct for this "misperceived" reduced excitatory input, the PV-positive GABAergic interneurons decrease the expression GAD67 as well as the $Ca^{2+}$ buffering protein, PV [189]).

## 5.8 PSYCHOSIS AS A DOWNSTREAM EVENT

While appearance of psychosis heralds the onset of schizophrenia, psychosis is not unique to schizophrenia and occurs in bipolar disorder, major depressive disorder, and Alzheimer's dementia. The central role of excessive stimulation of dopamine $D_2$ receptors in the pathology of psychosis is well established as essentially all antipsychotic drugs, with the exception of aripiprazole, a partial agonist, act by blocking dopamine $D_2$ receptors. While dysfunction of the dopamine system must be accounted for in any hypothesis about the etiology of schizophrenia, a primary deficit in dopaminergic neurotransmission does not explain many aspects of the schizophrenia prodrome, endophenotypes, and clinical course under treatment with currently available antipsychotics.

NMDAR antagonists have been shown to produce a hyperdopaminergic state in both experimental animals and humans [29, 190]. While the disinhibition of glutamatergic outputs appears to be widespread in the corticolimbic system, disinhibition of the glutamatergic output from the subiculum to the VTA appears to be critical for producing the hyperdopaminergic state with systemic treatment with dissociative anesthetics [188]. Thus, psychosis would be considered a "downstream" event. This interpretation of the pathophysiology of psychosis in schizophrenia has now received compelling support from a recent clinical trial that demonstrated that an mGluR2/3 agonist, which downregulates disinhibited glutamate release, exhibits antipsychotic effects roughly comparable to the atypical antipsychotic, olanzapine [191]. Preclinical studies demonstrated that activation of the mGluR2/3 receptor downregulated the excessive dopamine release caused by treatment with NMDAR antagonists [192].

## 5.9 CONCLUSION

While the role of dopamine in the pathophysiology of psychosis is secure, the inadequacy of antipsychotic medications to address the cognitive deficits and negative symptoms of schizophrenia suggest that dopamine $D_2$ receptor antagonism was not addressing the core pathophysiology of schizophrenia. Viewed from a circuit perspective, one can now appreciate that each of these neurotransmitters plays a distinct, contributory role to the overall phenotype of schizophrenia (Fig. 5.1). We propose that the NMDA receptors on the fast

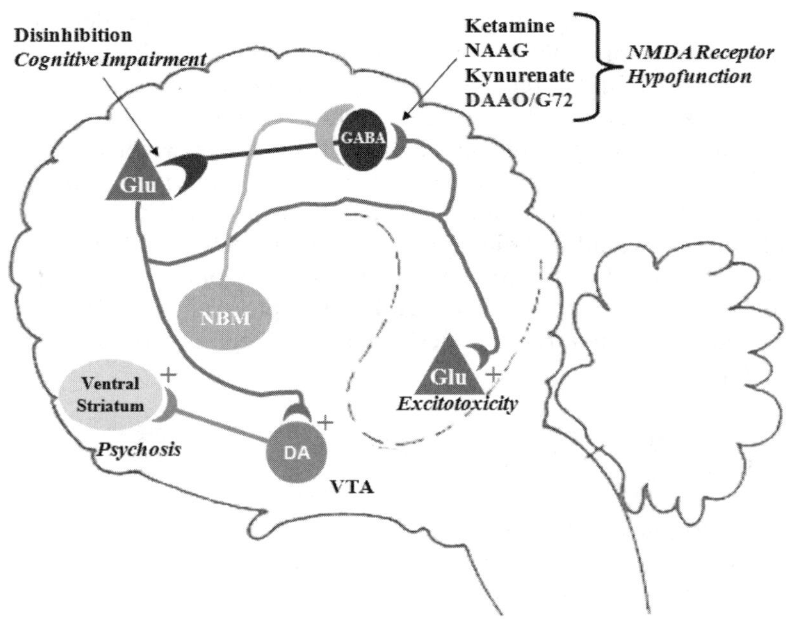


**FIGURE 5.1** Schematic representation of the primary synaptic circuitry affected in schizophrenia. Endogenous antagonists or reduce availability of glycine modulatory site agonists on the NMDA receptor cause reduced firing of the parvalbumen positive, recurrent inhibitory cortical interneurons. This results in disinhibition of pyramidal neurons, thereby driving subcortical dopamine (DA) release. Nucleus Basalis of Meynert (NBM) provides a cholinergic innervation to the GABAergic interneurons mediated by alpha-7 nicotinic receptors.

firing, PV-positive cortical GABAergic interneurons are hypofunctional secondary to elevated endogenous inhibitors, deficient co-agonists, or negative modulation. This neuron-selective NMDAR hypofunction results in reduced inhibitory feedback to pyramidal cells, causing increased excitatory output and disruption of the integrity of cortical columnar processing. In addition, hypofunction of NMDA receptors on the pyramidal neurons themselves may account for their smaller size, reduced dendritic complexity, and reduced number of spines. These primary functional abnormalities in the cortex (dishinibition and atrophy) would account for cognitive impairments and negative symptoms as supported by computational modeling [178, 193]. Consistent with this interpretation, default functional brain imaging in schizophrenia reveals hyperactivation and reduced task-related suppression in default regions in schizophrenia [194]. Disinhibition of the excitatory output of the subiculum would drive increased dopaminergic VTA neuronal activity and secondary psychosis.

Thus, the dysregulation of glutamtergic neurotransmission depends upon which neuronal components of the circuit are considered. Evidence supports hypofunction of NMDA receptors on cortical GABAergic and pyramidal neurons but excess glutamate release from the glutamatergic cortical efferents. Understanding of the pathologic circuit yields a much wider array of drug targets that might effectively address the cognitive impairments and negative symptoms neglected by current dopamine $D_2$ receptor blockers. For example, plausible targets would include agents that enhance NMDAR function such as GlyT1 inhibitors [195], glycine modulatory site agonists [196] or mGluR5 agonists [197], drugs that enhance $GABA_A$ receptor function [198], or drugs that attenuate glutamate release such as mGlur2/3 agonists or positive modulators [191].

## REFERENCES

1. Wu, E.Q., Birnbaum, H.G., Shi, L., Ball, D.E., Kessler, R.C., Moulis, M., Aggarwal, J. (2005). The economic burden of schizophrenia in the United States in 2002. *J Clin Psychiatry*, *66*, 1122–1129.
2. Seeman, P. (1987). Dopamine receptors and the dopamine hypothesis of schizophrenia. *Synapse*, *1*(2), 133–152.
3. Lieberman, J.A., Stroup, T.S., McEvoy, J.P., Swartz, M.S., Rosenheck, R.A., Perkins, D.O., Keefe, R.S., Davis, S.M., Davis, C.E., Lebowitz, B.D., Severe, J., Hsiao, J.K. (2005). Effectiveness of antipsychotic drugs in patients with chronic schizophrenia. *N Engl J Med*, *353*, 1209–1223.
4. Jones, P.B., Barnes, T.R., Davies, L., Dunn, G., Lloyd, H., Hayhurst, K.P., Murray, R.M., Markwick, A., Lewis, S.W. (2006). Randomized controlled trial of the effect on quality of life of second- vs first-generation antipsychotic drugs in schizophrenia: cost utility of the latest antipsychotic drugs in schizophrenia study (CUtLASS 1). *Arch Gen Psychiatry*, *63*(10), 1079–1087.
5. Sikich, L., Frazier, J.A., McClellan, J., Findling, R.L., Vitiello, B., Ritz, L., Ambler, D., Puglia, M., Maloney, A.E., Michael, E., De Jong, S., Slifka, K., Noyes, N., Hlastala, S., Pierson, L., McNamara, N.K., Delporto-Bedoya, D., Anderson, R., Hamer, R.M., Lieberman, J.A. (2008). Double-blind comparison of first- and second-generation antipsychotics in early-onset schizophrenia and schizo-affective disorder: findings from the treatment of early-onset schizophrenia spectrum disorders (TEOSS) study. *Am J Psychiatry*, *165*(11), 1420–1431.
6. Snyder, S.H. (1981). Dopamine receptors, neuroleptics, and schizophrenia. *Am J Psychiatry*, *138*, 460–464.
7. Seeman, P. (2002). Atypical antipsychotics: mechanism of action. *Can J Psychiatry*, *47*, 27–38.
8. Meltzer, H.Y. (1997). Treatment-resistant schizophrenia–the role of clozapine. *Curr Med Res Opin*, *14*, 1–20.
9. Davis, J.M., Chen, N., Glick, I.D. (2003). A meta-analysis of the efficacy of second-generation antipsychotics. *Arch Gen Psychiatry*, *60*, 553–564.

10. Evans, J.D., Bond, G.R., Meyer, P.S., Kim, H.W., Lysaker, P.H., Gibson, P.J., Tunis, S. (2004). Cognitive and clinical predictors of success in vocational rehabilitation in schizophrenia. *Schizophr Res*, *70*, 331–342.

11. Kirkpatrick, B., Buchanan, R.W., Ross, D.E., Carpenter, W.T., Jr (2001). Aseparate disease within the syndrome of schizophrenia. *Arch Gen Psychiatry*, *58*(2), 165–171.

12. Ho, B.C., Andreasen, N.C., Nopoulos, P., Arndt, S., Magnotta, V., Flaum, M. (2003). Progressive structural brain abnormalities and their relationship to clinical outcome: a longitudinal magnetic resonance imaging study early in schizophrenia. *Arch Gen Psychiatry*, *60*(6), 585–594.

13. Antonova, E., Kumari, V., Morris, R., Halari, R., Anilkumar, A., Mehrotra, R., Sharma, T. (2005). The relationship of structural alterations to cognitive deficits in schizophrenia: a voxel-based morphometry study. *Biol Psychiatry*, *58*(6), 457–467.

14. Mitelman, S.A., Brickman, A.M., Shihabuddin, L., Newmark, R.E., Hazlett, E.A., Haznedar, M.M., Buchsbaum, M.S. (2007). A comprehensive assessment of gray and white matter volumes and their relationship to outcome and severity in schizophrenia. *Neuroimage*, *37*(2), 449–462.

15. Hazlett, E.A., Buchsbaum, M.S., Haznedar, M.M., Newmark, R., Goldstein, K.E., Zelmanova, Y., Glanton, C.F., Torosjan, Y., New, A.S., Lo, J.N., Mitropoulou, V., Siever, L.J. (2008). Cortical gray and white matter volume in unmedicated schizotypal and schizophrenia patients. *Schizophr Res*, *101*(1–3), 111–123.

16. Pierri, J.N., Volk, C.L., Auh, S., Sampson, A., Lewis, D.A. (2001). Decreased somal size of deep layer 3 pyramidal neurons in the prefrontal cortex of subjects with schizophrenia. *Arch Gen Psychiatry*, *58*(5), 466–473.

17. Thune, J.J., Uylings, H.B., Pakkenberg, B. (2001). No deficit in total number of neurons in the prefrontal cortex in schizophrenics. *J Psychiatr Res*, *35*(1), 15–21.

18. Luby, E.D., Cohen, B.D., Rosenbaum, G., Gottlieb, J.S., Kelley, R. (1959). Study of a new schizophrenomimetic drug; sernyl. *AMA Arch Neurol Psychiatry*, *81*, 363–369.

19. Itil, T., Keskiner, A., Kiremitci, N., Holden, J.M. (1967). Effect of phencyclidine in chronic schizophrenics. *Can Psychiatr Assoc J*, *12*, 209–212.

20. Anis, N.A., Berry, S.C., Burton, N.R., Lodge, D. (1983). The dissociative anaesthetics, ketamine and phencyclidine, selectively reduce excitation of central mammalian neurones by N-methyl-aspartate. *Br J Pharmacol*, *79*(2), 565–575.

21. Fagg, G.E. (1987). Phencyclidine and related drugs bind to the activated N-methyl-D-aspartate receptor-channel complex in rat brain membranes. *Neurosci Lett*, *76*(2), 221–227.

22. Javitt, D.C., Zukin, S.R. (1991). Recent advances in the phencyclidine model of schizophrenia. *Am J Psychiatry*, *148*, 1301–1308.

23. Krystal, J.H., Karper, L.P., Seibyl, J.P., Freeman, G.K., Delaney, R., Bremner, J.D., et al. (1994). Subanesthetic effects of the noncompetitive NMDA antagonist, ketamine, in humans. Psychotomimetic, perceptual, cognitive, and neuroendocrine responses. *Arch Gen Psychiatry*, *51*, 199–214.

24. Lahti, A.C., Weiler, M.A., TamaraMichaelidis, B.A., Parwani, A., Tamminga, C.A. (2001). Effects of ketamine in normal and schizophrenic volunteers. *Neuropsychopharmacology*, *25*, 455–467.

25. Adler, C.M., Malhotra, A.K., Elman, I., Goldberg, T., Egan, M., Pickar, D., Breier, A. (1999). Comparison of ketamine-induced thought disorder in healthy volunteers and thought disorder in schizophrenia. *Am J Psychiatry*, *156*, 1646–1649.

26. Newcomer, J.W., Farber, N.B., Jevtovic-Todorovic, V., Selke, G., Melson, A.K., Hershey, T., Craft, S., Olney, J.W. (1999). Ketamine-induced NMDA receptor hypofunction as a model of memory impairment and psychosis. *Neuropsychopharmacology*, *20*, 106–118.

27. Holzman, P.S., Kringlen, E., Levy, D.L., Proctor, L.R., Haberman, S.J., Yasillo, N.J. (1977). Abnormal-pursuit eye movements in schizophrenia. Evidence for a genetic indicator. *Arch Gen Psychiatry*, *34*(7), 802–805.

28. Radant, A.D., Bowdle, T.A., Cowley, D.S., Kharasch, E.D., Roy-Byrne, P.P. (1998). Does ketamine-mediated N-methyl-D-aspartate receptor antagonism cause schizophrenia-like oculomotor abnormalities? *Neuropsychopharmacology*, *19*, 434–444.

29. Kegeles, L.S., Abi-Dargham, A., Zea-Ponce, Y., Rodenhiser-Hill, J., Mann, J.J., Van Heertum, R.L., Cooper, T.B., Carlsson, A., Laruelle, M. (2000). Modulation of amphetamine-induced striatal dopamine release by ketamine in humans: implications for schizophrenia. *Biol Psychiatry*, *48*, 627–640.

30. Braff, D., Stone, C., Callaway, E., Geyer, M., Glick, I., Bali, L. (1978). Prestimulus effects on human startle reflex in normals and schizophrenics. *Psychophysiology*, *15*(4), 339–343.

31. Braff, D.L., Geyer, M.A., Swerdlow, N.R. (2001). Human studies of prepulse inhibition of startle: normal subjects, patient groups,and pharmacological studies. *Psychopharmacology (Berl)*, *156*(2–3), 234–258.

32. Javitt, D.C., Doneshka, P., Zylberman, I., Ritter, W., Vaughan, H.G. Jr (1993). Impairment of early cortical processing in schizophrenia: an event-related potential confirmation study. *Biol Psychiatry*, *33*(7), 513–519.

33. Umbricht, D., Schmid, L., Koller, R., Vollenweider, F.X., Hell, D., Javitt, D.C. (2000). Ketamine-induced deficits in auditory and visual context-dependent processing in healthy volunteers: implications for models of cognitive deficits in schizophrenia. *Arch Gen Psychiatry*, *57*(12), 1139–1147.

34. Hulshoff, P.H.E., Kahn, R.S. (2008). What happens after the first episode? A review of progressive brain changes in chronically ill patients with schizophrenia. *Schizophr Bull*, *34*, 354–366.

35. Komuro, H., Rakic, P. (1993). Modulation of neuronal migration by NMDA receptors. *Science*, *260*(5104), 95–97.

36. Pearce, I.A., Cambray-Deakin, M.A., Burgoyne, R.D. (1987). Glutamate acting on NMDA receptors stimulates neurite outgrowth from cerebellar granule cells. *FEBS Lett*, *223*(1), 143–147.

37. Black, I.B. (1999). Trophic regulation of synaptic plasticity. *J Neurobiol*, *41*(1), 108–118.

38. Harris, E.W., Ganong, A.H., Cotman, C.W. (1984). Long-term potentiation in the hippocampus involves activation of N-methyl-D-aspartate receptors. *Brain Res*, *323*(1), 132–137.

39. Yasumatsu, N., Matsuzaki, M., Miyazaki, T., Noguchi, J., Kasai, H. (2008). Principles of long-term dynamics of dendritic spines. *J Neurosci*, *28*(50), 13592–13608.

40. Akbarian, S., Bunney, W.E. Jr, Potkin, S.G., Wigal, S.B., Hagman, J.O., Sandman, C.A., Jones, E.G. (1993). Altered distribution of nicotinamide-adenine dinucleotide phosphate-diaphorase cells in frontal lobe of schizophrenics implies disturbances of cortical development. *Arch Gen Psychiatry*, *50*(3), 169–177.

41. Sweet, R.A., Bergen, S.E., Sun, Z., Sampson, A.R., Pierri, J.N., Lewis, D.A. (2004). Pyramidal cell size reduction in schizophrenia: evidence for involvement of auditory feedforward circuits. *Biol Psychiatry*, *55*(12), 1128–1137.

42. Sweet, R.A., Henteleff, R.A., Zhang, W., Sampson, A.R., Lewis, D.A. (2009). Reduced dendritic spine density in auditory cortex of subjects with schizophrenia. *Neuropsychopharmacology*, *34*(2), 374–389.

43. Kuryatov, A., Laube, B., Betz, H., Kuhse, J. (1994). Mutational analysis of the glycine-binding site of the NMDA receptor: structural similarity with bacterial amino acid-binding proteins. *Neuron*, *12*(6), 1291–1300.

44. Johnson, J.W., Ascher, P. (1987). Glycine potentiates the NMDA response in cultured mouse brain neurons. *Nature*, *325*, 529–531.

45. Kleckner, N.W., Dingledine, R. (1988). Requirement for glycine in activation of NMDA receptors expressed in Xenopus oocytes. *Science*, *241*, 835–837.

46. Matsui, T., Sekiguchi, M., Hashimoto, A., Tomita, U., Nishikawa, T., Wada, K. (1995). Functional comparison of D-serine and glycine in rodents: the effect on cloned NMDA receptors and the extracellular concentration. *J Neurochem*, *65*, 454–458.

47. Schell, M.J., Molliver, M.E., Snyder, S.H. (1995). D-serine, an endogenous synaptic modulator: localization to astrocytes and glutamatestimulated release. *Proc Natl Acad Sci U S A*, *92*, 3948–3952.

48. Wolosker, H., Sheth, K.N., Takahashi, M., Mothet, J.P., Brady, J.R.O., Ferris, C.D. et al. (1999a). Purification of serine racemase: biosynthesis of the neuromodulator D-serine. *Proc Natl Acad Sci U S A*, *96*, 721–725.

49. Wolosker, H., Blackshaw, S., Snyder, S.H. (1999b). Serine racemase: a glial enzyme synthesizing D-serine to regulate glutamate-N-methyl-D-aspartate neurotransmission. *Proc Natl Acad Sci U S A*, *96*, 13409–13414.

50. Hashimoto, A., Nishikawa, T., Oka, T., Takahashi, K. (1993). Endogenous D-serine in rat brain: N-methyl-D-aspartate receptor-related distribution and aging. *J Neurochem*, *60*, 783–786.

51. Kapoor, R., Lim, K.S., Cheng, A., Garrick, T., Kapoor, V. (2006). Preliminary evidence for a link between schizophrenia and NMDA-glycine site receptor ligand metabolic enzymes, d-amino acid oxidase (DAAO) and kynurenine aminotransferase-1 (KAT-1). *Brain Res*, *1106*(1), 205–210.

52. Madeira, C., Freitas, M.E., Vargas-Lopes, C., Wolosker, H., Panizzutti, R. (2008). Increased brain D-amino acid oxidase (DAAO) activity in schizophrenia. *Schizophr Res*, *101*(1–3), 76–83.

53. Burnet, P.W., Eastwood, S.L., Bristow, G.C., Godlewska, B.R., Sikka, P., Walker, M., Harrison, P.J. (2008). D-amino acid oxidase activity and expression are increased in schizophrenia. *Mol Psychiatry*, *13*(7), 658–660.

54. Hashimoto, K., Engberg, G., Shimizu, E., Nordin, C., Lindström, L.H., Iyo, M. (2005). Reduced D-serine to total serine ratio in the cerebrospinal fluid of drug naive schizophrenic patients. *Prog Neuropsychopharmacol Biol Psychiatry*, *29*(5), 767–769.

55. Bendikov, I., Nadri, C., Amar, S., Panizzutti, R., De Miranda, J., Wolosker, H. et al. (2006). A CSF and postmortem brain study of D-serine metabolic parameters in schizophrenia. *Schizophr Res*, *90*, 41–51.

56. Kim, P.M., Aizawa, H., Kim, P.S., Huang, A.S., Wickramasinghe, S.R., Kashani, A.H., Barrow, R.K., Huganir, R.L., Ghosh, A., Snyder, S.H. (2005). Serine racemase: activation by glutamate neurotransmission via glutamate receptor interacting protein and mediation of neuronal migration. *Proc Natl Acad Sci U S A*, *102*(6), 2105–2110.

57. Robinson, M.B., Blakely, R.D., Couto, R., Coyle, J.T. (1987). Hydrolysis of the brain dipeptide N-acetyl-L-aspartyl-L-glutamate. Identification and characterization of a novel N-acetylated a-linked acidic dipeptidase activity from rat brain. *J Biol Chem*, *262*, 14498–14506.

58. Passani, L.A., Vonsattel, J.P., Coyle, J.T. (1997). Distribution of N-acetylaspartylglutamate immunoreactivity in human brain and its alteration in neurodegenerative disease. *Brain Res*, *772*, 9–22.

59. Bergeron, R., Coyle, J.T., Tsai, G., Greene, R.W. (2005). NAAG reduces NMDA receptor current in CA1 hippocampal pyramidal neurons of acute slices and dissociated neurons. *Neuropsychopharmacology*, *30*(1), 7–16.

60. Berger, U.V., Luthi-Carter, R., Passani, L.A., Elkabes, S., Black, I., Konradi, C., Coyle, J.T. (1999). Glutamate carboxypeptidase II is expressed by astrocytes in the adult rat nervous system. *J Comp Neurol*, *415*, 52–64.

61. Bischofberger, J., Schild, D. (1996). Glutamate and N-acetylaspartylglutamate block HVA calcium currents in frog olfactory bulb interneurons via an mGluR2/3-like receptor. *J Neurophysiol*, *76*, 2089–2092.

62. Wroblewska, B., Wroblewski, J.T., Pshenichkin, S., Surin, A., Sullivan, S.E., Neale, J.H. (1997). Nacetylaspartylglutamate selectively activates mGluR3 receptors in transfected cells. *J Neurochem*, *69*, 174–181.

63. Fricker, A.C., Mok, M.H., De La Flor, R., Shah, A.J., Woolley, M., Dawson, L.A., Kew, J.N. (2009). Effects of N-acetylaspartylglutamate (NAAG) at group II mGluRs and NMDAR. *Neuropharmacology*, *56*(6–7), 1060–1067.

64. Tsai, G., Passani, L.A., Slusher, B.S., Carter, R., Baer, L., Kleinman, J.E., Coyle, J.T. (1995). Abnormal excitatory neurotransmitter metabolism in schizophrenic brains. *Arch Gen Psychiatry*, *52*(10), 829–836.

65. Hakak, Y., Walker, J.R., Li, C., Wong, W.H., Davis, K.L., Buxbaum, J.D., et al. (2001). Genomewide expression analysis reveals dysregulation of myelination-related genes in chronic schizophrenia. *Proc Natl Acad Sci U S A*, *98*, 4746–4751.

66. Tkachev, D., Mimmack, M.L., Huffaker, S.J., Ryan, M., Bahn, S. (2007). Further evidence for altered myelin biosynthesis and glutamatergic dysfunction in schizophrenia. *Int J Neuropsychopharmacol*, *10*(4), 557–563.

67. Guilarte, T.R., Hammoud, D.A., McGlothan, J.L., Caffo, B.S., Foss, C.A., Kozikowski, A.P., Pomper, M.G. (2008). Dysregulation of glutamate carboxypeptidase II in psychiatric disease. *Schizophr Res*, *99*(1–3), 324–332.

68. Ghose, S., Chin, R., Gallegos, A., Roberts, R., Coyle, J., Tamminga, C. (2009). Localization of NAAG-related gene expression deficits to the anterior hippocampus in schizophrenia. *Schizophr Res*, *111*(1–3), 131–137. Epub 2009 Apr 28.
69. Birch, P.J., Grossman, C.J., Hayes, A.G. (1988). Kynurenic acid antagonises responses to NMDA via an action at the strychnine-insensitive glycine receptor. *Eur J Pharmacol*, *154*(1), 85–87.
70. Mayer, M.L., Westbrook, G.L., Vyklický, L. Jr. (1988). Sites of antagonist action on N-methyl-D-aspartic acid receptors studied using fluctuation analysis and a rapid perfusion technique. *J Neurophysiol*, *60*(2), 645–663.
71. Hilmas, C., Pereira, E.F., Alkondon, M., Rassoulpour, A., Schwarcz, R., Albuquerque, E.X. (2001). The brain metabolite kynurenic acid inhibits alpha7 nicotinic receptor activity and increases non-alpha7 nicotinic receptor expression: physiopathological implications. *J Neurosci*, *21*(19), 7463–7473.
72. Erhardt, S., Engberg, G. (2002). Increased phasic activity of dopaminergic neurones in the rat ventral tegmental area following pharmacologically elevated levels of endogenous kynurenic acid. *Acta Physiol Scand*, *175*(1), 45–53.
73. Schwarcz, R., Rassoulpour, A., Wu, H.Q., Medoff, D., Tamminga, C.A., Roberts, R.C. (2001). Increased cortical kynurenate content in schizophrenia. *Biol Psychiatry*, *50*, 521–530.
74. Erhardt, S., Blennow, K., Nordin, C., Skogh, E., Lindström, L.H., Engberg, G. (2001). Kynurenic acid levels are elevated in the cerebrospinal fluid of patients with schizophrenia. *Neurosci Lett*, *313*(1–2), 96–98.
75. Nilsson, L.K., Linderholm, K.R., Engberg, G., Paulson, L., Blennow, K., Lindström, L.H., Nordin, C., Karanti, A., Persson, P., Erhardt, S. (2005). Elevated levels of kynurenic acid in the cerebrospinal fluid of male patients with schizophrenia. *Schizophr Res*, *80*(2–3), 315–322.
76. Erhardt, S., Schwieler, L., Engberg, G. (2003). Kynurenic acid and schizophrenia. *Adv Exp Med Biol*, *527*, 155–165.
77. Dosemeci, A., Makusky, A.J., Jankowska-Stephens, E., Yang, X., Slotta, D.J., Markey, S.P. (2007). Composition of the synaptic PSD-95 complex. *Mol Cell Proteomics*, *6*(10), 1749–1760.
78. Ibrahim, H.M., Hogg, A.J. Jr, Healy, D.J., Haroutunian, V., Davis, K.L., Meador-Woodruff, J.H. (2000). Ionotropic glutamate receptor binding and subunit mRNA expression in thalamic nuclei in schizophrenia. *Am J Psychiatry*, *157*(11), 1811–1823.
79. Kristiansen, L.V., Meador-Woodruff, J.H. (2005). Abnormal striatal expression of transcripts encoding NMDA interacting PSD proteins in schizophrenia, bipolar disorder and major depression. *Schizophr Res*, *78*(1), 87–93.
80. Kristiansen, L.V., Beneyto, M., Haroutunian, V., Meador-Woodruff, J.H. (2006). Changes in NMDA receptor subunits and interacting PSD proteins in dorsolateral prefrontal and anterior cingulate cortex indicate abnormal regional expression in schizophrenia. *Mol Psychiatry*, *11*(8), 737–747. 705.
81. Ohnuma, T., Kato, H., Arai, H., Faull, R.L., McKenna, P.J., Emson, P.C. (2000). Gene expression of PSD95 in prefrontal cortex and hippocampus in schizophrenia. *Neuroreport*, *11*(14), 3133–3137.
82. Toyooka, K., Iritani, S., Makifuchi, T., Shirakawa, O., Kitamura, N., Maeda, K., Nakamura, R., Niizato, K., Watanabe, M., Kakita, A., Takahashi, H., Someya, T.,

Nawa, H. (2002). Selective reduction of a PDZ protein, SAP-97, in the prefrontal cortex of patients with chronic schizophrenia. *J Neurochem*, *83*(4), 797–806.

83. Huerta, I., McCullumsmith, R.E., Haroutunian, V., Giménez-Amaya, J.M., Meador-Woodruff, J.H. (2006). Expression of excitatory amino acid transporter interacting protein transcripts in the thalamus in schizophrenia. *Synapse*, *59*(7), 394–402.
84. Scarr, E., Beneyto, M., Meador-Woodruff, J.H., Dean, B. (2005). Cortical glutamatergic markers in schizophrenia. *Neuropsychopharmacology*, *30*(8), 1521–1531.
85. Porter, R.H., Eastwood, S.L., Harrison, P.J. (1997). Distribution of kainate receptor subunit mRNAs in human hippocampus, neocortex and cerebellum, and bilateral reduction of hippocampal GluR6 and KA2 transcripts in schizophrenia. *Brain Res*, *751*(2), 217–231.
86. Beneyto, M., Kristiansen, L.V., Oni-Orisan, A., McCullumsmith, R.E., Meador-Woodruff, J.H. (2007). Abnormal glutamate receptor expression in the medial temporal lobe in schizophrenia and mood disorders. *Neuropsychopharmacology*, *32*(9), 1888–1902.
87. Sokolov, B.P. (1998). Expression of NMDAR1, GluR1, GluR7, and KA1 glutamate receptor mRNAs is decreased in frontal cortex of "neuroleptic-free" schizophrenics: evidence on reversible up-regulation by typical neuroleptics. *J Neurochem*, *71*(6), 2454–2464.
88. Wilson, G.M., Flibotte, S., Chopra, V., Melnyk, B.L., Honer, W.G., Holt, R.A. (2006). DNA copy-number analysis in bipolar disorder and schizophrenia reveals aberrations in genes involved in glutamate signaling. *Hum Mol Genet*, *15*(5), 743–749.
89. Benes, F.M., Todtenkopf, M.S., Kostoulakos, P. (2001). GluR5,6,7 subunit immunoreactivity on apical pyramidal cell dendrites in hippocampus of schizophrenics and manic depressives. *Hippocampus*, *11*(5), 482–491.
90. Pickard, B.S., Malloy, M.P., Christoforou, A., Thomson, P.A., Evans, K.L., Morris, S.W., Hampson, M., Porteous, D.J., Blackwood, D.H., Muir, W.J. (2006). Cytogenetic and genetic evidence supports a role for the kainate-type glutamate receptor gene, GRIK4, in schizophrenia and bipolar disorder. *Mol Psychiatry*, *11*(9), 847–857.
91. Begni, S., Popoli, M., Moraschi, S., Bignotti, S., Tura, G.B., Gennarelli, M. (2002). Association between the ionotropic glutamate receptor kainate 3 (GRIK3) ser-310ala polymorphism and schizophrenia. *Mol Psychiatry*, *7*(4), 416–418.
92. Cardno, A.G., Gottesman, I.I. (2000). Twin studies of schizophrenia: from bow-and-arrow concordances to star wars Mx and functional genomics. *Am J Med Genet*, *97*(1), 12–17.
93. Tandon, R., Keshavan, M.S., Nasrallah, H.A. (2008). Schizophrenia, "just the facts" what we know in 2008. 2. Epidemiology and etiology. *Schizophr Res*, *102*(1–3), 1–18.
94. Shatz, C.J. (1990). Impulse activity and the patterning of connections during CNS development. *Neuron*, *5*, 745–756.
95. Scheetz, A.J., Constantine-Paton, M. (1994). Modulation of NMDA receptor function: implications for vertebrate neural development. *FASEB J*, *8*, 745–752.
96. Penn, A.A. (2001). Early brain wiring: activity-dependent processes. *Schizophr Bull*, *27*(3), 337–347.

97. Clancy, B., Darlington, R.B., Finlay, B.L. (2001). Translating developmental time across mammalian species. *Neuroscience*, *105*, 7–17.
98. Harris, L.W., Sharp, T., Gartlon, J., Jones, D.N., Harrison, P.J. (2003). Long-term behavioural, molecular and morphological effects of neonatal NMDA receptor antagonism. *Eur J Neurosci*, *18*, 1706–1710.
99. Takahashi, M., Kakita, A., Futamura, T., Watanabe, Y., Mizuno, M., Sakimura, K., Castren, E., Nabeshima, T., Someya, T., Nawa, H. (2006). Sustained brain-derived neurotrophic factor up-regulation and sensorimotor gating abnormality induced by postnatal exposure to phencyclidine: comparison with adult treatment. *J Neurochem*, *99*, 770–780.
100. Wang, C., McInnis, J., Ross-Sanchez, M., Shinnick-Gallagher, P., Wiley, J.L., Johnson, K.M. (2001). Long-term behavioral and neurodegenerative effects of perinatal phencyclidine administration: implications for schizophrenia. *Neuroscience*, *107*, 535–550.
101. Depoortère, R., Dargazanli, G., Estenne-Bouhtou, G., Coste, A., Lanneau, C., Desvignes, C., Poncelet, M., Heaulme, M., Santucci, V., Decobert, M., Cudennec, A., Voltz, C., Boulay, D., Terranova, J.P., Stemmelin, J., Roger, P., Marabout, B., Sevrin, M., Vigé, X., Biton, B., Steinberg, R., Françon, D., Alonso, R., Avenet, P., Oury-Donat, F., Perrault, G., Griebel, G., George, P., Soubrié, P., Scatton, B. (2005). Neurochemical, electrochemical, electrophysiological and pharmacological profiles of the selective inhibitor of the glycine transporter-1 SSR504734, a potential new type of antipsychotic. *Neuropsychopharmacology*, *30*, 1963–1985.
102. Stefani, M.R., Moghaddam, B. (2005). Transient N-methyl-D-aspartate receptor blockade in early development causes lasting cognitive deficits relevant to schizophrenia. *Biol Psychiatry*, *57*(4), 433–436.
103. Sircar, R. (2003). Postnatal phencyclidine-induced deficit in adult water maze performance is associated with N-methyl-D-aspartate receptor upregulation. *Int J Dev Neurosci*, *21*, 159–167.
104. Andersen, J.D., Pouzet, B. (2004). Spatial memory deficits induced by perinatal treatment of rats with PCP and reversal effect of D-serine. *Neuropsychopharmacology*, *29*, 1080–1090.
105. Beasley, C.L., Zhang, Z.J., Patten, I., Reynolds, G.P. (2002). Selective deficits in prefrontal cortical GABAergic neurons in schizophrenia defined by the presence of calcium-binding proteins. *Biol Psychiatry*, *52*(7), 708–715.
106. Zhang, Z.J., Reynolds, G.P. (2002). A selective decrease in the relative density of parvalbumin-immunoreactive neurons in the hippocampus in schizophrenia. *Schizophr Res*, *55*, 1–10.
107. Knable, M.B., Barci, B.M., Webster, M.J., Meador-Woodruff, J., Torrey, E.F., Stanley Neuropathology Consortium (2004). Molecular abnormalities of the hippocampus in severe psychiatric illness: postmortem findings from the Stanley Neuropathology Consortium. *Mol Psychiatry*, *9*(6), 609–620. 544.
108. Reynolds, G.P., Abdul-Monim, Z., Neill, J.C., Zhang, Z.J. (2004). Calcium binding protein markers of GABA deficits in schizophrenia—postmortem studies and animal models. *Neurotox Res*, *6*(1), 57–61.
109. Wang, C.Z., Yang, S.F., Xia, Y., Johnson, K.M. (2008). Postnatal phencyclidine administration selectively reduces adult cortical parvalbumin-containing interneurons. *Neuropsychopharmacology*, *33*(10), 2442–2455.

110. Abekawa, T., Ito, K., Nakagawa, S., Koyama, T. (2007). Prenatal exposure to an NMDA receptor antagonist, MK-801 reduces density of parvalbumin-immunoreactive GABAergic neurons in the medial prefrontal cortex and enhances phencyclidine-induced hyperlocomotion but not behavioral sensitization to methamphetamine in postpubertal rats. *Psychopharmacology (Berl)*, *192*(3), 303–316.

111. Bourgeois, J.P., Goldman-Rakic, P.S., Rakic, P. (1994). Synaptogenesis in the prefrontal cortex of rhesus monkeys. *Cereb Cortex*, *4*, 78–96.

112. Lewis, D.A. (1997). Development of the prefrontal cortex during adolescence: insights into vulnerable neural circuits in schizophrenia. *Neuropsychopharmacology*, *16*, 385–398.

113. Garey, L.J., Ong, W.Y., Patel, T.S., Kanani, M., Davis, A., Mortimer, A.M., Barnes, T.R., Hirsch, S.R. (1998). Reduced dendritic spine density on cerebral cortical pyramidal neurons in schizophrenia. *J Neurol Neurosurg Psychiatry*, *65*(4), 446–453.

114. Glantz, L.A., Lewis, D.A. (2008). Decreased dendritic spine density on prefrontal cortical pyramidal neurons in schizophrenia. *Arch Gen Psychiatry*, *57*(1), 65–73.

115. Segal, M., Andersen, P. (2000). Dendritic spines shaped by synaptic activity. *Curr Opin Neurobiol*, *10*(5), 582–586.

116. Gao, X.M., Sakai, K., Roberts, R.C., Conley, R.R., Dean, B., Tamminga, C.A. (2000). Ionotropic glutamate receptors and expression of N-methyl-D-aspartate receptor subunits in subregions of human hippocampus: effects of schizophrenia. *Am J Psychiatry*, *157*, 1141–1149.

117. Benes, F.M. (1989). Myelination of cortical-hippocampal relays during late adolescence. *Schizophr Bull*, *15*(4), 585–593.

118. Kubicki, M., Park, H., Westin, C.F., Nestor, P.G., Mulkern, R.V., Maier, S.E., Niznikiewicz, M., Connor, E.E., Levitt, J.J., Frumin, M., Kikinis, R., Jolesz, F.A., McCarley, R.W., Shenton, M.E. (2005). DTI and MTR abnormalities in schizophrenia: analysis of white matter integrity. *Neuroimage*, *26*(4), 1109–1118.

119. Kubicki, M., McCarley, R., Westin, C.F., Park, H.J., Maier, S., Kikinis, R., Jolesz, F.A., Shenton, M.E. (2007). A review of diffusion tensor imaging studies in schizophrenia. *J Psychiatr Res*, *41*(1–2), 15–30.

120. Ragland, J.D., Yoon, J., Minzenberg, M.J., Carter, C.S. (2007). Neuroimaging of cognitive disability in schizophrenia: search for a pathophysiological mechanism. *Int Rev Psychiatry*, *19*(4), 417–427.

121. Salter, M.G., Fern, R. (2005). NMDA receptors are expressed in developing oligodendrocyte processes and mediate injury. *Nature*, *438*(7071), 1167–1171.

122. Lindahl, J.S., Kjellsen, B.R., Tigert, J., Miskimins, R. (2008). In utero PCP exposure alters oligodendrocyte differentiation and myelination in developing rat frontal cortex. *Brain Res*, *1234*, 137–147.

123. International Schizophrenia Consortium (2008). Rare chromosomal deletions and duplications increase risk of schizophrenia. *Nature*, *455*(7210), 237–241. Epub 2008 Jul 30.

124. Allen, N.C., Bagade, S., McQueen, M.B., Ioannidis, J.P., Kavvoura, F.K., Khoury, M.J., Tanzi, R.E., Bertram, L. (2008). Systematic meta-analyses and field synopsis of genetic association studies in schizophrenia: the SzGene database. *Nat Genet*, *40*(7), 827–834.

125. Shi, J., Gershon, E.S., Liu, C. (2008b). Genetic associations with schizophrenia: meta-analyses of 12 candidate genes. *Schizophr Res*, *104*(1–3), 96–107.

126. Chumakov, I., Blumenfeld, M., Guerassimenko, O., Cavarec, L., Palicio, M., Abderrahim, H., Bougueleret, L., Barry, C., Tanaka, H., La Rosa, P., Puech, A., Tahri, N., Cohen-Akenine, A., Delabrosse, S., Lissarrague, S., Picard, F.P., Maurice, K., Essioux, L., Millasseau, P., Grel, P., Debailleul, V., Simon, A.M., Caterina, D., Dufaure, I., Malekzadeh, K., Belova, M., Luan, J.J., Bouillot, M., Sambucy, J.L., Primas, G., Saumier, M., Boubkiri, N., Martin-Saumier, S., Nasroune, M., Peixoto, H., Delaye, A., Pinchot, V., Bastucci, M., Guillou, S., Chevillon, M., Sainz-Fuertes, R., Meguenni, S., Aurich-Costa, J., Cherif, D., Gimalac, A., Van Duijn, C., Gauvreau, D., Ouellette, G., Fortier, I., Raelson, J., Sherbatich, T., Riazanskaia, N., Rogaev, E., Raeymaekers, P., Aerssens, J., Konings, F., Luyten, W., Macciardi, F., Sham, P.C., Straub, R.E., Weinberger, D.R., Cohen, N., Cohen, D. (2002). Genetic and physiological data implicating the new human gene G72 and the gene for D-amino acid oxidase in schizophrenia. *Proc Natl Acad Sci U S A*, *99*(21), 13675–13680.

127. Sacchi, S., Bernasconi, M., Martineau, M., Mothet, J.P., Ruzzene, M., Pilone, M.S., Pollegioni, L., Molla, G. (2008). pLG72 modulates intracellular D-serine levels through its interaction with D-amino acid oxidase: effect on schizophrenia susceptibility. *J Biol Chem*, *283*(32), 22244–22256.

128. Shi, J., Badner, J.A., Gershon, E.S., Liu, C. (2008a). Allelic association of G72/G30 with schizophrenia and bipolar disorder: a comprehensive meta-analysis. *Schizophr Res*, *98*(1–3), 89–97.

129. Hashimoto, K., Fukushima, T., Shimizu, E., Komatsu, N., Watanabe, H., Shinoda, N. et al. (2003). Decreased serum levels of D-serine in patients with schizophrenia: evidence in support of the N-methyl- D-aspartate receptor hypofunction hypothesis of schizophrenia. *Arch Gen Psychiatry*, *60*, 572–576.

130. Tsai, G., Yang, P., Chung, L.C., Lange, N., Coyle, J.T. (1998). D-serine added to antipsychotics for the treatment of schizophrenia. *Biol Psychiatry*, *44*, 1081–1089.

131. Heresco-Levy, U., Javitt, D.C., Ebstein, R., Vass, A., Lichtenberg, P., Bar, G., Catinari, S., Ermilov, M. (2005). D-serine efficacy as add-on pharmacotherapy to risperidone and olanzapine for treatment-refractory schizophrenia. *Biol Psychiatry*, *57*(6), 577–585.

132. Schumacher, J., Jamra, R.A., Freudenberg, J., Becker, T., Ohlraun, S., Otte, A.C., Tullius, M., Kovalenko, S., Bogaert, A.V., Maier, W., Rietschel, M., Propping, P., Nöthen, M.M., Cichon, S. (2004). Examination of G72 and D-amino-acid oxidase as genetic risk factors for schizophrenia and bipolar affective disorder. *Mol Psychiatry*, *9*(2), 203–207.

133. Liu, X., He, G., Wang, X., Chen, Q., Qian, X., Lin, W., Li, D., Gu, N., Feng, G., He, L. (2004). Association of DAAO with schizophrenia in the Chinese population. *Neurosci Lett*, *369*(3), 228–233.

134. Kapoor, R., Lim, K.S., Cheng, A., Garrick, T., Kapoor, V. (2006). Preliminary evidence for a link between schizophrenia and NMDA-glycine site receptor ligand metabolic enzymes, d-amino acid oxidase (DAAO) and kynurenine aminotransferase-1 (KAT-1). *Brain Res*, *1106*(1), 205–210.

135. Corvin, A., McGhee, K.A., Murphy, K., Donohoe, G., Nangle, J.M., Schwaiger, S., Kenny, N., Clarke, S., Meagher, D., Quinn, J., Scully, P., Baldwin, P., Browne, D.,

Walsh, C., Waddington, J.L., Morris, D.W., Gill, M. (2007). Evidence for association and epistasis at the DAOA/G30 and D-amino acid oxidase loci in an Irish schizophrenia sample. *Am J Med Genet B Neuropsychiatr Genet*, *144B*(7), 949–953.

136. Morita, Y., Ujike, H., Tanaka, Y., Otani, K., Kishimoto, M., Morio, A., Kotaka, T., Okahisa, Y., Matsushita, M., Morikawa, A., Hamase, K., Zaitsu, K., Kuroda, S. (2007). A genetic variant of the serine racemase gene is associated with schizophrenia. *Biol Psychiatry*, *61*(10), 1200–1203.

137. Goltsov, A.Y., Loseva, J.G., Andreeva, T.V., Grigorenko, A.P., Abramova, L.I., Kaleda, V.G., Orlova, V.A., Moliaka, Y.K., Rogaev, E.I. (2006). Polymorphism in the 5′-promoter region of serine racemase gene in schizophrenia. *Mol Psychiatry*, *11*(4), 325–326.

138. Fujii, K., Maeda, K., Hikida, T., Mustafa, A.K., Balkissoon, R., Xia, J., Yamada, T., Ozeki, Y., Kawahara, R., Okawa, M., Huganir, R.L., Ujike, H., Snyder, S.H., Sawa, A. (2006). Serine racemase binds to PICK1: potential relevance to schizophrenia. *Mol Psychiatry*, *11*(2), 150–157.

139. Hong, C.J., Liao, D.L., Shih, H.L., Tsai, S.J. (2004). Association study of PICK1 rs3952 polymorphism and schizophrenia. *Neuroreport*, *15*(12), 1965–1967.

140. Li, D., He, L. (2007). Association study between the NMDA receptor 2B subunit gene (GRIN2B) and schizophrenia: a HuGE review and meta-analysis. *Genet Med*, *9*(1), 4–8.

141. Hall, B.J., Ripley, B., Ghosh, A. (2007). NR2B signaling regulates the development of synaptic AMPA receptor current. *J Neurosci*, *27*(49), 13446–13456.

142. Williams, N.M., O'Donovan, M.C., Owen, M.J. (2005). Is the dysbindin gene (DTNBP1) a susceptibility gene for schizophrenia? *Schizophr Bull*, *31*(4), 800–805.

143. Numakawa, T., Yagasaki, Y., Ishimoto, T., Okada, T., Suzuki, T., Iwata, N., Ozaki, N., Taguchi, T., Tatsumi, M., Kamijima, K., Straub, R.E., Weinberger, D.R., Kunugi, H., Hashimoto, R. (2004). Evidence of novel neuronal functions of dysbindin, a susceptibility gene for schizophrenia. *Hum Mol Genet*, *13*, 2699–2708.

144. Talbot, K., Eidem, W.L., Tinsley, C.L., Benson, M.A., Thompson, E.W., Smith, R.J., Hahn, C.G., Siegel, S.J., Trojanowski, J.Q., Gur, R.E., Blake, D.J., Arnold, S.E. (2004). Dysbindin-1 is reduced in intrinsic, glutamatergic terminals of the hippocampal formation in schizophrenia. *J Clin Invest*, *113*, 1353–1363.

145. Weickert, C.S., Straub, R.E., McClintock, B.W., Matsumoto, M., Hashimoto, R., Hyde, T.M., Herman, M.M., Weinberger, D.R., Andkleinman, J.E. (2004). Human dysbindin (DTNBP1) gene expression in normal brain and in schizophrenic prefrontal cortex and midbrain. *Arch Gen Psychiatry*, *61*, 544–555.

146. Burdick, K.E., Lencz, T., Funke, B., Finn, C.T., Szeszko, P.R., Kane, J.M., Kucherlapati, R., Malhotra, A.K. (2006). Genetic variation in DTNBP1 influences general cognitive ability. *Hum Mol Genet*, *15*(10), 1563–1568.

147. Gornick, M.C., Addington, A.M., Sporn, A., Gogtay, N., Greenstein, D., Lenane, M., Gochman, P., Ordonez, A., Balkissoon, R., Vakkalanka, R., Weinberger, D.R., Rapoport, J.L., Straub, R.E. (2005). Dysbindin (DTNBP1, 6p22.3) is associated with childhood-onset psychosis and endophenotypes measured by the Premorbid Adjustment Scale (PAS). *J Autism Dev Disord*, *35*(6), 831–838.

148. Petryshen, T.L., Middleton, F.A., Kirby, A., Aldinger, K.A., Purcell, S., Tahl, A.R., Morley, C.P., McGann, L., Gentile, K.L., Rockwell, G.N., Medeiros, H.M.,

Carvalho, C., Macedo, A., Dourado, A., Valente, J., Ferreira, C.P., Patterson, N.J., Azevedo, M.H., Daly, M.J., Pato, C.N., Pato, M.T., Sklar, P. (2005). Support for involvement of neuregulin 1 in schizophrenia pathophysiology. *Mol Psychiatry*, *10*, 366–374.

149. Mei, L., Xiong, W.C. (2008). Neuregulin 1 in neural development, synaptic plasticity and schizophrenia. *Nat Rev Neurosci*, *9*(6), 437–452.

150. Bjarnadottir, M., Misner, D.L., Haverfield-Gross, S., Bruun, S., Helgason, V.G., Stefansson, H., Sigmundsson, A., Firth, D.R., Nielsen, B., Stefansdottir, R., Novak, T.J., Stefansson, K., Gurney, M.E., Andresson, T. (2007). Neuregulin1 (NRG1) signaling through Fyn modulates NMDA receptor phosphorylation: differential synaptic function in NRG1+/– knock-outs compared with wild-type mice. *J Neurosci*, *27*(17), 4519–4529.

151. Chen, Y.J., Johnson, M.A., Lieberman, M.D., Goodchild, R.E., Schobel, S., Lewandowski, N., Rosoklija, G., Liu, R.C., Gingrich, J.A., Small, S., Moore, H., Dwork, A.J., Talmage, D.A., Role, L.W. (2008). Type III neuregulin-1 is required for normal sensorimotor gating, memory-related behaviors, and corticostriatal circuit components. *J Neurosci*, *28*(27), 6872–6883.

152. Hahn, C.G., Wang, H.Y., Cho, D.S., Talbot, K., Gur, R.E., Berrettini, W.H., Bakshi, K., Kamins, J., Borgmann-Winter, K.E., Siegel, S.J., Gallop, R.J., Arnold, S.E. (2006). Altered neuregulin 1-erbB4 signaling contributes to NMDA receptor hypofunction in schizophrenia. *Nat Med*, *12*(7), 824–828.

153. Spokes, E.G., Garrett, N.J., Rossor, M.N., Iversen, L.L. (1980). Distribution of GABA in post-mortem brain tissue from control, psychotic and Huntington's chorea subjects. *J Neurol Sci*, *48*(3), 303–313.

154. Perry, E.K., Perry, R.H., Tomlinson, B.E. (1982). The influence of agonal status on some neurochemical activities of postmortem human brain tissue. *Neurosci Lett*, *29*(3), 303–307.

155. Spokes, E.G. (1979). An analysis of factors influencing measurements of dopamine, noradrenaline, glutamate decarboxylase and choline acetylase in human post-mortem brain tissue. *Brain*, *102*(2), 333–346.

156. Akbarian, S., Huang, H.S. (2006). Molecular and cellular mechanisms of altered GAD1/GAD67 expression in schizophrenia and related disorders. *Brain Res Rev*, *52*(2), 293–304.

157. Bu, D.F., Erlander, M.G., Hitz, B.C., Tillakaratne, N.J., Kaufman, D.L., Wagner-McPherson, C.B., Evans, G.A., Tobin, A.J. (1992). Two human glutamate decarboxylases, 65-kDa GAD and 67-kDa GAD, are each encoded by a single gene. *Proc Natl Acad Sci U S A*, *89*(6), 2115–2119.

158. Kaufman, D.L., Houser, C.R., Tobin, A.J. (1991). Two forms of the gamma-aminobutyric acid synthetic enzyme glutamate decarboxylase have distinct intraneuronal distributions and cofactor interactions. *J Neurochem*, *56*(2), 720–723.

159. Akbarian, S., Kim, J.J., Potkin, S.G., Hagman, J.O., Tafazzoli, A., Bunney, W.E. Jr, Jones, E.G. (1995). Gene expression for glutamic acid decarboxylase is reduced without loss of neurons in prefrontal cortex of schizophrenics. *Arch Gen Psychiatry*, *52*(4), 258–266.

160. Volk, D.W., Austin, M.C., Pierri, J.N., Sampson, A.R., Lewis, D.A. (2000). Decreased glutamic acid decarboxylase67 messenger RNA expression in a subset of

prefrontal cortical gamma-aminobutyric acid neurons in subjects with schizophrenia. *Arch Gen Psychiatry*, *57*(3), 237–245.

161. Heckers, S., Stone, D., Walsh, J., Shick, J., Koul, P., Benes, F.M. (2002). Differential hippocampal expression of glutamic acid decarboxylase 65 and 67 messenger RNA in bipolar disorder and schizophrenia. *Arch Gen Psychiatry*, *59*(6), 521–529.
162. Woo, T.U., Walsh, J.P., Benes, F.M. (2004). Density of glutamic acid decarboxylase 67 messenger RNA-containing neurons that express the N-methyl-D-aspartate receptor subunit NR2A in the anterior cingulate cortex in schizophrenia and bipolar disorder. *Arch Gen Psychiatry*, *61*(7), 649–657.
163. Volk, D., Austin, M., Pierri, J., Sampson, A., Lewis, D. (2001). GABA transporter-1 mRNA in the prefrontal cortex in schizophrenia: decreased expression in a subset of neurons. *Am J Psychiatry*, *158*, 256–265.
164. Conde, F., Lund, J.S., Jacobowitz, D.M., Baimbridge, K.G., Lewis, D.A. (1994). Local circuit neurons immunoreactive for calretinin, calbindin D-28k or parvalbumin in monkey prefrontal cortex: distribution and morphology. *J Comp Neurol*, *341*, 95–116.
165. Philpot, B.D., Lim, J.H., Brunjes, P.C. (1997). Activity-dependent regulation of calcium-binding proteins in the developing rat olfactory bulb. *J Comp Neurol*, *387*(1), 12–26.
166. Beasley, C.L., Reynolds, G.P. (1997). Parvalbumin-immunoreactive neurons are reduced in the prefrontal cortex of schizophrenics. *Schizophr Res*, *24*(3), 349–355.
167. Mirnics, K., Levitt, P., Lewis, D.A. (2006). Critical appraisal of DNA microarrays in psychiatric genomics. *Biol Psychiatry*, *60*(2), 163–176.
168. Lewis, D.A., Hashimoto, T. (2007). Deciphering the disease process of schizophrenia: the contribution of cortical GABA neurons. *Int Rev Neurobiol*, *78*, 109–131.
169. Hashimoto, T., Bazmi, H.H., Mirnics, K., Wu, Q., Sampson, A.R., Lewis, D.A. (2008). Conserved regional patterns of GABA-related transcript expression in the neocortex of subjects with schizophrenia. *Am J Psychiatry*, *165*(4), 479–489.
170. Reynolds, G.P., Czudek, C., Andrews, H.B. (1990). Deficit and hemispheric asymmetry of GABA uptake sites in the hippocampus in schizophrenia. *Biol Psychiatry*, *27*(9), 1038–1044.
171. Schleimer, S.B., Hinton, T., Dixon, G., Johnston, G.A. (2004). GABA transporters GAT-1 and GAT-3 in the human dorsolateral prefrontal cortex in schizophrenia. *Neuropsychobiology*, *50*(3), 226–230.
172. Woo, T.U., Whitehead, R.E., Melchitzky, D.S., Lewis, D.A. (1998). A subclass of prefrontal gamma-aminobutyric acid axon terminals are selectively altered in schizophrenia. *Proc Natl Acad Sci U S A*, *95*(9), 5341–5346.
173. Benes, F.M., Vincent, S.L., Marie, A., Khan, Y. (1996). Up-regulation of GABAA receptor binding on neurons of the prefrontal cortex in schizophrenic subjects. *Neuroscience*, *75*(4), 1021–1031.
174. Hanada, S., Mita, T., Nishino, N., Tanaka, C. (1987). [3H]muscimol binding sites increased in autopsied brains of chronic schizophrenics. *Life Sci*, *40*(3), 259–266.
175. Benes, F.M., Vincent, S.L., Alsterberg, G., Bird, E.D., SanGiovanni, J.P. (1992). Increased GABAA receptor binding in superficial layers of cingulate cortex in schizophrenics. *J Neurosci*, *12*(3), 924–929.

176. Volk, D.W., Pierri, J.N., Fritschy, J.M., Auh, S., Sampson, A.R., Lewis, D.A. (2002). Reciprocal alterations in pre- and postsynaptic inhibitory markers at chandelier cell inputs to pyramidal neurons in schizophrenia. *Cereb Cortex*, *12*(10), 1063–1070.

177. Impagnatiello, F., Guidotti, A.R., Pesold, C., Dwivedi, Y., Caruncho, H., Pisu, M.G., Uzunov, D.P., Smalheiser, N.R., Davis, J.M., Pandey, G.N., Pappas, G.D., Tueting, P., Sharma, R.P., Costa, E. (1998). A decrease of reelin expression as a putative vulnerability factor in schizophrenia. *Proc Natl Acad Sci U S A*, *95*(26), 15718–15723.

178. Grunze, H.C., Rainnie, D.G., Hasselmo, M.E., Barkai, E., Hearn, E.F., McCarley, R.W., et al. (1996). NMDA-dependent modulation of CA1 local circuit inhibition. *J Neurosci*, *16*, 2034–2043.

179. Sharp, F.R., Jasper, P., Hall, J., Noble, L., Sagar, S.M. (1991). MK-801 and ketamine induce heat shock protein HSP72 in injured neurons in posterior cingulate and retrosplenial cortex. *Ann Neurol*, *30*(6), 801–809.

180. Sharp, F.R., Butman, M., Koistinaho, J., Aardalen, K., Nakki, R., Massa, S.M., Swanson, R.A., Sagar, S.M. (1994). Phencyclidine induction of the hsp 70 stress gene in injured pyramidal neurons is mediated via multiple receptors and voltage gated calcium channels. *Neuroscience*, *62*(4), 1079–1092.

181. Li, Q., Clark, S., Lewis, D.V., Wilson, W.A. (2002). NMDA receptor antagonists disinhibit rat posterior cingulate and retrosplenial cortices: a potential mechanism of neurotoxicity. *J Neurosci*, *22*(8), 3070–3080.

182. Homayoun, H., Moghaddam, B. (2007). NMDA receptor hypofunction produces opposite effects on prefrontal cortex interneurons and pyramidal neurons. *J Neurosci*, *27*(43), 11496–11500.

183. Jodo, E., Suzuki, Y., Katayama, T., Hoshino, K.Y., Takeuchi, S., Niwa, S., Kayama, Y. (2005). Activation of medial prefrontal cortex by phencyclidine is mediated via a hippocampo-prefrontal pathway. *Cereb Cortex*, *15*(5), 663–669.

184. Pratt, J.A., Winchester, C., Egerton, A., Cochran, S.M., Morris, B.J. (2008). Modelling prefrontal cortex deficits in schizophrenia: implications for treatment. *Br J Pharmacol*, *153*(Suppl 1), S465–S470.

185. Kinney, J.W., Davis, C.N., Tabarean, I., Conti, B., Bartfai, T., Behrens, M.M. (2006). A specific role for NR2A-containing NMDA receptors in the maintenance of parvalbumin and GAD67 immunoreactivity in cultured interneurons. *J Neurosci*, *26*(5), 1604–1615.

186. Behrens, M.M., Ali, S.S., Dao, D.N., Lucero, J., Shekhtman, G., Quick, K.L., Dugan, L.L. (2007). Ketamine-induced loss of phenotype of fast-spiking interneurons is mediated by NADPH-oxidase. *Science*, *318*(5856), 1645–1647.

187. Zhang, Y., Behrens, M.M., Lisman, J.E. (2008). Prolonged exposure to NMDAR antagonist suppresses inhibitory synaptic transmission in prefrontal cortex. *J Neurophysiol*, *100*(2), 959–965.

188. Lisman, J.E., Coyle, J.T., Green, R.W., Javitt, D.C., Benes, F.M., Heckers, S., Grace, A.A. (2008). Circuit-based framework for understanding neurotransmitter and risk gene interactions in schizophrenia. *Trends Neurosci*, *31*(5), 234–242.

189. Lisman, J.E., Coyle, J.T., Green, R.W., Javitt, D.C., Benes, F.M., Heckers, S., Grace, A.A. (2008). Circuit-based framework for understanding neurotransmitter and risk gene interactions in schizophrenia. *Trends Neurosci*, *31*(5), 234–242.

190. Moghaddam, B., Adams, B.W. (1998). Reversal of phencyclidine effects by a group II metabotropic glutamate receptor agonist in rats. *Science*, *281*(5381), 1349–1352.

191. Patil, S.T., Zhang, L., Martenyi, F., Lowe, S.L., Jackson, K.A., Andreev, B.V., Avedisova, A.S., Bardenstein, L.M., Gurovich, I.Y., Morozova, M.A., Mosolov, S.N., Neznanov, N.G., Reznik, A.M., Smulevich, A.B., Tochilov, V.A., Johnson, B.G., Monn, J.A., Schoepp, D.D. (2007). Activation of mGlu2/3 receptors as a new approach to treat schizophrenia: a randomized Phase 2 clinical trial. *Nat Med*, *13*(9), 1102–1107.

192. Fell, M.J., Svensson, K.A., Johnson, B.G., Schoepp, D.D. (2008). Evidence for the role of metabotropic glutamate (mGlu)2 not mGlu3 receptors in the preclinical antipsychotic pharmacology of the mGlu2/3 receptor agonist (-)-(1R,4S,5S,6S)-4-amino-2-sulfonylbicyclo[3.1.0]hexane-4,6-dicarboxylic acid (LY404039). *J Pharmacol Exp Ther*, *326*(1), 209–217.

193. Vierling-Claassen, D., Siekmeier, P., Stufflebeam, S., Kopell, N. (2008). Modeling GABA alterations in schizophrenia: a link between impaired inhibition and altered gamma and beta range auditory entrainment. *J Neurophysiol*, *99*(5), 2656–2671.

194. Whitfield-Gabrieli, S., Thermenos, H.W., Milanovic, S., Tsuang, M.T., Faraone, S.V., McCarley, R.W., Shenton, M.E., Green, A.I., Nieto-Castanon, A., LaViolette, P., Wojcik, J., Gabrieli, J.D., Seidman, L.J. (2009). Hyperactivity and hyperconnectivity of the default network in schizophrenia and in first-degree relatives of persons with schizophrenia. *Proc Natl Acad Sci U S A*, *106*(4), 1279–1284.

195. Bergeron, R., Meyer, T.M., Coyle, J.T., Greene, R.W. (1998). Modulation of N-methyl-D-aspartate receptor function by glycine transport. *Proc Natl Acad Sci U S A*, *95*(26), 15730–15734.

196. Goff, D.C., Tsai, G., Manoach, D.S., Coyle, J.T. (1995). Dose-finding trial of D-cycloserine added to neuroleptics for negative symptoms in schizophrenia. *Am J Psychiatry*, *152*(8), 1213–1215.

197. Conn, P.J., Lindsley, C.W., Jones, C.K. (2009). Activation of metabotropic glutamate receptors as a novel approach for the treatment of schizophrenia. *Trends Pharmacol Sci*, *30*(1), 25–31.

198. Lewis, D.A., Cho, R.Y., Carter, C.S., Eklund, K., Forster, S., Kelly, M.A., Montrose, D. (2008). Subunit-selective modulation of GABA type A receptor neurotransmission and cognition in schizophrenia. *Am J Psychiatry*, *165*(12), 1585–1593.

# 6

# METABOTROPIC GLUTAMATE 2/3 RECEPTOR AGONISTS AND POSITIVE ALLOSTERIC MODULATORS OF METABOTROPIC GLUTAMATE RECEPTOR 2 AS NOVEL AGENTS FOR THE TREATMENT OF SCHIZOPHRENIA

GERARD J. MAREK, BRUCE J. KINON, DAVID L. MCKINZIE,
JEFFREY M. SCHKERYANTZ, AND JAMES A. MONN

## 6.1 INTRODUCTION

The origin of modern psychopharmacology can be traced to the discovery of the first clinically efficacious antipsychotic drug, chlorpromazine, in 1952. Following this watershed advance, several additional antipsychotic agents of the same (i.e., phenothiazine) class, as well as others derived from the butyrophenone scaffold (e.g., haloperidol, 1958), were discovered and widely utilized in the treatment of schizophrenia patients. Arvid Carlsson and his colleagues were the first to show that antipsychotics of both the phenothiazine and butyrophenone classes acted via blockade of dopamine (DA) receptors [1]. This hypothesis was further refined over a decade later by observations that all antipsychotic drugs potently block dopamine $D_2$-like receptors [2, 3]. Interest in moving to mechanisms of antipsychotic action other than dopamine $D_2$

*Targets and Emerging Therapies for Schizophrenia*, First Edition.
Edited by Jeffrey S. Albert and Michael W. Wood.

receptor blockade is based on three fundamental observations. First, $D_2$ receptor blockade is associated with treatment-emergent extrapyramidal symptoms in many patients. Second, patients treated with some antipsychotics that block dopamine $D_2$ receptors may have an increased risk of weight gain and changes in metabolic parameters. Third, although a modest improvement in the treatment of negative symptoms has been observed with a number of the second generation of antipsychotic drugs, some of these medications may have relatively little impact on the treatment of the cognitive symptoms associated with schizophrenia. These three features emphasize the need for new mechanisms of antipsychotic action for improvements in both the efficacy and safety domains.

Glutamate began to receive increasing focus with respect to schizophrenia beginning with the mid-1980s when ketamine, phencyclidine (PCP), and dizocilpine (MK-801) were first realized to be potent noncompetitive N-methyl-D aspartate (NMDA) receptor antagonists [4–6]. These channel-blocking NMDA receptor antagonists were known to induce psychotic symptoms in healthy adults and to faithfully reprise the symptoms experienced by schizophrenia patients during an acute episode [7–9]. A series of animal and patient studies converged on the suggestion that these uncompetitive NMDA receptor antagonists actually increased glutamatergic neurotransmission in the limbic forebrain, resulting in an increased activation of another postsynaptic ionotropic glutamate (iGluR) receptor, α-amino-3-hydroxy-5-methyl-4-isoxazolepropionic acid receptor AMPA receptors [10–14]. These observations imply that a novel antipsychotic drug acting on glutamate might suppress pathophysiologically increased glutamatergic neurotransmission.

## 6.2 METABOTROPIC GLUTAMATE RECEPTORS 2 AND 3: STRUCTURE, FUNCTION, AND LOCALIZATION

The eight known subtypes of metabotropic glutamate (mGlu) receptors comprise three groups of class C, 7-membrane spanning G-protein-coupled receptors based on differential structure, pharmacological characteristics, and signal transduction pathways [15–17]. All of the mGlu receptors have an external N-terminal "Venus fly trap" structure serving as the core for the glutamate recognition binding site to generally initiate signal transduction through homodimers. The group I mGlu receptors (mGlu1 and mGlu5) both have extensive central nervous system (CNS) localization to limbic-related regions and generally are coupled via $G_{q/11}$ proteins to either phospholipase C or phospholipase D and also activate cationic nonselective channels or inhibit $K^+$ channels that modulate firing patterns of neurons. These receptors predominantly have actions on the postsynaptic side of cells releasing glutamate; however, mGlu5 receptors are also present in presynaptic neurons and glial cells. The group II mGlu receptors (mGlu2 and mGlu3) are coupled via $G_i/G_o$ proteins to adenylyl cyclase in a negative modulatory fashion and also inhibit voltage operated calcium channels in many cell lines. The group II mGlu receptors also activate G protein inward-rectifying potassium (GIRK) channels and hyperpolarize neurons. The most prominent action of mGlu2 receptors is to decrease glutamate release via an autoreceptor function. Interestingly, mGlu2 autoreceptors appear outside of the synaptic release zone in the preterminal axons, unlike mGlu7 autoreceptors, which can be localized to the synapse. The mGlu3 receptors are localized on both presynaptic and postsynaptic neurons and are present throughout the brain in glia. The group III mGlu receptors (mGlu4, mGlu6, mGlu7, and mGlu8) are also coupled via $G_i/G_o$ proteins to adenylyl cyclase and inhibit stimulated concentrations of cyclic adenosine monophosphate (cAMP) formation and voltage-operated calcium channels in many cell lines. The mGlu receptors in this latter group function both as autoreceptors and as heteroceptors. The group II mGlu receptors will be the focus of the present chapter.

The crystal structure of the entire extracellular region of the mGlu3 receptor was solved recently [18]. This is important not only for understanding the molecular basis of agonist–receptor interactions but also for understanding how ligands can modulate dimer interactions through the cysteine-rich domain portion of the extracellular region shared in common between all three groups of mGlu receptors. This recent report also solved the structure of the extracellular Venus fly trap region of the mGlu7 receptor. Thus, with the previous groundbreaking report by this same group for the mGlu1 [19], examples of the crystal structure for the glutamate-binding region now exists for a representative protein within each mGlu receptor group. Such advances in visualizing three-dimensional representations of the mGlu receptor families will greatly aid both our understanding of ligand docking and medicinal chemistry in the pursuit of new pharmacological agents.

The mGlu2 receptor has an extensive localization throughout limbic-related sites relevant to understanding the pathophysiology and therapeutics for schizophrenia. In particular, dense distributions of mGlu2 receptor mRNA are found in the prefrontal cortex (PFC); the neocortex, dorsal and ventral striatum; midline and intralaminar thalamic nuclei; amygdala; hippocampus; entorhinal cortex; and medial mammillary bodies [20, 21]. Immunohistochemical work has suggested that mGlu2 receptors play a primary physiological role in axons of both glutamatergic and γ-aminobutyric acid (GABA)ergic neurons, although postsynaptic mGlu2 receptors are also found [22]. Colocalization experiments with antibodies directed at mGlu2 receptors and synapsin I have confirmed the widespread presynaptic expression of mGlu2 receptors in the forebrain regions such as the amygdala, hippocampus, oval nucleus of the bed nucleus of the stria terminalis, and the nucleus accumbens [21]; however, this strategy may miss the presumed extrasynaptic expression of mGlu2 receptors in preterminal axons as proposed for the PFC. In fact, lesions studies have suggested that mGlu2 receptors are present in the axons/terminals of long projection pathways such as the thalamocortical pathway originating in the midline and intralaminar thalamic nuclei of the thalamus (Fig. 6.1) [23]. Lesions

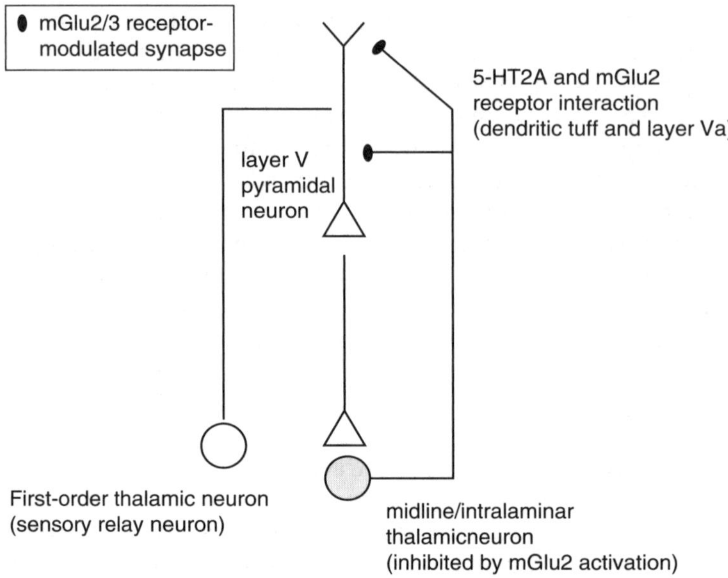


**FIGURE 6.1** Metabotropic glutamate 2 (mGlu2) receptors modulate the thalamocortical circuitry between the intralaminar and midline thalamic nuclei and layer V pyramidal neurons of the prefrontal cortex (PFC) and neocortex. One of the relatively few known robust somatodendritic actions of mGlu2 receptors is to hyperpolarize output neurons in the midline and intralaminar thalamic nuclei. These neurons send both superficial (layer I) and deep (layer Va) projections to the PFC and neocortex, which aligns with the richest distribution of 5-$HT_{2A}$ receptors. Activation of presynaptic mGlu2 receptors suppresses glutamate release in the PFC/neocortex induced by 5-$HT_{2A}$ receptors from multiple sources including the intralaminar and midline thalamic nuclei. These layer V pyramidal neurons then project back to the midline and intralaminar thalamic nuclei, which intimately involved in arousal and attention. The layer V pyramidal neurons do not project back to the first-order thalamic nuclei (e.g., thalamic sensory relay nuclei). The sensory thalamic neurons and the mediodorsal thalamic nucleus project to different cortical layers than do the midline and intralaminar thalamic nuclei. There is no evidence at the present time that mGlu2 or mGlu3 receptors modulate glutamate release from the terminals of the sensory relay neurons in adult animals. The other main neuronal action of mGlu3 receptors in this circuitry is the suppression of γ-aminobutyric acid (GABA) release from the terminals of the reticular nucleus of the thalamus (not shown). This ventrally located nucleus projects throughout the dorsal thalamus.

in the perforant pathway have revealed an important presynaptic role for mGlu2 in the trisynaptic pathways of the hippocampus, especially in the CA1-CA3 subfields and the medial perforant pathway (Fig. 6.2) [24, 25]. Ultrastructural studies using either mGlu2-preferring antibodies or other antibodies clearly labeling both mGlu2 and mGlu3 provide converging evidence consistent with a presynaptic localization for mGlu2 receptors throughout many regions of the hippocampus [24].

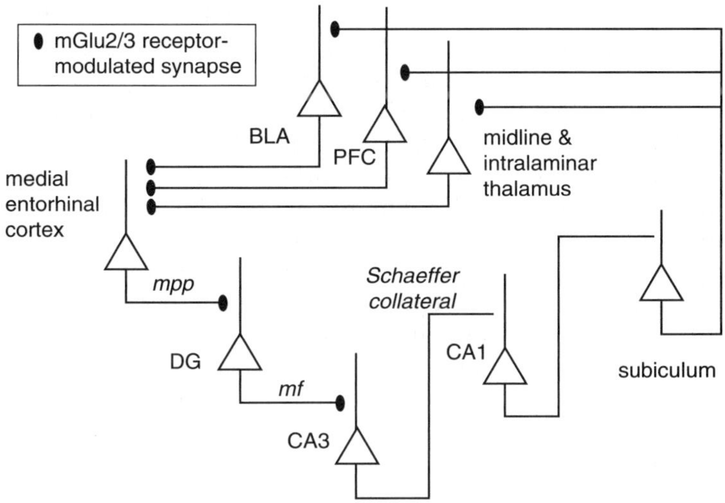


**FIGURE 6.2** Presynaptic metabotropic glutamate 2 (mGlu2) receptors modulate excitatory neurotransmission upon the principle output cells in a number of regions within the hippocampal formation. This is especially true of the medial perforant pathway (mpp) from the medial entorhinal cortex to the dentate gyrus granule cells. Presynaptic mGlu2 receptors also modulate glutamate release in the mossy fiber pathway (mf) from the dentate granule cells to the cornu ammonis (CA)3 pyramidal cells. While presynaptic mGlu2 receptors do not appear to directly modulate excitatory neurotransmission in the Schaeffer collaterals from the CA3 pyramidal cells to the CA1 pyramidal cells or from the CA1 to subicular neuron connection, mGlu2 activation may modulate glutamate release from one of the midline thalamic nuclei, the reunions nucleus, which projects to the medial entorhinal cortex, the CA1 region, and the subiculum (not shown). Not shown in this diagram are potential influences of mGlu3 receptors on γ-aminobutyric acid (GABA)ergic interneurons and astrocytes. Given both the prefrontal cortical projections to the medial entorhinal cortex and the projections of subicular/CA1 neurons to the prefrontal cortex, this provides potentially important sites by which cortical–hippocampal information processing may be modulated by mGlu2 receptors.

The mGlu3 receptor is distributed widely throughout the brain and, unlike the mGlu2 receptor, is known to be localized to glia as well as neurons [21, 26, 27]. In the neocortex, all pyramidal cells and nonpyramidal cells were found to be moderately or weakly labeled with the mGlu3 mRNA. Using antibodies recognizing mGlu3 receptors in mice with a deletion of mGlu2, relatively little labeling of the mGlu3 receptor was observed in cell bodies and dendritic shafts compared with previous observations with mGlu2 receptors [27]. Furthermore, even where mGlu3 mRNA is richly expressed (such as the GABAergic reticular nucleus of the thalamus), no prominent labeling for mGlu3 receptors was observed. Conversely, mGlu3 receptor labeling of glutamic acid decarboxylase (GAD)-positive axons and axon terminals was found in primary sensory thalamic nuclei, which themselves contain no GABAergic interneurons in the rodent [27].

One especially interesting feature for the mGlu3 receptor is the reported decreased dimeric/oligmeric mGlu3 levels in the PFC (Brodman area 10) of brains from schizophrenia patients compared with control subjects without psychiatric or neurological illness [28]. Furthermore, allelic variation in the gene for the mGlu3 receptor, *GRM3*, appears to alter cognition and prefrontal glutamate levels, and increases the risk for schizophrenia [29]. The involvement of mGlu3 receptors in schizophrenia has recently been reviewed [30].

Both mGlu2 and mGlu3 receptors are thought to be coupled via $G_i/G_o$ to an inhibition of adenylyl cyclase. The especially high affinity for glutamate (~41 nM) at human mGlu3 receptors transfected into rat glutamate transporter cells expressing the rat glutamate/aspartate transporter seems consistent with the necessary affinity of a glutamate receptor distant from the synaptic complex [31]. In contrast, the affinity of glutamate at human mGlu2 receptors in this cell line is approximately 12.8 μM, more than 300-fold higher and thus consistent with synaptic localization.

## 6.3 STRUCTURE–ACTIVITY RELATIONSHIPS FOR ORTHOSTERIC mGlu2 AND mGlu3 RECEPTOR AGONISTS

Extensive reviews of pharmacological agents acting at mGlu receptors have appeared [16, 32]. Orthosteric agonists acting at mGlu2 and mGlu3 receptors have been successfully identified by way of conformational restriction of the endogenous neurotransmitter, glutamate. The first of these agents, 1*S*,3*R*-1-aminocyclopentane-1,3-dicarboxylic acid (compound **1**; Table 6.1) [33–43], was an invaluable early research tool due to its lack of activity at iGlu receptors. However, the relatively weak (micromolar) potency and generally poor selectivity across other mGlu receptor subtypes (especially mGlu1 and mGlu5) has

**TABLE 6.1 Structure–Activity Relationship for Amino(hetero)cyclic Dicarboxylic Acids**

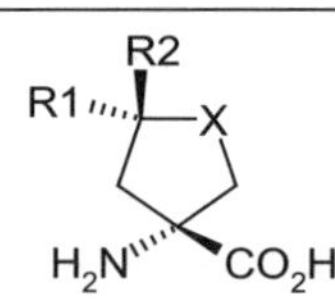


| No. | R1 | R2 | X | Common Name | mGlu2 $EC_{50}$ (μM) | mGlu3 $EC_{50}$ (μM) | Assay Format(s) | Reference |
|---|---|---|---|---|---|---|---|---|
| 1 | $CO_2H$ | H | $CH_2$ | *trans*-ACPD, 1*S*,3*R*-ACPD | 1–15 | 1–10 | IP; cAMP | [33–43] |
| 2 | $CO_2H$ | H | NH | 2*R*,4*R*-APDC | 0.2–0.4 | 0.4–3 | cAMP | [44–46] |
| 3 | $CO_2H$ | H | $NNH_2$ | 1-amino-APDC | 5 | 50 | cAMP | [47] |

limited the utility of this molecule, particularly given the discovery of later generation tools. Replacement of the cyclopentane ring system in **1** with a nitrogen-containing pyrrolidine ring resulted in 2*R*,4*R*-APDC (compound **2**; Table 6.1), a relatively potent ($EC_{50}$ ~300–500 nM) agonist for mGlu2 and mGlu3 receptors devoid of activity at other mGlu receptor subtypes at concentrations of up to 100 μM [44–46]. To date, structure–activity relationship (SAR) studies conducted on both compounds **1** and **2** have been unsuccessful in enhancing agonist potency or selectivity at mGlu2 and mGlu3 receptors. Target potency notwithstanding, a novel modification of compound **2** led to the identification of 1-amino-APDC (compound **3**; Table 6.1), which, while possessing diminished agonist potency at both mGlu2 and mGlu3 receptors compared with compound **2**, is interesting as it appears to behave as a partial agonist (~50% maximal efficacy) at each of these receptors [47]. The *in vivo* functional implications of this partial agonist *in vitro* pharmacological profile remain to be determined.

A second and highly valuable chemical scaffold for targeting mGlu2 and mGlu3 receptors arose out of the systematic exploration of cyclopropane-constrained analogs of glutamate [48–51]. Of the eight isomeric analogs prepared in this SAR, only the 2*S*,1′*S*,2′*S*-isomer (L-CCG-1; compound **4**, Table 6.2) was found to possess both excellent agonist potency at mGlu2 and mGlu3 ($EC_{50}$ ~300–500 nM) receptors and a high degree of selectivity over iGlu receptors. Although not entirely selective within the mGlu family (agonist activity at both group I and III receptors at concentrations between 1 and 10 μM) [52] , this agent has been used widely to study mGlu2 and mGlu3 receptor function *in vitro*. (2*S*,1′*R*,2′*R*,3′*R*)-2-(2,3-dicarboxycyclopropyl) glycine (DCG-IV; compound **5**; Table 6.2), designed as a hybrid of L-CCG-I and the NMDA-selective cyclopropane isomer L-CCG-IV [53], and demonstrates greater potency for mGlu2 and mGlu3 receptors ($EC_{50}$ ~ 10–50 nM) and selectivity over mGlul and mGlu5 subtypes but possesses significant agonist activity at NMDA receptors [52–56], and antagonist activity at each (mGlu4, mGlu6, mGlu7, and mGlu8 receptors) of the group III mGlu subtypes [52]. Later generation compounds within this structural motif include the C3′-difluorinated analog L-$F_2$CCG-I (compound **6**; Table 6.2) [57, 58] and a number of 3′-substituted variants (e.g., compounds **7–10**; Table 6.2), the latter of which appear to possess both excellent mGlu2 and mGlu3 agonist potency and selectivity [59–64]. Certain other (C3′ aryl- and arylalkyl-substituted) analogs (e.g., compound **11**) have been reported to possess potent antagonist activity at these receptor subtypes [65, 66].

A significant advance in the identification of useful orthosteric agonists for studying mGlu2 and mGlu3 receptors occurred with the discovery of the conformationally constrained glutamate analog (+)-2-aminobicyclo[3.1.0]hexane-2,6-dicarboxylic acid, LY354740 (compound **12**; Tables 6.3 and 6.4) [67, 68]. This molecule displays excellent binding and functional agonist potency at both mGlu2 and mGlu3 subtypes ($EC_{50}$ ~10–50 nM), a wide selectivity margin over other mGlu and iGlu subtypes, and sufficient brain penetration following

**TABLE 6.2 Structure–Activity Relationship for C3′-substituted Carboxycyclopropylglycines**

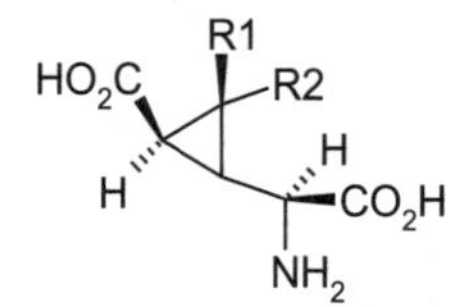


| No. | R1 | R2 | Common Name | mGlu2 $EC_{50}$ (μM) *or $IC_{50}$ (μM)* | mGlu3 $EC_{50}$ (μM) | Assay Format(s) | Reference |
|---|---|---|---|---|---|---|---|
| 4 | H | H | L-CCG-I | 0.3–0.5 | 0.4–0.6 | cAMP; IP in Gqi9 expressing cells | [48–52] |
| 5 | H | $CO_2H$ | DCG-IV | 0.3–0.4 | 0.1–0.2 | Spinal neuron electrophys; IP stimulation in Gqi9 expressing cells | [52–56] |
| 6 | F | F | L-$F_2$-CCG1 | 0.2 | – | Spinal neuron electrophys | [57, 58] |
| 7 | H | Me | | 0.008 | 0.038 | cAMP | [59] |
| 8 | H | $CH_2OH$ | | 0.004 | 0.007 | cAMP | [63] |
| 9 | H | $CH_2OCH_3$ | *cis*-MCG-I | 1.5–3.8 | – | cAMP; Spinal neuron electrophys | [58–61] |
| 10 | H | CN | | 0.19 | 0.064 | cAMP | [64] |
| 11 | H | Ph | PCCG-4 | *8* | – | cAMP | [65, 66] |

**TABLE 6.3 Structure–Activity Relationship for Amino(hetero)bicyclo[3.1.0]hexane-Dicarboxylic Acids**

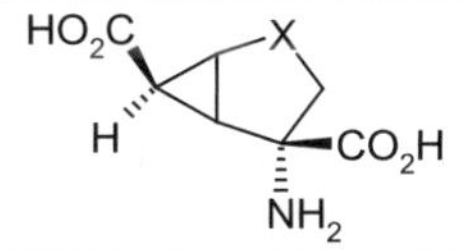


| No. | X | Common Name | mGlu2 $EC_{50}$ (μM) | mGlu3 $EC_{50}$ (μM) | Assay Format | Reference |
|---|---|---|---|---|---|---|
| 12 | $CH_2$ | LY354740 | 0.011 | 0.038 | cAMP | [67, 68] |
| 13 | O | LY379268 | 0.003 | 0.005 | cAMP | [69] |
| 14 | S | LY389795 | 0.004 | 0.008 | cAMP | [69] |
| 15 | SO | LY404040 | 0.000,09 | 0.001 | cAMP | [70, 71] |
| 16 | $SO_2$ | LY404039 | 0.023 | 0.048 | cAMP | [70, 71] |

systemic dosing. Replacement of the C4-methylene in compound **12** with either oxygen (LY379268, compound **13**; Table 6.3) or sulfur (LY389795, compound **14**; Table 6.3) resulted in additional potent, selective mGlu2/3 receptor agonists that demonstrated good oral bioavailability in rodents [69]. Oxidation of the sulfur atom in compound **14** resulted in both sulfoxide (compound **15**; Table 6.3) and sulfone (compound **16**; Table 6.3) derivatives [70] that retain these desirable pharmacological and pharmacokinetic attributes [70, 71]. Substitution about the bicyclic ring system of compound **12** has led to several additional mGlu2 and mGlu3 agonists (e.g., compounds **17**, **19**, **23**, **25**, **27**, **28**, and **32**; Table 6.4) [72–74], mGlu2 and mGlu3 antagonists (e.g., compounds **18**, **20**, **21**, **26**, and **29–31**; Table 6.4) [72–76], and a single example of a molecule (compound **22**) that appears to functionally discriminate between mGlu2 and mGlu3 receptors, displaying agonist activity at mGlu2 but antagonist activity at mGlu3 [73]. Of the potent and selective mGlu2 and mGlu3 agonists prepared to date, the most thoroughly explored in preclinical animal models are compounds **12**, **13**, **16**, and **32**. Importantly, orally active prodrugs (compounds **33** and **34**, Fig. 6.3) of **12** and **16** have advanced to proof-of-concept efficacy studies in humans, and compound **32** is reportedly in early clinical development.

## 6.4 STRUCTURE–ACTIVITY RELATIONSHIPS FOR POSITIVE ALLOSTERIC MODULATORS (PAMS) OF mGLU2 RECEPTORS

A more recent approach toward enhancing mGlu2 receptor function has been to augment the potency of the endogenous neurotransmitter (glutamate) at mGlu2 receptors via an allosteric mechanism. High-throughput screening technologies were combined with functional assays in cells expressing recombinant mGlu2 receptors to allow for the discovery of novel PAMs and negative

**TABLE 6.4 Structure–Activity Relationship for Substituted 2-Aminobicyclo[3.1.0]hexane-2,6-dicarboxylic Acids**

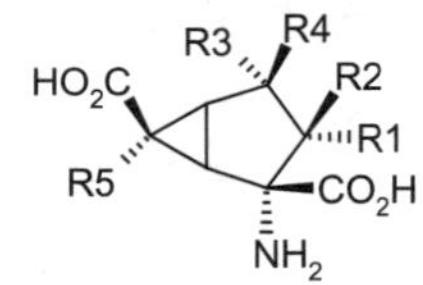


| No. | R1 | R2 | R3 | R4 | R5 | Common Name | mGlu2 $EC_{50}$ (μM) or $IC_{50}$ (μM) | mGlu3 $EC_{50}$ (μM) or $IC_{50}$ (μM) | Assay Format(s) | Reference |
|---|---|---|---|---|---|---|---|---|---|---|
| 12 | H | H | H | H | H | LY354740 | 0.011 | 0.038 | cAMP | [67, 68] |
| 17 | F | H | H | H | H | MGS0008 | 0.029 | 0.045 | cAMP | [72] |
| 18 | H | F | H | H | H | | *17* | – | cAMP | [72] |
| 19 | H | H | H | H | F | | 0.017 | 0.081 | cAMP | [72] |
| 20 | F | F | H | H | H | | *36.2* | – | cAMP | [72] |
| 21 | H | Me | H | H | H | | *2* | *10* | cAMP | [73] |
| 22 | H | H | Me | H | H | LY541850 | 0.16 | *1* | cAMP | [73] |
| 23 | H | H | H | Me | H | | 0.045 | 0.034 | cAMP | [73] |
| 24 | H | H | H | H | Me | | >100 | – | cAMP | [72] |
| 25 | OH | H | H | H | H | | 0.098 | – | GTPγS | [74] |
| 26 | H | OH | H | H | H | HYDIA | *1.0* | – | GTPγS; cAMP; GIRK | [74] |
| 27 | H | H | H | OH | F | | 0.021 | – | cAMP | [72] |
| 28 | $NH_2$ | H | H | H | H | | 0.20 | – | GTPγS | [74] |
| 29 | H | OMe | | | | | *0.229* | – | cAMP | [75] |
| 30 | H | OBn | | | | | *0.131* | – | cAMP | [75] |
| 31 | H | O-(3,4-diCl)Bn | | | F | MGS0039 | *0.020* | *0.024* | cAMP | [75] |
| 32 | H | H | =O | | F | MGS0028 | 0.00057 | 0.0021 | cAMP | [72] |

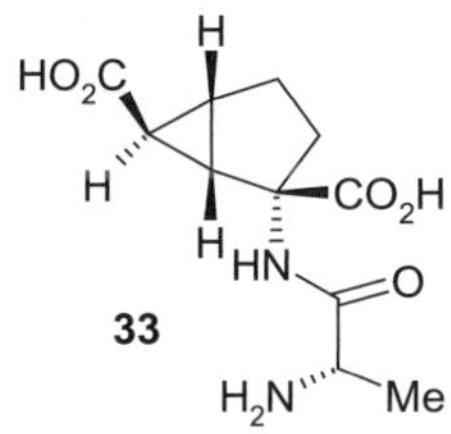
33

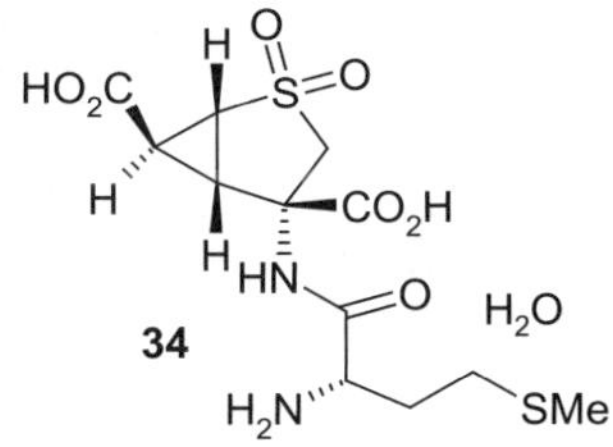
34

**FIGURE 6.3** Chemical structures of LY544344 (compound **33**) and LY2140023 monohydrate (compound **34**); orally bioavailable prodrugs of LY354740 (compound **12**); and LY404039 (compound **16**), respectively.

allosteric modulators (NAMs), which interact with site(s) distinct from the glutamate binding domain. To date this, method has been useful in identifying a diverse range of mGlu2 PAMs [77–79]. Although a convincing advantage for PAMs versus orthosteric agonists has yet to be fully established, there are both structural and pharmacological arguments in favor of the former. From a structural perspective, all of the competitive (orthosteric) agonists of mGlu2 receptors are conformationally restricted derivatives of glutamate and generally lack selectivity over the closely related mGlu3 receptor, presumably due to the highly conserved amino acid sequence in the orthosteric binding site. As glutamate analogs, issues associated with synthetic complexity, intestinal absorption, and brain penetration can be encountered. Conversely, PAMs benefit from a diverse set of chemical platforms providing opportunities for modulating potency, selectivity, physicochemical, pharmacokinetic, and pharmacodynamic properties. Additionally, while orthosteric agonists provide continuous activation of mGlu2 and mGlu3 receptors, which can theoretically lead to receptor desensitization and downregulation [80], the activity of mGlu2 PAMs is only anticipated in the presence of physiologically released glutamate. Consequently, a PAM with no inherent agonist activity may lead to an effective treatment of disorders associated with glutamatergic hyperactivity without risk of possible receptor overstimulation and/or development of behavioral tolerance as has been observed in the case of orthosteric agonist **13** [81]. It should be noted, however, that this potential advantage of mGlu2 receptor PAMs remains speculative.

A high-throughput functional screen in which test compounds and a submaximal concentration of glutamate (10% of maximal glutamate) are added simultaneously to a stable cell line co-expressing mGlu2 receptors coupled to a promiscuous G protein, that is, $G_{\alpha16}$, is a common method of identifying mGlu2 PAMs. In fact, compound LY181837 N-(4-phenoxyphenyl)-N-(3-pyridinylmethyl)ethan-sulfonamide (compound **35**; Table 6.5), the first reported subtype-selective mGlu2 PAM, was identified with this technique [82, 83]. Changes in intracellular levels of calcium were measured using fluorescence

**TABLE 6.5 Select Examples of Pyridylmethylsulphonamide Class of Molecules**

| No. | Common Name | Compound | mGlu2 $EC_{50}$ (μM)[a] | Reference |
|---|---|---|---|---|
| 35 | orthopyridylmethyl sulfonamide class | 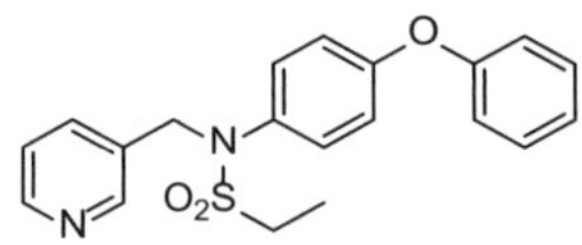 | 1.50 | [82] |
| 36 | 4-MMPTS | 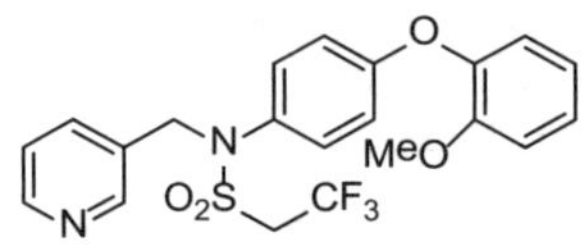 | 0.27 | [82, 84] |
| 37 | cyPPTS | 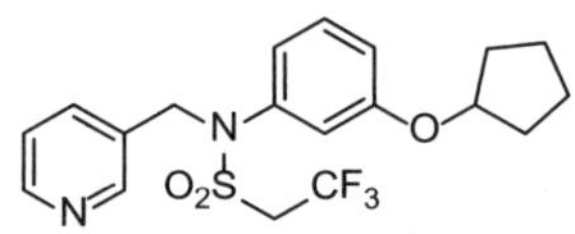 | 0.024 | [82, 84] |
| 38 | 2,2,2-TEMPS | 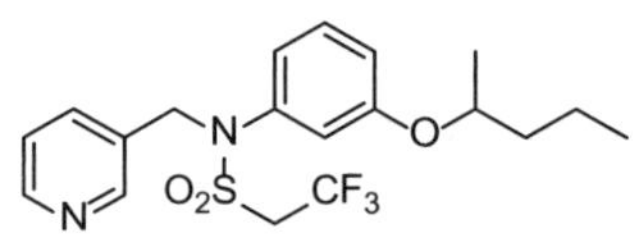 | 0.014 | [83, 84] |
| 39 | CBiPES | 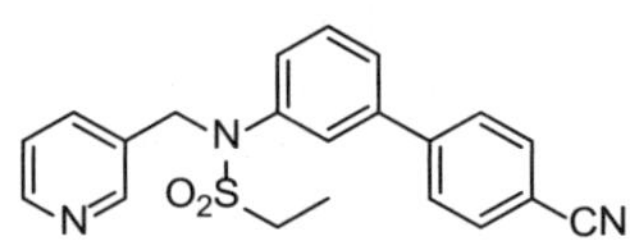 | 0.093 | [83, 84] |

[a]Potentiation $EC_{50}$ determined in the presence of a submaximal amount of glutamate using fluorescence detection of changes in intracellular calcium.

in a dose-responsive manner with an $EC_{50}$ defined as the concentration of test compound needed to generate 50% of the maximal (30 μM) glutamate response. Compound LY181837 did not activate the mGlu2 receptor when dosed alone (i.e., no intrinsic agonist activity), but provided a concentration-dependent potentiation of the submaximal glutamate response with a calculated $EC_{50}$ of 1.5 μM. This class of compounds as well as those of the hydroxyacetophenone class has been extensively reviewed [77] and will not be discussed in detail in this review with the exception of compounds **36**, 4-MMPTS, ($EC_{50}$ = 0.27 μM), **37**, cyPPTS ($EC_{50}$ = 0.024 μM), **38**, 2,2,2-TEMPS ($EC_{50}$ = 0.014 μM), **39**, CBiPES, ($EC_{50}$ = 0.0.093 μM), and **48**, BINA ($EC_{50}$ = 0.11 μM), which have exhibited activity in rodent models of anxiety and schizophrenia and as such are considered valuable tools in the study of mGlu2 pharmacology (*vide infra*) (Tables 6.6 and 6.8) [82, 84–86].

Another important class of molecules to emerge as selective mGlu2 PAMs contains the indanone ring system [87]. Indanone **40** is reported to have an $EC_{50}$ of 600 nM with a maximum potentiation value of 86% (Table 6.6). However, this compound has poor bioavailability, which was improved by removing the

**TABLE 6.6 Structure–Activity Relationship for the Phenyltetrazolyl Indalones**

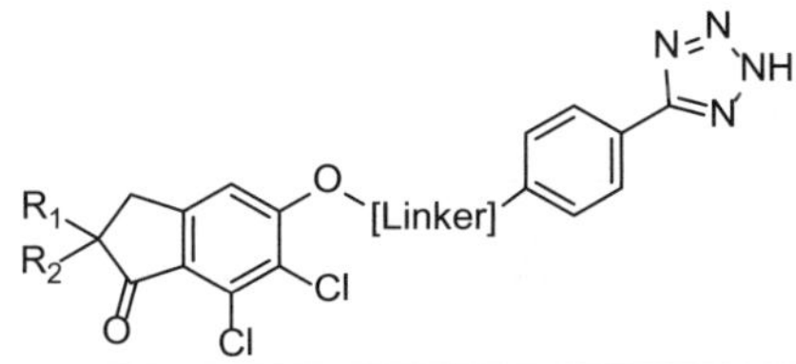


| No. | $R_1$ | $R_2$ | [Linker] | mGlu2 $EC_{50}$ (μM)[a] | % Potentiation | Reference |
|---|---|---|---|---|---|---|
| 40 | cyclopentyl | $CH_3$ | -$CH_2$CONH- | 0.60 | 86% | [87] |
| 41 | cyclopentyl | $CH_3$ | -$CH_2$- | 0.22 | 85% | |
| 42 | cyclopentyl | H | -$CH_2$- | 0.12 | 80% | |
| 43 | propyl | H | -$CH_2$- | 0.28 | 57% | |

[a]Concentration of compound required to activate 50% of [$^{35}$S]GTPγS in the presence of an $EC_{10}$ concentration of glutamate.

**TABLE 6.7 Structure–Activity Relationship for the Thiopyridyl Indalones**

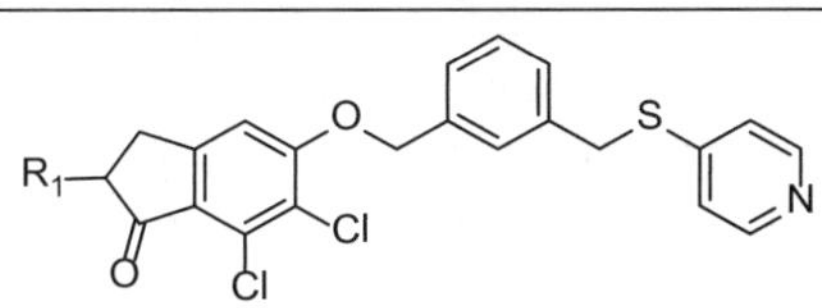


| No. | $R_1$ | mGlu2 $EC_{50}$ (μM)[a] | % Potentiation | Reference |
|---|---|---|---|---|
| 44 | cyclopentyl | 0.56 | 114% | [87] |
| 45 | propyl | 0.19 | 169% | |

[a]Concentration of compound required to activate 50% of [$^{35}$S]GTPγS in the presence of an $Ec_{10}$ concentration of glutamate.

amide in the linker region of the molecule. This structural change resulted in compound **41**, which benefits from 65% bioavailability and an $EC_{50}$ of 223 nM with a maximal potentiator efficacy of 85%. Resolving compound **41** into its respective enantiomers documented the potency resided in the (-) isomer (i.e., an $EC_{50}$ = 122 nM, 90% maximal potentiation, structure not shown).

Further SAR around the indanone nucleus revealed that lipophilic alkyl groups were optimal for both potency and efficacy. In addition, removal of the methyl group α to the ketone afforded compound **42** with a twofold increase in potency ($EC_{50}$ = 122 nM, 80% potentiation). Other modifications of the lipophilic region of the indanone led to a straight chain propyl group providing compound **43** ($EC_{50}$ = 282 nM and a 57% potentiation) (Table 6.6). The tetrazole moiety in these molecules was identified as a hinderance to effective brain penetration and a replacement was sought. Toward this end, a thio-pyridyl group was incorporated, leading to compound **44** with an $EC_{50}$ of 562 nM (Table 6.7). Replacing the cyclopentyl group with a propyl group gave agent

**TABLE 6.8 Structure–Activity Relationship for the Biphenyl-indanones**

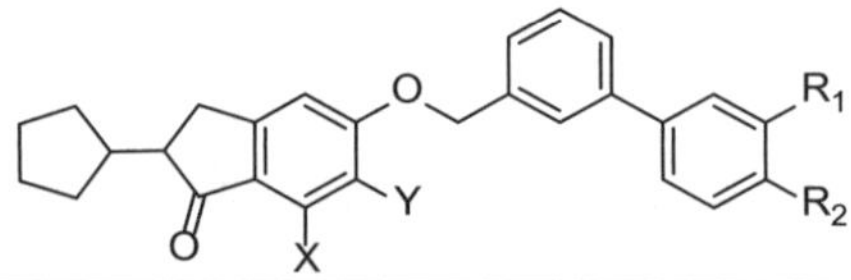


| No. | Common Name | X | Y | $R_1$ | $R_2$ | mGlu2 $EC_{50}$ (μM)[a] | % Pot. | Ref. |
|---|---|---|---|---|---|---|---|---|
| 46 | | Cl | Cl | H | $CO_2H$ | 0.24 | 98% | [88] |
| 47 | | $CH_3$ | $CH_3$ | $CO_2H$ | H | 0.069 | 118% | |
| 48 | BINA | $CH_3$ | $CH_3$ | H | $CO_2H$ | 0.11 | 114% | |
| 49 | | Cl | $CH_3$ | $CO_2H$ | H | 0.064 | 122% | |

[a]Concentration of compound required to activate 50% of [$^{35}$S]GTPγS in the presence of an $EC_{10}$ concentration of glutamate.

**45** with an $EC_{50}$ of 186 nM and a maximal potentiation at 169%. Despite relatively low overall exposure, compound **45** exhibited a favorable brain to plasma ratio of 1.08:1 and *in vivo* activity in the ketamine locomotor assay was demonstrated following intraperitoneal (i.p.) dosing.

The combination of incorporating a bi-phenyl linker with the indanone ring system and replacing the tetrazole functionality with a carboxylic acid led to a series of selective mGlu2 potentiators [85, 88]. Properties possessed by this class of potentiators are good potencies, ranging from 64 to 220 nM, high maximal potentiator efficacy values (greater than 98%), and desirable brain (B) to plasma (P) ratios (B/P > 0.33) (Table 6.8). In addition, these compounds also demonstrated high brain exposure levels (>3 μM). The most promising compound reported to date from this SAR is (3′-((2-cyclopentyl-6,7-dimethyl-1-oxo-2,3-dihydro-1H-inden-5-yloxy)methyl)biphenyl-4-carboxylic acid (compound **48**, BINA), which exhibits *in vivo* activity following systemic dosing [85, 86, 88].

Benzazoles have been reported as another set of mGlu2 PAMS [89]. The two most optimal benzazole variants in regard to potency were the benzotriazole and indole ring systems. However, the benzotriazole containing molecules (structures not shown) also had potentiator activity at the mGlu3 receptor and SAR was therefore focused on the indole series. With compounds incorporating the indole ring system it was found that large lipophilic side-chains like neopentyl or methylene cyclohexyl were preferred for potency (compounds **50** and **51**, respectively, Table 6.9). Compounds **50** and **51** both contain the butyloxy linker between the two terminal aromatic regions while compounds **52** and **53** employ a more rigid benzyl linkage. Although this linker modification slightly improved the mGlu2 PAM potency, it is worth noting that it led to inferior brain to plasma ratios (B/P < 0.01) even though plasma levels were high (>7 μM) when dosed i.p. at 20 mg/kg. The most promising compound disclosed in this series proved to be compound **50** ($EC_{50}$ = 559 nM, 98% maximal potentiation), which demonstrated central penetration and activity

**TABLE 6.9 Structure–Activity Relationship for the Phenyltetrazolylindoles**

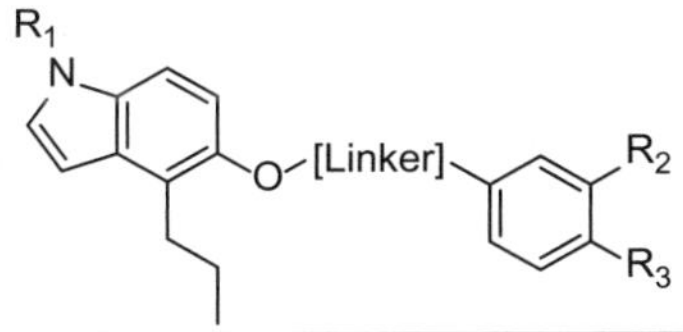


| No. | $R_1$ | $R_2$ | $R_3$ | [Linker] | mGlu2 $EC_{50}$ (μM)[a] | % Potentiation | Reference |
|---|---|---|---|---|---|---|---|
| 50 | neopentyl | H | tetrazole | 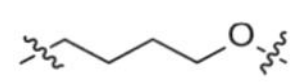 | 0.56 | 98% | [89] |
| 51 | methylene cyclohexyl | H | tetrazole | 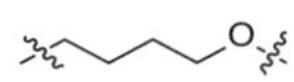 | 0.23 | 101% | |
| 52 | neopentyl | H | tetrazole | 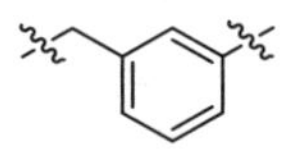 | 0.32 | 94% | |
| 53 | neopentyl | tetrazole | H | 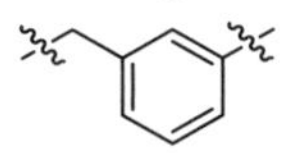 | 0.13 | 107% | |

[a]Concentration of compound required to activate 50% of [$^{35}$S]GTPγS in the presence of an $EC_{10}$ concentration of glutamate.

in the ketamine-induced hyperlocomotion assay following systemic dosing at 40 mg/kg.

The N-methylbenzimidazole compound **54** (Table 6.10) has been identified as an mGlu2 PAM (mGlu2 $EC_{50}$ = 27 nM), although neither its mGlu receptor selectivity nor its effects at mGlu2 in the absence of glutamate were reported [90]. Because compound **54** possessed suboptimal pharmacokinetic parameters (*r*CLh > 65.7 mL/min/kg, [predicted hepatic clearance from a rat liver microsomal stability assay], bioavailability <2%), structural modifications at the termini of the 3,6-disubstituted-azabicyclohexane core were pursued. Attempts to replace the N-methyl benzimidazole with alternative heterocycles like benzothiazoles or quinolines had detrimental effects on the mGlu2 PAM activity. However, halogens and small alkyl groups are tolerated in the phenyl ring with the *para*-disposed functionalities (i.e., compound **55**) providing enhanced microsomal stability and lower predicted intrinsic human clearance rates (*h*-CLh, 7 mL/min/kg for compound **55**) while maintaining potency (mGlu2 $EC_{50}$ = 26 nM). In an attempt to improve water solubility, a mildly basic functionality (pyridine nitrogen) was incorporated into either the aromatic ring or the benzimidazole system, leading to compounds **56** through **58** possessing excellent mGlu2 receptor potentiator potencies ($EC_{50} \leq 30$ nM) and desired pharmacokinetic properties.

Another set of compounds containing the N-methylbenzimidazole functionality has been disclosed as selective mGlu2 receptor potentiators [91]. Compound **59** (Table 6.11), identified through a high-throughput screen

**TABLE 6.10 Structure–Activity Relationship for 3,6-disubstituted-3-aza-bicyclo [3.1.0]hexanes**

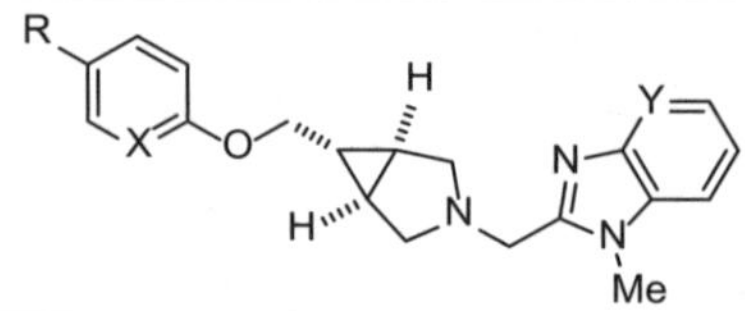


| No. | R | X | Y | mGlu2 $EC_{50}$ (nM)[a] | Reference |
|---|---|---|---|---|---|
| 54 | H | CH | CH | 27 | [90] |
| 55 | Cl | CH | CH | 26 | |
| 56 | Cl | N | CH | 26 | |
| 57 | $CF_3$ | N | CH | 30 | |
| 58 | $CF_3$ | CH | N | 20 | |

[a]Potentiation $EC_{50}$ determined in the presence of a submaximal amount of glutamate using fluorescence detection of changes in intracellular calcium.

**TABLE 6.11 Structure–Activity Relationship for the Piperazinyl and Piperdinyl N-methylbenzimidazoles**

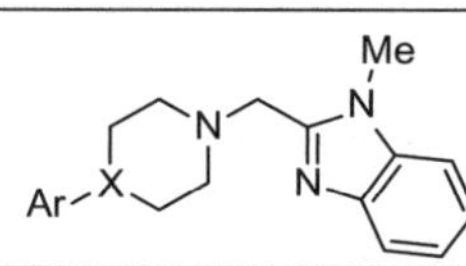


| No. | X | Ar | mGlu2 $EC_{50}$ (uM)[a] | % Pot. | Dopaminergic Activity (Ki) $D_2$ µM | $D_3$ µM | $D_4$ µM | Ref. |
|---|---|---|---|---|---|---|---|---|
| 59 | CH | 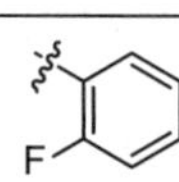 | 0.13 | 91 | 0.04 | 0.13 | – | [91] |
| 60 | CH | 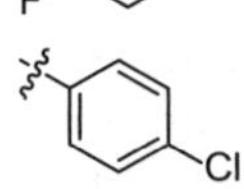 | 0.80 | 91 | 0.016 | 0.32 | 0.063 | |
| 61 | N | 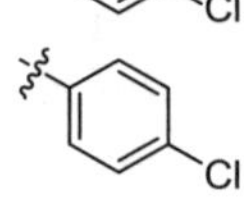 | 0.79 | – | >10 | >10 | 0.13 | |
| 62 | N | 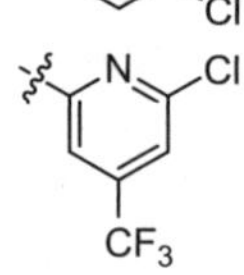 | 0.079 | 71 | >5.0 | >5.0 | 0.63 | |
| 63 | N | 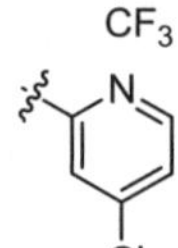 | 0.13 | 69 | >10 | >10 | 2.5 | |

[a]Potentiation $EC_{50}$ determined in the presence of a submaximal amount of glutamate using fluorescence detection of changes in intracellular calcium.

(HTS), had an $EC_{50}$ of 126 nM at mGlu2 and no appreciable agonist or antagonist activity at the group I mGlu receptors ($EC_{50}$ > 15 μM). This compound did, however, possess dopaminergic off-target activity (dopamine $D_2$ $IC_{50}$ = 40 nM, $D_3$ = 126 nM). SAR about the phenyl ring showed modest improvements in potencies for mGlu2 but did little to diminish the dopaminergic activity. The *para*-chloro analog **60** illustrates this point (mGlu2 $EC_{50}$ = 80 nM, dopamine $D_2$ $IC_{50}$ = 16 nM, $D_3$ = 320 nM, $D_4$ = 63 nM). Replacing the piperadine ring system in compound **60** with a piperazine as in compound **61** lowered $D_2$ and $D_3$ antagonist activity, but the $D_4$ activity still persisted. Further optimization of the arylpiperazine moiety identified compounds GSK1331258 **62** and GSK1331268 **63**, both of which exhibited significantly reduced dopaminergic activity. In general, the compounds in this series potentiated an $EC_{20}$ of glutamate to 70% to 100% of a glutamate $EC_{100}$ response. Selectivity for compounds **62** and **63** was assessed against a panel of mGlu receptors (i.e., subtypes 1, 4, and 5) and other CNS-related receptors (i.e., histaminergic, seratonergic, and adrenergic) with no appreciable activity identified. Compounds **62** and **63** also exhibited good *in vitro* metabolic stability, moderate clearance, and acceptable bioavailability, warranting further *in vivo* studies in behavioral models of schizophrenia.

In an interesting approach toward identifying new mGlu2 PAMs, researchers undertook a three-dimensional shape and electrostatic similarity comparison with a previously known pyridone core active at mGlu2 [92]. This computer-assisted scaffold-hopping technique identified the imidazopyridine ring system as one of the best ranking hits (Fig. 6.4). Using the previous pyridone SAR as a guide (see compound **64**), the researchers attached arylpiperazinyl or substituted aryl groups to the southwest portion of the new system, leading to compounds with acceptable mGlu2 receptor potentiator potency (Table 6.12). In both cases, the 2,2,2-trifluoroethyl substituent in the northeastern domain led to increases in potency and improved metabolic stability relative to simple alkyl groups at this site. The arylimidazolopyridines were generally more potent than their arylpiperazinyl-substituted imidazolopyridine counterparts and also more potent than the aforementioned pyridone compound **64**. Compare compound **66** with compound **65** and **64**. Compounds **65** and **66** showed no significant agonist or antagonist activity against mGlu receptors 1–8, indicating that the imidazopyridine core is a satisfactory starting point as a selective mGlu2 receptor PAM.

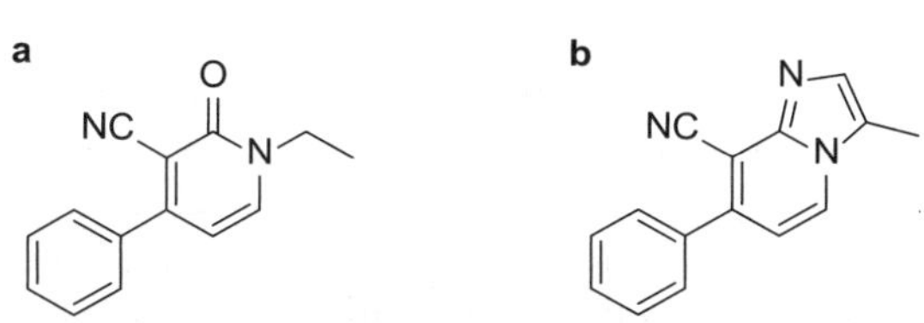


**FIGURE 6.4** (a) Pyridone query fragment and (b) imidazopyridine hit fragment.

**TABLE 6.12 Structure–Activity Relationship for the Imidazopyridines**

| No. | Structure | mGlu2 $EC_{50}$ (μM)[a] | % Pot. | Reference |
|---|---|---|---|---|
| 64 | 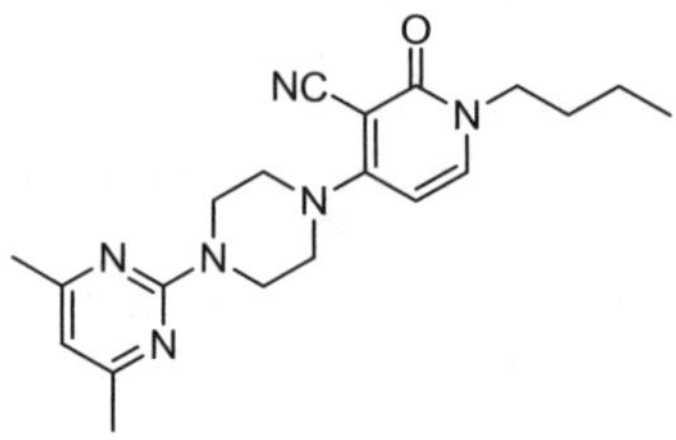 | 0.63 | 235 | [92] |
| 65 | 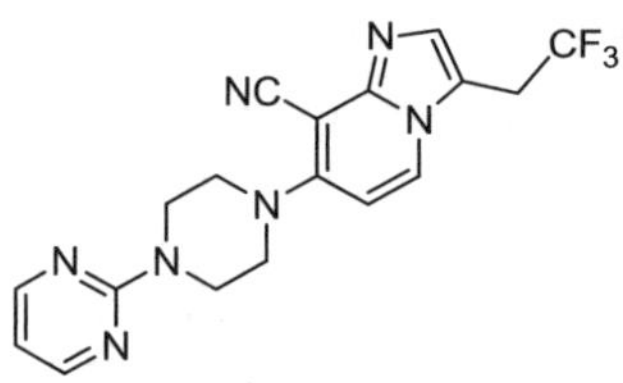 | 0.85 | 231 | |
| 66 | 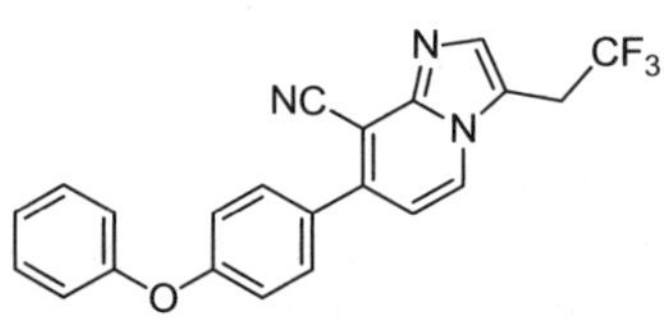 | 0.19 | 200 | |

[a]Concentration of compound required to activate 50% of [$^{35}$S]GTPγS in the presence of an $EC_{20}$ concentration of glutamate.

A FLIPR-based HTS and some structural detective work identified the oxazolidinone compound **67** (Table 6.13) as an mGlu2 PAM with an $EC_{50}$ of 117 nM [93]. Further optimization about the oxazolidinone ring as well as the ether linkage resulted in the very potent agent **68** possessing an $EC_{50}$ of 5 nM. However, the significant lipophilic character and high *in vitro* microsomal clearance of this compound (*c*LogP = 5.12, *r*CLh = 14.7 mL/min/mg) were the basis for the incorporation of a basic amine moiety into the cycloalkyl ether portion of the molecule. Although this structural modification reduced microsomal clearance to acceptable levels, it resulted in significantly reduced mGlu2 receptor PAM activity as in compound **69** (>12 μM). Therefore, an alternative approach wherein the alkyl ether functionality was replaced with a substituted phenyl ring to create a bi-phenyl as in compound **70** (mGlu2 $EC_{50}$ = 76 nM) was carried out. Extensive SAR in this bi-phenyl series was undertaken to balance acceptable physicochemical and pharmacokinetic properties with mGlu2 PAM potency. Additionally, alleviating off-target activity (5-$HT_{2A}$) became necessary. The most optimized compound to emerge from this undertaking was oxazolidinone **71**. Compound **71** exhibited an mGlu2 receptor $EC_{50}$ of 30 nM, good rat bioavailability 64%, and decreased methamphetamine-induced hyperlocomotion in mice with a minimal effective dose of 10 mg/kg s.c. Compound **71**, however, exhibits high rat clearance (102 mL/min/kg), a moderate volume of distribution (4.7 L/kg), a short half-life ($T_{1/2}$ = 0.8 hour),

**TABLE 6.13 Structure–Activity Relationship for the Oxazolidinones**

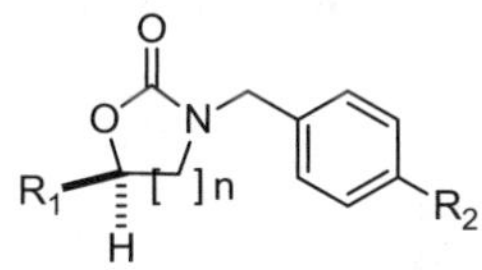

| No. | n | $R_1$ | $R_2$ | mGlu2 $EC_{50}$ (μM)[a] | Reference |
|---|---|---|---|---|---|
| 67 | 2 | H | 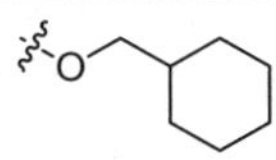 | 0.120 | [93] |
| 68 | 1 | Me | 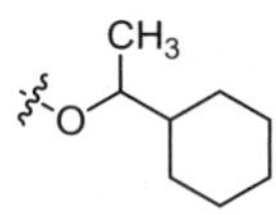 | 0.005 | |
| 69 | 1 | Me | 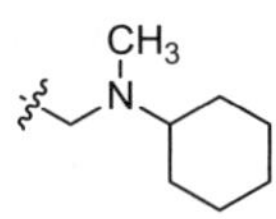 | >12 | |
| 70 | 1 | Me | 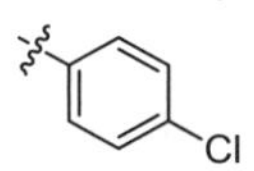 | 0.076 | |
| 71 | 1 | Me | 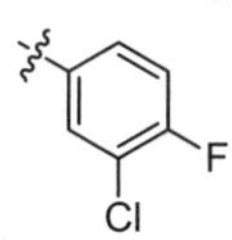 | 0.030 | |

[a]Potentiation $EC_{50}$ determined in the presence of a submaximal amount of glutamate using fluorescence detection of changes in intracellular calcium.

and a 5-$HT_{2A}$ $K_i$ of 2100 nM, suggesting that further optimization is probably necessary for a compound from this series to achieve clinical relevance.

The development of mGlu2 allosteric modulators is at an earlier stage than the mGlu2 and mGlu3 orthosteric agonists, although there are some indications that allosteric mGlu2 receptor PAMs have entered clinical development. The years from 2006 to 2010 have seen a noteworthy increase in the number of mGlu2 PAM disclosures in the scientific and patent [79] literature, underscoring the interest in this mechanism for activating the mGlu2 receptor. Additionally, these disclosures reveal the remarkable breadth of chemical diversity recognized by the allosteric site (or sites) of this receptor. Likewise, the reported efficacy in rodent models of schizophrenia and anxiety to date lends target validity for the mGlu2 allosteric mechanism.

## 6.5 ELECTROPHYSIOLOGICAL PROPERTIES OF ORTHOSTERIC mGlu2 AND mGlu3 RECEPTOR AGONISTS

A number of mGlu2 and mGlu3 receptor agonists have been examined in the medial PFC using *in vitro* brain slice preparation. When recording from layer

V pyramidal cells, spontaneous (i.e., not due to electrically evoked stimulation) synaptic currents are induced by brief bath applications of 5-HT in contrast to electrically evoked potentials induced by stimulation of the white matter deep to the cortex. Activation of 5-$HT_{2A}$ receptors mediates the 5-HT-induced excitatory postsynaptic currents (EPSCs) [94]. Interestingly, the potency of the mGlu2 and mGlu3 receptor agonist LY354740 to suppress these 5-HT-induced EPSCs ($EC_{50}$ = 83 nM) is about threefold greater than the potency of LY354740 in attenuating the early electrically evoked EPSPs ($EC_{50}$ = 249 nM). Conversely, the mGlu2 and mGlu3 antagonist LY341495 appears to be approximately threefold more potent in blocking the suppressant action of LY354740 at the early electrically evoked EPSP than the spontaneous 5-HT-induced EPSCs [95]. The suppression of 5-HT-induced EPSCs by mGlu2 and mGlu3 agonists appears to be mediated by a presynaptic mechanism as (1) the mGlu2 and mGlu3 antagonist LY341495 increased the frequency of 5-HT-induced EPSCs; (2) the mGlu2 and mGlu3 agonist had no effect on inward currents in layer V pyramidal cells induced by AMPA after exposure of the slices to tetrodotoxin to block sodium channels; and (3) thalamic lesions decreased the frequency of 5-HT-induced EPCS by approximately 50% and also decreased the density of [$^3$H]LY354740 binding by approximately 20%. Experiments with a thalamocortical slice preparation have confirmed the presence of functional presynaptic mGlu2 receptors in this pathway [96]. Like LY354740, compound LY404039 (the active constituent of oral prodrug LY2140023 monohydrate) potently suppressed 5-HT-induced EPSCs in layer V pyramidal cells [71]. More recently, an mGlu2 receptor potentiator has been shown to suppress 5-HT-induced EPSCs recorded from layer V pyramidal cells, confirming the importance of mGlu2 receptors on this response [86]. Like many of the brain regions recorded from, and consistent with, a presynaptic locus of action, changes in the membrane potential or input resistance generally are not observed following short bath applications of orthosteric mGlu2 and mGlu3 agonists [96, 97]. However, this interpretation does not rule out the possibility of postsynaptic effects that might not be measured during recordings from the cell body due to technical space-clamp issues.

Presynaptic actions of mGlu2 and mGlu3 agonists are seen in a number of different areas that involve circuitry that is thought to be involved in the pathophysiology and/or treatment of schizophrenia, such as the hippocampus-related circuitry. Both LY354740 and DCG-IV were found to suppress glutamate release from stimulation of the medial perforant pathway leading to the dentate gyrus [98]. Kilbride and colleagues speculated that the slightly lower potency and efficacy of LY354740 in suppressing activity in the lateral perforant pathway than the medial perforant pathway might relate to a different density of mGlu2 or mGlu3 receptors. A presynaptic locus of action for the mGlu2 and mGlu3 agonists in these pathways was confirmed by concentration-dependent changes in paired-pulse depression/facilitation. Converging data from immunohistochemical, electron microscopic, differential cation dependence of ligand-binding, and lesion studies have suggested that mGlu2 receptors play a primary presynaptic role in the medial perforant pathway from the neurons originating in the entorhinal cortex and projecting to the dentate gyrus midmolecular layer/CA1 lacunosum moleculare (Fig. 6.2) [24, 25, 27, 99, 100].

Presynaptic actions of mGlu2 and mGlu3 receptors are found at various synapses in the basal ganglia circuitry [101]. Both mGlu2 and mGlu3 may be localized to corticostriatal afferents originating largely from layer VI pyramidal cells and terminating in either the caudate–putamen or the nucleus accumbens [71, 101–103]. Presynaptic actions have also been identified for mGlu2 agonism in suppressing excitatory synaptic currents in the globus pallidus, with activity likely originating in the subthalamic nucleus [104]. Not only does activation of mGlu2 and mGlu3 receptors suppress synaptic excitation of substantia nigra pars reticulate neurons, but DA modulates the action of group II and group III mGlu receptors in this region [105, 106].

The rodent thalamus is characterized by a marked heterogeneity of mGlu receptor mRNA and protein expression. However, these distinct patterns of mGlu receptor mRNA and protein expression in different types of thalamic nuclei appear to be biologically relevant given the unique physiological roles that these distinct types of thalamic nuclei play [20, 22, 107–109]. Many, but not all, studies have suggested that schizophrenia patients may possess a reduced thalamic volume. The mediodorsal thalamic nucleus is the thalamic structure most commonly shown to be decreased in size. Concentration-dependent suppression by LY379268 and a lack of activity for the putative modestly selective mGlu3 agonist N-acetylaspartylglutamate (NAAG) suggest that activation of mGlu2 receptors is responsible for the suppression of corticogeniculate activity in the ferret dorsal geniculate nucleus [110]. In contrast to the corticogeniculate pathway, the activation of the retinogeniculate pathway was not suppressed by the mGlu2 and mGlu3 agonist LY379268. Consistent with a robust mGlu3 mRNA expression in the reticular nucleus of the thalamus (RTn), suppression by LY379268 and NAAG of the GABAergic inhibitory postsynaptic channels appears to be mediated by a presynaptic mGlu3 acting as a heteroceptor, although suggested to have a surprising low potency for this subtype (i.e., $EC_{50} = 3.3\ \mu M$) [111].

The thalamus appears to be one region where the principal cells in select nuclei may be modulated by mGlu2 receptor activation both in the terminal arbor and in the somatodendritic region. As discussed earlier, activation of prefrontal cortical mGlu2 receptors appears to suppress glutamate release in the PFC from terminals with their cells of origin in the midline and intralaminar thalamic nuclei (Fig. 6.1). Findings from a recent report, coupled with the localization of mGlu2 mRNA and protein in the midline and intralaminar thalamic nuclei and lack of mGlu3 receptor mRNA, suggest that activation of mGlu2 receptors induces a robust hyperpolarization of principle cells from one of the midline thalamic nuclei, the paraventricular nucleus of the thalamus [112]. This robust postsynaptic effect of mGlu2 receptor activation in a higher order thalamic nuclei differs from the lack of postsynaptic effects of mGlu2 and mGlu3 receptor activation in sensory thalamic nuclei such as the ventrobasal thalamic nucleus or the dorsal lateral geniculate nucleus [110, 111, 113]. The apparent robust postsynaptic effect of mGlu2 activation in the higher order midline thalamic nuclei appears to be relatively unusual compared with widespread presynaptic effects of mGlu2 activation at suppressing excitatory amino acid release.

The extended amygdala is another brain region involved in the modulation of fear, anxiety, and stress. Excitatory neurotransmission at both the basolateral amygdala (BLA)-central nucleus projection of the amygdala synapse and within the bed nucleus of the stria terminalis (BNST) is highly sensitive to the presynaptic suppressant actions of LY354740 [114, 115]. A different study that compared presynaptic versus postsynaptic effects in both the BLA and the BNST found that LY354740 did not elicit postsynaptic effects at concentrations that decreased excitatory neurotransmission via presynaptic effects. For example, LY354740 was only weakly potent at inducing a tetrodotoxin-insensitive membrane hyperpolarization ($EC_{50}$~2 μM) from neurons of the BLA compared with a 90% inhibition of spontaneous excitatory postsynaptic activity at a 1-μM LY354740 concentration [116]. Furthermore, only about half of neurons in the BNST were directly inhibited by LY354740, compared with neurons in the BLA, where hyperpolarization was induced by LY354740 in all 30 tested cells. Electron microscopic surveys in these two regions uncovered correlations to the electrophysiological data, as mGlu2- and mGlu3-like labeling was observed in 22.5% and 9.5% of dendritic shafts and spines in the BLA and BNST, respectively. Thus, the presynaptic effects of mGlu2 and mGlu3 agonists in the amygdala are at least 10 times more potent and also are more efficacious than postsynaptic effects.

Taken together, the most salient electrophysiological action of mGlu2 receptors is the suppression of excitatory synaptic transmission in brain slices from a variety of regions that are thought to be involved in the pathophysiology and treatment of schizophrenia, such as the PFC, dorsal and ventral striatum, thalamus, hippocampus, and amygdala (Table 6.14). *In vivo* recordings in awake, freely moving rats where systemically administered LY354740 reversed the excitation of deep layer pyramidal cells of the medial PFC (prelimbic area) induced by MK-801 [117] appear to provide a bridge between the slice electrophysiology and behavioral experiments described later in this chapter. A more recent report that systemic LY354740, like haloperidol and clozapine, reverses the excitation of orbitofrontal cortical deep layer pyramidal cells induced by MK-801 extends the bridge between *in vitro* and behavioral pharmacological results [118].

## 6.6 ELECTROPHYSIOLOGICAL PROPERTIES OF mGLU2 RECEPTOR POSITIVE ALLOSTERIC MODULATORS

One of the more remarkable features of mGlu2 PAMs is the frequency dependence of these effects in some systems compared with orthosteric mGlu2 and

**TABLE 6.14 Potency and Efficacy of mGlu2 and mGlu3 Agonists in Suppression of Evoked Glutamatergic Excitatory Synaptic Responses in Different Brain Slice Preparations**

| Preparation | Drug | $EC_{50}$ (nM) | Maximal Inhibition (%) | LY341495 $pA_2$ | Reference |
|---|---|---|---|---|---|
| mPFC (5-HT-induced EPSCs) | LY354740 | 89 | 88 | 7.27 | [95] |
| | LY354740 | 137 | 89 | | [162] |
| | LY379268 | 231 | | | [95] |
| | LY404039 | 82 | 86 | | [71] |
| mPFC (electrically evoked EPSPs) | LY354740 | 235 | 78 | 7.9 | [95] |
| | LY379268 | 276 | | | [95] |
| | LY379268 | 29 | ~20 | | [97] |
| | LY404039 | 148 | 78 | | Eli Lilly, data on file |
| Fronto-parietal (5HT EPSCs) | LY354740 | 398 | ~60 | | [95] |
| Hippocampus (MPP-DG) | LY354740 | 115 | 80 | | [98] |
| | LY354740 | 77 | 90 | 7.9 | [163] |
| Hippocampus (LPP-DG) | LY354740 | 230 | 50 | | [98] |
| Hippocampus (MPP-CA1 LMol | LY354740 | 32 | 80 | 8.0 | [163] |
| Caudate–putamen (corticostriatal) | LY354740 | 20 | ~80 | | [71] |
| | LY404039 | 141 | ~70 | | [71] |
| N. Accumbens (PrL-n accumbens) | LY354740 | 33 | 60 | | [103] |
| Amygdala (BLA-CeA) | LY354740 | 2 | 68 | | [114] |
| Bed nucleus stria/terminalis (BNST) | LY354740 | 6 | 55 | | [115] |
| Thalamus (cortico-geniculate EPSCs | LY379268 | 9 | 50 | | [110] |
| Substantia nigra (STN-SNr) | LY354740 | 75 | 69 | | [105] |

mGlu3 agonists. For example, the efficacy of the mGlu2 PAM cyPPTS in suppressing electrically evoked responses in the corticostriatal pathway was dependent on stimulus frequency unlike the orthosteric mGlu2 and mGlu3 agonist LY379268 [84]. Another mGlu2 receptor PAM, BINA, was found to attenuate the frequency of 5-HT-induced EPSCs recorded from layer V pyramidal cells of the medial PFC [86]. The dependence of this effect on potentiating mGlu2 receptors was confirmed by blocking this action with the mGlu2 and mGlu3 antagonist LY341495. The mGlu2 PAM LY487379 modulates the medial perforant pathway-dentate gyrus (middle third of the molecular layer) synapse only when sufficient ambient glutamate concentrations are present in the neuropil. Thus, the mGlu2 PAM had no effect by itself, but did result in an approximately threefold leftward shift in the concentration–response relationship in assessing the suppressant action of the mGlu2 and mGlu3 agonist DCG-IV [119]. BINA also modulated excitatory neurotransmission in hippocampal afferents through the medial perforant pathway [85]. Thus, these initial experiments suggest that mGlu2 PAMs offer promise in reprising critical aspects of mGlu2 and mGlu3 agonist physiology in areas such as the PFC, striatum, and hippocampus.

## 6.7 NEUROCHEMICAL EFFECTS OF ORTHOSTERIC mGLU2 AND mGLU3 AGONISTS

Schizophrenia patients are thought to possess both a hypodopaminergic prefrontal cortical profile and a hyperdopaminergic subcortical profile [120]. Several mGlu2 and mGlu3 agonists have been found to increase DA turnover in cortical regions. Rodent studies found that LY404039 increased both extracellular DA levels and DA turnover in the medial PFC similar to clozapine; however, unlike clozapine, it also increased 5-HT turnover as measured by the metabolite 5-HIAA:5-HT ratio [121]. Previously, LY379268 had also been found to increase both DA and serotonin turnover in the medial PFC [122]. In the same study, clozapine was found to increase PFC DA turnover as well. Furthermore, the effects of behaviorally active doses of LY379268 on monoamine turnover were blocked by the administration of the mGlu2 and mGlu3 antagonist LY341495.

Important interactions between NMDA receptor antagonists and mGlu2 and mGlu3 agonists have also been examined during *in vivo* dialysis experiments. LY354740 was found to suppress PCP-induced increase in glutamate in the PFC without altering the PCP-induced increase in prefrontal cortical or ventral striatal DA [123]. LY379268 was found by another group to decrease ketamine-induced increases in glutamate in the PFC and nucleus accumbens, but without altering ketamine-induced changes in DA [124]. In other studies, the mGlu2/3 agonist was found to decrease MK-801-induced increases in extracellular levels of norepinephrine (NE), but not DA, in a manner that parallels alterations in locomotor behavior [125]. Furthermore, the suppression by LY379268 of the ketamine-induced increase in extracellular NE in the ventral hippocampus was suggested to depend on the suppression of glutamate release by the mGlu2 and mGlu3 agonist in the medial PFC [126]. The mGlu2 and mGlu3 agonist LY379268 has also been found to decrease extracellular levels of GABA measured in the reticular nucleus of the rat thalamus [21], a finding consistent with previously noted electrophysiological studies suggesting involvement of an mGlu3 heteroreceptor on GABAergic terminals in this brain structure [111]. Overall, these findings suggest that mGlu2 and mGlu3 agonists may enhance dopaminergic neurotransmission in the PFC and that their antagonism of the behavioral effects of psychotomimetic drugs is not due simply to decreasing extracellular DA concentrations.

## 6.8 BEHAVIORAL PHARMACOLOGY OF ORTHOSTERIC mGLU2 AND mGLU3 AGONISTS

Symptoms of schizophrenia are traditionally defined within three domain clusters: positive symptoms, negative symptoms, and cognitive deficits. To date, positive symptoms are best managed with current monoamine-based medications. As a result, the most validated animal models for detecting putative antipsychotic mechanisms tend to reflect efficacy for treating positive symptoms in schizophrenia. Positive symptoms appear to be associated most closely with mesolimbic hyperdopaminergia and are pharmacologically mimicked through the administration of DA agonists. Examples of common animal models for positive symptoms of schizophrenia include amphetamine- or cocaine-induced locomotor activity in rats or mice, and apomorphine-induced climbing in mice. These mGlu2 and mGlu3 agonists have generally proven effective against DA agonist-induced hyperactivity [121, 127, 128]. However, unlike the profile of monoamine-based antipsychotics, mGlu2 and mGlu3 agonists appear to be more potent in blocking of PCP- versus amphetamine-induced behaviors [129, 130].

Another predictive animal model of antipsychotic efficacy is the conditioned avoidance response assay (CAR) [131]. Although potency of antipsychotic compounds in this assay correlates well with dopamine $D_2$ receptor occupancy at therapeutic doses in humans, activity in CAR does not depend on direct $D_2$ binding. For instance, the muscarinic agonist xanomeline was shown by Shannon and colleagues [132] to be efficacious in multiple animal models of schizophrenia, including CAR, and was recently reported to be efficacious in schizophrenia patients [133]. Similarly, mGlu2 and mGlu3 agonists exhibit an antipsychotic-like profile in CAR [121, 134].

The ability of agents to attenuate locomotor stimulation produced by other psychotomimetics such as 5-$HT_{2A}$ agonists and NMDA antagonists are also believed to reflect antipsychotic-like activity and debate exists as to whether activity against these mechanisms indicates a cortical site of action and serves to identify compounds with an "atypical-like" antipsychotic profile. Several investigators have demonstrated acute efficacy of multiple mGlu2 and mGlu3 agonists in reversing hyperactivity induced by noncompetitive NMDA antagonists such as PCP, ketamine, and MK-801 [70, 123, 124, 135, 136]. Regarding 5-$HT_{2A}$–mGlu2 and mGlu3 interactions, Gewirtz and Marek [137] first reported that LY354740 blocked head shake behavior in rats induced by the 5-$HT_{2A}$ agonist ±1-(2,5-dimethoxy-4-iodophenyl)-2-aminopropane (DOI). This finding was replicated in mice with mGlu2 and mGlu3 LY354740 and LY379268 [138]. Moreover, a recent combination study with LY379268 and the 5-$HT_{2A}$ antagonist M100907 indicated greater efficacy of the combination in blocking locomotor and neurochemical effects of MK-801 as compared with either compound administered alone [139].

Efficacy following repeat dosing of mGlu2 and mGlu3 agonists has been mixed. Cartmell and colleagues [140] found that oral administration of

LY379268 was equally efficacious in reversing PCP-induced hyperactivity following either acute or 4 days of daily dosing, whereas tolerance was observed to the motor-disrupting effects measured in the rotorod assay. Conversely, systemic dosing of LY379268 was ineffective against PCP-stimulating effects following 7 [81] or 8 days of dosing [141]. Regarding chronic dosing effects of PCP in sensitization paradigms, mGlu2 and mGlu3 agonists appear to block the expression of PCP-induced sensitization (i.e., enhanced locomotor response following repeat dosing). For instance, LY379268 blocked the sensitized response to PCP on the 10th day of dosing; however, co-administration of LY379268 during the 9 days of PCP treatment failed to block the development of sensitization when PCP was tested alone on day 10 [142]. A similar blockade of the expression of amphetamine sensitization by LY379268 was observed in a study by Kim and Vezina [128]. Unfortunately, the ability of LY379268 to alter development of sensitization was not assessed.

Although acute dosing of mGlu2 and mGlu3 agonists consistently blocks the locomotor-stimulating effects of NMDA antagonists, several laboratories have been unable to demonstrate reversal of other NMDA antagonist-induced pharmacological effects. For example, Schreiber et al. [143] using LY354740, and Imre et al. [144] using LY379268, failed to attenuate prepulse inhibition disruptions by PCP or ketamine—or by amphetamine [145]. Mixed data also exist regarding the ability of mGlu2 and mGlu3 to reverse the subjective effects of PCP. Winter et al. [146] found that LY379268 partially reversed PCP (and the 5-$HT_{2A}$ agonist LSD) drug discrimination; however, Schreiber et al. [143] failed to attenuate drug discrimination cues of PCP with LY354740. These data indicate that mGlu2 and mGlu3 agonists do not impact the full pharmacological spectrum of NMDA antagonist effects. This conclusion is supported by a clinical study by Krystal and colleagues [147], which found that LY354740 attenuated specific ketamine-induced aspects (e.g., working memory deficits) while having no effect on other ketamine responses such as psychotic-like symptoms.

The above findings showing that LY354740 had relatively specific effects against ketamine-induced cognitive deficits are intriguing and, at least, are suggestive that mGlu2 and mGlu3 agonists may have therapeutic benefits in improving cognitive and negative symptoms associated with schizophrenia. Unfortunately, little preclinical work exists exploring the effects of mGlu2 and mGlu3 agonists on cognitive functioning. In rats, LY354740 administered alone disrupted multiple working and spatial memory tasks, including delayed matching and nonmatching to sample and Morris water maze learning [25]. Similarly, Spinelli et al. [148] reported deficits in marmoset monkeys on sustained-attention accuracy in the five-choice serial reaction test (5-CSRT) following LY354740 administration. The apparent cognitive disrupting effects of mGlu2 and mGlu3 receptor agonism are countered by reports of cognitive-restoring effects in rodents impaired by PCP. For instance, LY379268 attenuated PCP-induced anticipatory and perseverative response errors in mice testing in the five-choice serial reaction task *(5-CSRT) [149]. Conversely,

Amitai and Markou reported that LY379268 exacerbated PCP-induced disruption of 5-CSRT performance in rats [150]. In a developmental model of schizophrenia, LY354740 restored social novelty discrimination deficits in adult rats induced by repeated early postnatal PCP treatments [151]. These results suggest that the effects of mGlu2 and mGlu3 agonists may be dependent on the level of glutamatergic tone.

To delineate the mechanisms mediating the actions of mGlu2 and mGlu3 agonists, pharmacology studies have been conducted using mice lacking the genes for mGlu2 and mGlu3 receptors. Spooren et al. [152] first reported that the mGlu2 receptor is key in mediating the PCP-reversing effects of mGlu2 and mGlu3 agonists by demonstrating that the ability of LY314582 (racemate of LY354740) to suppress PCP-induced hyperactivity was lost in mGlu2 receptor knockout mice. More recently, Woolley and colleagues [153] reported that LY379268 blocked both PCP- and amphetamine-induced hyperactivity in mGlu3 receptor knockout mice and wild-type controls but was ineffective in mGlu2 receptor knockout mice. Fell et al. [154] replicated these findings using the mGlu2/3 agonist LY404039 and also showed that the efficacy of clozapine and risperidone were not dependent on mGlu2 or mGlu3 receptor integrity. These studies demonstrating target-specific effects of mGlu2 and mGlu3 agonists are nicely supported by other mutant mouse studies showing that LY379268 attenuated the spontaneous hyperactivity phenotype of mice lacking the glial glutamate and aspartate transporter, which is likely a consequence of elevated glutamate tone [155]. Finally, activity of mGlu2 and mGlu3 agonists does not appear to be dependent on DA system integrity; DA-deficient mice resulting from a lack of tyrosine hydroxylase and mice lacking dopamine $D_2$ receptors both show normal responses to NMDA antagonist-induced hyperactivity [154, 156].

## 6.9 BEHAVIORAL PHARMACOLOGY OF mGlu2 RECEPTOR POSITIVE ALLOSTERIC MODULATORS

There is increasing interest in PAMs for the mGlu receptor group II receptor family. At least theoretically, compounds that demonstrate affinity for allosteric binding sites may have advantages over orthosteric agents in terms of a lower propensity to produce receptor desensitization (where agonists are concerned) due to their phasic, use-dependent mechanism, and the potential for developing compounds with greater receptor subtype selectivity [157, 158].

A number of PAMs have been identified (e.g., CBiPES; 4-MPPTS; 2,2,2-TEMPS; and BINA) that, similar to orthosteric mGlu2 and mGlu3 agonists, block the locomotor-stimulating effects of NMDA antagonists [79, 81, 85, 87, 89, 126]. Positive mGlu2 allosteric modulators also have been shown to reverse amphetamine-stimulated activity and 5-$HT_{2A}$ agonist-induced head twitch behavior [81, 86, 97]. One reported differentiable pharmacological feature between orthosteric and allosteric ligands is the apparent ability of mGlu2 receptor allosteric compounds to reverse prepulse inhibition deficits induced by amphetamine using 4-MPPTS [81] or by PCP using BINA [85]. A recent paper also demonstrated that BINA reversed the neuronal metabolic signal of PCP using blood-oxygen-level dependent functional magnetic resonance imaging (BOLD fMRI) methods in rats, suggesting a possible translatable biomarker for clinical evaluation [159]. Finally, additional evidence for a beneficial influence of positive mGlu2 receptor modulation within the domain of cognition comes from a study by Harich and colleagues [151], who found that the mGlu2 potentiator 4-MPPTS facilitated social discrimination deficits in rats that received early postnatal PCP administrations, an effect found also with the orthosteric mGlu2 and mGlu3 agonist LY354740.

Taken together, the *in vivo* pharmacological effects of PAMs for the mGlu2 receptor have largely recapitulated findings reported with orthosteric mGlu2 and mGlu3 agonists. Two reports have also extended the therapeutic findings of mGlu2 potentiators to include reversal of PCP- and amphetamine-induced prepulse inhibition deficits. As stated earlier, there are no reported successes of orthosteric mGlu2 and mGlu3 agonists normalizing pharmacological disruptions of prepulse inhibition. Further studies need to be conducted to delineate the source of this potentially important distinction.

## 6.10 CLINICAL ASPECTS OF ORTHOSTERIC mGLU2 AND mGLU3 RECEPTOR AGONISTS

The preclinical pharmacological profile of mGlu2 and mGlu3 agonists demonstrate therapeutic features that are consistent with clinically effective antipsychotics and suggest that ligands targeting this mechanism may provide therapeutic potential for treating the symptoms of schizophrenia. LY2140023 monohydrate is the methionine amide prodrug of the mGlu2 and mGlu3 agonist LY404039 that has enhanced intestinal absorption following oral administration in humans. Once absorbed, LY2140023 monohydrate is efficiently hydrolyzed to produce the active mGlu2 and mGlu3 agonist LY404039. Two Phase II, 4-week, multicenter, randomized, double-blind, placebo-controlled, and active comparator-controlled trials were conducted with LY2140023 monohydrate.

Study 1 [160], a proof-of-concept study, examined the efficacy and safety of LY2140023 monohydrate in acutely ill patients suffering with a recent exacerbation of chronic schizophrenia. In this study, a total of 196 patients were enrolled and randomly assigned to receive LY2140023 monohydrate (40 mg BID), placebo, or olanzapine (15 mg daily) in a 3:2:1 ratio. All patients were hospitalized, withdrawn from any pretrial antipsychotic medications, and treated in a double-blind manner for 4 weeks. The dose of LY2140023 monohydrate was determined from early phase clinical and toxicology studies to be safe and also to provide CNS exposure in humans that is equivalent to CNS exposure that blocked PCP-induced hyperactivity in rats.

Treatment with LY2140023 monohydrate or olanzapine resulted in statistically significant improvements in Positive and Negative Syndrome Scale (PANSS) total scores as well as in other outcome measures such as Clinical Global Impression—Severity (CGI-S) scores and PANSS positive and negative subscores compared with placebo. The LY2140023 monohydrate group and the olanzapine group showed rapid onset of efficacy, with statistically significant effects manifesting at week 1. Significant improvements in all efficacy measures were sustained at subsequent weeks after week 1 through the end of the study. After 4 weeks of treatment, both the LY2140023 monohydrate group (32.0%) and the olanzapine group (41.2%) showed significantly greater response rates (25% or more decrease from baseline in PANSS total score) than the placebo group (3.2%).

LY2140023 monohydrate was generally well tolerated. Common treatment-emergent adverse events (incidence >3% in all patients assigned to LY2140023 monohydrate) included insomnia, affect lability, nausea, headache, somnolence, and increase in blood creatine phosphokinase. Notably, there were no significant elevations in serum prolactin levels or significant treatment-emergent extrapyramidal motor signs with any of the three treatments, suggesting that LY2140023 monohydrate did not have a clinically discernible effect on $D_2$ receptors. LY2140023 monohydrate was not associated with any significant weight change compared with placebo or any clinically significant change in vital signs, electrocardiograms, or laboratory analytes.

Study 2 [161] was designed to replicate the findings of the first study and to examine efficacy over an expanded dose range of LY2140023 monohydrate (5, 20, 40, or 80 mg BID). In this 4-week inpatient study, patients with an acute exacerbation of chronic schizophrenia (N = 669) were randomized (2:2:2:2:2:1) to receive double-blind each of the 4 LY2140023 monohydrate doses, placebo, or olanzapine (15 mg/day). Unlike study 1, efficacy results were inconclusive: none of the four LY2140023 monohydrate doses was significantly more efficacious than placebo, nor was olanzapine (15 mg/day) as measured by baseline-to-endpoint mean change in the PANSS total score. A larger-than-anticipated effect in the placebo group was observed (14.6-point reduction in the PANSS total score) and could explain this lack of an efficacy finding. As in study 1, LY2140023 monohydrate was generally well tolerated, although five convulsions were reported in four patients, who all recovered fully without any sequelae. Convulsions did not appear related to dose or time on LY2140023 monohydrate treatment. Common treatment-emergent adverse events (incidence >3% in all patients assigned to LY2140023 monohydrate) included insomnia, increased eosinophil count, anxiety, nausea, agitation, and headache. There were no clinically significant changes in extrapyramidal motor symptoms, prolactin, weight, vital signs, laboratory analytes, or electrocardiogram for patients treated with LY2140023 monohydrate.

Further study is needed to better understand the long-term safety and efficacy of LY2140023 monohydrate. Moreover, a comprehensive understanding of factors leading to a greater-than-anticipated placebo response in schizophrenia trials is necessary to mitigate this challenge to new drug development.

## 6.11 SUMMARY AND CONCLUSIONS

The appearance over the past 15 years of highly optimized pharmacological tools, representing both orthosteric and allosteric mechanisms, has enabled extensive preclinical characterization of mGlu2 and mGlu3 receptors under both physiologic and pathophysiologic conditions. Emerging from this basic preclinical work, important progress has been made toward the clinical validation of these receptors as therapeutic targets for the treatment of schizophrenia.

Treating schizophrenia through stimulation of inhibitory autoreceptors on glutamatergic pyramidal neurons may open a new vista of achievable therapeutic outcomes associated with the normalization of glutamatergic tone in relation to diverse cortical networks and associated neurotransmitters. Improvement in negative symptoms and cognitive impairment may be amenable to this intervention, as well as a reduction in the comorbid substance abuse that diminishes most therapeutic gains possible in this disorder. In addition, it may also provide the extraordinary opportunity to implement a therapeutic modality that may have little intrinsic activity during periods of clinical remission yet be available to prevent or mitigate illness exacerbation associated with glutamatergic dysregulation.

Furthermore, the promise of a new antipsychotic medication that, unlike all currently approved agents, does not bind to monoamine receptors offers the possibility of providing patients a medicament with a lower risk of treatment-emergent adverse events that can include extrapyramidal motor dysfunction, elevated serum prolactin, weight gain, sedation, and orthostatic hypotension.

## REFERENCES


1. Carlsson, A., Lindquist, M. (1963). Effect of chlorpromazine and haloperidol on formation of 3-methoxytyramine and normetanephrine in mouse brain. *Acta Pharmacol Toxicol (Copenh)*, *20*, 140–144.
2. Creese, I., Burt, D.R., Snyder, S.H. (1976). Dopamine receptor binding predicts clinical and pharmacological potencies of antischizophrenic drugs. *Science*, *192*, 481–483.
3. Seeman, P., Lee, T., Chau-Wong, M., Wong, K. (1976). Antipsychotic drug doses and neuroleptic/dopamine receptors. *Nature*, *261*, 717–719.
4. Anis, N.A., Berry, S.C., Burton, N.R., Lodge, D. (1983). The dissociative anesthetics, ketamine and phencyclidine, selectively reduce excitations of central mammalian neurons by N-methyl-aspartate. *Br J Pharmacol*, *79*, 565–575.

5. Wong, E.H., Kemp, J.A., Priestley, T., Knight, A.R., Woodruff, G.N., Iversen, L.L. (1986). The anticonvulsanat MK-801 is a potent N-methyl-D-aspartate antagonist. *Proc Natl Acad Sci U S A*, *83*, 7104–7108.

6. Lodge, D. (2009). The history of the pharmacology and cloning of ionotropic glutamate receptors and the development of idiosyncratic nomenclature. *Neuropharmacology*, *56*, 6–21.

7. Luby, E.D., Cohen, B.D., Rosenbaum, G., Gottlieb, J.S., Kelly, R. (1959). Study of a new schizophrenomimetic drug—Sernyl. *Arch Neurol Psychiatry*, *81*, 363–369.

8. Tamminga, C.A. (1998). Schizophrenia and glutamatergic transmission. *Crit Rev Neurobiol*, *12*, 21–36.

9. Krystal, J.H., Belger, A. (1999). Therapeutic implications of the hyperglutamatergic effects of NMDA antagonists. *Neuropsychopharmacology*, *21*, S143–S157.

10. Lahti, A.C., Koffel, B., LaPorte, D., Tamminga, C.A. (1995). Subanesthetic doses of ketamine stimulate psychosis in schizophrenia. *Neuropsychopharmacology*, *13*, 9–19.

11. Moghaddam, B., Adams, B., Verma, A., Daly, D. (1997). Activation of glutamatergic neurotransmission by ketamine: a novel step in the pathway from the NMDA receptor blockade to dopaminergic and cognitive disruptions associated with the prefrontal cortex. *J Neurosci*, *17*, 2921–2927.

12. Duncan, G.E., Miyamoto, S., Leipzig, J.N., Lieberman, J.A. (1999). Comparison of brain metabolic activity patterns induced by ketamine, MK-801 and amphetamine in rats: support for NMDA receptor involvement in responses to subanesthetic dose of ketamine. *Brain Res*, *843*, 171–183.

13. Anand, A., Charney, D.S., Oren, D.A., Berman, R.M., Hu, X.S., Cappiello, A., Krystal, J.H. (2000). Attenuation of the neuropsychiatric effects of ketamine with lamotrigine. *Arch Gen Psychiatry*, *57*, 270–276.

14. Holcomb, H.H., Lahti, A.C., Medoff, D.R., Cullen, T., Tamminga, C.A. (2005). Effects of noncompetitive NMDA receptor blockade on anterior cingulate cerebral blood flow in volunteers with schizophrenia. *Neuropsychopharmacology*, *30*, 2275–2282.

15. Conn, P.J., Pin, J.P. (1997). Pharmacology and functions of metabotropic glutamate receptors. *Annu Rev Pharmacol Toxicol*, *37*, 205–237.

16. Schoepp, D.D., Jane, D.E., Monn, J.A. (1999). Pharmacological agents acting at subtypes of metabotropic glutamate receptors. *Neuropharmacology*, *38*, 1431–1476.

17. Pin, J.P., Archer, F. (2002). The metabotropic glutamate receptors: structure, activation mechanism, and pharmacology. *Curr Drug Targets CNS Neurol Disord*, *1*, 297–317.

18. Muto, T., Tsuchiya, D., Morikawa, K., Jingami, H. (2007). Structures of the extracellular regions of the group II/III metabotropic glutamate receptors. *Proc Natl Acad Sci U S A*, *104*, 3759–3764.

19. Kunishima, N., Shimada, Y., Tsuji, Y., Sato, T., Yamamoto, M., Kumasaka, T., Nakanishi, S., Jingami, H., Morikawa, K. (2000). Structural basis of glutamate recognition by a dimeric metabotropic glutamate receptor. *Nature*, *407*, 971–977.

20. Ohishi, H., Shigemoto, R., Nakanishi, S., Mizuno, N. (1993a). Distribution of the messenger RNA for a metabotropic glutamate receptor, mGluR2, in the central nervous system of the rat. *Neuroscience*, *53*, 1009–1018.

21. Gu, G., Lorrain, D.S., Wei, H., Cole, R.L., Zhang, X., Daggett, L.P., Schaffhauser, H., Bristow, L.J., Lechner, S.M. (2008). Distribution of metabotropic glutamate 2 and 3 receptors in the rat forebrain: implication in emotional responses and central disinhibition. *Brain Res*, *1197*, 47–62.
22. Ohishi, H., Neki, A., Mizuno, N. (1997). Distribution of a metabotropic glutamate receptor, mGluR2, in the central nervous system of the rat and mouse: an immunohistochemical study with a monoclonal antibody. *Neurosci Res*, *30*, 65–82.
23. Marek, G.J., Wright, R.A., Gewirtz, J.C., Schoepp, D.D. (2001). A major role for thalamocortical afferents in serotonergic hallucinogen receptor function in the rat neocortex. *Neuroscience*, *105*, 379–392.
24. Shigemoto, R., Kinoshita, A., Wada, E., Nomura, S., Ohishi, H., Takada, M., Flor, P.J., Neki, A., Abe, T., Nakanishi, S., Mizuno, N. (1997). Differential presynaptic localization of metabotropic glutamate receptor subtypes in the rat hippocampus. *J Neurosci*, *17*, 7503–7522.
25. Higgins, G.A., Ballard, T.M., Kew, J.N.C., Richards, J.G., Kemp, J.A., Adam, G., Woltering, T., Nakanishi, S., Mutel, V. (2004). Pharmacological manipulation of mGlu2 receptors influences cognitive performance in the rodent. *Neuropharmacology*, *46*, 907–917.
26. Ohishi, H., Shigemoto, R., Nakanishi, S., Mizuno, N. (1993b). Distribution of the mRNA for a metabotropic glutamate receptor (mGluR3) in the rat brain: an in situ hybridization study. *J Comp Neurol*, *335*, 252–266.
27. Tamaru, Y., Nomura, S., Mizuno, N., Shigemoto, R. (2001). Distribution of metabotropic glutamate receptor mGlu3 in the mouse CNS: differential location relative to pre- and postsynaptic sites. *Neuroscience*, *106*, 481–503.
28. Corti, C., Crepaldi, L., Mion, S., Roth, A.L., Xuereb, J.H., Ferraguti, F. (2007). Altered dimerization of metabotropic glutamate receptor 3 in schizophrenia. *Biol Psychiatry*, *62*, 747–755.
29. Egan, M.F., Straub, R.E., Goldberg, T.E., Yakub, I., Callicott, J.H., Hairiri, A.R., Mattay, V.S., Bertolino, A., Hyde, T.M., Shannon-Weickert, C., AkilM, C.J., Vakkalanka, R.K., Balkissoon, R., Gibbs, R.A., Kleinman, J.E., Weinberger, D.R. (2004). Variation in GRM3 affects cognition, prefrontal glutamate, and risk for schizophrenia. *Proc Natl Acad Sci U S A*, *101*, 12604–12609.
30. Harrison, P.J., Lyon, L., Sartorius, L.J., Burnett, P.W.J., Lane, T.A. (2008). The group II metabotropic glutamate receptor 3 (mGluR3, mGlu3, GRM3): expression, function and involvement in schizophrenia. *J Psychopharmacol*, *22*, 308–322.
31. Johnson, B.G., Wright, R.A., Arnold, M.B., Wheeler, W.J., Ornstein, P.L., Schoepp, D.D. (1999). [$^3$H]-LY341495 as a novel antagonist radioligand for group II metabotropic glutamate (mGlu) receptors: characterization of binding to membranes of mGlu receptor subtype expressing cells. *Neuropharmacology*, *38*, 1519–1529.
32. Schoepp, D.D., Monn, J.A. (2002). *Pharmacology of Metabotropic Glutamate Receptors (in Glutamate and GABA Receptors and Transporters)*. New York: Taylor and Francis, Inc., pp. 151–186.
33. Palmer, E., Monaghan, D.T., Cotman, C.W. (1989). Trans-ACPD, a selective agonist of the phosphoinositide-coupled excitatory amino acid receptor. *Eur J Pharmacol*, *166*, 585–587.
34. Desai, M.A., Conn, P.J. (1990). Selective activation of phosphoinositide hydrolysis by a rigid analogue of glutamate. *Neurosci Lett*, *109*, 157–162.

35. Manzoni, O., Fagni, L., Pin, J.P., Rassendren, F., Poulat, F., Sladeczek, F., Bockaert, J. (1990). (trans)-1-Amino-cyclopentyl-1,3-dicarboxylate stimulates quisqualate phosphoinositide-coupled receptors but not ionotropic glutamate receptors in striatal neurons and xenopus oocytes. *Mol Pharmacol*, *38*, 1–6.

36. Schoepp, D.D., Johnson, B.G., True, R.A., Monn, J.A. (1991a). Comparison of (1S,3R)-1-aminocyclopentane-1,3-dicarboxylic acid (1S,3R-ACPD)- and 1R,3S-ACPD-stimulated brain phosphoinositide hydrolysis. *Eur J Pharmacol*, *207*, 351–353.

37. Schoepp, D.D., Johnson, B.G., Salhoff, C.R., McDonald, J.W., Johnston, M.V. (1991b). In vitro and in vivo pharmacology of trans- and cis-(±)-1-amino-1,3-cyclopentanedicarboxylic acid: dissociation of metabotropic and ionotropic excitatory amino acid receptor effects. *J Neurochem*, *56*, 1789–1796.

38. Tanabe, Y., Masu, M., Ishii, T., Shigemoto, R., Nakanishi, S. (1992). A family of metabotropic glutamate receptors. *Neuron*, *8*, 169–179.

39. Tanabe, Y., Nomura, A., Masu, M., Shigemoto, R., Mizuno, N., Nakanishi, S. (1993). Signal transduction, pharmacological properties, and expression patterns of two rat metabotropic glutamate receptors, mGluR3 and mGluR4. *J Neurosci*, *13*, 1372–1378.

40. Flor, P.J., Lindauer, K., Puttner, I., Rüegg, D., Lukic, S., Knöpfel, T., Kuhn, R. (1995). Molecular cloning, functional expression and pharmacological characterization of the human metabotropic glutamate receptor type 2. *Eur J Neurosci*, *7*, 622–629.

41. Gomeza, J., Mary, S., Brabet, I., Parmentier, M.-L., Restituito, S., Bockaert, J., Pin, J.-P. (1996). Coupling of metabotropic glutamate receptors 2 and 4 to $G_{\alpha 15}$, $G_{\alpha 16}$, and chimeric $G_{\alpha q/i}$ proteins: characterization of new antagonists. *J Pharmacol Exp Ther*, *50*, 923–930.

42. Schoepp, D.D., Johnson, B.G., Monn, J.A. (1992). Inhibition of cyclic AMP formation by a selective metabotropic glutamate receptor agonist. *J Neurochem*, *58*, 1184–1186.

43. Cartmell, J., Curtis, A.R., Kemp, J.A., Kendall, D.A., Alexander, S.P.H. (1993). Subtypes of metabotropic excitatory amino acid receptor distinguished by stereoisomers of the rigid glutamate analogue, 1-aminocyclopentane-1,3-dicarboxylate. *Neurosci Lett*, *153*, 107–110.

44. Schoepp, D.D., Johnson, B.G., Salhoff, C.R., Valli, M.J., Desai, M.A., Burnett, J.P., Mayne, N.G., Monn, J.A. (1995). Selective inhibition of forskolin-stimulated cyclic AMP formation in rat hippocampus by a novel mGluR agonist, 2R,4R-4-aminopyrrolidine-2,4-dicarboxylate. *Neuropharmacology*, *34*, 843–850.

45. Monn, J.A., Valli, M.J., Johnson, B.G., Salhoff, C.R., Wright, R.A., Howe, T., Bond, A., Lodge, D., Spangle, L.A., Paschal, J.W., Campbell, J.B., Griffey, K., Tizzano, J.P., Schoepp, D.D. (1996). Synthesis of the four isomers of 4-aminopyrrolidine-2,4-dicarboxylate: identification of a potent, highly selective, and systemically active agonist for metabotropic glutamate receptors negatively coupled to adenylate cyclase. *J Med Chem*, *39*, 2990–3000.

46. Schoepp, D.D., Salhoff, C.R., Wright, R.A., Johnson, B.G., Burnett, J.P., Belagaje, R., Wu, S., Monn, J.A. (1996). The novel metabotropic glutamate receptor agonist 2R,4R-APDC potentiates stimulation of phosphoinositide hydrolysis in the rat hippocampus by 3,5-dihydroxyphenylglycine: evidence for a synergistic interaction between group 1 and group 2 receptors. *Neuropharmacology*, *35*, 1661–1672.

47. Kozikowski, A.P., Araldi, G.L., Tückmantel, W., Pshenichkin, S., Surina, E.J., Wroblewski, T. (1999). 1-Amino-ACPD, a partial agonist of group II metabotropic glutamate receptors with neuroprotective properties. *Bioorg Med Chem Lett*, *9*, 1721–1726.

48. Yamanoi, K., Ohfune, Y. (1988). Syntheses of trans- and cis-α-(carboxycyclopropyl) glycines. Novel neuroinhibitory amino acids as L-glutamate analogue. *Tetrahedron Lett*, *29*, 1181–1184.

49. Nakagawa, Y., Saitoh, K., Ishihara, T., Ishida, M., Shinozaki, H. (1990). (2S,3S,4S)-α-(Carboxycyclopropyl)glycine is a novel agonist of metabotropic glutamate receptors. *Eur J Pharmacol*, *184*, 205–206.

50. Shimamoto, K., Ishida, M., Shinozaki, H., Ohfune, Y. (1991). Synthesis of four diastereomeric L-2-(carboxycyclopropyl)glycines. Conformationally constrained L-glutamate analogs. *J Org Chem*, *56*, 4167–4176.

51. Hayashi, Y., Tanabe, Y., Aramori, I., Masu, M., Shimamoto, K., Ohfune, Y., Nakanishi, S. (1992). Agonist analysis of 2-(carboxycyclopropyl)glycine isomers for cloned metabotropic glutamate receptor subtypes expressed in Chinese hamster ovary cells. *Br J Pharmacol*, *107*, 539–543.

52. Brabet, I., Parmentier, M.-L., De Colle, C., Bockaert, J., Acher, F., Pin, J.-P. (1998). Comparative effect of L-CCG-I, DCG-IV and γ-carboxy-L-glutamate on all cloned metabotropic glutamate receptor subtypes. *Neuropharmacology*, *37*, 1043–1051.

53. Ohfune, Y., Shimamoto, K., Ishida, M., Shinozaki, H. (1993). Synthesis of L-2-(2,3-dicarboxycyclopropyl)glycines. Novel conformationally restricted glutamate analogues. *Biomed Chem Lett*, *3*, 15–18.

54. Ishida, M., Saitoh, T., Shimamoto, K., Ohfune, Y., Shinozaki, H. (1993). A novel metabotropic glutamate receptor agonist: marked depression of monosynaptic excitation in the newborn rat isolated spinal cord. *Br J Pharmacol*, *109*, 1169–1177.

55. Wilsch, V.W., Pidoplichko, V.I., Opitz, T., Shinozaki, H., Reymann, K.G. (1994). Metabotropic glutamate receptor agonist DCG-IV as NMDA receptor agonist in immature in immature rat hippocampus. *Eur J Pharmacol*, *262*, 287–291.

56. Uyama, Y., Ishida, M., Shinozaki, H. (1997). DCG-IV, a potent metabotropic glutamate receptor agonist, as an NMDA receptor agonist in the rat cortical slice. *Brain Res*, *752*, 327–330.

57. Shibuya, A., Sato, A., Taguchi, T. (1998). Preparation of difluoro analogs of CCGs and their pharmacological evaluations. *Bioorg Med Chem Lett*, *8*, 1979–1984.

58. Saitoh, T., Ishida, M., Shinozaki, H. (1998). Potentiation of DL-α-aminopimelate of the inhibitory action of a novel mGluR agonist (L-$F_2$CCG-I) on monosynaptic excitation in the rat spinal cord. *Br J Pharmacol*, *123*, 771–779.

59. Ishida, M., Saitoh, T., Nakamura, Y., Kataoka, K., Shinozaki, H. (1994). A novel metabotropic glutamate receptor agonist: (2S,1′S,2′R,3′R)-2-(2-carboxy-3-methoxymethylcyclopropyl)glycine (cis-MCG-I). *Eur J Pharmacol*, *268*, 267–270.

60. Ishida, M., Saitoh, T., Tsuji, K., Nakamura, Y., Kataoka, K., Shinozaki, H. (1995). Novel agonists for metabotropic glutamate receptors: trans- and cis-2-(2-carboxy-3-methoxymethylcyclopropyl)glycine (trans- and cis-MCG-I). *Neuropharmacology*, *34*, 821–827.

61. Shimamoto, K., Ohfune, Y. (1993). Inversion of cis-substituted α-cyclopropyl acyl anion. Stereoselective entry to the synthesis of a potent metabotropic glutamate agonist, (2S,1′S,2′S)-2-(carboxycyclopropyl)glycine (L-CCG-I), and its 3′-substituted analogues. *SynLett*, 919–920.

62. Collado, I., Pedregal, C., Mazon, A., Espinosa, J.F., Blanco-Urgoiti, J., Schoepp, D.D., Wright, R.A., Johnson, B.G., Kingston, A.E. (2002). (2S,1′S,2′S,3′R)-2-(2′-Carboxy-3′-methylcyclopropyl) glycine is a potent and selective metabotropic group 2 receptor agonist with anxiolytic properties. *J Med Chem*, *45*, 3619–3629.

63. Collado, I., Pedregal, C., Bueno, A.B., Marcos, A., Gonzalez, R., Blanco-Urgoiti, J., Perez-Castells, J., Schoepp, D.D., Wright, R.A., Johnson, B.G., Kingston, A.E., Moher, E.D., Hoard, D.W., Griffey, K.I., Tizzano, J.P. (2004). (2S, 1′S, 2′R, 3′R)-2-(2′-Carboxy-3′-hydroxymethylcyclopropyl) glycine is a highly potent group 2 and 3 metabotropic glutamate receptor agonist with oral activity. *J Med Chem*, *47*, 456–466.

64. Gonzalez, R., Collado, I., Lopez De Uralde, B., Marcos, A., Martin-Cabrejas, L.M., Pedregal, C., Blanco-Urgoiti, J., Perez-Castells, J., Fernandez, M.A., Andis, S.L., Johnson, B.G., Wright, R.A., Schoepp, D.D., Monn, J.A. (2005). C3′-cis-substituted carboxycyclopropyl glycines as metabotropic glutamate 2/3 receptor agonists: synthesis and SAR studies. *Bioorg Med Chem*, *13*, 6556–6570.

65. Pellicciari, R., Marinozzi, M., Natalini, B., Costantino, G., Luneia, R., Giogi, G., Moroni, F., Thomsen, C. (1996). Synthesis and pharmacological characterization of all sixteen stereoisomers of 2-(2′-carboxy-3′-phenylcyclopropyl)glycine. Focus on (2S,1′S,2′S,3′R)-2-(2′-carboxy-3′phenylcyclopropyl)glycine, a novel and selective group II metabotropic glutamate receptors agonist. *J Med Chem*, *39*, 2259–2269.

66. Pellicciari, R., Costantino, G., Marinozzi, M., Macchiarulo, A., Amori, L., Flor, P.J., Gasparini, F., Kuhn, R., Urwyler, S. (2001). Design, synthesis and preliminary evaluation of novel 3′-substituted carboxycyclopropylglycines as antagonists at group 2 metabotropic glutamate receptors. *Bioorg Med Chem Lett*, *11*, 3179–3182.

67. Monn, J.A., Valli, M.J., Massey, S.M., Wright, R.A., Salhoff, C.R., Johnson, B.G., Howe, T., Alt, C.A., Rhodes, G.A., Robey, R.L., Griffey, K.R., Tizzano, J.P., Kallman, M.J., Helton, D.R., Schoepp, D.D. (1997). Design, synthesis and pharmacological characterization of (+)-2-aminobicyclo[3.1.0]hexane-2,6-dicarboxylic Acid (LY354740): a potent, selective and orally active group 2 metabotropic glutamate receptor agonist possessing anticonvulsant and anxiolytic properties. *J Med Chem*, *40*, 528–537.

68. Schoepp, D.D., Johnson, B.G., Wright, R.A., Salhoff, C.R., Mayne, N.G., Wu, S., Cockerham, S.L., Burnett, J.P., Belagaje, R., Bleakman, D., Monn, J.A. (1997). LY354740 is a potent and highly selective group II metabotropic glutamate receptor agonist in cells expressing human glutamate receptors. *Neuropharmacology*, *36*, 1–11.

69. Monn, J.A., Valli, M.J., Massey, S.M., Hansen, M.M., Kress, T.J., Wepsiec, J.P., Harkness, A.R., Grutsch, J.L. Jr, Wright, R.A., Johnson, B.G., Andis, S.L., Kingston, A.E., Tomlinson, R., Lewis, R., Griffey, K.R., Tizzano, J.P., Schoepp, D.D. (1999). Synthesis, pharmacological characterization and molecular modeling of heterobicyclic amino acids related to LY354740: identification of LY379268 and LY389795: two

new potent, selective and systemically active agonists for group II metabotropic glutamate receptors. *J Med Chem*, *42*, 1027–1040.

70. Monn, J.A., Valli, M.J., Massey, S.M., Henry, S.S., Stephenson, G.A., Bures, M., Herin, M., Catlow, J., Giera, D., Wright, R.A., Johnson, B.G., Andis, S.L., Kingston, A.E., Schoepp, D.D. (2007). Synthesis and metabotropic glutamate receptor activity of S-oxidized variants of LY389795: identification of potent, selective and orally bioavailable agonists for mGlu2/3 receptors. *J Med Chem*, *50*, 233–240.
71. Rorick-Kehn, L.M., Johnson, B.G., Burkey, J.L., Wright, R.A., Calligaro, D.O., Marek, G.J., Nisenbaum, E.S., Catlow, J.T., Kingston, A.E., Giera, D., Herin, M.F., Monn, J.A., McKinzie, D.L., Schoepp, D.D. (2007). Pharmacological and pharmacokinetic properties of a structurally novel, potent, and selective metabotropic glutamate 2/3 receptor agonist: in vitro characterization of agonist (-)-(1R,4S,5S,6S)-4-Amino-2-sulfonylbicyclo[3.1.0]-hexane-4,6-dicarboxylic acid (LY404039). *J Pharmacol Exp Ther*, *321*, 308–317.
72. Nakazato, A., Kumagai, T., Sakagami, K., Yoshikawa, R., Suzuki, Y., Shigeyuki, C., Ito, H., Taguchi, T., Nakanishi, S., Okuyama, S. (2000). Synthesis, SARs, and pharmacological characterization of 2-amino-3 or 6-fluorobicyclo[3.1.0]hexane-2,6-dicarboxylic acid derivatives as potent, selective, and orally active group II metabotropic glutamate receptor agonists. *J Med Chem*, *43*, 4893–4909.
73. Dominguez, C., Prieto, L., Valli, M.J., Massey, S.M., Bures, M., Wright, R.A., Johnson, B.G., Andis, S.L., Kingston, A., Schoepp, D.D., Monn, J.A. (2005). Methyl substitution of 2-aminobicyclo[3.1.0]hexane-2,6-dicarboxylate (LY354740) determines functional activity at metabotropic glutamate receptors: identification of a subtype selective mGlu2 receptor agonist. *J Med Chem*, *48*, 3605–3612.
74. Woltering, T.J., Adam, G., Huguenin, P., Wichmann, J., Kolczewski, S., Gatti, S., Bourson, A., Kew, J.N.C., Richards, G., Kemp, J.A., Mutel, V., Knoflach, F. (2008). Asymmetric synthesis and receptor pharmacology of the group II mGlu receptor ligand (1S,2R,3R,5R,6S)-2-amino-3-hydroxy-bicyclo[3.1.0]hexane-2,6-dicarboxylic acid- HYDIA. *ChemMedChem*, *3*, 323–335.
75. Nakazato, A., Sakagami, K., Yasuhara, A., Ohta, H., Yoshikawa, R., Itoh, M., Nakamura, M., Chaki, S. (2004). Synthesis, in vitro pharmacology, structure-activity relationships, and pharmacokinetics of 3-alkoxy-2-amino-6-fluorobicyclo[3.1.0] hexane-2,6-dicarboxylic acid derivatives as potent and selective group II metabotropic glutamate receptor antagonists. *J Med Chem*, *47*, 4570–4587.
76. Yasuhara, A., Sakagami, K., Yoshikawa, R., Chaki, S., Nakamura, M., Nakazato, A. (2006). Synthesis, in vitro pharmacology, and structure-activity relationships of 2-aminobicyclo[3.1.0]hexane-2,6-dicarboxylic acid derivatives as mGluR2 antagonists. *Bioorg Med Chem*, *14*, 3405–3420.
77. Rudd, M.T., McCauley, J.A. (2005). Positive allosteric modulators of the metabotropic glutamate receptor subtype 2 (mGluR2). *Curr Top Med Chem*, *5*, 869–884.
78. Gasparini, F., Spooren, W. (2007). Allosteric modulators for mGlu receptors. *Curr Neuropharmacol*, *5*, 187–194.
79. Fraley, M.E. (2009). Positive allosteric modulators of the metabotropic glutamate receptor 2 for the treatment of schizophrenia. *Expert Opin Ther Pat*, *19*, 1–17.
80. Freedman, N.J., Lefkowitz, R.J. (1996). Desensitization of G protein-coupled receptors. *Recent Prog Horm Res*, *51*, 319–353.

81. Galici, R., Echemendia, N.G., Rodriquez, A.L., Conn, P.J. (2005). A selective allosteric potentiator of metabotropic glutamate (mGlu) 2 receptors has effects similar to an orthosteric mGlu2/3 receptor agonist in mouse models predictive of antipsychotic activity. *J Pharmacol Exp Ther*, *315*, 1181–1187.

82. Johnson, M.P., Baez, M., Jagdmann, G.E. Jr, Britton, T.C., Large, T.H., Callagaro, D.O., Tizzano, J.P., Monn, J.A., Schoepp, D.D. (2003). Discovery of allosteric potentiators for the metabotropic glutamate 2 receptor: synthesis and subtype selectivity of N-(4-(2-methoxyphenoxy)phenyl)-N-(2,2,2-trifluoroethylsulfonyl)pyrid-3-ylmethyl-amine. *J Med Chem*, *46*, 3189–3192.

83. Barda, D.A., Wang, Z.Q., Britton, T.C., Henry, S.S., Jagdmann, G.E., Coleman, D.S., Johnson, M.P., Andis, S.L., Schoepp, D.D. (2004). SAR study of a subtype selective allosteric potentiator of metabotropic glutamate 2 receptor, N-(4-phenoxyphenyl)-N-(3-pyridinylmethyl)ethanesulfonamide. *Bioorg Med Chem Lett*, *14*, 3099–3102.

84. Johnson, M.P., Barda, D., Britton, T.C., Emkey, R., Hornback, W.J., Jagdmann, G.E., McKinzie, D.L., Nisenbaum, E.S., Tizanno, J.P., Schoepp, D.D. (2005). Metabotropic glutamate 2 receptor potentiators: receptor modulation, frequency-dependent synaptic activity, and efficacy in preclinical anxiety and psychosis model(s). *Psychopharmacology*, *179*, 271–283.

85. Galici, R., Jones, C.K., Hemstapat, K., Nong, Y., Echemendia, N.G., Williams, L.C., de Paulis, T., Conn, P.J. (2006). Biphenyl-indanone A, a positive allosteric modulator of the metabotropic glutamate receptor subtype 2, has antipsychotic- and anxiolytic-like effects in mice. *J Pharmacol Exp Ther*, *318*, 173–185.

86. Benneyworth, M.A., Xiang, Z., Smith, R.L., Garcia, E.E., Conn, P.J., Sanders-Bush, E. (2007). A selective positive allosteric modulator of metabotropic glutamate receptor subtype 2 blocks a hallucinogenic drug model of psychosis. *Mol Pharmacol*, *72*, 477–484.

87. Pinkerton, A.B., Cube, R.V., Hutchinson, J.H., James, J.K., Gardner, M.F., Rowe, B.A., Schaffhauser, H., Rodriguez, D.E., Cambell, U.C., Daggett, L.P., Vernier, J.M. (2005). Allosteric potentiators of the metabotropic glutamate receptor 2 (mGlu2). Part 3: identification and biological activity of indanone containing mGlu2 receptor potentiators. *Bioorg Med Chem Lett*, *15*, 1565–1571.

88. Bonnefous, C., Vernier, J.M., Hutchinson, J.H., Gardner, M.F., Cramer, M., James, J.K., Rowe, B.A., Daggett, L.P., Schaffhauser, H., Kamenecka, T.M. (2005). Biphenyl-indanones: allosteric potentiators of the metabotropic glutamate subtype 2 receptor. *Bioorg Med Chem Lett*, *15*, 4354–4358.

89. Govek, S.P., Bonnefous, C., Hutchinson, J.H., Kamenecka, T., McQuiston, J., Pracitto, R., Zhao, L.X., Gardner, M.F., James, J.K., Daggett, L.P., Rowe, B.A., Schaffhauser, H., Bristow, L.J., Campbell, U.C., Rodriguez, D.E., Vernier, J.M. (2005). Benzazoles as allosteric potentiators of metabotropic glutamate receptor 2 (mGluR2): efficacy in an animal model for schizophrenia. *Bioorg Med Chem Lett*, *15*, 4068–4072.

90. Zhang, L., Rogers, B.N., Duplantier, A.J., McHardy, S.F., Efremov, I., Berke, H., Qian, W., Zhang, A.Q., Maklad, N., Candler, J., Doran, A.C., Lazzaro, J.T., Ganong, A.H. (2008). 3-(Imidazolylmethyl)-3-aza-bicyclo[3.1.0]hexan-6-yl)methyl ethers: a novel series of mGluR2 positive allosteric modulators. *Bioorg Med Chem Lett*, *18*, 5493–5496.

91. D'Alessandro, P.L., Corti, C., Roth, A., Ugolini, A., Sava, A., Montanari, D., Bianchi, F., Garland, S., Powney, B., Koppe, E.L., Rocheville, M., Osborne, G., Perez, P., De La Fuente, J., De Los Frailes, M., Smith, P.W., Branch, C., Nash, D., Watson, S.P. (2010). The identification of structurally novel, selective, orally bioavailable positive modulators of mGluR2. *Bioorg Med Chem Lett*, *20*, 759–762.

92. Tresadern, G., Cid, J.M., Macdonald, G.J., Vega, J.A., de Lucas, A.I., Garcia, A., Matesanz, E., Linares, M.L., Oehlrich, D., Lavreysen, H., Biesmans, I., Trabanco, A.A. (2010). Scaffold hopping from pyridones to imidazo[1,2-a]pyridines. New positive allosteric modulators of metabotropic glutamate 2-receptor. *Bioorg Med Chem Lett*, *20*, 175–179.

93. Duplantier, A.J., Efremov, I., Candler, J., Doran, A.C., Ganong, A.H., Hass, J.A., Hanks, A.N., Kraus, K.G., Lazzaro, J.T., Lu, J., Maklad, N., McCarthy, S.A., O'Sullivan, T.J., Siuciak, J.A., Sprracklin, D.K., Zhang, L. (2009). 3-Benzyl-1,3-oxazolidin-2-ones as mGluR2 positive allosteric modulators: hit-to-lead and lead optimization. *Bioorg Med Chem Lett*, *19*, 2524–2529.

94. Aghajanian, G.K., Marek, G.J. (1997). Serotonin induces excitatory postsynaptic potentials in apical dendrites of neocortical pyramidal cells. *Neuropharmacology*, *36*, 589–599.

95. Marek, G.J., Wright, R.A., Schoepp, D.D., Monn, J.A., Aghajanian, G.K. (2000). Physiological antagonism between 5-hydroxytryptamine$_{2A}$and group II metabotropic glutamate receptors in prefrontal cortex. *J Pharmacol Exp Ther*, *292*, 76–87.

96. Mateo, Z., Porter, J.T. (2007). Group II metabotropic glutamate receptors inhibit glutamate release at thalamocortical synapses in the developing somatosensory cortex. *Neuroscience*, *146*, 1062–1072.

97. Zhai, Y., George, C.A., Zhai, J., Nisenbaum, E.S., Johnson, M.P., Nisenbaum, L.K. (2003). Group II metabotropic glutamate receptor modulation of DOI-induced c-fos mRNA and excitatory responses in the cerebral cortex. *Neuropsychopharmacology*, *28*, 45–52.

98. Kilbride, J., Huang, L.Q., Rowan, M.J., Anwyl, R. (1998). Presynaptic inhibitory action of the group II metabotropic glutamate receptor agonists, LY354740 and DCG-IV. *Eur J Pharmacol*, *356*, 149–157.

99. Malherbe, P., Richards, J.G., Broger, C., Zenner, M.-T., Messer, J., Kratzeisen, C., Nakanishi, S., Mutel, V. (2005). Opposite effects of Zn on the *in vitro* binding of [$^3$H]LY354740 to recombinant and native metabotropic glutamate 2 and 3 receptors. *J Neurochem*, *94*, 150–160.

100. Richards, G., Messer, J., Malherbe, P., Pink, R., Brockhaus, M., Stadler, H., Wichmann, J., Schaffhauser, H., Mutel, V. (2005). Distribution and abundance of metabotropic glutamate receptor subtype 2 in rat brain revealed by [$^3$H]LY354740 binding in vitro and quantitative radioautoradiography: correlation with the sites of synthesis, expression, and agonist stimulation of [$^{35}$S]GTP$\gamma$S binding. *J Comp Neurol*, *487*, 15–27.

101. Conn, P.J., Battaglia, G., Marino, M.J., Nicoletti, F. (2005). Metabotropic glutamate receptors in the basal ganglia motor circuit. *Nat Rev Neurosci*, *6*, 787–798.

102. Lovinger, D.M., McCool, B.A. (1995). Metabotropic glutamate receptor-mediated presynaptic depression at corticostriatal synapses involves mGluR2 or 3. *J Neurophysiol*, *73*, 1076–1083.

103. Robbe, D., Alonso, G., Chaumont, S., Bockaert, J., Manzoni, O. (2002). Role of P/Q-$Ca^{2+}$ channels in metabotropic glutamate receptor 2/3-dependent presynaptic long-term depression at nucleus accumbens synapses. *J Neurosci*, *22*, 4346–4356.

104. Poisik, O., Raju, D.V., Verreault, M., Rodriquez, A., Abeniyi, O.A., Conn, P.J., Smith, Y. (2005). Metabotropic glutamate receptor 2 modulates excitatory synaptic transmission in the rat globus pallidus. *Neuropharmacology*, *49*, 57–69.

105. Bradley, S.R., Marino, M.J., Wittmann, M., Rouse, S.T., Awad, H., Levey, A.I., Conn, P.J. (2000). Activation of group II metabotropic glutamate receptors inhibits synaptic excitation of the substantia nigra pars reticulata. *J Neurosci*, *20*, 3085–3094.

106. Wittmann, M., Marino, M.J., Conn, P.J. (2002). Dopamine modulates the function of group II and group III metabotropic glutamate receptors in the substantia nigra pars reticulata. *J Pharmacol Exp Ther*, *302*, 433–441.

107. Guillery, R.W. (1995). Anatomical evidence concerning the role of the thalamus in corticocortical communication: a brief review. *J Anat*, *187*, 583–592.

108. Sherman, S.M., Guillery, R.W. (1996). Functional organization of thalamocortical relays. *J Neurophysiol*, *76*, 1367–1395.

109. Neto, F.L., Schadrack, J., Berthele, A., Zieglgansberger, W., Tolle, T.R., Castro-Lopes, J.M. (2000). Differential distribution of metabotropic glutamate receptor subtype mRNAs in the thalamus of the rat. *Brain Res*, *854*, 93–105.

110. Alexander, G.M., Godwin, D.W. (2005). Presynaptic inhibition of corticothalamic feedback by metabotropic glutamate receptors. *J Neurophysiol*, *94*, 163–175.

111. Turner, J.P., Salt, T.E. (2003). Group II and III metabotropic glutamate receptors and the control of the nucleus reticularis thalami input to rat thalamocortical neurons *in vitro*. *Neuroscience*, *122*, 459–469.

112. Hermes, M.L., Kolaj, M. (2009). *Activation of Pre- and Postsynaptic Group II Metabotropic Glutamate Receptors Reduce the Excitability of Midline Thalamic Neurons*. Chicago: Society for Neuroscience. 2009 Neuroscience Meeting Planner.

113. Turner, J.P., Salt, T.E. (1999). Group III metabotropic glutamate receptors control corticothalamic synaptic transmission in the rat thalamus *in vitro*. *J Physiol*, *519*, 2, 481–491.

114. Neugebauer, V., Zinebi, F., Russell, R., Gallagher, J.P., Shinnick-Gallagher, P. (2000). Cocaine and kindling alter the sensitivity of group II and group III metabotropic glutamate receptors in the central amygdala. *J Neurophysiol*, *84*, 759–770.

115. Grueter, B.A., Winder, D.G. (2005). Group II and III metabotropic glutamate receptors suppress excitatory synaptic transmission in the dorsolateral bed nucleus of the stria terminalis. *Neuropsychopharmacology*, *30*, 1302–1311.

116. Muly, E.C., Mania, I., Guo, J.-D., Rainnie, D.G. (2007). Group II metabotropic glutamate receptors in anxiety circuitry: correspondence of physiological response and subcellular distribution. *J Comp Neurol*, *505*, 682–700.

117. Homayoun, H., Jackson, M.E., Moghaddam, B. (2005). Activation of metabotropic glutamate 2/3 receptors reverses the effects of NMDA receptor hypofunction on prefrontal cortex unit activity in awake rats. *J Neurophysiol*, *93*, 1989–2001.

118. Homayoun, H., Moghaddam, B. (2008). Orbitofrontal cortex neurons as a common target for classic and glutamateric antipsychotic drugs. *Proc Natl Acad Sci U S A*, *105*, 18041–18046.

119. Schaffhauser, H., Rowe, B.A., Morales, S., Chavez-Noriega, L.E., Yin, R., Jachec, C., Rao, S.P., Bain, G., Pinkerton, A.B., Vernier, J.-M., Bristow, L.J., Varney, M.A., Daggett, L.P. (2003). Pharmacological characterization and identification of amino acids involved in the positive modulation of metabotropic glutamate receptor subtype 2. *Mol Pharmacol*, *64*, 798–810.

120. Abi-Dargham, A. (2004). Do we still believe in the dopamine hypothesis? New data bring new evidence. *Int J Neuropsychopharmacol*, *7*(Suppl 1), S1–S5.

121. Rorick-Kehn, L.M., Johnson, B.G., Knitowski, K.M., Salhoff, C.R., Witkin, J.M., Perry, K.W., Griffey, K.I., Tizzano, J.P., Monn, J.A., McKinzie, D.L., Schoepp, D.D. (2007). In vivo pharmacological characterization of the structurally novel, potent, selective mGlu2/3 receptor agonist LY404039 in animal models of psychiatric disorders. *Psychopharmacology*, *193*, 121–136.

122. Cartmell, J., Perry, K.W., Salhoff, C.R., Monn, J.A., Schoepp, D.D. (2000). The potent, selective mGlu2/3 receptor agonist LY379268 increases extracellular levels of dopamine, 3,4-dihydroxyphenylacetic acid, homovanillic acid, and 5-hydroxyindole3-acetic acid in the medial prefrontal cortex of the freely moving rat. *J Neurochem*, *75*, 1147–1154.

123. Moghaddam, B., Adams, B.W. (1998). Reversal of phencyclidine effects by a group II metabotropic glutamate receptor agonists in rats. *Science*, *281*, 1349–1352.

124. Lorrain, D.S., Baccei, C.S., Bristow, L.J., Anderson, J.J., Varney, M.A. (2003a). Effects of ketamine and N-methyl-D-aspartate on glutamate and dopamine release in the rat prefrontal cortex: modulation by a group II selective metabotropic glutamate receptor agonist LY379268. *Neuroscience*, *117*, 697–706.

125. Swanson, C.J., Schoepp, D.D. (2003). A role for noradrenergic transmission in the actions of phencyclidine and the antipsychotic and antistress effects of mGlu2/3 receptor agonists. *Ann N Y Acad Sci*, *1003*, 309–317.

126. Lorrain, D.S., Schaffhauser, H., Campbell, U.C., Baccei, C.S., Correa, L.D., Rowe, B., Rodriquez, D.E., Anderson, J.J., Varney, M.A., Pinkerton, A.B., Vernier, J.M., Bristow, L.J. (2003b). Group II mGlu receptor activation suppresses norepinephrine release in the ventral hippocampus and locomotor responses to acute ketamine challenge. *Neuropsychopharmacology*, *28*, 1622–1632.

127. Fell, M.J., Svensson, K.A., Johnson, B.G., Schoepp, D.D. (2008). Evidence for the role of metabotropic glutamate (mGlu)2 but not mGlu3 receptors in the preclinical antipsychotic pharmacology of the mGlu2/3 receptor agonist (-)-(1R,4S,5S,6S)-4-amino-2-sulfonylbicyclo[3.1.0]hexane-4,6-dicarboxylic acid (LY404039). *J Pharmacol Exp Ther*, *326*, 209–217.

128. Kim, J.H., Vezina, P. (2002). The mGlu2/3 receptor agonist LY379268 blocks the expression of locomotor sensitization by amphetamine. *Pharmacol Biochem Behav*, *73*, 333–337.

129. Cartmell, J., Monn, J.A., Schoepp, D.D. (1999). The metabotropic glutamate 2/3 receptor agonists LY354740 and LY379268 selectively attenuate phencyclidine versus d-amphetamine motor behaviors in rats. *J Pharmacol Exp Ther*, *291*, 161–170.

130. Cartmell, J., Monn, J.A., Schoepp, D.D. (2000). The mGlu(2/3) receptor agonist LY379268 selectively blocks amphetamine ambulations and rearing. *Eur J Pharmacol*, *400*, 221–224.

131. Wadenberg, M.G., Hicks, P.B. (1999). The conditioned avoidance response test re-evaluated: is it a sensitive test for the detection of potentially atypical antipsychotics? *Neurosci Biobehav Rev*, *23*, 851–862.

132. Shannon, H.E., Rasmussen, K., Bymaster, F.P., Hart, J.C., Peters, S.C., Swedberg, M.D., Jeppesen, L., Sheardown, M.J., Sauerberg, P., Fink-Jensen, A. (2000). Xanomeline, an M(1)/M(4) preferring muscarinic cholinergic receptor agonist, produces antipsychotic-like activity in rats and mice. *Schizophr Res*, *42*, 249–259.

133. Shekhar, A., Potter, W.Z., Lightfoot, J., Lienemann, J., Dube, S., Mallinckrodt, C., Bymaster, F.P., McKinzie, D.L., Felder, C.C. (2008). Selective muscarinic receptor agonist xanomeline as a novel treatment approach for schizophrenia. *Am J Psychiatry*, *165*, 1033–1039.

134. Takamori, K., Hirota, S., Chaki, S., Tanaka, M. (2003). Antipsychotic action of selective group II metabotropic glutamate receptor agonist MGS0008 and MGS0028 on conditioned avoidance responses in the rat. *Life Sci*, *73*, 1721–1728.

135. Cartmell, J., Monn, J.A., Schoepp, D.D. (2000). Attenuation of specific PCP-evoked behaviors by the potent mGlu2/3 receptor agonist, LY379268 and comparison with the atypical antipsychotic, clozapine. *Psychopharmacology*, *148*, 423–429.

136. Rorick-Kehn, L., Perkins, E.J., Knitowki, K.M., Hart, J.C., Johnson, B.G., Schoepp, D.D., McKinzie, D.L. (2006). Improved bioavailability of the mGlu2/3 receptor agonist LY354740 using a prodrug strategy: in vivo pharmacology of LY544344. *J Pharmacol Exp Ther*, *316*, 905–913.

137. Gewirtz, J.C., Marek, G.J. (2000). Behavioral evidence for interactions between a hallucinogenic drug and group II metabotropic glutamate receptors. *Neuropsychopharmacology*, *23*, 569–576.

138. Klodzinska, A., Bijak, M., Tokarski, K., Pilc, A. (2002). Group II mGlu receptor agonists inhibit behavioral and electrophysiological effects of DOI in mice. *Pharmacol Biochem Behav*, *73*, 327–332.

139. Uslaner, J.M., Smith, S.M., Huszar, S.L., Pachmerhiwala, R., Hinchliffe, R.M., Vardigan, J.D., Hutson, P.H. (2009). Combined administratino of an mGlu2/3 receptor agonist and a 5-HT 2A receptor antagonist markedly attenuate the psychomotor-activating and neurochemical effects of psychostimulants. *Psychopharmacology (Berl)*, *206*, 641–651.

140. Cartmell, J., Monn, J.A., Schoepp, D.D. (2000). Tolerance to the motor impairment, but not reversal of PCP-induced motor activities by oral administration of the mGlu2/3 receptor agonist, LY379268. *Naunyn Schmiedebergs Arch Pharmacol*, *361*, 39–46.

141. Imre, G., Fokkema, D.S., Ter Horst, G.J. (2006a). Subchronic administration of LY379268 does not modify ketamine-evoked behavior and neuronal activity in rats. *Eur J Pharmacol*, *544*, 77–81.

142. Clark, M., Johnson, B.G., Wright, R.A., Monn, J.A., Schoepp, D.D. (2002). Effects of the mGlu2/3 receptor agonist LY379268 on motor activity in phencyclidine-sensitized rats. *Pharmacol Biochem Behav*, *73*, 339–346.

143. Schreiber, R., Lowe, D., Voerste, A., De Vry, J. (2000). LY354740 affects startle responding but not sensorimotor gating or discriminative effects of phencyclidine. *Eur J Pharmacol*, *388*, R3–R4.

144. Imre, G., Salomons, A., Jongsma, M., Fokkema, D.S., Den Boer, J.A., Ter Horsts, G.J. (2006). Effects of the mGluR2/3 agonist LY379268 on ketamine-evoked behaviors and neurochemical changes in the dentate gyrus of the rat. *Pharmacol Biochem Behav*, *84*, 392–399.

145. Satow, A., Maehara, S., Ise, S., Hikichi, H., Fukushima, M., Suzuki, G., Kimura, T., Tanak, T., Ito, S., Kawamoto, H., Ohta, H. (2008). Pharmacological effects of the metabotropic glutamate receptor 1 antagonist compared with those of the metabotropic glutamate receptor 5 antagonist and metabotropic glutamate receptor 2/3 agonist in rodents: detailed investigations with a selective allosteric metabotropic glutamate receptor 1 antagonist, FTIDC [4-[1-(2-fluoropyridine-3-yl)-5-methyl-1H-1,2,3-triazol-4-yl]-N-isopropyl-N-methyl-3,6-dihydropyridine-1(2H)-carboxamide]. *J Pharmacol Exp Ther*, *326*, 577–586.
146. Winter, J.C., Eckler, J.R., Rabin, R.A. (2004). Serotonergic/glutamatergic interactions: the effects of mGlu2/3 receptor ligands in rats trained with LSD and PCP as discriminative stimuli. *Psychopharmacology*, *172*, 233–240.
147. Krystal, J.H., Abi-Saab, W., Perry, E., D'Souza, D.C., Liu, N., Gueorguieva, R., McDougall, L., Hunsberger, T., Belger, A., Levine, L., Breier, A. (2005). Preliminary evidence of attenuation of the disruptive effects of the NMDA glutamate receptor antagonist, ketamine, on working memory by pretreatment with the group II metabotropic glutamate receptor agonist, LY354740, in healthy human subject. *Psychopharmacology (Berl)*, *179*, 303–309.
148. Spinelli, S., Ballard, T., Gatti-McArthur, S., Richards, G.J., Kapps, M., Woltering, T., Wichmann, J., Stadler, H., Feldon, J., Pryce, C.R. (2005). Effects of the mGluR2/3 agonist LY354740 on computerized tasks of attention and working memory in marmoset monkeys. *Psychopharmacology*, *179*, 292–302.
149. Greco, B., Invernizzi, R.W., Carli, M. (2005). Phencyclidine-induced impairment in attention and response control depends on the background genotype of mice: reversal by the mGlu(2/3) receptor agonist LY379268. *Psychopharmacology*, *179*, 68–76.
150. Amitai, N., Markou, A. (2010). Effects of metabotropic glutamate receptor 2/3 agonism and antagonism on schizophrenia-like cognitive deficits induced by phencyclidine in rats. *Eur J Pharmacol*, *639*, 67–80. [Epubl]: PMID: 20371228.
151. Harich, S., Gross, G., Bespalov, A. (2007). Stimulation of the metabotropic glutamate 2/3 receptor attenuates social novelty discrimination deficits induced by neonatal phencyclidine treatment. *Psychopharmacology (Berl)*, *192*, 511–519.
152. Spooren, W.P., Gasparini, F., van der Putten, H., Koller, M., Nakanishi, S., Kuhn, R. (2000). Lack of effect of LY314582 (a group 2 metabotropic glutamate receptor agonist) on phencyclidine-induced locomotor activity in metabotropic glutamate receptor 2 knockout mice. *Eur J Pharmacol*, *397*, R1–R2.
153. Woolley, M.L., Pemberton, D.J., Bate, S., Corti, C., Jones, D.N. (2008). The mGlu2 but not the mGlu3 receptor mediates the actions of the mGluR2/3 agonist, LY379268, in mouse models predictive of antipsychotic activity. *Psychopharmacology (Berl)*, *196*, 431–440.
154. Fell, M.J., Johnson, B.G., Falcone, J.F., Perry, K.W., Barth, V.N., Rash, K.S., Monn, J.A., Schoepp, D.D., McKinzie, D.L., Nelson, D.L., Marek, G.J., Svensson, K.A. (2008). *In vivo Neurochemical and Behavioral Evidence for Lack of direct Dopamine D2 Receptor Mediated Actions of mGluR2/3 Agonists, Program No. 155.7.* Washington, DC: Society for Neuroscience, 2008 Neuroscience Meeting Planner. Online.
155. Karlsson, R.M., Tanaka, K., Heilig, M., Holmes, A. (2008). Loss of glial glutamate and aspartate transporter (excitatory amino acid transporter 1) causes locomotor

hyperactivity and exaggerated responses to psychotomimetics: rescue by haloperidol and metabotropic glutamate 2/3 agonists. *Biol Psychiatry*, *64*, 810–814.

156. Chartoff, E.H., Heusner, C.L., Palmiter, R.D. (2005). Dopamine is not required for the hyperlocomotor response to NMDA receptor antagonists. *Neuropsychopharmacology*, *30*, 1324–1333.

157. Bridges, T.M., Lindsley, C.W. (2008). G-protein-coupled receptors: from classical modes of modulation to allosteric mechanisms. *ACS Chem Biol*, *19*, 530–541.

158. May, L.T., Leach, K., Sexton, P.M., Christopoulos, A. (2007). Allosteric modulation of G protein-coupled receptors. *Annu Rev Pharmacol Toxicol*, *47*, 1–51.

159. Hackler, E.A., Byun, N.E., Jones, C.K., Williams, J.M., Baheza, R., Sengupta, S., Grier, M.D., Avison, M., Conn, P.J., Gore, J.C. (2010). Selective potentiation of the metabotropic glutamate receptor subtype 2 blocks the phencyclidine-induced hyperlocomotion and brain activation. *Neuroscience*, *168*, 209–218. [Epub] PMID: 20350588.

160. Patil, S.T., Zhang, L., Martenyi, F., Lowe, S.L., Jackson, K.A., Andreev, B.V., Avedisova, A.S., Bardenstein, L.M., Gurovich, I.Y., Morozova, M.A., Mosolov, S.N., Neznanov, N.G., Reznik, A.M., Smulevich, A.B., Tochilov, V.A., Johnson, B.G., Monn, J.A., Schoepp, D.D. (2007). Activation of mGlu2/3 receptors as a new approach to treat schizophrenia: a randomized Phase 2 clinical trial. *Nat Med*, *13*, 1102–1107.

161. Kinon, B.J., Zhang, L., Millen, B.A., Osuntokun, O.O., Williams, J.E., Kollack-Walker, S., Jackson, K., Kryzhanovskaya, L., Jarkova, N., and the HBBI Study Group (2011) A multicenter, inpatient, phase 2, double-blind, placebo-controlled dose ranging study of LY2140023 monohydrate in patients with DSM-IV schizophrenia. *J Clin Psychopharmacol*, *31*(3), 349–355.

162. Zhang, C., Marek, G.J. (2007). Group III metabotropic glutamate receptor agonists selectively suppress excitatory synaptic currents in the rat prefrontal cortex induced by 5-hydroxytryptamine$_{2A}$ receptor activation. *J Pharmacol Exp Ther*, *320*, 437–447.

163. Kew, J.N., Ducarre, J.M., Pflimlin, M.C., Mutel, V., Kemp, J.A. (2001). Activity-dependent presynaptic autoinhibition by group II metabotropic glutamate receptors at the perforant path inputs to the dentate gyrus and CA1. *Neuropharmacology*, *40*, 20–27.

# 7

# AMPA RECEPTOR POSITIVE MODULATORS

John A. Morrow, John K.F. Maclean, and Craig Jamieson

## 7.1 INTRODUCTION

L-glutamate is the major excitatory neurotransmitter in the mammalian central nervous system (CNS) and exerts its physiological effects through two functionally distinct receptor families. The metabotropic (G-protein coupled) receptors are responsible for mediating slow metabolic responses whereas the ionotropic (ligand-gated ion channels) mediate the fast synaptic response to extracellular L-glutamate. The ionotropic glutamate receptors are divided into three subclasses on the basis of molecular and pharmacological differences and are named after the agonists that were originally identified to selectively activate them: α-amino-3-hydroxy-5-methyl-4-isoxazole-propionic acid (AMPA), *N*-methyl-D-aspartate (NMDA), and 2-carboxy-3-carboxymethyl-4-isopropenylpyrrolidine (kainate) [1,2]. AMPA receptors mediate the majority of fast excitatory amino acid transmission in the CNS and also participate in forms of synaptic plasticity that are thought to underlie learning and memory. Although the importance of AMPA receptors in brain physiology is widely recognized, no drugs that have been designed to specifically modulate AMPA receptors are currently used in clinical practice. Considerable effort has been focused on identification of AMPA receptor antagonists as neuroprotectant agents to ameliorate the degenerative effects of excess glutamate release

*Targets and Emerging Therapies for Schizophrenia*, First Edition.
Edited by Jeffrey S. Albert and Michael W. Wood.

resulting from stroke or epilepsy; however, such compounds have not progressed because of side effects such as ataxia, sedation, and memory impairment. More recently, there has been a growing appreciation of the utility of positive allosteric modulators of the AMPA receptor as a means of increasing glutamatergic function while avoiding excitotoxic effects of direct agonists. Several classes of potent, selective, and centrally active AMPA receptor positive modulators have now been described and have been shown to enhance synaptic transmission, long-term potentiation (LTP), and increase the expression on neurotrophic factors. As such, the potential therapeutic utility of these molecules is being investigated for a variety of clinical indications including schizophrenia, depression, Alzheimer's disease, and Parkinson's disease.

Schizophrenia is a heterogeneous disorder that is characterized by positive symptoms, negative symptoms, and cognitive deficits. Although prominence is often given to positive symptoms such as delusions and hallucinations, which appear more dramatic and often characterize relapses, disability results particularly from negative symptoms and cognitive deficits. These features are more chronic and inflexible and have a greater impact on long-term prognosis. Treatment of schizophrenia is predominantly by drugs whose primary mechanism is dopamine receptor $D_2$ antagonism. Although the newer atypical antipsychotics have superior side effect profiles and tolerability (e.g., rarely causing extrapyramidal symptoms [EPS], reduced prolactin secretion) compared with the older typical antipsychotics, all of these treatments only have proven efficacy for the treatment of positive symptoms of schizophrenia. Despite appropriate treatment with these drugs, many schizophrenia patients continue to display pronounced cognitive impairment. As such, major unmet medical needs include the effective treatment of both negative symptoms and cognitive dysfunction. Perhaps the most important rationale for focusing on cognitive impairments as a treatment target is that persistent cognitive deficits represent some of the core features of the disorder (i.e., they represent a fundamental aspect of the illness) and have a substantial impact on the outcome of schizophrenia [3, 4].

This chapter summarizes our current understanding of the pharmacology and the potential clinical utility of AMPA receptor potentiators and provides an overview of new chemical entities that have recently been disclosed. We will discuss the advances that have been made in our understanding of how these molecules interact with the AMPA receptor and focus on the preclinical and indeed emerging clinical evidence that suggests that AMPA receptor potentiators will serve as a promising new therapy for the treatment of schizophrenia, and in particular, the cognitive impairments associated with this disorder.

## 7.2 AMPA RECEPTOR STRUCTURE AND FUNCTION

AMPA receptor subunits are encoded by four separate genes (GluR1 to 4, also sometimes referred to as GluRA to D), each encoding proteins approximately 900 amino acids long with about 70% sequence identity between each of the polypeptides (notwithstanding alternate splicing; see below). These subunits share the same basic molecular architecture comprising four domains: (1) a large N-terminal domain that shares weak amino acid sequence homology with bacterial periplasmic binding proteins; (2) the extracellular ligand binding core, which consists of two subdomains designated S1 and S2; (3) a transmembrane domain comprising three transmembrane regions, TM1, TM3, and TM4 together with the re-entrant loop TM2; and (4) an intracellular C-terminal domain of varying lengths (Fig. 7.1). The ligand binding core of the AMPA receptor is important for determining pharmacological specificity as well as key biophysical properties such as desensitization and deactivation. This is particularly evident from studies where exchanging ligand binding domains (LBDs) between the AMPA GluR3 and kainate GluR6 receptors also exchanged their concomitant pharmacological properties [5, 6]. More recently, the X-ray crystal structure of full-length GluR2, and numerous high-resolution structures of the GluR2 S1S2 LBDs, have provided a unique insight

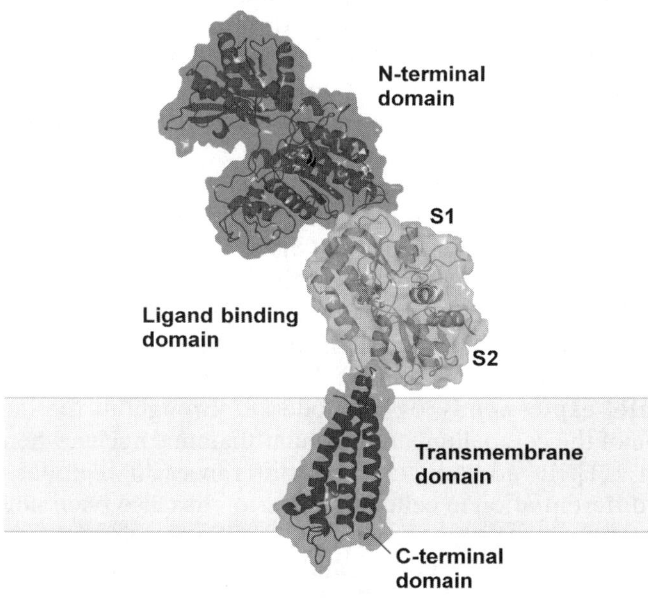


**FIGURE 7.1** Schematic illustration of the domain structure of a monomeric AMPA receptor peptide, modeled from PDB entry 3KG2 [118]. The functional receptor is tetrameric, each monomer comprising extracellular N-terminal and ligand binding domains (LBDs), a transmembrane region, and an intracellular C-terminal domain of varying sizes. Positive allosteric modulators have been shown to interact at the LBD, a bilobed clamshell structure (lobes labeled S1 and S2) [8]. Sequence differences relevant to flip/flop splice variation are localized between the carboxyl-terminal portion of the LBD and the final transmembrane helix. Figures prepared using Coot [194] and PyMol [195].

into the mechanism underlying receptor desensitization and deactivation as well as the mode of action of agonists, antagonists, and positive allosteric modulators [2, 7, 8].

The intracellular C-terminal domain of AMPA receptors has been demonstrated to be the interaction site for a variety of intracellular proteins including PDZ-domain containing proteins and the ATPase N-ethylmaleimide-sensitive factor (NSF), many of which are involved in receptor trafficking and synaptic plasticity [9, 10].

All four AMPA receptor subunits undergo alternative splicing of 38 amino acid encoding exons in the S2 extracellular subdomain. The two splice variants, termed flip and flop, differ by less than 10 amino acid residues and modify the kinetic and pharmacological properties of the channel, with flip receptors displaying slower rates of desensitization than their corresponding flop receptor splice variants [11] as well as differential sensitivity to the allosteric modulator cyclothiazide [12]. Further diversity of AMPA receptors arises from RNA editing, most notably the Gln/Arg site located in the pore region (TM2) of the GluR2 gene subunit. The majority of native GluR2 subunits in adult animals are thought to contain the edited Arg variant, which is characterized by significantly reduced calcium permeability, decreased single channel conductance, and reduced rectification [13–15]. A further Arg/Gly RNA editing site is located in the S2 subdomain of the GluR2, GluR3, and GluR4 subunits with the Gly form exhibiting an acceleration in the kinetics of recovery from desensitization [16].

A number of studies employing a variety of techniques such as *in situ* hybridization, receptor autoradiography, and immunocytochemistry have demonstrated that AMPA receptor subunits exhibit a distinct yet overlapping expression pattern in the mammalian brain. Studies in both rodents [17–19] and macaques [20] show the same general pattern, with relatively high levels of expression of GluR1, GluR2, and GluR3 in the hippocampus, outer layers of the cortex, amygdala, basal ganglia, lateral septum, and olfactory regions, whereas GluR4 expression is low to moderate throughout the rat CNS, with the exception of the cerebellum and reticular thalamic nuclei, where levels are much higher [21]. In addition to these differences in regional expression, remarkable differentiation in cellular expression has also been noted in many studies. For instance, in the hippocampus, GluR4 expression is restricted to the CA1 region, whereas GluR1, GluR2, and GluR3 are expressed in CA1, CA3, and dentate gyrus. Furthermore, while the GluR1-3 flip mRNAs are expressed at high levels in these hippocampal regions, GluR1-3 flop mRNAs are expressed highly only in CA1 and dentate gyrus, with GluR1-2 nearly absent and GluR3 expression considerably lower in CA3 [19, 20, 22, 23]. Interestingly, AMPA receptors are not only expressed in neurons but also in glial cells [24, 25], where they appear to be implicated in excitotoxicity [26, 27].

Expression of AMPA receptor subunit splice variants is also subject to developmental regulation with flip subunits predominating before birth and continuing to be expressed through to adulthood in rats. Flop subunit expression on the other hand is low prior to the eighth postnatal day, after which they are upregulated to about the same level as the flip variants in adult animals [28, 29].

The four AMPA receptor subunits co-assemble to form heterotetrameric complexes comprising an ion channel through which sodium and, with the exception of receptors containing the edited GluR2 subunit, calcium ions enter the cell upon receptor activation. Collectively, the heterogeneity of AMPA receptor subunit expression across the brain, together with the differences conferred by heteromeric subunit combinations, RNA editing, and splice variant composition, contributes to pharmacological as well as biophysical (e.g., kinetics of desensitization and deactivation) variability in the properties of AMPA receptors. In turn, this leads to considerable heterogeneity in AMPA-mediated synaptic responses across the brain. The kinetics of desensitization and deactivation are key functional properties of AMPA receptors that shape the amplitude and duration of synaptic responses to glutamate. Desensitization is the process of ion channel closure with agonist remaining bound to the receptor and, in contrast to NMDA receptors, occurs extremely rapidly and profoundly within 10 milliseconds of receptor activation. An insight into the mechanism underlying AMPA receptor desensitization has been provided by high-resolution X-ray crystallographic studies with a solubilized S1S2 LBD construct that suggest that rearrangements in receptor subunit interactions uncouple the ion channel gate from the LBD following binding of the agonist [30]. Deactivation is the process of channel inactivation following the dissociation of glutamate and is typically measured as the decay of agonist-induced current following removal of agonist. Again, in contrast to NMDA receptors, this occurs in an extremely rapid time scale (1–2 milliseconds) and probably reflects, among other things, the relatively low affinity that glutamate has for the AMPA receptor. Both desensitization and deactivation can be regulated by allosteric modulators of the AMPA receptor, which interact at a site remote from agonist binding and influence either agonist binding itself or the conformational changes associated with receptor gating or desensitization [31]. Modulation of these receptor properties by positive allosteric modulators may have potential therapeutic utility for a wide variety of CNS disorders associated with diminished glutamatergic signaling such as schizophrenia.

## 7.3 AMPA RECEPTOR MODULATION AND THE GLUTAMATE HYPOTHESIS OF SCHIZOPHRENIA

The glutamate hypothesis of schizophrenia was originally based on the observation that noncompetitive NMDA receptor antagonists such as ketamine and phencyclidine (PCP) induce schizophrenia-like symptoms in normal individuals and exacerbate positive and negative symptoms in patients with schizophrenia [32–35]. This has led to the evolution of a number of novel therapeutic strategies for the treatment of schizophrenia based on augmenting NMDA receptor-mediated neurotransmission. Activation of NMDA receptors requires glutamate, which binds to the NR2 subunits, and co-agonism by either glycine [36] or D-serine [37], which binds to the NR1 subunits. Furthermore, an additional characteristic of NMDA receptors is their blockade at resting membrane potential by extracellular $Mg^{2+}$. This block is relieved by membrane depolarization that is mediated by activation of AMPA receptors that colocalize with the NMDA receptor, thereby permitting NMDA receptor activation. This has been supported by experimental studies on synaptic transmission [38].

It has been observed that many excitatory synapses, particularly early in development, appear to contain only NMDA receptors. Since these receptors are blocked by extracellular $Mg^{2+}$ and are thereby unable to contribute to the generation of postsynaptic responses, these have been termed "silent synapses" [39, 40]. Activity-dependent recruitment of AMPA receptors to the postsynaptic membrane is considered to allow these previously silent NMDA receptors to participate as functional components of neural networks [41]. Recent studies in adult hippocampal pyramidal neurons have demonstrated that delivery of AMPA receptors to the postsynaptic membrane occurs via two distinct mechanisms in a subunit specific manner. AMPA receptors consisting of heteromeric combination of GluR2/3 subunits are continuously recycled in a constitutive manner while receptors consisting of GluR1/2 subunit combinations are recruited in an activity-dependent manner [10, 42, 43]. Activity-dependent recruitment of AMPA receptors is one of the mechanisms underlying forms of synaptic plasticity such as LTP, a use-dependent increase in synaptic function that is considered to underlie learning and memory formation [42, 44].

Thus, agents that enhance glutamatergic transmission such as positive modulators of the AMPA receptor may hold promise in the treatment of schizophrenia. Furthermore, given that disability in schizophrenia results particularly from negative symptoms and cognitive deficits that are more chronic and inflexible in nature and have a greater impact on long-term prognosis than the more dramatic positive symptoms, the central role of AMPA receptors in potentiating NMDA receptor function, and indeed in cognition, suggests that they may be abnormal in schizophrenia.

Although most research has focused on the role of NMDA receptors in schizophrenia, it has yet to be established whether NMDA receptor hypofunction is attributable to NMDA receptor function per se or indeed regulation of NMDA receptor signaling. This raises the possibility that deficits in AMPA receptor-mediated signaling may be a contributing factor to glutamatergic hypofunction in schizophrenia. Thus, a number of investigations have been performed in recent years to attempt to understand how these receptors may be altered in schizophrenia.

### 7.3.1 Alterations of AMPA Receptors in Schizophrenia

Despite increasing recent focus on the glutamate system in schizophrenia, in contrast to the dopamine system, our understanding of the expression levels and regulation of glutamate receptors in schizophrenia has been hampered by the lack of suitable positron emission tomography (PET) and single photon emission computed tomography (SPECT) ligands to perform *in vivo* imaging studies [45]. Thus, all studies to date have had to rely on postmortem brain tissue where AMPA receptor expression has been investigated using a variety of techniques including receptor binding, *in situ* hybridization, and quantitative polymerase chain reaction (qPCR) to determine AMPA receptor subunit mRNA levels and immunocytochemistry to determine levels of subunit protein expression. Such investigations suffer from a number of limitations. Perhaps most importantly, a limitation that affects all postmortem studies in schizophrenia is that the majority of patients have been exposed to antipsychotic drug medication [46]. Furthermore, mRNA quality can be affected by age, postmortem interval, and brain pH [47, 48], although most studies are increasingly attempting to control for these factors.

Examination of AMPA receptor expression in temporal lobe regions has revealed a consistent pattern, with most studies showing a decrease in the expression of subunit mRNAs, proteins, and ligand binding sites [49, 50]. A series of investigations has shown a marked reduction of GluR1 and GluR2 transcripts in multiple hippocampal subfields (dentate gyrus, CA3, CA4, and subiculum) [51]. The splicing pattern of GluR2 mRNA was also found to be altered in hippocampal structures with a preferential reduction in the flop variant in comparison to flip [52]. Reductions in AMPA receptor levels in medial temporal lobe structures, albeit to a lesser extent than noted at the mRNA level, were also observed at the protein level by immunocytochemical analysis, with GluR1 significantly reduced in the parahippocampal gyrus and combined GluR2/3 immunoreactivity reduced in most hippocampal subfields but particularly in CA4 [53]. Some receptor binding studies have also demonstrated a decrease in AMPA receptor density in the hippocampus as demonstrated by a reduction in [$^3$H]CNQX or [$^3$H]AMPA binding [54, 55]. Other studies, however, have failed to detect any changes in medial temporal lobe AMPA receptor levels in schizophrenic brains, which may be due to differences in subject cohorts or antipsychotic drug treatment or to methodological reasons such as technique sensitivity [56, 57].

Studies assessing AMPA subunit expression in the dorsolateral prefrontal cortex (DLPFC) in schizophrenic brains have been somewhat equivocal, with reports of no change in AMPA receptor binding or subunit mRNA levels [58–60], increased GluR1 and GluR4 mRNA levels [61], or a decrease in GluR2 expression [62, 63]. Interestingly, one group that found no change in AMPA receptor levels in the dorsolateral prefrontal cortex (DLPFC) when performing regional analysis using qPCR [58] were able to demonstrate increased GluR1 levels in discrete cell populations (layer II/II and layer V pyramidal cells) from the same subjects as determined by a combination of laser capture microdissection and qPCR [64]. Thus, the equivocality of data in many of these studies is possibly a result of subtle alterations in subunit expression at the cellular level in specific neuronal populations in any given region.

Determination of AMPA receptor expression and binding in other brain regions has identified minimal or no meaningful changes in striatal subregions (caudate, putamen, and nucleus accumbens) [59, 65], although, again, there are exception to these findings with a decrease in [$^3$H]CNQX binding noted in one study [66]. In another study, GluR1 and GluR3 mRNA was significantly lower in thalamic nuclei while GluR2, GluR4, and [$^3$H]AMPA binding remained unchanged [67].

Given the importance of AMPA receptor trafficking to mechanisms underlying synaptic plasticity, some focus has also recently been paid to the study of intracellular signaling pathways to determine whether problems with receptor trafficking mechanisms rather than with AMPA receptors per se might underlie abnormalities in glutamatergic signaling in schizophrenia. Trafficking of AMPA receptors in the postsynaptic cell occurs through several integrated pathways and is mediated by intracellular proteins in the postsynaptic density (PSD) that interact with the carboxy termini of the AMPA receptor subunits via PDZ domains, motifs of approximately 90 amino acids that play a role in receptor trafficking and localization in the synapse. A recent study examining expression of four AMPA receptor-associated PSD proteins (NSF, PICK1, syntenin, and stargazin) found that the expression of two of these, PICK1 and stargazin, were altered in schizophrenic brains in comparison with controls [63]. Decreased expression of PICK1 and increased expression of stargazin in the DLPFC in schizophrenia were demonstrated with both changes restricted to large cells in cortical layer III. These changes were accompanied by decreases in GluR2 and GluR4 mRNA levels, although not GluR1 or GluR2 mRNA levels, or AMPA receptor binding in the DLPFC. PICK1 has been shown to be involved in the exocytosis of GluR2-containing receptors to the plasma membrane [68–70], while stargazin is a member of the transmembrane AMPA receptor regulatory protein (TARP) family of auxiliary subunits, which are not only involved in AMPA receptor trafficking but also act as positive allosteric modulators of AMPA receptor ion channel function [71].

In summary, despite the inconsistency across reports, the available evidence points to abnormal expression of AMPA receptors in schizophrenic brains that appears specific to the hippocampus. However, the relevance of these changes to schizophrenia remains to be established. Indeed, it is still unclear whether they are intrinsically pathological or represent a compensatory or maladaptive response to a primary abnormality elsewhere in the system (glutamate or not). Although postmortem observations cannot really address these questions, they do support the hypothesis of abnormal glutamatergic neurotransmission in schizophrenia and further suggest that novel strategies that target AMPA receptors may be of therapeutic utility in this illness.

## 7.4 AMPA RECEPTOR POSITIVE MODULATORS: CHEMISTRY AND PHARMACOLOGY

The Eli Lilly Corporation has had an interest in AMPA positive modulators for a number of years. A novel series of sulfonamide-based modulators exemplified by compound **1** (Fig. 7.2), which had an $EC_{50}$ at GluR4 flip of 19.6 μM, was identified through high-throughput screening [72]. Using parallel chemistry, the initial hit was rapidly optimized to furnish entities such as compound **2** (LY404187; Fig. 7.2), which demonstrated significantly improved potency at GluR4 flip ($EC_{50}$ = 0.29 μM). As discussed later, LY404187 has become an important tool compound in further elucidating the role of AMPA receptors in neurological disorders.

Subsequent work has shown that LY404187 is GluR2 and GluR4 preferring (GluR2 flip $EC_{50}$ = 0.15 μM, GluR3 flip $EC_{50}$ = 1.66 μM, GluR1 flip $EC_{50}$ = 5.65 μM) [73]. In addition, LY404187 was shown to have around 10-fold selectivity for flip versus flop receptors (GluR2 flop $EC_{50}$ = 1.44 μM). From a broader selectivity perspective, LY404187 does not activate other ionotropic glutamate receptors such as kainate or NMDA, nor does it have any effect on voltage-gated potassium, sodium, or calcium channels [38].

Using electrophysiology in Purkinje neurons, compounds in this class were shown to be at least 1000-fold more potent than the first reported series of AMPA receptor modulators disclosed by Cortex (CX516, **22**; Fig. 7.3). Mechanistically, LY404187 is considered to be a blocker of desensitization or more specifically, to potentiate AMPA receptor activity by allowing faster recovery from desensitization [74]. When studied in prefrontal cortex pyramidal neurons from a slice preparation, LY404187 in a concentration dependent manner enhanced glutamatergic synaptic AMPA receptor dependent excitatory postsynaptic potentials (EPSPs) in terms of both amplitude and duration [38].

Given that LY404187 and related compounds show robust potentiation of AMPA receptors using *in vitro* preparations, they would be expected to demonstrate similar actions *in vivo*, provided they were sufficiently CNS penetrant. Intravenous (i.v.) administration of both LY392098 (**10**; Fig. 7.2) and LY404187 demonstrated a dose-dependent increase in firing rate on hippocampal neurons, with $ED_{50}$ values of 10 ± 2 μg/kg and 12 ± 1 μg/kg for LY392098 and LY404187, respectively [75]. Thus, the *in vivo* effects of the sulfonamide-based AMPA receptor modulators were significantly more potent than observed with the benzamide compound CX516 (**22**; Fig. 7.3), with an $ED_{50}$ of 5 ± 2 mg/kg in the same assay (see Fig. 7.4). One surprising aspect of this study was the apparent lack of selectivity between AMPA and NMDA responses on the hippocampal neurons, given that selectivity is observed *in vitro*, although the enhancement of the AMPA response is significantly greater than the NMDA response. Co-administration with an AMPA antagonist (LY300168) reversed the effect of LY392098 on both AMPA- and NMDA-mediated currents in hippocampal neurons, whereas co-administration with an NMDA antagonist (ketamine) only resulted in a significant reduction in the NMDA-mediated response. These data indicated that the potentiation of firing in response to NMDA by an AMPA receptor modulator is in fact an indirect effect through action at the AMPA receptor.

A noninvasive brain imaging study utilizing pharmacological magnetic resonance imaging (phMRI) technology to assess changes in blood oxygen

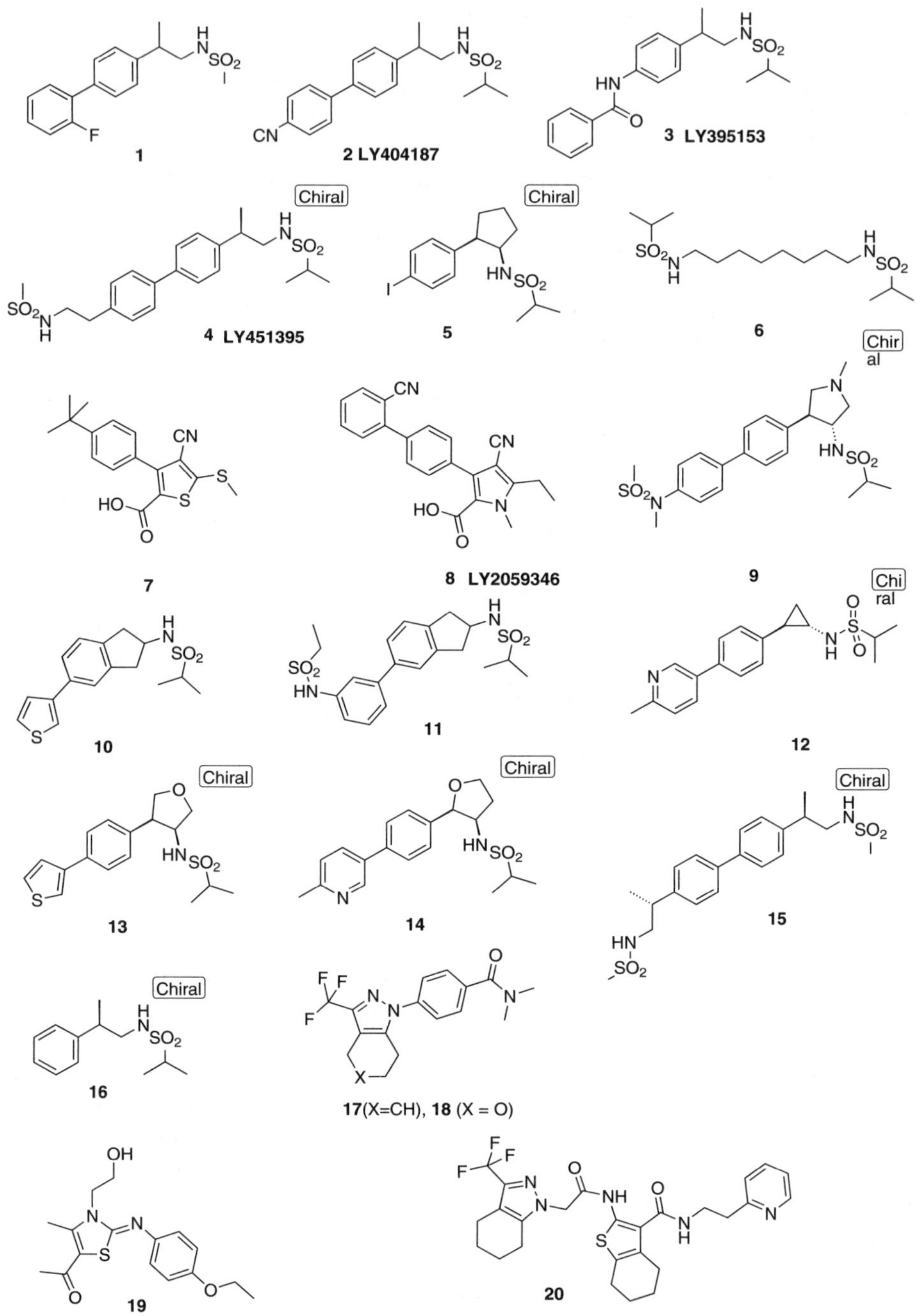


**FIGURE 7.2** The structures of selected AMPA receptor positive modulators.

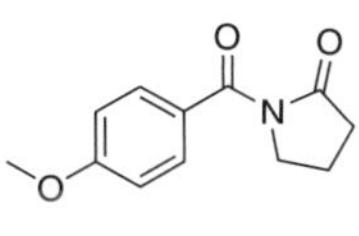

**21 Aniracetam**

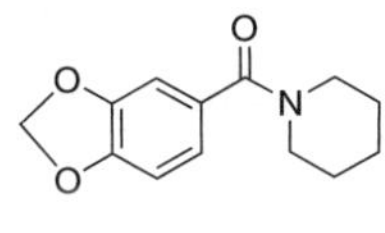

**22 1-BCP**

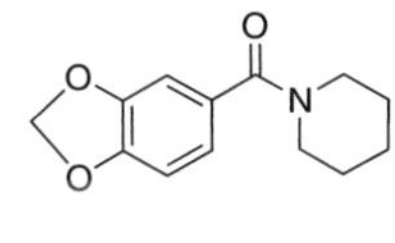

**23 BDP-5**

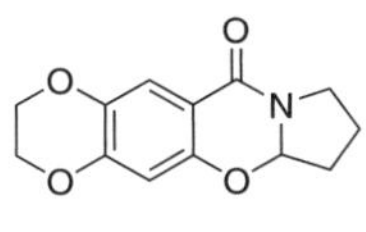

**24 CX614**

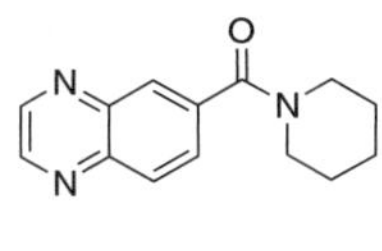

**25 CX516**

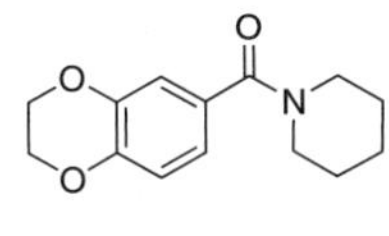

**26 CX546**

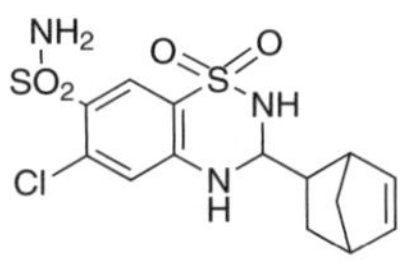

**27 Cyclothiazide**

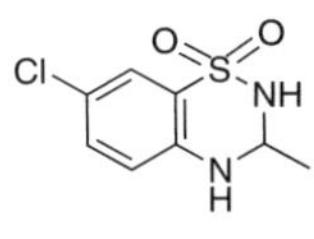

**28 IDRA21**

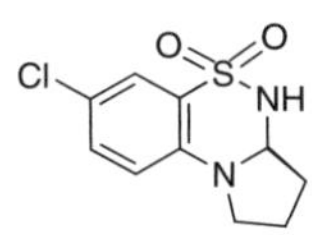

**29 S18986**

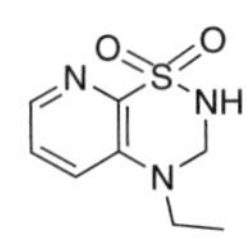

**30**

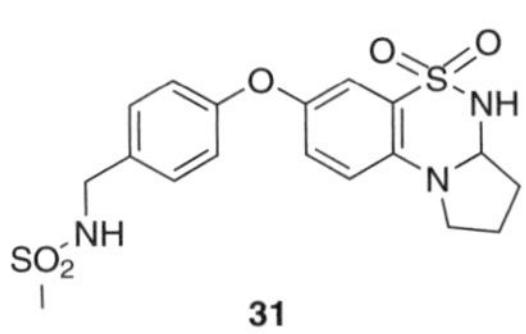

**31**

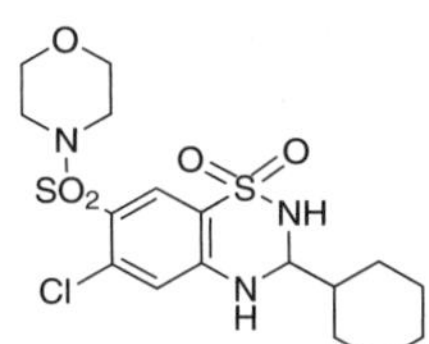

**32**

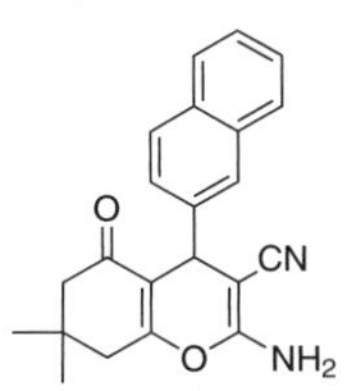

**33**

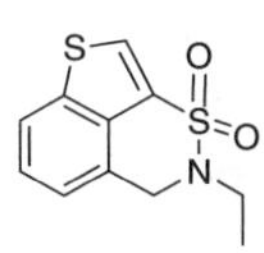

**34**

**FIGURE 7.3** The structures of selected AMPA receptor positive modulators.

level-dependent (BOLD) contrast as a marker of neuronal activity examined the effect of LY404187 in the anesthetized rat. LY 404187 produced significant increases in BOLD contrast in several brain regions including the hippocampus, lateral and medial habenula, and superior and inferior colliculi [76]. Again, these responses, which were interpreted as increases in excitatory neurotransmission, could be reversed by administration of an AMPA receptor antagonist [76]. The effects of LY404187 observed in brain imaging are mirrored in the modulation of growth factors such as brain-derived neurotrophic factor (BDNF). Early data from Lilly demonstrated that LY392098, either alone or in combination with AMPA, elicited an increase in BDNF mRNA and protein levels in neuronal cultures [77]. More recent studies have suggested

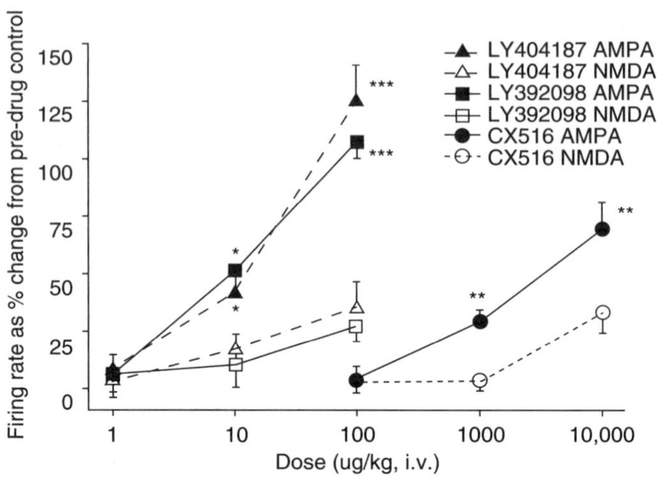


**FIGURE 7.4** Dose response data on sulfonamides LY404187 and LY392098 and the benzamide CX516 as potentiators of AMPA and NMDA on hippocampal neurons. Each data point is the mean value ± SEM from 4–8 neurons. The enhancement of the AMPA response was significantly greater than that of the NMDA responses at 10 μg/kg (*$P < 0.05$) and 100 (***$P < 0.001$) of LY392098 and LY404187 and at 1 and 10 mg/kg of CX516 (**$P < 0.01$). Full details of experimental conditions and data are available in Reference [75]. Figure reproduced from Reference [75]. Copyright (2001) with permission from Elsevier.

that subchronic treatment of rats with LY404187 produced an increase in BDNF expression that was most profound in the dentate gyrus [78]. These effects on BDNF have provided pivotal evidence for pursuing AMPA receptor potentiators for indications such as depression [79] and Parkinson's disease [80].

Building on the promising preclinical data generated around LY404187 and LY392098, Lilly has developed a series of bis-sulfonamide derivatives such as compound **4** (LY451395; Fig. 7.2). Although little preclinical data have been published on these compounds to date, LY451395 has progressed to clinical studies (see Section 7.7).

Further structure–activity relationship (SAR) studies on the sulfonamide template have also been reported [81–83]. For example, changing the linker system to insert an amide spacer resulted in compound **3** (Fig. 7.2), which when tested in a radioligand binding assay using a cortical neuron membrane preparation had an $IC_{50}$ of 0.17 μM. Constrained analogs of LY404187 have also been prepared, resulting in compounds of the type 5 (Fig. 7.2) [84]. Such entities show potency around 10-fold greater than the related open-chain analogs (e.g., 5 GluR4 $EC_{50}$ = 23 nM). Deletion analogs such as **6** (Fig. 7.2) have also been claimed by Lilly as AMPA receptor positive modulators; however, to date no development has been reported for compounds in this series [81].

More recently, the Lilly Corporation has disclosed an unrelated series of AMPA potentiators based on a heterocyclic acid scaffold. LY2059346 (8; Fig. 7.2) [85–87] was identified through optimization of a HTS-derived hit (7; Fig. 7.2) and is claimed to be highly potent as a positive modulator at different isoforms and splice variants ($EC_{50}$ = 56 nM [GluR4 flip], 53 nM [GluR4 flop], 82 nM [GluR2 flip], 73 nM [GluR2 flop]). No further data have been published on this compound to date.

GlaxoSmithKline has also disclosed their interest in the area of AMPA receptor modulators with numerous patent applications on various series of compounds, some of which are structurally related to LY404187 [88–90]. From this work, a clinical candidate has emerged, GSK729327, which is reported to be in Phase I clinical trials for cognitive impairment associated with schizophrenia [91]. Only limited biological characterization has been claimed; however, it is likely that compounds of this type are of lower potency compared with the entities claimed previously by the Lilly group (e.g., 9 $EC_{50}$ = 1.6 μM, 10 $EC_{50}$ = 10 μM, 11 $EC_{50}$ = 3 μM at the GluR2 flip receptor; Fig. 7.2) [88–90]. Subsequent compounds [92–94] have focused on developing SAR at the sulfonamide linker region (e.g., 12–14; Fig. 7.2), although no biological activity has been reported to date.

Another sulfonamide-based modulator that has appeared in the literature is the biaryl bis-sulfonamide (15; Fig. 7.2) which is formally related to LY451395 (4) [95]. This dimeric sulfonamide was designed from consideration of the X-ray crystal structure of the LBD of the AMPA receptor. Electrophysiological characterization showed that these dimeric systems exhibited significantly greater potency than their monomeric precursors typified by **16** (Fig. 7.2) (**15**, oocyte $EC_{50}$ = 0.73 ± 0.13 μM; 16, oocyte $EC_{50}$ = 195 ± 13 μM) [96]. The binding mode of this compound is discussed in detail below.

Other series of interest from GlaxoSmithKline include compounds of the type **17–19** (Fig. 7.2), which represent a unique structural class to the sulfonamide series discussed earlier [97–99]. A direct comparison of these newer templates is not possible as no detailed biological data is yet in the public domain. One additional chemotype that has emerged in the patent literature is the series of pyrazazolealkanamide substituted thiophene compounds (**20**; Fig. 7.2) from Organon [100]. Again, only limited biological data are available, thereby preventing a direct comparison with the Lilly sulfonamide series.

The first class of compounds to be investigated as AMPA positive allosteric modulators was among the benzamide series. This class of compound emerged from the observation that aniracetam (**21**; Fig. 7.3) is able to potentiate AMPA transmission in the hippocampus [101], although with potency in the millimolar range. Aniracetam is well tolerated and is approved in certain European countries for the treatment of mild cognitive impairment associated with Alzheimer's disease. Other notable earlier modulators included 1-BCP (**22**) and BDP-5 (**23**). A number of related compounds (referred to as AMPAkines) that possess greater potency have been developed by Cortex Pharmaceuticals (CX516, **25**; CX546, **26**; and CX614, **24**; Fig. 7.3). For example, CX516 (or

Ampalex) has an $EC_{50}$ in a hippocampal slice preparation of 150 μM as measured by patch clamp electrophysiology in cultured hippocampal neurons [102]. CX614 has been shown to have somewhat higher potency than CX516, for example, exhibiting $EC_{50}$'s in the range 19–37 μM across recombinant GluR1-3 receptors [103].

Although both CX516 and CX546 have a very high degree of chemical similarity, they have been shown to have different effects on receptor kinetics when studied on patches excised from pyramidal cells in the CA1 area of the hippocampus [102]. CX516 has only modest effects on desensitization, whereas CX546 has been shown to be a complete blocker. Both compounds had effects on deactivation, but again CX546 proved to be more effective at prolonging deactivation. Biostructural data would be invaluable for elucidating the differences in mode of action for these apparently similar compounds. Competition experiments using modulation of fluorowillardiine binding have shown partial overlap with the CX614 and cyclothiazide binding sites, thereby indicating a degree of commonality [103]. Interestingly, electrophysiological experiments in the same study demonstrated that CX614 has effects on both deactivation and desensitization, which may offer some insight into the binding mode of the compound.

Like the Lilly biarylsulfonamide compounds, CX546 and CX516 are active in hippocampal slice preparations, typically increasing the amplitude and duration of field excitatory postsynaptic potentials (fEPSPs). Again, a difference was observed between the two compounds, with CX516 increasing response amplitudes but only minimally prolonging the response duration. In contrast, CX546 significantly increased the response duration but had a more modest effect on response amplitude [104]. By comparison, CX614 increased both amplitude and duration of fEPSPs in the hippocampal slice [103].

Both CX546 and CX516 have been shown to have an effect on synaptic plasticity by facilitating induction of hippocampal long-term potentiation (LTP). In this paradigm, LTP is induced using short theta-burst stimulation at 200-millisecond intervals, with four bursts being sufficient to enhance the amplitude and slope by over 50% compared with the baseline response. With fewer bursts, the potentiation becomes smaller. When CX546 and CX516 are present during stimulation, the maximal response is achieved with fewer bursts [105], thereby demonstrating that AMPA receptor potentiators can lower the threshold required for LTP induction. Given that LTP is thought to be a functional correlate for memory encoding, it then follows that compounds that facilitate this process (such as CX516, CX546, and indeed aniracetam) could find utility in enhancing memory (see Section 7.6.1).

The relationship between positive modulators of the AMPA receptor and BDNF is again reinforced with the benzamide series. For example, treatment of organotypic hippocampal cultures with CX614 led to substantial increases (up to 10-fold) in BDNF mRNA [106]. Similarly, when CX546 was administered i.v. (30 mg/kg) to aged rats and mice over a period of 5 days, elevation of BDNF was observed at the mRNA level in the hippocampus [107]. Although a connection exists between AMPA positive modulator activity and BDNF for various classes of compound, it is not clear to what extent this mechanism mediates the behavioral effects associated with AMPA positive modulators. Intriguingly, O'Neill and co-workers at Lilly claim to have identified a series of AMPA receptor modulators (structures not revealed) that have the typical pharmacology at cloned native receptors but do not enhance BDNF levels in cultured cells [108]. Comparing this class of compound with the biarylsulfonamides and benzamides in relevant behavioral paradigms could offer some insight into the role of BDNF in exerting the positive mnemonic effects of AMPA receptor positive modulators.

Another major series of AMPA positive modulator that has received attention in the literature are the benzothiadiazines. Such compounds are broadly based on cyclothiazide (27; Fig. 7.3) which has been studied extensively as a positive modulator of the AMPA receptor, giving a twofold potentiation (EC2x) of the AMPA current at a concentration of 1.6 μM [109]. Another well-known compound related to cyclothiazide is IDRA-21 (28). Probably the best characterized member of this series is the Servier compound S18986 (29; Fig. 7.3), which showed an EC2x of 60 μM [110] in AMPA-induced current when applied to *Xenopus oocytes* expressing recombinant AMPA receptors. In this series, only the (S)-enantiomer was shown to be effective as an AMPA positive modulator. Despite having lower potency than cyclothiazide, S18986 differs in that it can penetrate the blood–brain barrier, thereby enabling *in vivo* investigation [111]. In this respect, S18986 has been shown to elevate acetylcholine levels in the hippocampus as well as being effective in various tests predictive of cognition enhancing activity (see below). Interestingly, in one study where S18986 was administered chronically to aged rats, levels of BDNF mRNA were not significantly different from basal levels [112]. This contrasts with previous *in vitro* studies that showed enhancement of (S)-AMPA-mediated BDNF mRNA and protein expression in cultured rat neurons [113].

Analog derived from S18986 have been shown to have superior levels of potency (e.g., **30**; Fig. 7.3) EC2x = 8.8 μM) [109]. Subsequent patent applications from Servier have demonstrated how the benzothiadiazine template can be further functionalized to furnish analogs such as compound **31** (Fig. 7.3) [114].

Neurosearch have also reported analogues that are structurally related to CTZ as exemplified by **32** (Fig. 7.3) [115]. Such compounds have been shown to potentiate AMPA mediated currents in mouse neocortical neurons. Furthermore, by way of *in vivo* electrophysiology, 31 (Fig. 7.3) was shown to enhance AMPA-induced spike activity in the hippocampus when dosed at 10 mg/kg i.v. in rat.

A number of more structurally diverse compounds have appeared in the literature in recent years including benzopyran derivatives from CoCensys [116] (33, Fig. 7.3), EC2x = 1.6 μM) and Boehringer Ingleheim's benzothiazine analogs [117] (**34**, Fig. 7.3; no data reported).

### 7.4.1 Biostructural Approaches to Understanding the Action of AMPA Receptor Modulators

Unusually for an ion channel, biostructural data have significantly impacted on both the progress of AMPA-directed drug design and the understanding of structure–function relationships in AMPA receptors. While electron microscopy [118, 119] demonstrated that the AMPA receptor exists as a dimer-of-dimers, the recent publication of the structure of a full-length tetrameric AMPA receptor is a significant milestone and provides detailed insights into receptor structure and gating, and suggests mechanisms that underlie activation, desensitization, and deactivation of the channel (Fig. 7.5a) [8].

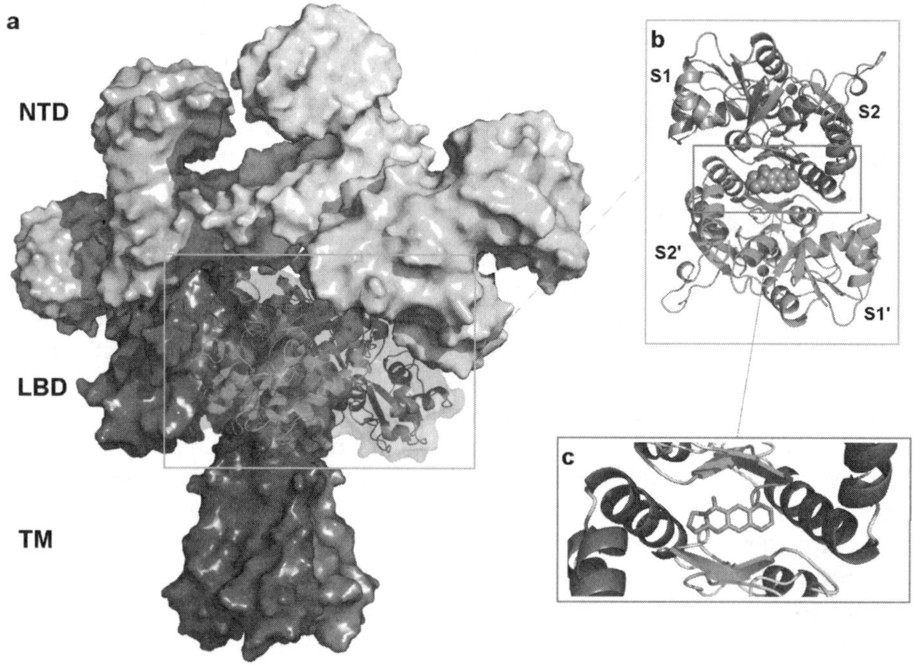


**FIGURE 7.5** Tetrameric AMPA receptor structure, modeled from PDB entry 3KG2 [8, 118]. (a) Colors discriminate individual monomers (green, cyan, purple, orange). One ligand binding domain (LBD) dimer is shown as a transparent surface. (b) Ribbon structure of the complex between the AMPA LBD dimer and the positive modulator CX614, viewed down the twofold symmetry axis relating the monomers. CX614 binds across the symmetry axis. Agonist (glutamate) binding sites are shown as magenta spheres—the agonist and allosteric binding sites are clearly distinct. (c) Close-up view of the binding site for positive allosteric modulators. As the site spans a symmetry axis, a ligand can bind in two equivalent orientations, related by rotation about the axis. A single orientation is shown here for clarity. TM, transmembrane domain; NTD, amino terminal domain. (See color insert.)

AMPA biostructural efforts have built on seminal work by the Keinänen [120] and Gouaux [121] groups. The former exploited the modular nature of the AMPA receptor (Fig. 7.1) and excised the extracellular LBD as a soluble construct. This was more complex than simply defining the domain boundaries, as the AMPA LBD is composed of two distinct lobes (termed S1 and S2) separated by 175 residues. The development of a soluble construct involved the replacement of the intervening residues by a linker peptide, methodology that was optimized by the Gouaux group to arrive at a construct (S1S2) suitable for X-ray crystallography. Subsequent investigations have shown that S1S2 is an excellent model system with pharmacology analogous to the native receptor. It forms dimers both in solution and in crystal structures, and it has rather elegantly been demonstrated that the observed conformation of S1S2 represents the nondesensitized state of the receptor [30].

The first AMPA X-ray structure was determined in 1998, confirming predictions that the LBD formed a clamshell that closed around the orthosteric ligand binding site. There has been a wealth of subsequent work, with 82 AMPA LBD structures (from the GluR2, 3, and 4 isoforms) now deposited in the Protein Data Bank. In addition, similar constructs have been exploited to generate multiple LBD structures for kainate and NMDA glutamate receptor subtypes. These provide significant insights into receptor–ligand interactions both at the orthosteric (agonist) and at the allosteric (positive allosteric modulator) ligand binding sites. The majority of the available structures represent the nondesensitized form of the LBD, the state with which allosteric modulators are presumed to interact.

The general fold of the GluR2 LBD clamshell has been described in detail elsewhere [122]. As outlined earlier, the LBD is composed of two distinct peptides, S1 and S2, which form the lobes of the clamshell, and which move relative to one another to open and close upon ligand binding. Two of these clamshells pack together back-to-back to form the dimeric LBD functional unit (Fig. 7.5b) in which the central hinge regions come close together. The majority of the contacts in the dimer are formed by the S1 lobes, with few contacts from S2 [30]. The flip/flop splice variants manifest themselves at the C-terminal end of the S2 domain. As shown in Figure 7.5b,c, the C-terminal portion of S2 frames a deep twofold symmetric cavity at the dimer interface. This is the positive allosteric modulator binding site, the base of which is formed by residues from S1, but numerous S2 residues also contribute; crucially these include residues (on helices J and K) which are part of the flip/flop cassette, and which are implicated in flip/flop selectivity of allosteric binders.

Most of the GluR2 structures focus on the agonist site, and there are numerous examples that demonstrate the binding of antagonists, full agonists, and partial agonists. The degree of closure of the clamshell upon ligand binding has been convincingly linked [123] to the current amplitude induced by the corresponding ligand in wild-type AMPA receptors. To date, there are 13 disclosed crystal structures of AMPA positive modulators bound to the GluR2 dimer, which represent three of the broad structural classes already described.

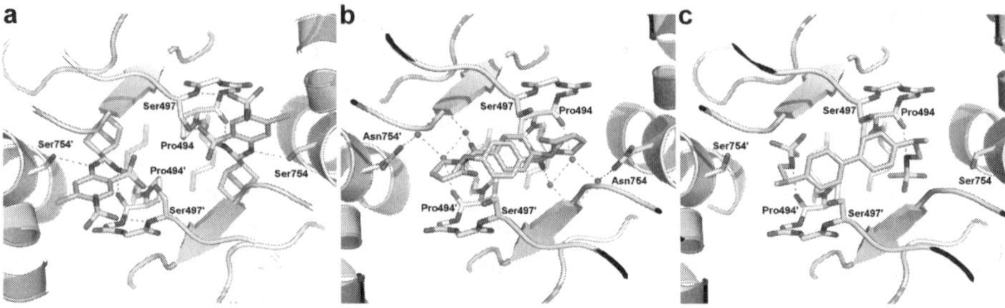


**FIGURE 7.6** Binding modes of the benzothiadiazine (a), benzamide (b), and arylsulfonamide (c) classes of AMPA modulators. Two equivalent, symmetry-related orientations are shown for (a) and (b), while only one orientation is shown for the symmetric ligand (c). **a:** Binding mode of cyclothiazide (**25**; Fig. 7.3), which forms hydrogen bonds with the side chains of Ser497 and Ser754, and with main chain atoms of Pro494 and Ser497. The norbornyl moiety is buried within a hydrophobic pocket, displacing a network of solvent molecules. **b:** Binding mode of aniracetam (**21**; Fig. 7.3), in which the two possible orientations span the symmetry axis and therefore overlap. Aniracetam makes no hydrophilic interactions with protein atoms, and forms just one hydrogen bond with a network of solvent molecules occupying the buried hydrophobic pocket. **c:** Binding mode of the aryl sulfonamide compound (**15**; Fig. 7.2). The sulphonamide occupies a hydrophobic pocket, displacing a network of solvent molecules in a similar way to cyclothiazide, while the sulphonamide NH forms a hydrogen bond with the carbonyl of Pro494. (See color insert.)

The first AMPA positive modulator structure disclosed was that of cyclothiazide (**25**; Fig. 7.3) in 2002 [30]. Cyclothiazide was shown to bind at a site entirely distinct from that occupied by agonists/antagonists, and subsequent crystal structures from the benzamide (21, 24; Fig. 7.3) and arylsulfonamide (15; Fig. 7.2) classes confirmed a common allosteric binding pocket for these modulators.

Cyclothiazide is observed at two symmetrically equivalent sites (Fig. 7.6a). The benzothiadiazide ring forms hydrogen bonds with Pro494 and Ser754 from one monomer; the exocyclic sulphonamide is also hydrogen-bonded to Ser497; and the norbornyl moiety occupies a hydrophobic pocket formed by residues from both monomers. There are additional hydrogen bonds to solvent molecules and contacts both with hydrophobic and with hydrophilic surfaces.

Cyclothiazide modulation is highly sensitive to the flip/flop splice variation, and specifically to the residue at position 754. Flop splice variants, containing Asn754, are not modulated by cyclothiazide, while flip variants, containing Ser754, are highly sensitive. The cyclothiazide crystal structure was generated using a flop construct with an additional Asn754Ser point mutation. Comparison with native flop structures (e.g., Fig. 7.4b) demonstrates that the presence of Asn754 modulates the shape of the binding site such that it is no longer complementary to cyclothiazide.

The co-crystal structures of two representatives from the benzamide class (aniracetam and CX614) have also been disclosed [124]. Although the mechanism of action of the benzamide class is distinct from that of the benzothiadiazides, they share a common binding site (Fig. 7.6b). While cyclothiazide is observed in two positions at the extremes of the allosteric site, single molecules of aniracetam and CX614 bind across the twofold axis at the center of the site, and occlude just 20% of the volume occupied by cyclothiazide. In contrast to cyclothiazide, interactions between aniracetam/CX614 and the receptor are predominantly hydrophobic, the most significant contacts with Pro494 and Ser497. The only hydrogen bond observed in either structure is an interaction between the ligand carbonyl and a cluster of water molecules occupying the hydrophobic pocket that accommodates the norbornyl group of cyclothiazide. Although compounds from this class display a wide range of $EC_{50}$ values, it is likely that all members interact with the receptor in approximately the same manner. The significantly better binding of CX614 relative to aniracetam probably reflects its greater size (increased lipophilic contacts) and increased rigidity (reduced entropic penalty upon binding).

Most recently, the binding mode of an arylsulfonamide (15; Fig. 7.2) was predicted [125] and later confirmed [96] by X-ray crystallography (Fig. 7.6c). LY451395 (**4**; Fig. 7.2), and presumably the other compounds in the arylsulfonamide class, can be expected to share this binding mode, overlapping significantly with both the benzamide and the thiadiazide binding sites, consistent with previous predictions [125, 126] based on their intermediate pharmacology. The biaryl motif spans the central part of the binding pocket, making hydrophobic contacts with the saddle formed by Pro494 and Pro494′, while the flexible aliphatic linker allows the two sulfonamide moieties to curl into the small hydrophobic pockets on either side. Interestingly, the methylsulfonamide of 15 overlaps with neither of the sulfonamides of cyclothiazide, instead behaving as a hydrophobic group overlaying with the norbornyl motif.

While these compound classes occupy approximately the same binding pocket, their pharmacology is distinct. A tentative explanation has been proposed [124] based on the structures from the benzamide class, and this remains consistent with subsequent data. Briefly, this model attempts to separate the processes of receptor deactivation and desensitization. Both appear to involve conformational changes in the LDB of the receptor, and although they involve common elements, they can be decoupled both structurally and pharmacologically.

Deactivation requires the opening of the clamshell structure to release agonist. In the back-to-back GluR2 dimer, the hinge regions of each clamshell come together near the center of the allosteric pocket (Fig. 7.5b). Thus, modulators that occupy the central region of the allosteric pocket serve to stabilize the closed-cleft agonist bound state, reducing the extent of receptor deactivation. A biostructural understanding of the desensitized state of the AMPA receptor has proven considerably more elusive, but desensitized states of GluR2 have been trapped out and characterized using disulfide tethers [127].

These structures reveal that the transition from nondesensitized to desensitized states require a rotation of one monomer relative to another, normal to the plane of the dimer interface. Such a conformational change essentially deletes the conventional allosteric binding pocket; thus, any compound that occupies that pocket will serve to stabilize the nondesensitized state and will reduce receptor desensitization.

Potentiation by positive modulators of the AMPA receptor is therefore a combination of effects on receptor deactivation and desensitization. Modulators occupying the central part of the binding site, close to the clamshell hinge (e.g., **21**, **24**; Fig. 7.3), will slow receptor deactivation, while those that do not (e.g., 25; Fig. 7.3) will predominantly inhibit desensitization. This discrimination nicely reflects the different pharmacological profiles exhibited by the benzamide and benzothiadiazide classes. Specifically, compounds that largely affect deactivation are generally low-potency modulators and are well tolerated, whereas compounds such as cyclothiazide, which predominantly affect desensitization, have much higher potency at the receptor. Compound classes with binding modes combining elements of these two extremes demonstrate intermediate pharmacological profiles (e.g., arylsulfonamides **1–6**, **9–14**; Fig. 7.2), which may provide a more acceptable balance between potency and tolerability.

## 7.5 PRECLINICAL EVIDENCE FOR THE USE OF AMPA RECEPTOR MODULATORS IN SCHIZOPHRENIA: TESTS PREDICTIVE OF ANTIPSYCHOTIC-LIKE ACTIVITY

The preclinical assessment of antipsychotic-like activity for a number of AMPA receptor positive modulators has depended on tests purported to be models of psychosis such as the attenuation of stereotypic behavior (e.g., exploration, locomotion) induced by psychostimulants such as methamphetamine and NMDA receptor channel blockers (e.g., MK-801 and PCP). Although these stereotypic behaviors are considered to model the psychotomimetic effects of these drugs in human subjects, these tests can only really be said to have predictive validity for functional dopamine receptor $D_2$ antagonism rather than antipsychotic efficacy per se.

The AMPAkine CX564 (also referred to as BDP 29) was demonstrated to counteract the stereotypic rearing activity elicited by methamphetamine in rats [128]. Another study with this compound that examines the effect of i.p. administration on c-fos expression in rat brains found that AMPAkine CX564 induced a significant decrease in c-fos activity in the striatum and an increase in the somatosensory cortex with a general overall increase in the ratio of cortical to striatal labeling [129]. In contrast, methamphetamine induced a marked increase in the striatum, with an increase also noted in the orbitofrontal cortex but with an overall reduction in the ratio of cortical to striatal labeling [129]. These results were taken to suggest that facilitation of glutamatergic transmission in the brain may have effects that are opposite to those resulting from enhanced dopaminergic transmission and possibly account for the attenuation of the behavioral stereotypy of methamphetamine with CX564. In other studies, CX516 failed to show any significant effect against methamphetamine or MK-801-induced locomotor activity when given alone [130, 131] but did enhance the inhibitory effect of clozapine and, to a lesser extent, haloperidol against methamphetamine-induced locomotor activity. A pharmacokinetic interaction was ruled out with each of these drugs [131]. Also, no exacerbation of haloperidol-induced catalepsy was noted, indicating that the interaction is specific for the antipsychotic-like effect with a reduced likelihood for exacerbating extrapyramidal side effects with this combination. Another report demonstrated that CX546 and CX614 were able to reduce methamphetamine-induced circling behavior in rats with unilateral 6-hydroxydopamine lesions of the ascending nigro-striatal dopamine system and had been additionally sensitized to methamphetamine [132] This was accompanied by an increase in c-fos expression in the parietal sensorimotor neocortex with hemispheric asymmetry of cortical activation less pronounced in the AMPAkine co-treatment group as compared with the methamphetamine-alone group [132]. Further evidence supporting the ability of AMPA modulators to counteract dopaminergic hyperactivity comes from studies with dopamine transporter (DAT) knockout mice. These mice exhibit marked changes in dopamine homeostasis resulting in a persistent hyperdopaminergic tone and pronounced locomotor hyperactivity [133]. Aniracetam and the AMPAkines CX516, CX546, CX672, and CX776 were shown to significantly suppress hyperactivity in these mice. Neither aniracetam nor CX516 had any corresponding effects on striatal dopamine levels, thereby suggesting a lack of direct effect of these compounds on striatal dopaminergic tone in the modulatory effect of these drugs on locomotor activity [133].

Another test that is widely reported to possess high predictive validity for antipsychotic efficacy is the selective suppression of conditioned avoidance response (CAR) behavior (i.e., a conditioned response that anticipates the occurrence of an aversive stimulus) in the rat. This test is widely used to differentiate antipsychotics from other drug classes such as anxiolytics and antidepressants, which act as negative controls, and is also regarded as a valid test to detect potentially novel antipsychotics as well as supporting various augmentation strategies. Furthermore, the ability of antipsychotic drugs to suppress CAR has been shown to be closely related to clinical potency with respect to the treatment of psychosis. In one such study, CX516, while being found to be ineffective on its own, significantly potentiated the suppression of CAR induced by threshold doses of risperidone, olanzapine, and clozapine without causing additional motor disturbances [134]. This specific augmentation of antipsychotic-like activity is in agreement with the findings described earlier where CX516 potentiated the effects of antipsychotic drugs in the methamphetamine activity test [131]. Again, a pharmacokinetic interaction was ruled out as a possible explanation of the augmentation induced by CX516 upon antipsychotic efficacy.

Although all of the tests described above are generally accepted to have predictive validity for antipsychotic action, animal models of behavioral endophenotypes of schizophrenia such as prepulse inhibition (PPI) and latent inhibition (LI) are regarded as important preclinical tools in that they have face validity for evaluating antipsychotic-like action of novel pharmacological compounds [135]. PPI is a measure of sensorimotor gating and refers to the attenuation of the startle response by a weak stimulus (prepulse) appearing a short time before a startle stimulus. LI is a well-established phenomenon that reflects an organism's ability to learn and filter out irrelevant stimuli. Deficits in both PPI and LI have been reported in schizophrenia [136, 137]. Although disruption of PPI and LI in rodents by psychotomimetic drugs can be ameliorated by antipsychotic drugs [135], the only data to so far show the positive effects of an AMPA modulator comes from a study using mGluR5 knockout mice [138]. The absence of mGluR5 in these mice was shown to cause NMDA receptor hypofunction and result in stable and profound disruption in both PPI and LI. These impairments were both restored by CX546 showing that in this experimental system at least, facilitation of AMPA receptor function was able to overcome a functional deficit of the glutamatergic system [138]. Aniracetam was also shown to ameliorate the deficit in PPI although its effect was much less pronounced than that of CX546. While these effects were claimed to be antipsychotic-like, previous studies had shown that the observed PPI deficit in mGluR5 knockout mice was resistant to antipsychotics following acute administration [139] although a recent study has shown that clozapine was effective following chronic administration [140] Nevertheless, while the predictive validity of this model for testing the effects of existing antipsychotic drugs has been questioned, it cannot be ruled out that this model may be more relevant for the development of antipsychotic compounds with novel mechanisms of action working through the glutamate system.

In summary, a limited amount of data from a few traditional animal models suggests that some AMPA receptor positive modulators may have antipsychotic-like activity on their own while others only potentiate the effect of existing clinically effective antipsychotic drugs. This may reflect methodological differences between labs. However, a major limitation in the overall assessment of these studies is that many have been performed with AMPA receptor positive modulators with distinct mechanisms of action in terms of their pharmacological and biophysical effects on AMPA receptor function. These differences, coupled with observations that some of these compounds (e.g., CX516 and CX546) have been shown to have different effects across different brain regions [141], suggest that therapeutic selectivity may arise from the distinct regional brain distribution of the AMPA receptor subunits [31] Given this level of complexity, it is a real possibility that the therapeutic potential of such compounds could be very different. Thus, a clearer understanding of the therapeutic utility of positive AMPA receptor modulators as antipsychotic agents and the optimal pharmacological profile that may be required as such will likely require a systematic comparison of compounds with distinct pharmacological properties over a wide range of behavioral tests.

While there may be insufficient preclinical data—and indeed, clinical data [142] (see Section 7.7)—to support the therapeutic potential of AMPA receptor positive modulators as antipsychotic agents (i.e., for the treatment of positive symptoms of schizophrenia), in view of the well-documented positive cognitive effects of these compounds it may be anticipated that they will serve as a promising adjunctive therapy for cognitive impairment, and perhaps even the negative symptoms associated with schizophrenia, which are widely acknowledged to be poorly treated by existing antipsychotic therapies.

## 7.6 TARGETING COGNITION IN SCHIZOPHRENIA

The development of novel pharmacological approaches for the treatment of cognitive impairment in schizophrenia is currently a major focus in academic and pharmaceutical industry laboratories. Indeed, the National Institute of Mental Health (NIMH) has established the Measurement and Treatment Research to Improve Cognition in Schizophrenia (MATRICS) initiative (http://www.matrics.ucla.edu) to facilitate these efforts. This project has been designed to identify the core cognitive impairments in schizophrenia, identify promising targets for drug development, and establish a battery of preclinical and clinical tests to assess the effectiveness of potential cognitive-enhancing agents. Among the achievements to date are the identification of the seven primary cognitive domains that are affected in schizophrenia: attention/vigilance, speed of processing, working memory, verbal learning and memory, visual learning and memory, reasoning and problem solving, and social cognition [4].

Among the targets that have been considered as leading candidates with therapeutic utility for the treatment of cognitive impairments are glutamatergic agents including those that act at either metabotropic or ionotropic glutamate receptors [143] and, given their well-documented positive cognitive effects, prominent among these are positive modulators of the AMPA receptor.

### 7.6.1 Preclinical Evidence Supporting the Cognition-Enhancing Effects of AMPA Receptor Positive Modulators

Given the prominent role that AMPA receptors have been demonstrated to play in forms of synaptic plasticity, such as LTP, which have been considered to underlie forms of memory encoding, it is perhaps not surprising that significant effort has been focused on the development of positive modulators of the AMPA receptor as cognition enhancers. Indeed, the positive effects of a number of these compounds have been well documented over the last few years across a variety of cognitive domains in both rodent and nonhuman primates in normal and deficit models [144–147].

For instance, the cognitive enhancing effects of pyrrolidinones such as aniracetam and piracetam, originally developed as nootropic drugs over 30 years ago, was recognized long before these compounds were identified as weak positive allosteric modulators of the AMPA receptor [148]. Aniracetam has been extensively studied in a range of animal models of learning and memory where, for example, it was found to improve short-term working memory and long-term spatial memory in the delayed nonmatching to sample [149] and maze tasks [150, 151], respectively. Furthermore, aniracetam was found to ameliorate cognitive deficits induced by the benzodiazepine alprazolam [152], scopolamine [153–155], apomorphine [156], cerebral ischemia [157], and cortical lesions [158].

Subsequent generations of AMPA receptor positive modulators such as IDRA-21, CX516, CX717, and S18986 have been subject to quite extensive studies across a variety of cognitive domains in rodent and nonhuman primates. Extensive use has been made of the eight-arm radial maze, a test of spatial learning and memory where the retention of information derived from extra-maze spatial cues is required in relation to the unexplored arms of a maze in order to gain a reward. CX516 (also referred to as BA-74 and BDP-12 in some of the earliest reports) was shown to enhance retention of information as demonstrated by the drug-treated animals being more likely than controls to enter maze arms that had not been entered in an earlier acquisition phase [159]. In a further study by the same group, CX516 was subsequently shown to improve both acquisition and memory retention in middle aged rats (12–18 months old) to levels equivalent to those found in young adults in the radial maze task [160]. CX516 was also shown to selectively increase hippocampal spatial cell firing as demonstrated by electrophysiological recordings from freely moving animals engaged in a delayed match to sample task. A related benzamide compound, CX554 (BDP-20), was also shown to ameliorate age-related deficits in 19- to 21-month old rats in the radial maze task with an increased potency over CX516 that reflected the differences in potency of these two compounds from *in vitro* measurements of AMPA receptor function [161]. Improvements in radial maze performance were observed with the benzamide compounds BDP-5 [162] and 1-BCP [163], with compound exposure in the brain in each case consistent with levels required to modulate AMPA-mediated currents *in vitro*. Improvements in spatial learning and memory with AMPA receptor positive modulators have also been observed in the Morris water maze where a rat or mouse must learn to swim to a hidden escape platform using visual cues placed around the pool. Improvements in memory acquisition were observed with 1-BCP in this test [163]. The benzothiadiazine derivative IDRA-21, while also enhancing performance in normal animals with a potency greater than that of aniracetam, also reversed amnestic effects of alprazolam, scopolamine, and NBQX [153]. Among the few reports to have emerged so far on biarylpropylsulfonamides in measures of cognition, LY404187 and LY451395 were reported to enhance performance of rats in the water maze and acquisition and retention in the radial arm maze [74, 146].

LY451646 (the active enantiomer of LY404187) was shown to decrease the total number of errors on the fourth day of testing in a dose-dependent manner. A recent report has also demonstrated that chronic (4 months) administration with the benzothiadiazine S18986 ameliorated aged-related deficits in spatial learning and memory as determined in a Y-maze test [112]. This was accompanied by a significant attenuation in the decline of forebrain cholinergic neurons and midbrain dopaminergic neurons.

AMPA receptor positive modulators have also been reported to have positive effects on cognitive function in nonspatial memory tests such as the novel object recognition task. This is a nonrewarded ethologically relevant paradigm based on the spontaneous exploratory behavior of mice or rats that measures a form of episodic memory and is dependent on the integrity of the perirhinal cortex [164]. An animal is presented with two identical objects in an arena. Following a delay, the animal is reintroduced into the area where one of the objects presented in the first trial is replaced by a new object. Animals that are able to recognize the original object from the first trial will spend more time exploring the novel object. In this task, S18986 was shown to enhance recognition memory following either 3-day or 7-day administration, and this procognate activity was mediated by facilitating retrieval and not acquisition of memory information [165]. Furthermore, despite a relatively short half-life in plasma and brain (around 1 hour), S18986 remained active for up to 4 hours post administration in this task [165], and a subsequent study showed that this effect was lost by 6 hours [166]. Interestingly, in this last study, whose aim was to determine the optimal dosing regimen with S18986, 1 mg/kg QD for 3 days was found to be more effective at enhancing object recognition memory than 0.3 mg/kg TID over the same period [166]. The authors concluded that despite its short half life, S18986 was able to facilitate a sustained improvement in recognition memory without the requirement for multiple administrations to achieve an optimal efficacy. It was proposed that these long lasting effects may be due to the triggering of downstream electrophysiological and/or neurochemical adaptive pathways.

Effects on short term working memory have been investigated using the delayed nonmatching to sample task (DNMS), which assesses working memory in an operant conditioning chamber. In this task, the animal is presented with one of two levers which, when pressed, initiates a delay phase of varied time intervals (typically up to 40 seconds) and is then followed by a choice phase where the animal must press the original sample lever in a delayed matching to sample (DMTS) task and the opposite (nonmatching) lever in a DNMS task in order to gain a reward. By increasing the delay between the sample phase and the choice phase, the choice accuracy typically declines as a function of this retention interval. In a seminal study by Hampson et al. [167] using the DNMS task, CX516 was administered to rats once every 2 days over a 17-day drug administration period. The CX516-treated animals displayed a marked and progressive increase in performance over the drug administration period (see Fig. 7.7), with significantly improved task accuracy at the longer delay

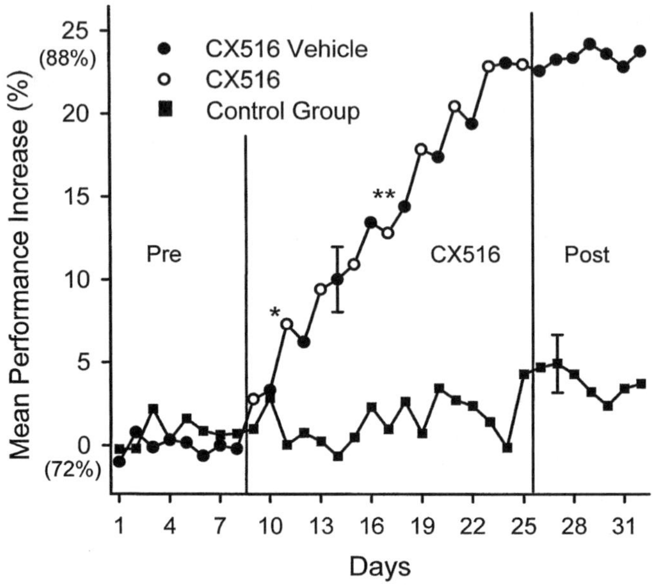


**FIGURE 7.7** CX516 enhances short-term memory in the delayed nonmatching to sample (DNMS) task in rats. Animals were treated with vehicle for 8 days prior to entering the drug phase of the study in which CX516 (35 mg/kg) was administered on alternate days for 16 days. Mean DNMS performance over all trials was calculated for each individual session and transformed to percent increase over baseline performance. Each point is the mean performance over all animals within each group that day. The error bar indicates the largest SEM across all days. Pre, CX516, and Post indicate drug administration on alternate days (open circles). On all other days (closed circles) animals received vehicle only. The control group received vehicle on all 32 days. Asterisks indicate significant increases from the control group on that day (*$P < 0.01$; **$P < 0.001$). Full details of experimental conditions and data are available in Reference [167]. Figure reproduced with permission from the Society for Neuroscience. Copyright (1998) Society for Neuroscience.

intervals particularly evident. Interestingly, a carry-over effect was noted with improved performance maintained on nondrug days. Furthermore, CX516-treated animals maintained their improved performance for up to 7 days after the drug testing period. These studies were performed while monitoring hippocampal CA1 and CA3 neuronal activity through the use of chronically implanted electrodes and showed that improved performance on the task was correlated with increased firing by subpopulations of task-related neurons [168]. The protracted nature of the pro-cognate effects of CX516 is particularly striking given the short plasma half-life (15–20 minutes). Similar effects were also observed with IDRA-21 in a delayed matching task in nonhuman primates similar to the rodent task but where monkeys are trained to remember which color key as opposed to which lever has been pressed [169]. Although

IDRA-21 (dosed once every 3 days) improved performance in both young and aged monkeys, the optimal dose for individual monkeys varied significantly. The improvement in task accuracy was maintained for up to 48 hours after a single dose administration, which, given the short half-life of this compound (<1 hour), indicates that, as with CX516 in the DNMS task [167], a pharmacokinetic/pharmacodynamic disconnect may exist. Although the nature of the protracted mnemonic effects with these compounds is not clear, it was suggested that animals under the influence of these drugs are able to develop new ways of mastering the task [167].. The implications are that the optimal dosing regimen with such compounds may be once every 2 or 3 days as opposed to maintaining steady-state levels of drug exposure around the clock.

Finally, a highly significant study to emerge recently was the demonstration that CX717 was able to improve cognitive performance in sleep-deprived monkeys performing the DMTS [170]. PET imaging that was performed while the animals were carrying out this task showed that CX717 was able to normalize increases in temporal lobe activity and decreases in frontal cortical activity induced by sleep deprivation.

Collectively, these data show that multiple classes of AMPA receptor positive modulators such as the benzamides (aniracetam, CX516, CX546), benzothiadiazines (IDRA-21, S18986), and biarylsulfonamides (LY404187, LY451395) facilitate memory performance in a number of preclinical tests. Furthermore, a number of these tests fall into categories that may map onto cognitive domains that are impaired in schizophrenia as identified by the MATRICS consortium, with for example, DNMS, novel object recognition, and maze tasks potentially mapping onto cognitive domains such as working memory, visual learning and memory, and reasoning and problem solving, respectively [171]. However, caution is required in the interpretation of these results since they have been derived, for the most part, in experiments with healthy animals, some with age-related or sleep deprivation-induced cognitive deficits. None of these can really be considered models of schizophrenia, and indeed the neurobiological substrates underlying the deficits resulting from old age or sleep deprivation may well be different from those present in schizophrenia. Testing compounds in animals with no apparent mental illness is only the first step in the process of defining the potential utility of such compounds in a patient population, and as with the cognitive domains themselves, animal modeling of the deficits apparent in schizophrenia patients is especially challenging because of the very nature of the impairments. Thus, there is a genuine need to encourage development of animal models that express a deficit that resembles that seen in the patients, that is, some level of face and construct validity. In this respect, the development of animal models involving subchronic PCP treatment may be of interest since they appear to mimic several symptoms domains of schizophrenia including cognitive deficits in models such as reversal learning [172], attentional set shifting [173], and novel object recognition [174]. Indeed, a recent study has demonstrated that both CX516 and CX547 were able reverse subchronic PCP-induced disruption of object memory in the novel object recognition task [175], thereby providing further evidence that AMPA modulation may represent a mechanism for the treatment of cognitive deficits in schizophrenia.

## 7.7 CLINICAL STUDIES WITH AMPA RECEPTOR MODULATORS

The potential therapeutic utility of AMPA receptor modulators is being explored for a number of indications including major depression, Parkinson's disease, alcohol intoxication, respiratory depression, and Alzheimer's disease as well as schizophrenia [78, 147, 176–179]. Clinical data, however, are still quite limited, with only a few compounds, CX516, CX717, Org 24448 (farampator), and LY451395, having progressed to Phase II trials. Indeed, of these, the only AMPA positive modulator with published clinical data for schizophrenia is CX516, a relatively low potency compound with suboptimal pharmacokinetic properties. Early studies with this compound in human volunteers provided encouraging data to suggest that it would have a positive effect on memory performance. A transient improvement in the delayed recall of nonsense syllables was demonstrated following administration of a single 900 mg dose of CX516 in elderly subjects (aged >65 years) [180] and following single CX516 doses ranging from 600 to 1200 mg in younger subjects [181]. CX516 also produced small, but statistically significant, improvements in a series of cognitive tasks measuring visual, olfactory, and visiospatial memory following repeated administration of 300 mg in a group of healthy males (aged 25–35 years) [182].

To date, three double-blind studies have been published on the clinical effects of CX516 in schizophrenia. A limited study by Marenco et al. [183] failed to observe any antipsychotic effect of CX516 monotherapy at dosages of between 300 and 900 mg three times daily for 2–4 weeks on four partially refractory schizophrenia patients withdrawn from antipsychotic treatment. More encouraging data was initially provided by Goff et al. [184], who reported on a preliminary 4-week placebo controlled add-on study in 19 patients treated with clozapine. CX516 at doses of 900–1200 mg three times daily was associated with improvements in measures of attention and memory with the effects persisting for up to 2 weeks after completion of the trial. However, a more comprehensive follow-up study examining the effect of add-on treatment with CX516 (900 mg three times daily) or placebo on a total of 105 schizophrenia patients treated with clozapine, olanzapine, or risperidone failed to show any effect on any measure of cognition or for symptoms of schizophrenia [185]. Further development of CX516 has since been terminated and results from clinical studies with more optimal compounds are eagerly awaited. For instance, the Schering-Plough/Cortex compound farampator (Org 24448) has been selected for the National Institute of Mental Health-supported Treatment Units for Research on Neurocognition and Schizophrenia (TURNS) program, which aims to provide an infrastructure for conducting clinical trials of pharmacological agents for enhancing cognition in patients with schizophrenia (see http://www.turns.ucla.edu). Recent data from a double-blind placebo-controlled study performed with 16 healthy, elderly volunteers has shown that a single dose of farampator (500 mg) was effective at improving working memory and information processing but appeared to impair episodic memory [186].

Following up on the demonstration that CX717 was able to improve cognitive performance in sleep-deprived monkeys [170], Cortex Pharmaceuticals have reported that CX717 had an alerting effect on sleep deprivation trials in healthy young men and produced some attenuation of cognitive deficits. However, in a double-blind placebo-controlled trial in 48 volunteers undergoing four consecutive nights of simulated night shift work, CX717 was not effective in reversing performance and alertness deficits when tested at doses between 200 and 1000 mg [187].

Initial clinical studies with the AMPA receptor potentiator LY451395 indicated that it was safe and well tolerated in human volunteers at doses of 1 mg or 5 mg with levels of drug being quantifiable in cerebrospinal fluid (CSF) [95]. In a subsequent, double-blind, placebo-controlled Phase II clinical study on 181 patients with Alzheimer's disease, LY451395 (administered 0.2 mg BID for 28 days and 1.0 mg BID thereafter up to a maximum of 8 weeks) failed to have any effect on cognitive outcome as measured by the Alzheimer's Disease Assessment Scale-Cognitive Subscale (ADAS-Cog) [188]. It is worth noting, however, that this study did show improvements in neuropsychiatric symptoms as measured by the Neuropsychiatric Inventory (NPI) rating scale.

Overall, the clinical studies that have been performed thus far have delivered mixed results. Although there is some promising data to suggest that AMPA receptor positive modulators may have some utility to improve cognition, the precise reasons for the apparent lack of efficacy in a number of these studies is presently unknown and may be due to a number of factors. Some of these compounds (e.g., CX516) have suboptimal pharmacokinetic properties and are probably not the best tools to establish proof-of-concept for AMPA receptor positive modulators in the clinic. In other cases, as suggested by the authors of the study with LY451395 [188], the doses that have been used may not have been optimal. Indeed, perhaps one of the key issues facing clinical development of AMPA receptor potentiators is the lack of suitable biomarkers for dose prediction in humans. Although measuring drug levels in CSF may give an indication of exposure in the brain, proof of target engagement (i.e., interaction of the drug with the AMPA receptor) is still lacking. This is typically achieved through the use of PET ligands to measure receptor occupancy of a given experimental compound; however, such tools do not yet exist for the AMPA receptor [45].

Using indirect measures of target engagement such as imaging technologies can potentially provide translational data to guide dose prediction in clinical proof-of-concept studies. Indeed, pharmacological magnetic resonance imaging (phMRI) has been used in rodents to demonstrate the dose-dependent central effects of LY404187 on neuronal activity in specific brain regions [76]. Furthermore, the increase in BOLD contrast with LY404187 was blocked by the AMPA receptor antagonist LY293558 [76]. This methodology is translatable to functional magnetic resonance imaging (fMRI) studies in humans and, more importantly, provides a readout by which the mechanism of action of the compound can be further investigated.

## 7.8 CONCLUSION

Substantial progress has been made in recent years in our understanding of the pharmacology and biophysical properties of AMPA receptors. Furthermore, a growing body of preclinical evidence demonstrating the effects of AMPA receptor positive modulators on synaptic plasticity and cognition has led to such compounds being explored for clinical indications such as cognitive deficits associated with a variety of neurological and psychiatric disorders. To date there are insufficient data to support the clinical potential of AMPA receptor positive modulators for the treatment of the psychotic symptoms of schizophrenia, although clinical data from compounds with more optimal pharmacokinetic properties will be required to establish this unequivocally. However, it may be anticipated that AMPA receptor positive modulators will serve as promising adjunctive therapy to atypical antipsychotic treatment for the treatment of cognitive impairment associated with schizophrenia. While this approach is being explored with compounds such as farampator, a number of issues remain that will require significant experimental investigation. For instance, it will be important to understand how the administration of AMPA positive modulators and antipsychotic drugs in combination will impact on their respective therapeutic properties. Furthermore, in view of the pharmacokinetic/pharmacodynamic disconnect that appears to exist with regard to the protracted mnemonic effects that have been observed with CX516 [167] and IDRA-21 [169], the optimal dosing regimen with AMPA receptor positive modulators may require refinement since a conventional regimen maintaining steady-state levels of drug exposure around the clock may not be necessary. AMPA receptor positive modulators have been better tolerated than would have been expected given the link with excitotoxicity that has been associated with excessive activation of ionotropic glutamate receptors [189, 190]. In fact, AMPA receptor positive modulators appear to have relatively few adverse effects at therapeutically relevant doses, and indeed, have been shown to protect neurons against neurotoxic insults [141, 191, 192]. These seemingly paradoxical findings have been linked to the induction by AMPA receptor positive modulators of growth factors, such as BDNF, which is known to possess neuroprotective properties [193].

A wide variety of AMPA receptor positive modulators have emerged in recent years, showing distinct actions on recombinant and native AMPA receptors with respect to potency, efficacy, and mechanism. This, together with the complexity of AMPA receptors arising from heteromeric subunit composition and region-specific subunit expression in the brain, presents a challenge for the identification of compounds with the most optimal therapeutic profile. Nevertheless, a number of compounds have progressed to the clinic for cognitive disorders, and more specifically, for schizophrenia. Although preliminary data have proved somewhat equivocal, the expectation is that compounds with an optimal balance between efficacy, safety, and pharmacokinetic properties will have the potential to provide a breakthrough in the treatment of schizophrenia.

## REFERENCES


1. Kew, J.N.C., Kemp, J.A. (2005). Ionotropic and metabotropic glutamate receptor structure and pharmacology. *Psychopharmacology*, *179*, 4–29.
2. Mayer, M.L., Armstrong, N. (2004). Structure and function of glutamate receptor ion channels. *Annual Review of Physiology*, *66*, 161–181.
3. Green, M.F. (1996). What are the functional consequences of neurocognitive deficits in schizophrenia? *The American Journal of Psychiatry*, *153*, 321–330.
4. Green, M.F., Nuechterlein, K.H., Gold, J.M., Barch, D.M., Cohen, J., Essock, S., Fenton, W.S., Frese, F., Goldberg, T.E., Heaton, R.K., Keefe, R.S.E., Kern, R.S., Kraemer, H., Stover, E., Weinberger, D.R., Zalcman, S., Marder, S.R. (2004). Approaching a consensus cognitive battery for clinical trials in schizophrenia: the NIMH-MATRICS conference to select cognitive domains and test criteria. *Biological Psychiatry*, *56*, 301–307.
5. Stern-Bach, Y., Russo, S., Neuman, M., Rosenmund, C. (1998). A point mutation in the glutamate binding site blocks desensitization of AMPA receptors. *Neuron*, *21*, 907–918.
6. Stern-Bach, Y., Bettler, B., Hartley, M., Sheppard, P.O., O'Hara, P.J., Heinemann, S.F. (1994). Agonist selectivity of glutamate receptors is specified by two domains structurally related to bacterial amino acid-binding proteins. *Neuron*, *13*, 1345–1357.
7. Mayer, M.L. (2006). Glutamate receptors at atomic resolution. *Nature*, *440*, 456–462.
8. Sobolevsky, A.I., Rosconi, M.P., Gouaux, E. (2009). X-ray structure, symmetry and mechanism of an AMPA-subtype glutamate receptor. *Nature*, *462*, 745–756.
9. Shepherd, J.D., Huganir, R.L. (2007). The cell biology of synaptic plasticity: AMPA receptor trafficking. *Annual Review of Cell and Developmental Biology*, *23*, 613–643.
10. Greger, I.H., Esteban, J.A. (2007). AMPA receptor biogenesis and trafficking. *Current Opinion in Neurobiology*, *17*, 289–297.
11. Mosbacher, J., Schoepfer, R., Monyer, H., Burnashev, N., Seeburg, P.H., Ruppersberg, J.P. (1994). A molecular determinant for submillisecond desensitization in glutamate receptors. *Science*, *266*, 1059–1062.
12. Partin, K.M., Patneau, D.K., Mayer, M.L. (1994). Cyclothiazide differentially modulates desensitization of alpha-amino-3-hydroxy-5-methyl-4-isoxazolepropionic acid receptor splice variants. *Molecular Pharmacology*, *46*, 129–138.

13. Burnashev, N., Zhou, Z., Neher, E., Sakmann, B. (1995). Fractional calcium currents through recombinant GluR channels of the NMDA, AMPA and kainate receptor subtypes. *The Journal of Physiology*, *485*(Pt 2), 403–418.
14. Burnashev, N., Monyer, H., Seeburg, P.H., Sakmann, B. (1992). Divalent ion permeability of AMPA receptor channels is dominated by the edited form of a single subunit. *Neuron*, *8*, 189–198.
15. Hume, R.I., Dingledine, R., Heinemann, S.F. (1991). Identification of a site in glutamate receptor subunits that controls calcium permeability. *Science*, *253*, 1028–1031.
16. Lomeli, H., Mosbacher, J., Melcher, T., Hoger, T., Geiger, J.R., Kuner, T., Monyer, H., Higuchi, M., Bach, A., Seeburg, P.H. (1994). Control of kinetic properties of AMPA receptor channels by nuclear RNA editing. *Science*, *266*, 1709–1713.
17. Boulter, J., Hollmann, M., O'Shea-Greenfield, A., Hartley, M., Deneris, E., Maron, C., Heinemann, S. (1990). Molecular cloning and functional expression of glutamate receptor subunit genes. *Science*, *249*, 1033–1037.
18. Keinanen, K., Wisden, W., Sommer, B., Werner, P., Herb, A., Verdoorn, T.A., Sakmann, B., Seeburg, P.H. (1990). A family of AMPA-selective glutamate receptors. *Science*, *249*, 556–560.
19. Sommer, B., Keinanen, K., Verdoorn, T.A., Wisden, W., Burnashev, N., Herb, A., Kohler, M., Takagi, T., Sakmann, B., Seeburg, P.H. (1990). Flip and flop: a cell-specific functional switch in glutamate-operated channels of the CNS. *Science*, *249*, 1580–1585.
20. Beneyto, M., Meador-Woodruff, J.H. (2004). Expression of transcripts encoding AMPA receptor subunits and associated postsynaptic proteins in the macaque brain. *The Journal of Comparative Neurology*, *468*, 530–554.
21. Petralia, R.S., Wenthold, R.J. (1992). Light and electron immunocytochemical localization of AMPA-selective glutamate receptors in the rat brain. *The Journal of Comparative Neurology*, *318*, 329–354.
22. Park, Y., Jang, C.G., Yang, K.H., Loh, H.H., Ma, T., Ho, I.K. (2003). Regional specific increases of [3H]AMPA binding and mRNA expression of AMPA receptors in the brain of [mu]-opioid receptor knockout mice. *Molecular Brain Research*, *113*, 116–123.
23. Rosa, M.L.N.M., GuimarπEs, F.S., Pearson, R.C.A., Del Bel, E.A. (2002). Effects of single or repeated restraint stress on GluR1 and GluR2 flip and flop mRNA expression in the hippocampal formation. *Brain Research Bulletin*, *59*, 117–124.
24. Gallo, V., Russell, J.T. (1995). Excitatory amino acid receptors in glia: different subtypes for distinct functions? *Journal of Neuroscience Research*, *42*, 1–8.
25. Garcia-Barcina, J.M., Matute, C. (1998). AMPA-selective glutamate receptor subunits in glial cells of the adult bovine white matter. *Brain Research. Molecular Brain Research*, *53*, 270–276.
26. Park, E., Liu, Y., Fehlings, M.G. (2003). Changes in glial cell white matter AMPA receptor expression after spinal cord injury and relationship to apoptotic cell death. *Experimental Neurology*, *182*, 35–48.
27. Yoshioka, A., Bacskai, B., Pleasure, D. (1996). Pathophysiology of oligodendroglial excitotoxicity. *Journal of Neuroscience Research*, *46*, 427–437.

28. Monyer, H., Seeburg, P.H., Wisden, W. (1991). Glutamate-operated channels: developmentally early and mature forms arise by alternative splicing. *Neuron*, *6*, 799–810.
29. Stine, C.D., Lu, W., Wolf, M.E. (2001). Expression of AMPA receptor flip and flop mRNAs in the nucleus accumbens and prefrontal cortex after neonatal ventral hippocampal lesions. *Neuropsychopharmacology*, *24*, 253–266.
30. Sun, Y., Olson, R., Horning, M., Armstrong, N., Mayer, M., Gouaux, E. (2002). Mechanism of glutamate receptor desensitization. *Nature*, *417*, 245–253.
31. Black, M.D. (2005). Therapeutic potential of positive AMPA modulators and their relationship to AMPA receptor subunits. A review of preclinical data. *Psychopharmacology*, *179*, 154–163.
32. Coyle, J.T., Tsai, G. (2004). NMDA receptor function, neuroplasticity, and the pathophysiology of schizophrenia. *International Review of Neurobiology*, *59*, 491–515.
33. Coyle, J.T., Tsai, G., Goff, D. (2003). Converging evidence of NMDA receptor hypofunction in the pathophysiology of schizophrenia. *Annals of the New York Academy of Sciences*, *1003*, 318–327.
34. Krystal, J.H., Karper, L.P., Seibyl, J.P., Freeman, G.K., Delaney, R., Bremner, J.D., Heninger, G.R., Bowers, M.B., Jr, Charney, D.S. (1994). Subanesthetic effects of the noncompetitive NMDA antagonist, ketamine, in humans. Psychotomimetic, perceptual, cognitive, and neuroendocrine responses. *Archives of General Psychiatry*, *51*, 199–214.
35. Millan, M.J. (2005). N-Methyl-d-aspartate receptors as a target for improved antipsychotic agents: novel insights and clinical perspectives. *Psychopharmacology*, *179*, 30–53.
36. Johnson, J.W., Ascher, P. (1987). Glycine potentiates the NMDA response in cultured mouse brain neurons. *Nature*, *325*, 529–531.
37. Mothet, J.P., Parent, A.T., Wolosker, H., Brady, R.O., Jr, Linden, D.J., Ferris, C.D., Rogawski, M.A., Snyder, S.H. (2000). D-serine is an endogenous ligand for the glycine site of the N-methyl-D-aspartate receptor. *Proceedings of the National Academy of Sciences of the United States of America*, *97*, 4926–4931.
38. Baumbarger, P.J., Muhlhauser, M., Zhai, J., Yang, C.R., Nisenbaum, E.S. (2001). Positive modulation of alpha-amino-3-hydroxy-5-methyl-4-isoxazole propionic acid (AMPA) receptors in prefrontal cortical pyramidal neurons by a novel allosteric potentiator. *The Journal of Pharmacology and Experimental Therapeutics*, *298*, 86–102.
39. Isaac, J.T., Crair, M.C., Nicoll, R.A., Malenka, R.C. (1997). Silent synapses during development of thalamocortical inputs. *Neuron*, *18*, 269–280.
40. Takumi, Y., Ramirez-Leon, V., Laake, P., Rinvik, E., Ottersen, O.P. (1999). Different modes of expression of AMPA and NMDA receptors in hippocampal synapses. *Nature Neuroscience*, *2*, 618–624.
41. Feldman, D.E., Knudsen, E.I. (1998). Experience-dependent plasticity and the maturation of glutamatergic synapses. *Neuron*, *20*, 1067–1071.
42. Esteban, J.A. (2003). AMPA receptor trafficking: a road map for synaptic plasticity. *Molecular Interventions*, *3*, 375–385.

43. Shi, S., Hayashi, Y., Esteban, J.A., Malinow, R. (2001). Subunit-specific rules governing AMPA receptor trafficking to synapses in hippocampal pyramidal neurons. *Cell*, *105*, 331–343.
44. Lisman, J., Raghavachari, S. (2006). A unified model of the presynaptic and postsynaptic changes during LTP at CA1 synapses. *Science's STKE*, *2006*, re11.
45. Bressan, R.A., Pilowsky, L.S. (2000). Imaging the glutamatergic system in vivo—relevance to schizophrenia. *European Journal of Nuclear Medicine*, *27*, 1723–1731.
46. Torrey, E.F., Webster, M., Knable, M., Johnston, N., Yolken, R.H. (2000). The Stanley Foundation Brain Collection and Neuropathology Consortium. *Schizophrenia Research*, *44*, 151–155.
47. Barton, A.J.L., Pearson, R.C.A., Najlerahim, A., Harrison, P.J. (1993). Pre-and postmortem influences on brain RNA. *Journal of Neurochemistry*, *61*, 1–11.
48. Harrison, P.J., Heath, P.R., Eastwood, S.L., Burnet, P.W.J., McDonald, B., Pearson, R.C.A. (1995). The relative importance of premortem acidosis and postmortem interval for human brain gene expression studies: selective mRNA vulnerability and comparison with their encoded proteins. *Neuroscience Letters*, *200*, 151–154.
49. Meador-Woodruff, J.H., Healy, D.J. (2000). Glutamate receptor expression in schizophrenic brain. *Brain Research Reviews*, *31*, 288–294.
50. Harrison, P.J., Law, A.J., Eastwood, S.L. (2003). Glutamate receptors and transporters in the hippocampus in schizophrenia. *Annals of the New York Academy of Sciences*, *1003*, 94–101.
51. Eastwood, S.L., McDonald, B., Burnet, P.W., Beckwith, J.P., Kerwin, R.W., Harrison, P.J. (1995). Decreased expression of mRNAs encoding non-NMDA glutamate receptors GluR1 and GluR2 in medial temporal lobe neurons in schizophrenia. *Brain Research. Molecular Brain Research*, *29*, 211–223.
52. Eastwood, S.L., Burnet, P.W., Harrison, P.J. (1997). GluR2 glutamate receptor subunit flip and flop isoforms are decreased in the hippocampal formation in schizophrenia: a reverse transcriptase-polymerase chain reaction (RT-PCR) study. *Brain Research. Molecular Brain Research*, *44*, 92–98.
53. Eastwood, S.L., Kerwin, R.W., Harrison, P.J. (1997). Immunoautoradiographic evidence for a loss of alpha-amino-3-hydroxy-5-methyl-4-isoxazole propionate-preferring non-N-methyl-D-aspartate glutamate receptors within the medial temporal lobe in schizophrenia. *Biological Psychiatry*, *41*, 636–643.
54. Kerwin, R., Patel, S., Meldrum, B. (1990). Quantitative autoradiographic analysis of glutamate binding sites in the hippocampal formation in normal and schizophrenic brain post mortem. *Neuroscience*, *39*, 25–32.
55. Gao, X.M., Sakai, K., Roberts, R.C., Conley, R.R., Dean, B., Tamminga, C.A. (2000). Ionotropic glutamate receptors and expression of N-Methyl-D-Aspartate receptor subunits in subregions of human hippocampus: effects of schizophrenia. *The American Journal of Psychiatry*, *157*, 1141–1149.
56. Breese, C.R., Freedman, R., Leonard, S.S. (1995). Glutamate receptor subtype expression in human postmortem brain tissue from schizophrenics and alcohol abusers. *Brain Research*, *674*, 82–90.
57. Beneyto, M., Kristiansen, L.V., Oni-Orisan, A., McCullumsmith, R.E., Meador-Woodruff, J.H. (2007). Abnormal glutamate receptor expression in the medial

temporal lobe in schizophrenia and mood disorders. *Neuropsychopharmacology*, *32*, 1888–1902.

58. O'Connor, J.A., Muly, E.C., Arnold, S.E., Hemby, S.E. (2007). AMPA receptor subunit and splice variant expression in the DLPFC of schizophrenic subjects and rhesus monkeys chronically administered antipsychotic drugs. *Schizophrenia Research*, *90*, 28–40.
59. Healy, D.J., Haroutunian, V., Powchik, P., Davidson, M., Davis, K.L., Watson, S.J., Meador-Woodruff, J.H. (1998). AMPA receptor binding and subunit mRNA expression in prefrontal cortex and striatum of elderly schizophrenics. *Neuropsychopharmacology*, *19*, 278–286.
60. Scarr, E., Beneyto, M., Meador-Woodruff, J.H., Dean, B. (2005). Cortical glutamatergic markers in schizophrenia. *Neuropsychopharmacology*, *30*, 1521–1531.
61. Dracheva, S., McGurk, S.R., Haroutunian, V. (2005). mRNA expression of AMPA receptors and AMPA receptor binding proteins in the cerebral cortex of elderly schizophrenics. *Journal of Neuroscience Research*, *79*, 868–878.
62. Vawter, M.P., Crook, J.M., Hyde, T.M., Kleinman, J.E., Weinberger, D.R., Becker, K.G., Freed, W.J. (2002). Microarray analysis of gene expression in the prefrontal cortex in schizophrenia: a preliminary study. *Schizophrenia Research*, *58*, 11–20.
63. Beneyto, M., Meador-Woodruff, J.H. (2006). Lamina-specific abnormalities of AMPA receptor trafficking and signaling molecule transcripts in the prefrontal cortex in schizophrenia. *Synapse*, *60*, 585–598.
64. O'Connor, J.A., Hemby, S.E. (2007). Elevated GRIA1 mRNA expression in Layer II/III and V pyramidal cells of the DLPFC in schizophrenia. *Schizophrenia Research*, *97*, 277–288.
65. Freed, W.J., Dillon-Carter, O., Kleinman, J.E. (1993). Properties of [3H]AMPA binding in postmortem human brain from psychotic subjects and controls: increases in caudate nucleus associated with suicide. *Experimental Neurology*, *121*, 48–56.
66. Noga, J.T., Wang, H. (2002). Further postmortem autoradiographic studies of AMPA receptor binding in schizophrenia. *Synapse*, *45*, 250–258.
67. Ibrahim, H.M., Hogg, A.J., Jr, Healy, D.J., Haroutunian, V., Davis, K.L., Meador-Woodruff, J.H. (2000). Ionotropic glutamate receptor binding and subunit mRNA expression in thalamic nuclei in schizophrenia. *The American Journal of Psychiatry*, *157*, 1811–1823.
68. Gardner, S.M., Takamiya, K., Xia, J., Suh, J.G., Johnson, R., Yu, S., Huganir, R.L. (2005). Calcium-permeable AMPA receptor plasticity is mediated by subunit-specific interactions with PICK1 and NSF. *Neuron*, *45*, 903–915.
69. Liu, S.J., Cull-Candy, S.G. (2005). Subunit interaction with PICK and GRIP controls Ca2+ permeability of AMPARs at cerebellar synapses. *Nature Neuroscience*, *8*, 768–775.
70. Lu, W., Ziff, E.B. (2005). PICK1 interacts with ABP/GRIP to regulate AMPA receptor trafficking. *Neuron*, *47*, 407–421.
71. Suzuki, E., Kessler, M., Arai, A.C. (2008). The fast kinetics of AMPA GluR3 receptors is selectively modulated by the TARPs gamma4 and gamma8. *Molecular and Cellular Neurosciences*, *38*, 117–123.

72. Ornstein, P.L., Zimmerman, D.M., Arnold, M.B., Bleisch, T.J., Cantrell, B., Simon, R., Zarrinmayeh, H., Baker, S.R., Gates, M., Tizzano, J.P., Bleakman, D., Mandelzys, A., Jarvie, K.R., Ho, K., Deverill, M., Kamboj, R.K. (2000). Biarylpropylsulfonamides as novel, potent potentiators of 2-amino-3- (5-methyl-3-hydroxyisoxazol-4-yl)-propanoic acid (AMPA) receptors. *Journal of Medicinal Chemistry*, *43*, 4354–4358.
73. Miu, P., Jarvie, K.R., Radhakrishnan, V., Gates, M.R., Ogden, A., Ornstein, P.L., Zarrinmayeh, H., Ho, K., Peters, D., Grabell, J., Gupta, A., Zimmerman, D.M., Bleakman, D. (2001). Novel AMPA receptor potentiators LY392098 and LY404187: effects on recombinant human AMPA receptors in vitro. *Neuropharmacology*, *40*, 976–983.
74. Quirk, J.C., Nisenbaum, E.S. (2002). LY404187: a novel positive allosteric modulator of AMPA receptors. *CNS Drug Reviews*, *8*, 255–282.
75. Vandergriff, J., Huff, K., Bond, A., Lodge, D. (2001). Potentiation of responses to AMPA on central neurones by LY392098 and LY404187 in vivo. *Neuropharmacology*, *40*, 1003–1009.
76. Jones, N., O'Neill, M.J., Tricklebank, M., Libri, V., Williams, S.C., Jones, N., O'Neill, M.J., Tricklebank, M., Libri, V., Williams, S.C.R. (2005). Examining the neural targets of the AMPA receptor potentiator LY404187 in the rat brain using pharmacological magnetic resonance imaging. *Psychopharmacology*, *180*, 743–751.
77. Legutko, B., Li, X., Skolnick, P. (2001). Regulation of BDNF expression in primary neuron culture by LY392098, a novel AMPA receptor potentiator. *Neuropharmacology*, *40*, 1019–1027.
78. O'Neill, M.J., Witkin, J.M. (2007). AMPA receptor potentiators: application for depression and Parkinson's disease. *Current Drug Targets*, *8*, 603–620.
79. Li, X., Tizzano, J.P., Griffey, K., Clay, M., Lindstrom, T., Skolnick, P. (2001). Antidepressant-like actions of an AMPA receptor potentiator (LY392098). *Neuropharmacology*, *40*, 1028–1033.
80. O'Neill, M.J., Murray, T.K., Whalley, K., Ward, M.A., Hicks, C.A., Woodhouse, S., Osborne, D.J., Skolnick, P. (2004). Neurotrophic actions of the novel AMPA receptor potentiator, LY404187, in rodent models of Parkinson's disease. *European Journal of Pharmacology*, *486*, 163–174.
81. Zarrinmayeh, H., Bleakman, D., Gates, M.R., Yu, H., Zimmerman, D.M., Ornstein, P.L., McKennon, T., Arnold, M.B., Wheeler, W.J., Skolnick, P. (2001). [3H]N-2-(4-(N-benzamido)phenyl)propyl-2-propanesulfonamide: a novel AMPA receptor potentiator and radioligand. *Journal of Medicinal Chemistry*, *44*, 302–304.
82. Arnold, M.B., Bleisch, T.J., Cuff, G.W., Ornstein, P.L., Zimmerman, D.M. (2001). Preparation of [[[(methylsulfonamido)ethyl]phenyl]phenyl]propyl sulfonamide derivatives with glutamate receptor function potentiating activity. Eli Lilly and Company, WO2001090057.
83. Knobelsdorf, J.A., Shepherd, T.A., Tromiczak, E.G., Zarrinmayeh, H., Zimmerman, D.M. (2001). Preparation of sulfonamide derivatives useful for potentiating glutamate receptor function in a mammal. Eli Lilly and Company, WO2001096289.
84. Shepherd, T.A., Aikins, J.A., Bleakman, D., Cantrell, B.E., Rearick, J.P., Simon, R.L., Smith, E.C., Stephenson, G.A., Zimmerman, D.M., Mandelzys, A., Jarvie, K.R., Ho, K., Deverill, M., Kamboj, R.K. (2002). Design and synthesis of a novel series of 1,2-disubstituted cyclopentanes as small, potent potentiators of 2-amino-

3-(3-hydroxy-5-methyl-isoxazol-4-yl)propanoic acid (AMPA) receptors. *Journal of Medicinal Chemistry*, *45*, 2101–2111.

85. Albaugh, P.A., Dominguez-Manzanares, E., Hong, J.E., Hornback, W.J., Jiang, D., Ornstein, P.L., Thompson, M.L., Tromiczak, E.G., Wu, Z., Zarrinmayeh, H., Zimmerman, D.M., Castano, M.A.M., Huffman, L.G., Miller, W.D. (2004). Preparation of pyrrole and pyrazole derivatives as potentiators of glutamate receptors. Eli Lilly and Company, WO2005040110.
86. Castano Mansanet, A.M., Dominguez-Manzanares, E., Escribano, A.M., Fernandez, M.C., Hornback, W.J., Jimenez-Aguado, A.M., Tromiczak, E.G., Wu, Z., Zarrinmayeh, H., Zimmerman, D.M. (2005). Preparation of thiophene and furan compounds for potentiating glutamate receptor function. Eli Lilly and Company, WO2005070916.
87. Zarrinmayeh, H., Tromiczak, E., Zimmerman, D.M., Rankl, N., Ho, K.H., Dominguez, E., Casta±O, A., Escribano, A., Fernandez, C., Jimenez, A., Hornback, W.J., Nisenbaum, E.S. (2006). A novel class of positive allosteric modulators of AMPA receptors: design, synthesis, and structure-activity relationships of 3-biphenyl-4-yl-4-cyano-5-ethyl-1-methyl-1H-pyrrole-2-carboxylic acid, LY2059346. *Bioorganic & Medicinal Chemistry Letters*, *16*, 5203–5206.
88. Thewlis, K.M., Ward, S.E. (2005). Preparation of N-pyrrolidinyl sulfonamides that potentiate glutamate receptor for use against schizophrenia. Glaxo Group Limited. WO2006015827.
89. Bradley, D.M., Thewlis, K.M., Ward, S.E. (2006). Preparation of N-indan-2-yl and related sulfonamides that potentiate glutamate receptor for use against schizophrenia. Glaxo Group Limited. WO2006015828.
90. Ward, S.E., Thewlis, K.M. (2005). Preparation of N-indan-2-yl and related sulfonamides that potentiate glutamate receptor for use against schizophrenia. Glaxo Group Limited. WO2006015829.
91. GSK (2008). GSK Pipeline update.
92. Andreotti, D., Ward, S.E. (2007). Preparation of N-[2-phenyltetrahydrofuran-3-yl]-2-propanesulfonamide derivatives as glutamate receptor modulators. Glaxo Group Limited. WO2007090841.
93. Andreotti, D., Arista, L., Cardullo, F., Spada, S., Thewlis, K.M., Ward, S.E. (2006). Preparation of N-arylcyclopropyl isopropylsulfonamides which potentiate glutamate receptor and uses thereof in medicine. Glaxo Group Limited. WO2006087169.
94. Thewlis, K.M., Ward, S.E. (2007). Preparation of 4-phenyl-3-(isopropylsulfonylamino) tetrahydrofuran derivatives as glutamate receptor modulators for treatment of schizophrenia. Glaxo Group Limited. WO2007090840.
95. Jhee, S.S., Chappell, A.S., Zarotsky, V., Moran, S.V., Rosenthal, M., Kim, E., Chalon, S., Toublanc, N., Brandt, J., Coutant, D.E., Ereshefsky, L. (2006). Multiple-dose plasma pharmacokinetic and safety study of LY450108 and LY451395 (AMPA receptor potentiators) and their concentration in cerebrospinal fluid in healthy human subjects. *Journal of Clinical Pharmacology*, *46*, 424–432.
96. Kaae, B.H., Harpsøe, K., Kastrup, J.S., Sanz, A.C., Pickering, D.S., Metzler, B., Clausen, R.P., Gajhede, M., Sauerberg, P., Liljefors, T., Madsen, U. (2007). Structural proof of a dimeric positive modulator bridging two identical AMPA receptor-binding sites. *Chemistry & Biology*, *14*, 1294–1303.

97. Bradley, D.M., Chan, W.N., Thewlis, K.M., Ward, S.E. (2007). Preparation of pyranopyrazoles and pyrazolopyridines as AMPA receptor potentiators. Glaxo Group Limited. WO2008053031.

98. Bradley, D.M., Chan, W.N., Harrison, S., Hughes, O., Miller, D.D., Neesom, J., Thewlis, K.M., Ward, S.E. (2007). (Arylimino)dihydrothiazoles as AMPA receptor modulators and their preparation, pharmaceutical compositions and use in the treatment of schizophrenia and cognition impairment. Glaxo Group Limited. WO2007122241.

99. Bradley, D.M., Chan, W.N., Harrison, S., Thatcher, R., Thewlis, K.M., Ward, S.E. (2007). Preparation 3-(trifluoromethyl)-4,5,6,7-tetrahydro-1H-indazole derivatives and their potential uses as glutamate receptor in particular AMPA receptor. Glaxo Group Limited. WO2007107539.

100. Gillen, K.J., Jamieson, C., Maclean, J.K.F., Moir, E.M., Rankovic, Z. (2008). Preparation of pyrazolealkanamide substituted thiophenes as AMPA potentiators. Organon, N. V. WO2008003452.

101. Ito, I., Tanabe, S., Kohda, A., Sugiyama, H. (1990). Allosteric potentiation of quisqualate receptors by a nootropic drug aniracetam. *The Journal of Physiology*, *424*, 533–543.

102. Arai, A.C., Xia, Y.F., Rogers, G., Lynch, G., Kessler, M. (2002). Benzamide-type AMPA receptor modulators form two subfamilies with distinct modes of action. *The Journal of Pharmacology and Experimental Therapeutics*, *303*, 1075–1085.

103. Arai, A.C., Kessler, M., Rogers, G., Lynch, G. (2000). Effects of the potent ampakine CX614 on hippocampal and recombinant AMPA receptors: interactions with cyclothiazide and GYKI 52466. *Molecular Pharmacology*, *58*, 802–813.

104. Arai, A., Kessler, M., Rogers, G., Lynch, G. (1996). Effects of a memory-enhancing drug on DL-alpha-amino-3-hydroxy-5-methyl-4-isoxazolepropionic acid receptor currents and synaptic transmission in hippocampus. *The Journal of Pharmacology and Experimental Therapeutics*, *278*, 627–638.

105. Arai, A.C., Xia, Y.-F., Suzuki, E. (2004). Modulation of AMPA receptor kinetics differentially influences synaptic plasticity in the hippocampus. *Neuroscience*, *123*, 1011–1024.

106. Lauterborn, J.C., Truong, G.S., Baudry, M., Bi, X., Lynch, G., Gall, C.M. (2003). Chronic elevation of brain-derived neurotrophic factor by ampakines. *The Journal of Pharmacology and Experimental Therapeutics*, *307*, 297–305.

107. Lauterborn, J.C., Lynch, G., Vanderklish, P., Arai, A., Gall, C.M. (2000). Positive modulation of AMPA receptors increases neurotrophin expression by hippocampal and cortical neurons. *The Journal of Neuroscience*, *20*, 8–21.

108. O'Neill, M.J., Messenger, M.J., Lakics, V., Murray, T.K., Karran, E.H., Szekeres, P.G., Nisenbaum, E.S., Merchant, K.M. (2007). Neuroreplacement, growth factor, and small molecule neurotrophic approaches for treating Parkinson's disease. *International Review of Neurobiology*, *77*, 179–217.

109. Pirotte, B., Podona, T., Diouf, O., de Tullio, P., Lebrun, P., Dupont, L., Somers, F., Delarge, J., Morain, P., Lestage, P., Lepagnol, J., Spedding, M. (1998). 4H-1,2,4-Pyridothiadiazine 1,1-dioxides and 2,3-dihydro-4H-1,2, 4-pyridothiadiazine 1,1-dioxides chemically related to diazoxide and cyclothiazide as powerful positive allosteric modulators of (R/S)-2-amino-3-(3-hydroxy-5-methylisoxazol-4-yl)

propionic acid receptors: design, synthesis, pharmacology, and structure-activity relationships. *Journal of Medicinal Chemistry*, *41*, 2946–2959.

110. Desos, P., Serkiz, B., Morain, P., Lepagnol, J., Cordi, A. (1996). Enantioselective synthesis of a pyrrolo-benzothiadiazine derivative S 18986, a new AMPA receptor positive modulator. *Bioorganic & Medicinal Chemistry Letters*, *6*, 3003–3008.
111. Bourasset, F., Bernard, K., Munoz, C., Genissel, P., Scherrmann, J.M. (2005). Neuropharmacokinetics of a new α-amino-3-hydroxy-5-methyl-4-isoxazole propionic acid (AMPA) modulator, S18986 [(S)-2,3-dihydro-[3,4]cyclopentano-1,2,4-benzothiadiazine-1,1-dioxide], in the rat. *Drug Metabolism and Disposition*, *33*, 1137–1143.
112. Bloss, E.B., Hunter, R.G., Waters, E.M., Munoz, C., Bernard, K., McEwen, B.S. (2008). Behavioral and biological effects of chronic S18986, a positive AMPA receptor modulator, during aging. *Experimental Neurology*, *210*, 109–117.
113. Lockhart, B.P., Rodriguez, M., Mourlevat, S., Peron, P., Catesson, S., Villain, N., Galizzi, J.P., Boutin, J.A., Lestage, P. (2007). S18986: a positive modulator of AMPA-receptors enhances (S)-AMPA-mediated BDNF mRNA and protein expression in rat primary cortical neuronal cultures. *European Journal of Pharmacology*, *561*, 23–31.
114. Desos, P., Cordi, A., Lestage, P. (2004). Derivatives of benzothiazine and benzothiadiazine, process for their preparation, and pharmaceutical compositions containing them as AMPA receptor modulators. Les Laboratoires Servier, EP1486503.
115. Gouliaev, A.H., Larsen, M., Varming, T., Mathiesen, C., Johansen, T.H., Scheel-Kruger, J., Olsen, G.M., Nielsen, E.O. (1999). Preparation of benzothiadiazines, quinazolines, and other aryl-fused heterocycles as positive AMPA-receptor modulators for treatment of memory and learning disorders. Neurosearch, WO9942456.
116. Konkoy, C.S., Fick, D.B., Cai, S.X., Lan, N.C., Keana, J.F.W. (2000). Substituted 5-oxo-5,6,7,8-tetrahydro-4H-1-benzopyrans and benzothiopyrans and their use as potentiators of AMPA. Cocensys, Inc. WO2000075123.
117. Winter, K., Weiser, T., Blech, S.M., Ceci, A. (2001). Preparation of azaacenaphthylene dioxides and related compounds as positive allosteric AMPA receptor modulators (PAARM). Boehringer Ingelheim, Pharma K. G. WO2001057045.
118. Nakagawa, T., Cheng, Y., Ramm, E., Sheng, M., Walz, T. (2005). Structure and different conformational states of native AMPA receptor complexes. *Nature*, *433*, 545–549.
119. Tichelaar, W., Safferling, M., KeinΣNen, K., Stark, H., Madden, D.R. (2004). The three-dimensional structure of an ionotropic glutamate receptor reveals a dimer-of-dimers assembly. *Journal of Molecular Biology*, *344*, 435–442.
120. Kuusinen, A., Arvola, M., Keinänen, K. (1995). Molecular dissection of the agonist binding site of an AMPA receptor. *The EMBO Journal*, *14*, 6327–6332.
121. Chen, G.Q., Sun, Y., Jin, R., Gouaux, E. (1998). Probing the ligand binding domain of the GluR2 receptor by proteolysis and deletion mutagenesis defines domain boundaries and yields a crystallizable construct. *Protein Science*, *7*, 2623–2630.
122. Armstrong, N., Sun, Y., Chen, G.Q., Gouaux, E. (1998). Structure of a glutamate-receptor ligand-binding core in complex with kainate. *Nature*, *395*, 913–917.
123. Jin, R., Banke, T.G., Mayer, M.L., Traynelis, S.F., Gouaux, E. (2003). Structural basis for partial agonist action at ionotropic glutamate receptors. *Nature Neuroscience*, *6*, 803–810.

124. Jin, R., Clark, S., Weeks, A.M., Dudman, J.T., Gouaux, E., Partin, K.M. (2005). Mechanism of positive allosteric modulators acting on AMPA receptors. *The Journal of Neuroscience*, *25*, 9027–9036.

125. Harpsoe, K., Liljefors, T., Balle, T. (2008). Prediction of the binding mode of biarylpropylsulfonamide allosteric AMPA receptor modulators based on docking, GRID molecular interaction fields and 3D-QSAR analysis. *Journal of Molecular Graphics & Modelling*, *26*, 874–883.

126. Morrow, J.A., Maclean, J.K., Jamieson, C. (2006). Recent advances in positive allosteric modulators of the AMPA receptor. *Current Opinion in Drug Discovery & Development*, *9*, 571–579.

127. Armstrong, N., Jasti, J., Beich-Frandsen, M., Gouaux, E. (2006). Measurement of conformational changes accompanying desensitization in an ionotropic glutamate receptor. *Cell*, *127*, 85–97.

128. Larson, J., Quach, C.N., LeDuc, B.Q., Nguyen, A., Rogers, G.A., Lynch, G. (1996). Effects of an AMPA receptor modulator on methamphetamine-induced hyperactivity in rats. *Brain Research*, *738*, 353–356.

129. Palmer, L.C., Hess, U.S., Larson, J., Rogers, G.A., Gall, C.M., Lynch, G. (1997). Comparison of the effects of an ampakine with those of methamphetamine on aggregate neuronal activity in cortex versus striatum. *Brain Research. Molecular Brain Research*, *46*, 127–135.

130. Vanover, K.E. (1997). Effects of AMPA receptor positive modulators on amphetamine- and dizocilpine-induced locomotion. *European Journal of Pharmacology*, *332*, 115–119.

131. Johnson, S.A., Luu, N.T., Herbst, T.A., Knapp, R., Lutz, D., Arai, A., Rogers, G.A., Lynch, G. (1999). Synergistic interactions between ampakines and antipsychotic drugs. *The Journal of Pharmacology and Experimental Therapeutics*, *289*, 392–397.

132. Hess, U.S., Whalen, S.P., Sandoval, L.M., Lynch, G., Gall, C.M. (2003). Ampakines reduce methamphetamine-driven rotation and activate neocortex in a regionally selective fashion. *Neuroscience*, *121*, 509–521.

133. Gainetdinov, R.R., Mohn, A.R., Bohn, L.M., Caron, M.G. (2001). Glutamatergic modulation of hyperactivity in mice lacking the dopamine transporter. *Proceedings of the National Academy of Sciences of the United States of America*, *98*, 11047–11054.

134. Olsen, C.K., Kreilgaard, M., Didriksen, M. (2006). Positive modulation of glutamatergic receptors potentiates the suppressive effects of antipsychotics on conditioned avoidance responding in rats. *Pharmacology, Biochemistry, and Behavior*, *84*, 259–265.

135. Geyer, M.A., Ellenbroek, B. (2003). Animal behavior models of the mechanisms underlying antipsychotic atypicality. *Progress in Neuro-Psychopharmacology & Biological Psychiatry*, *27*, 1071–1079.

136. Swerdlow, N.R., Light, G.A., Cadenhead, K.S., Sprock, J., Hsieh, M.H., Braff, D.L. (2006). Startle gating deficits in a large cohort of patients with schizophrenia: relationship to medications, symptoms, neurocognition, and level of function. *Archives of General Psychiatry*, *63*, 1325–1335.

137. Gray, N.S., Pilowsky, L.S., Gray, J.A., Kerwin, R.W. (1995). Latent inhibition in drug naive schizophrenics: relationship to duration of illness and dopamine D2 binding using SPET. *Schizophrenia Research*, *17*, 95–107.

138. Lipina, T., Weiss, K., Roder, J. (2006). The ampakine CX546 restores the prepulse inhibition and latent inhibition deficits in mGluR5-deficient mice. *Neuropsychopharmacology*, *32*, 745–756.

139. Brody, S.A., Conquet, F., Geyer, M.A. (2004). Effect of antipsychotic treatment on the prepulse inhibition deficit of mGluR5 knockout mice. *Psychopharmacology (Berl)*, *172*, 187–195.

140. Gray, L., Van Den, Buuse, M., Scarr, E., Dean, B., Hannan, A.J. (2009). Clozapine reverses schizophrenia-related behaviours in the metabotropic glutamate receptor 5 knockout mouse: association with N-methyl-d-aspartic acid receptor up-regulation. *The International Journal of Neuropsychopharmacology*, *12*, 45–60.

141. Arai, A.C., Kessler, M. (2007). Pharmacology of ampakine modulators: from AMPA receptors to synapses and behavior. *Current Drug Targets*, *8*, 583–602.

142. Goff, D.C., Lamberti, J.S., Leon, A.C., Green, M.F., Miller, A.L., Patel, J., Manschreck, T., Freudenreich, O., Johnson, S.A. (2007). A placebo-controlled add-on trial of the ampakine, CX516, for cognitive deficits in schizophrenia. *Neuroreport*, *33*, 465–472.

143. Buchanan, R.W., Freedman, R., Javitt, D.C., Abi-Dargham, A., Lieberman, J.A. (2007). Recent advances in the development of novel pharmacological agents for the treatment of cognitive impairments in schizophrenia. *Schizophrenia Bulletin*, *33*, 1120–1130.

144. Lynch, G. (2004). AMPA receptor modulators as cognitive enhancers. *Current Opinion in Pharmacology*, *4*, 4–11.

145. Lynch, G. (2006). Glutamate-based therapeutic approaches: ampakines. *Current Opinion in Pharmacology*, *6*, 82–88.

146. O'Neill, M.J., Bleakman, D., Zimmerman, D.M., Nisenbaum, E.S. (2004). AMPA receptor potentiators for the treatment of CNS disorders. *Current Drug Targets. CNS and Neurological Disorders*, *3*, 181–194.

147. O'Neill, M.J., Dix, S. (2007). AMPA receptor potentiators as cognitive enhancers. *IDrugs*, *10*, 185–192.

148. Copani, A., Genazzani, A., Aleppo, G., Casabona, G., Canonico, L., Scapagnini, U., Nicoletti, F. (1992). Nootropic drugs positively modulate Alpha-Amino-3-Hydroxy-5-Methyl-4-Isoxazolepropionic acid-sensitive glutamate receptors in neuronal cultures. *Journal of Neurochemistry*, *58*, 1199–1204.

149. Pontecorvo, M.J., Evans, H.L. (1985). Effects of aniracetam on delayed matching-to-sample performance of monkeys and pigeons. *Pharmacology, Biochemistry, and Behavior*, *22*, 745–752.

150. Rao, Y., Xiao, P., Xu, S.T. (2001). Effects of intrahippocampal aniracetam treatment on Y-maze avoidance learning performance and behavioral long-term potentiation in dentate gyrus in rat. *Neuroscience Letters*, *298*, 183–186.

151. Martin, J.R., Cumin, R., Aschwanden, W., Moreau, J.L., Jenck, F., Haefely, W.E. (1992). Aniracetam improves radial maze performance in rats. *Neuroreport*, *3*, 81–83.

152. Thompson, D.M., Guidotti, A., DiBella, M., Costa, E. (1995). 7-Chloro-3-methyl-3,4-dihydro-2H-1,2,4-benzothiadiazine S,S-dioxide (IDRA 21), a congener of aniracetam, potently abates pharmacologically induced cognitive impairments in patas monkeys. *Proceedings of the National Academy of Sciences of the United States of America*, *92*, 7667–7671.

153. Zivkovic, I., Thompson, D.M., Bertolino, M., Uzunov, D., DiBella, M., Costa, E., Guidotti, A. (1995). 7-Chloro-3-methyl-3-4-dihydro-2H-1,2,4 benzothiadiazine S,S-dioxide (IDRA 21): a benzothiadiazine derivative that enhances cognition by attenuating DL-alpha-amino-2,3-dihydro-5-methyl-3-oxo-4- isoxazolepropanoic acid (AMPA) receptor desensitization. *The Journal of Pharmacology and Experimental Therapeutics*, *272*, 300–309.

154. Nakamura, K., Kurasawa, M., Tanaka, Y. (1998). Scopolamine model of delirium in rats and reversal of the performance impairment by aniracetam. *Drug Development Research*, *43*, 85–97.

155. Bartolini, L., Risaliti, R., Pepeu, G. (1992). Effect of scopolamine and nootropic drugs on rewarded alternation in a T-maze. *Pharmacology, Biochemistry, and Behavior*, *43*, 1161–1164.

156. Nakamura, K., Kurasawa, M., Tanaka, Y. (1998). Apomorphine-induced hypoattention in rats and reversal of the choice performance impairment by aniracetam. *European Journal of Pharmacology*, *342*, 127–138.

157. Ohno, M., Yamamoto, T., Kitajima, I., Ueki, S. (1990). WEB 1881 FU ameliorates impairment of working memory induced by scopolamine and cerebral ischemia in the three-panel runway task. *Japanese Journal of Pharmacology*, *54*, 53–60.

158. Zajaczkowski, W., Danysz, W. (1997). Effects of D-cycloserine and aniracetam on spatial learning in rats with entorhinal cortex lesions. *Pharmacology, Biochemistry, and Behavior*, *56*, 21–29.

159. Granger, R., Staubli, U., Davis, M., Perez, Y., Nilsson, L., Rogers, G.A., Lynch, G. (1993). A drug that facilitates glutamatergic transmission reduces exploratory activity and improves performance in a learning-dependent task. *Synapse (New York, N.Y.)*, *15*, 326–329.

160. Granger, R., Deadwyler, S.A., Davis, M., Moskovitz, B., Kessler, M., Rogers, G., Lynch, G. (1996). Facilitation of glutamate receptors reverses an age-associated memory impairment in rats. *Synapse*, *22*, 332–337.

161. Davis, C.M., Moskovitz, B., Nguyen, M.A., Tran, B.B., Arai, A., Lynch, G., Granger, R. (1997). A profile of the behavioral changes produced by facilitation of AMPA-type glutamate receptors. *Psychopharmacology (Berl)*, *133*, 161–167.

162. Staubli, U., Perez, Y., Xu, F., Rogers, G., Ingvar, M., Stone-Elander, S., Lynch, G. (1994). Centrally active modulators of glutamate receptors facilitate the induction of long-term potentiation in vivo. *Proceedings of the National Academy of Sciences of the United States of America*, *91*, 11158–11162.

163. Staubli, U., Rogers, G., Lynch, G. (1994). Facilitation of glutamate receptors enhances memory. *Proceedings of the National Academy of Sciences of the United States of America*, *91*, 777–781.

164. Winters, B.D., Bussey, T.J. (2005). Glutamate receptors in perirhinal cortex mediate encoding, retrieval, and consolidation of object recognition memory. *The Journal of Neuroscience*, *25*, 4243–4251.

165. Lebrun, C., Pilliere, E., Lestage, P. (2000). Effects of S 18986-1, a novel cognitive enhancer, on memory performances in an object recognition task in rats. *European Journal of Pharmacology*, *401*, 205–212.

166. Bertaina-Anglade, V., Drieu La Rochelle, C., Munoz, C., Morain, P., Bernard, K. (2007). Comparison of single vs. multiple administrations of the AMPA receptors modulator S 18986 in the object recognition task in rats. *Fundamental & Clinical Pharmacology*, *21*, 349–354.

167. Hampson, R.E., Rogers, G., Lynch, G., Deadwyler, S.A. (1998). Facilitative effects of the ampakine CX516 on short-term memory in rats: enhancement of delayed-nonmatch-to-sample performance. *The Journal of Neuroscience*, *18*, 2740–2747.

168. Hampson, R.E., Rogers, G., Lynch, G., Deadwyler, S.A. (1998). Facilitative effects of the ampakine CX516 on short-term memory in rats: correlations with hippocampal neuronal activity. *The Journal of Neuroscience*, *18*, 2748–2763.

169. Buccafusco, J.J., Weiser, T., Winter, K., Klinder, K., Terry, A.V. (2004). The effects of IDRA 21, a positive modulator of the AMPA receptor, on delayed matching performance by young and aged rhesus monkeys. *Neuropharmacology*, *46*, 10–22.

170. Porrino, L.J., Daunais, J.B., Rogers, G.A., Hampson, R.E., Deadwyler, S.A. (2005). Facilitation of task performance and removal of the effects of sleep deprivation by an ampakine (CX717) in nonhuman primates. *PLoS Biology*, *3*, e299.

171. Hagan, J.J., Jones, D.N.C. (2005). Predicting drug efficacy for cognitive deficits in schizophrenia. *Schizophrenia Bulletin*, *31*, 830–853.

172. Abdul-Monim, Z., Reynolds, G.P., Neill, J.C. (2006). The effect of atypical and classical antipsychotics on sub-chronic PCP-induced cognitive deficits in a reversal-learning paradigm. *Behavioural Brain Research*, *169*, 263–273.

173. McLean, S.L., Beck, J.P., Woolley, M.L., Neill, J.C. (2008). A preliminary investigation into the effects of antipsychotics on sub-chronic phencyclidine-induced deficits in attentional set-shifting in female rats. *Behavioural Brain Research*, *189*, 152–158.

174. Grayson, B., Idris, N.F., Neill, J.C. (2007). Atypical antipsychotics attenuate a sub-chronic PCP-induced cognitive deficit in the novel object recognition task in the rat. *Behavioural Brain Research*, *184*, 31–38.

175. Damgaard, T., Larsen, D.B., Hansen, S.L., Grayson, B., Neill, J.C., Plath, N. Positive modulation of alpha-amino-3-hydroxy-5-methyl-4-isoxazolepropionic acid (AMPA) receptors reverses sub-chronic PCP-induced deficits in the novel object recognition task in rats. (2010) *Behavioural Brain Research*, *207*, 144–150.

176. Jones, N., Messenger, M.J., O'Neill, M.J., Oldershaw, A., Gilmour, G., Simmons, R.M.A., Iyengar, S., Libri, V., Tricklebank, M., Williams, S.C.R. (2007). AMPA receptor potentiation can prevent ethanol-induced intoxication. *Neuropsychopharmacology*, *33*, 1713–1723.

177. Ren, J., Poon, B.Y., Tang, Y., Funk, G.D., Greer, J.J. (2006). Ampakines alleviate respiratory depression in rats. *American Journal of Respiratory and Critical Care Medicine*, *174*, 1384–1391.

178. Marenco, S., Weinberger, D.R. (2006). Therapeutic potential of positive AMPA receptor modulators in the treatment of neuropsychiatric disorders. *CNS Drugs*, *20*, 173–185.

179. Zarate, J., Manji, H.K. (2008). The role of AMPA receptor modulation in the treatment of neuropsychiatric diseases. *Experimental Neurology*, *211*, 7–10.

180. Lynch, G., Granger, R., Ambros-Ingerson, J., Davis, C.M., Kessler, M., Schehr, R. (1997). Evidence that a positive modulator of AMPA-type glutamate receptors improves delayed recall in aged humans. *Experimental Neurology*, *145*, 89–92.

181. Lynch, G., Kessler, M., Rogers, G., Ambros-Ingerson, J., Granger, R., Schehr, R.S. (1996). Psychological effects of a drug that facilitates brain AMPA receptors. *International Clinical Psychopharmacology*, *11*, 13–19.

182. Ingvar, M., Ambros-Ingerson, J., Davis, M., Granger, R., Kessler, M., Rogers, G.A., Schehr, R.S., Lynch, G. (1997). Enhancement by an ampakine of memory encoding in humans. *Experimental Neurology*, *146*, 553–559.

183. Marenco, S., Egan, M.F., Goldberg, T.E., Knable, M.B., McClure, R.K., Winterer, G., Weinberger, D.R. (2002). Preliminary experience with an ampakine (CX516) as a single agent for the treatment of schizophrenia: a case series. *Schizophrenia Research*, *57*, 221–226.

184. Goff, D.C., Leahy, L., Berman, I., Posever, T., Herz, L., Leon, A.C., Johnson, S.A., Lynch, G. (2001). A placebo-controlled pilot study of the ampakine CX516 added to clozapine in schizophrenia. *Journal of Clinical Psychopharmacology*, *21*, 484–487.

185. Goff, D.C., Lamberti, J.S., Leon, A.C., Green, M.F., Miller, A.L., Patel, J., Manschreck, T., Freudenreich, O., Johnson, S.A. (2008). A placebo-controlled add-on trial of the ampakine, CX516, for cognitive deficits in schizophrenia. *Neuropsychopharmacology*, *33*, 465–472.

186. Wezenberg, E., Verkes, R.J., Ruigt, G.S., Hulstijn, W., Sabbe, B.G. (2007). Acute effects of the ampakine farampator on memory and information processing in healthy elderly volunteers. *Neuropsychopharmacology*, *32*, 1272–1283.

187. Wesensten, N.J., Reichardt, R.M., Balkin, T.J. (2007). Ampakine (CX717) effects on performance and alertness during simulated night shift work. *Aviation, Space, and Environmental Medicine*, *78*, 937–943.

188. Chappell, A.S., Gonzales, C., Williams, J., Witte, M.M., Mohs, R.C., Sperling, R., Chappell, A.S., Gonzales, C., Williams, J., Witte, M.M., Mohs, R.C., Sperling, R. (2007). AMPA potentiator treatment of cognitive deficits in Alzheimer disease. *Neurology*, *68*, 1008–1012.

189. Arundine, M., Tymianski, M. (2004). Molecular mechanisms of glutamate-dependent neurodegeneration in ischemia and traumatic brain injury. *Cellular and Molecular Life Sciences*, *61*, 657–668.

190. Doble, A. (1999). The role of excitotoxicity in neurodegenerative disease: implications for therapy. *Pharmacology & Therapeutics*, *81*, 163–221.

191. Dicou, E., Rangon, C.M., Guimiot, F., Spedding, M., Gressens, P. (2003). Positive allosteric modulators of AMPA receptors are neuroprotective against lesions induced by an NMDA agonist in neonatal mouse brain. *Brain Research*, *970*, 221–225.

192. Murray, T.K., Whalley, K., Robinson, C.S., Ward, M.A., Hicks, C.A., Lodge, D., Vandergriff, J.L., Baumbarger, P., Siuda, E., Gates, M., et al. (2003). LY503430, a novel alpha-amino-3-hydroxy-5-methylisoxazole-4-propionic acid receptor potentiator with functional, neuroprotective and neurotrophic effects in rodent models of Parkinson's disease. *The Journal of Pharmacology and Experimental Therapeutics*, *306*, 752–762.

193. Siegel, G.J., Chauhan, N.B. (2000). Neurotrophic factors in Alzheimer's and Parkinson's disease brain. *Brain Research Reviews*, *33*, 199–227.

194. Emsley, P., Cowtan, K. (2008). Coot: model-building tools for molecular graphics. *Acta Crystallographica. Section D, Biological Crystallography*, *60*, 2126–2132.

195. DeLano, W.L. (2008). The PyMOL molecular graphics system.

# 8

# PROGRESS IN THE EXPLORATION AND DEVELOPMENT OF GlyT1 INHIBITORS FOR SCHIZOPHRENIA

JEFFREY S. ALBERT AND MICHAEL W. WOOD

## 8.1 BACKGROUND

This review includes a brief historical perspective and discusses recent developments in the exploration of glycine transporter 1 (GlyT1) inhibitors primarily for treatment of schizophrenia. Schizophrenia affects about 1% of the world's population and is thus more prevalent than Alzheimer's disease or diabetes. Adequate treatments are available to treat the positive symptoms of schizophrenia in many patients. However, those treatments have reportedly tended to produce side effects, and it has been reported that they do not treat the negative symptoms or cognitive deficits of the disorder [1]. Currently, several molecular targets are being explored that aim to address these shortcomings. Preclinical evidence continues to accumulate in support of the glutamatergic hypothesis for schizophrenia. According to this model, the disease is associated with deficits in N-methyl-D-aspartate receptor (NMDAR) neurotransmission. Early pharmacological approaches that sought to restore NMDAR function by direct NMDAR antagonism reportedly failed because they were all neurotoxic. As a result, attention shifted to indirect methods to stimulate NMDAr neurotransmission. Among these various approaches, GlyT1 inhibitors are known to robustly increase NMDAR function in electrophysiological studies and therefore have promise for disease treatment. Early

*Targets and Emerging Therapies for Schizophrenia*, First Edition.
Edited by Jeffrey S. Albert and Michael W. Wood.

classes of GlyT1 inhibitors were associated with severe neurological side effects in rodents, and thus this approach also seemed at risk. However, continued commitment to this target led to the identification of new compound classes with reduced side effect liabilities [2], and several compounds have advanced to Phase II clinical studies and beyond. Several reviews discuss the exploration and evaluation of GlyT1 inhibitors [3–8]. This chapter will focus on recent developments and on pharmacological characterization of different compound classes.

## 8.2 THE NMDAR HYPOFUNCTION MODEL

Although the etiology of schizophrenia remains poorly understood, a longstanding hypothesis is that excessive dopaminergic neurotransmission plays a key role in the origin of positive symptoms. Indeed, there is no evidence that existing neuroleptics do not act, at least in part, as $D_2$ receptor antagonists. Moreover, the therapeutic efficacy of these agents can generally be correlated with their $D_2$ receptor affinity [9]. However, hyperactive subcortical dopaminergic neurotransmission cannot fully explain the range of symptoms of the disease, nor do $D_2$ antagonists treat the disease completely. More recently, an alternative hypothesis has emerged implicating disrupted glutamatergic neurotransmission. NMDAR hypofunction in certain brain regions is believed to underlie the basic mechanistic deficit responsible for the disease symptoms. In particular, it has been argued that a loss of NMDA receptor function on γ-aminobutyric acid (GABA)ergic interneurons in the cortex leads to dysregulated and excessive glutamatergic activation of pyramidal neurons. In line with this hypothesis, excessive activation leads to increased cortico-cortical activation that may drive negative and cognitive symptoms, and increased outflow to subcortical structures that may drive the positive symptom domains of schizophrenia [10]. The NMDAR hypofunction model is supported, in part, by the observation that NMDA receptor blockers, such as phencyclidine and ketamine, produce symptoms analogous to schizophrenia in humans [11]. Furthermore, NMDAR hypofunction is now a standard preclinical model of the disease. Therapeutic strategies to enhance NMDAR neurotransmission directly are likely to fail because direct, robust activation is reported to induce neurodegeneration. Consequently, alternative therapeutic approaches to stimulating NMDAR activity have been investigated. Among the possibilities, inhibition of GlyT1 appears to be promising.

### 8.2.1 The Regulation of Neuronal Glycine

NMDAR activation requires the binding of both glutamate and glycine as requsite agonists [12]. Although other subunits influence the affinity of the complex for glycine, glycine binding requires extensive interaction with the NR1 subunit of the heteromeric complex [13]. In the glutamatergic synapse

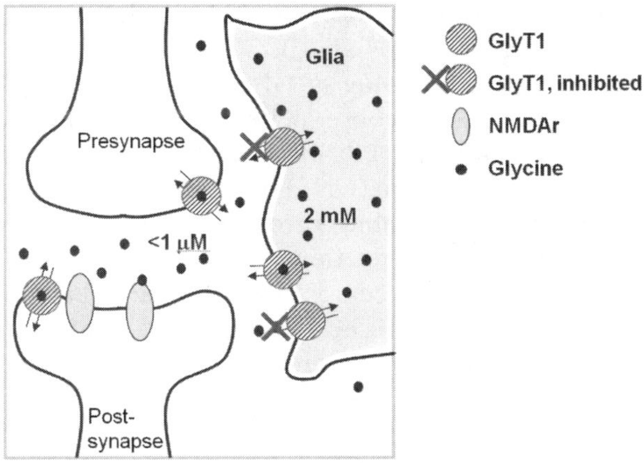


**FIGURE 8.1** Illustration of the role of GlyT1 and effect on NMDAR neurotransmission. GlyT1 acts to maintain a low concentration of glycine (<1 μM) at the synapse. Inhibition of GlyT1 leads to increased synaptic glycine and, thus, increased interaction of that synaptic glycine with NMDAR.

the glutamate concentration is tightly controlled by its vesicular release and uptake at the presynaptic terminal. In contrast, glycine appears to be regulated by other mechanisms based on the lack of evidence of vesicular packaging of glycine in cortical neurons. The source of glycine appears to be from interstitial fluid (glycine concentration ~10 μM), or the surrounding glial cells (glycine concentration ~2 mM). Within the cortex, the concentration of glycine is regulated by GlyT1 [14], which acts to transport glycine in and out of the synaptic region. In this manner, cortical glycine levels may be regulated more similarly to a classical hormone, rather than as a classical neurotransmitter. The synaptic concentration of glycine is typically maintained at less than 1 μM (Fig. 8.1). At this concentration, the NMDAR glycine site is believed to be subsaturated since the affinity for glycine is in the range of 0.1–5 μM, depending on the makeup of the NR2 subunit [14–17]. Inhibiting the uptake of glycine out of the synapse through GlyT1 blockade results in the accumulation of synaptic glycine and concomitant increase in NMDAR neurotransmission.

## 8.3 EXPRESSION AND GENETICS

### 8.3.1 Localization and Homology

GlyT1 is a $Na^+/Cl^-$ dependent glycine transporter and is related to the family of monoamine and amino acid transporters including GlyT2, DAT, SERT, and NET. At least six human GlyT1 isoforms have been reported. Among the most prominent, GlyT1a is present in both periphery and brain, while GlyT1b and

GlyT1c are brain-restricted. However, no pharmacological differences have been detected among the isoforms and no isoform-selective inhibitors have been reported. The closest homolog is GlyT2; however, GlyT1 and GlyT2 share only 50% homology. As a consequence, essentially all reported inhibitors are very selective for either GlyT1 or GlyT2. GlyT1 is predominantly found in the central nervous system (CNS) on glial cells and is highly expressed in regions where inhibitory signaling through glycine receptors exists (e.g., spinal cord and brainstem). However, there is evidence that GlyT1 is expressed in cortical pyramidal neurons where it is closely colocalized with NMDAR [4, 18, 19]. The predominance of published data suggests that glycinergic neurotransmission does not occur in the forebrain [20–23]. The combination of observations of GlyT1 (and GlyR) localization by autoradiography and immunohistochemistry at the tissue and cellular levels suggest that GlyT1 may play different roles in different brain regions. In caudal regions, where GlyT1 expression appears to be restricted to glia and is colocalized with GlyT2, GlyT1 may act to clear extrasynaptic glycine from glycinergic terminals. In rostral regions, where GlyT1 is expressed in glia and neurons and is colocalized with NMDAR, it may act as the primary clearance mechanism for synaptic glycine from glutamatergic terminals. Given its broad distribution, there may even be a gradient of relative function from caudal to rostral regions (see Table 8.1). The functional implications of these observations will be considered later. GlyT1 localization has been examined several times in rodents with different radioligands including [$^3$H]-NFPS [24] (**1**), [$^{35}$S]-ACPBB [25] (**2**), [$^3$H]-SB73399 [26] (**3**), and [$^3$H]-GSK931145 [26] (**4**), and results typically show wide distribution throughout the brain, with relative levels as follows: brainstem > cerebellum > thalamus > cortex. Although the presumed site of action for GlyT1 inhibitors in the treatment of schizophrenia is the cortex, there is also high expression in the spinal cord. The GlyT1 inhibitors Org25935 [27] (**5**) and ALX-5407 [28] (**1**) have been reported to have potent antinociceptive effects in rodent models. This is consistent with expression of GlyT1 in the spinal cord (although GlyT2 inhibitors are also reportedly active in these models [27, 28]).

### 8.3.2 GlyT1 Knockouts and Knockdowns

Mice having complete GlyT1 knockouts appear normal at birth; however, they show severely depressed motor skills, have breathing deficits, and die during the first postnatal day [29]. Heterozygous GlyT1 knockdown animals have 50% reduction of glycine uptake activity in membrane preparations but are otherwise fully viable. These animals have increased NMDAR activity and higher sensitivity to blockers of the NMDAR channel pore (e.g., MK-801), and show improvement in cognitive and psychosis tests [30–33]. These observations are all consistent with a model where the reduced GlyT1 activity leads to higher synaptic glycine levels and concomitant NMDAR potentiation.

**TABLE 8.1 Comparison of Roles of GlyT1 in Extremes of Rostral and Caudal Brain Regions and the Ligands Used in Labeling GlyT1**

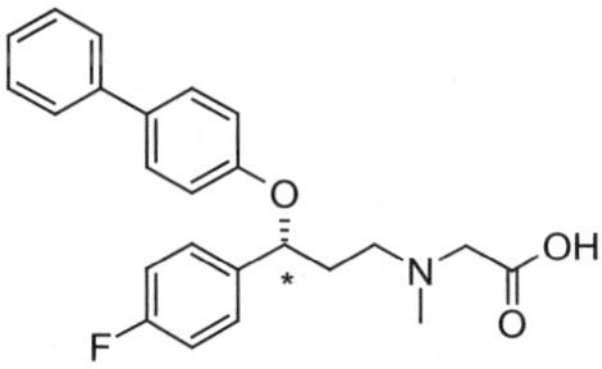

**1**
NFPS: RS mixture
Alx-5407: R isomer

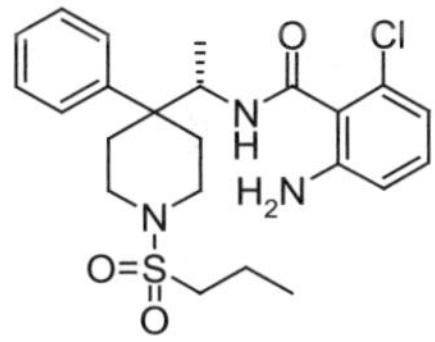

**2**
ACPPB

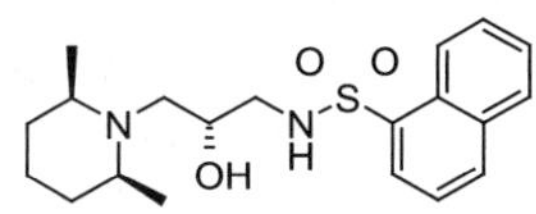

**3**
SB733993

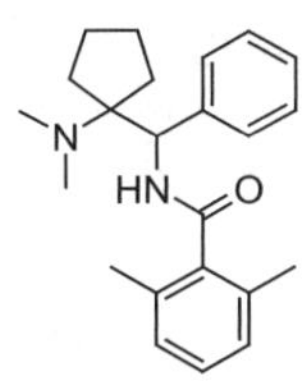

**4**
GSK931145

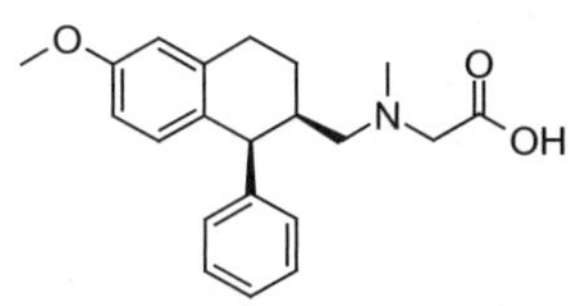

**5**
Org25935
SCH-900435

Summary of Data Examining Relative GlyT1, GlyT2, and GlyR Expression Implies That GlyT1 Plays Different Roles across These Regions

| | Cortex (rostral) | Hindbrain (caudal) |
|---|---|---|
| GlyT1 density | Low | High |
| Cellular localization | Glial and neuronal | Glial |
| Glutamate terminal localization | Co-localized with NMDAR | Not present |
| Glycinergic neurotransmission | None | Dense innervation |
| GlyT2 expression | None (no redundancy) | Dense (functional redundancy) |
| Primary role | Modulating NMDA function | Terminating GlyR function |

## 8.4 SUPPORT FOR GlyT1 AS A THERAPEUTIC TARGET FOR SCHIZOPHRENIA

### 8.4.1 Preclinical *In Vitro* and Mechanistic Support

Extensive literature exists reporting activity of various GlyT1 inhibitors in multiple *in vivo* models related to psychosis [6, 34–36]. As a representative illustration, Sanofi-Aventis's SSR504734 is among the most thoroughly studied compounds. This compound has been reported to (1) increase potentiation of glycine in PFC [37, 38], (2) inhibit MK-801- or phencyclidine (PCP)-induced elevation of locomotor activity (LMA) [34, 35], and (3) increase NMDAR-evoked excitatory postsynaptic currents (eEPSCs) and enhance long-term potentiation (LTP) in the hippocampus [37]. Evidence in support of GlyT1 for cognitive symptoms is also increasing. SSR504734 was reported to improve social recognition deficits induced by chronic, neonatal administration of PCP in rats [37] and improve working memory function in nondisrupted C57BL/6 mice [39]. A compound that shares a structural relationship with SSR504734 was reported to reverse prepulse inhibition (PPI) deficits in DBA/2J mice [35]. Recent studies report contradictory connections between the NMDAR hypofunction and dopamine hyperfunction models such that some GlyT1 inhibitors enhance hyperdopaminergic behaviors. Administration of SSR504734 (**6**) potentiated the amphetamine-induced increase in LMA and further reduced the apomorphine-induced reduction in LMA (Fig. 8.2). This may provide evidence that increased cortical NMDAR function alone cannot reverse the effects of pharmacological agents that stimulate subcortical dopamine pathways [34].

### 8.4.2 GlyT1 Inhibitors Increase Central Levels of Glycine

As discussed earlier, the concentration of glycine is regulated at less than 1 μM concentration in the synaptic region of glutamatergic nerves despite much higher levels (about 2 mM) in the surrounding glia. Inhibiting GlyT1 increases synaptic glycine levels, and this excess glycine can spill over into the extrasynaptic space. Although it is generally not possible to measure the glycine levels that are actually present in a synapse, it is relatively routine to measure the increased levels (the spillover) by microdialysis in various regions of the brain or cerebrospinal fluid (CSF) in different species. Various studies in rodent with different GlyT1 inhibitors have reported that central glycine levels can be increased by 150–300% of basal levels and higher [8, 40–43]. In these cases, the actual synaptic glycine levels could be different and could vary according to brain region [40].

In a nonpeer-reviewed meeting report, Organon reported effects on central glycine levels using microdialysis studies in rat and cynomolgus monkey due to administration of Org25935 [44] (**5**). At 10 μmol/kg po in rat, the compound reportedly reached concentrations in the brain of up to 143 ng/g and increased striatal glycine levels by about 148% over basal. The compound reportedly was administered to monkey at up to 2 mg/kg/day for 3 weeks and reached levels of up to 22 ng/g in the CSF (glycine elevation was not reported). In another nonpeer-reviewed 2006 report to shareholders, Organon discussed results from administering Org25935 (**5**) (16 mg single dose) to five human volunteers. Drug concentrations reportedly reached about 15–20 ng/mL in the CSF, and glycine levels increased from approximately 4–10 nmol/mL by about two- to threefold in the CSF. This same compound (redesignated as SCH-900435) was reportedly in Phase II clinical studies by Merck in 2010. Overall, drug and glycine monitoring in the CSF appears to be a promising clinical

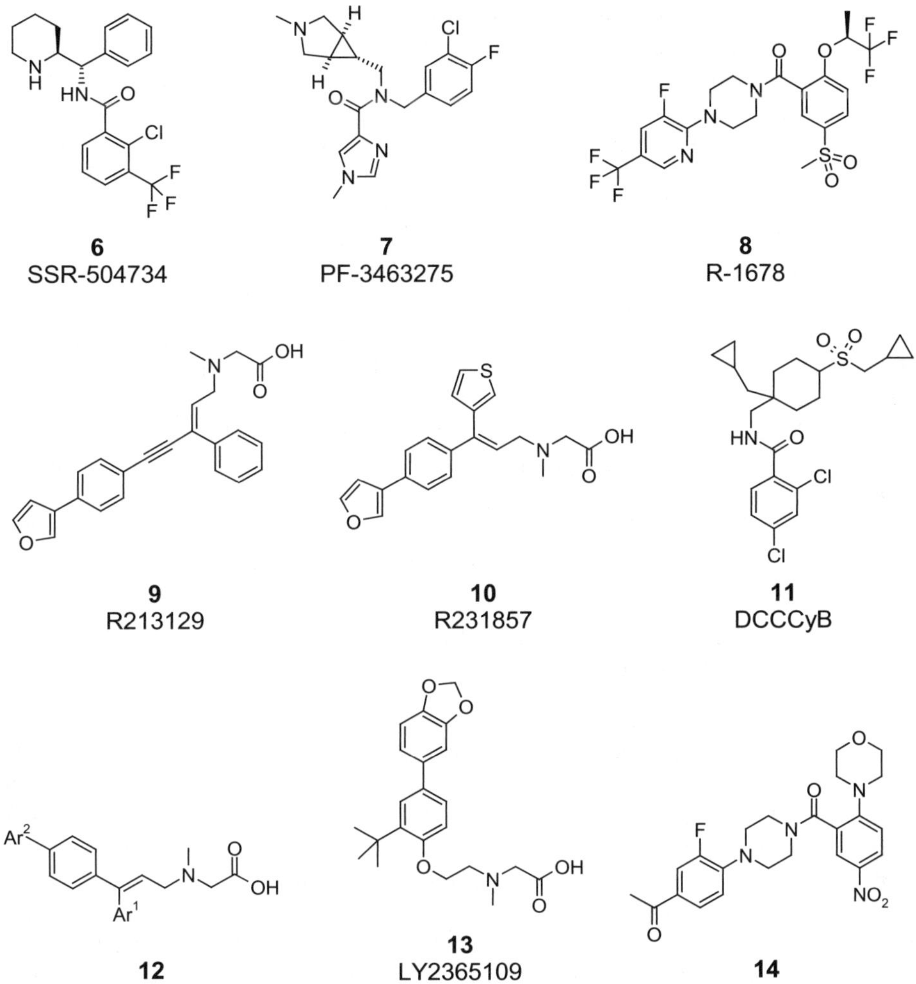


**FIGURE 8.2** A selection of GlyT1 inhibitors.

biomarker. It should be noted, however, that while CSF glycine levels are measureable and do indicate a consequence of GlyT1 inhibition, increased CSF glycine concentrations may actually represent a disruption of glycinergic neurotransmission in more caudal brain regions. In fact, modulation of cortical glycine near the presumed NMDAR targets may occur in a dose range below where the changes in CSF levels occur.

### 8.4.3 Reversal of PCP-Induced Neuronal Activation in Rat Using fMRI

Phencyclidine is a known negative NMDAR modulator that elicits psychotic and dissociative symptoms that are similar to the symptoms of schizophrenia.

Using functional magnetic resonance imaging (fMRI) a team from GSK reported that administration of PCP to rat resulted in sustained activation of specific cortico-limbo-thalamic circuits, and further, that this activation could be reversed by co-administration of GlyT1 inhibitor SSR504734 (**6**) (10 mg/kg) [45]. This effect is believed to arise because the GlyT1 inhibitor increases synaptic glycine, thus increasing occupancy of glycine at the glycine-B binding site on NMDAR, and thereby results in a higher proportion of NMDA channels activated upon synaptic release of glutamate. A similar reversal of PCP-induced neuronal activation was reported from administration of D-serine (1 g/kg) in place of SSR504734. Like glycine, D-serine binds to the NMDAR glycine-B binding site and acts as a co-agonist. Taken together, these studies provide evidence for the linkage between GlyT1 inhibitors and their effects on specific neuronal circuitry that are believed to be potentially important in schizophrenia and also offer a foundation for developing clinical translational tools. Continuing advances in imaging approaches, for example, through magnetic resonance detection of glycine [46, 47] and functional neuroimaging [48], will likely find increased application as less invasive translational tests that also enable researchers to focus on the brain regions of most interest (e.g., cortex).

### 8.4.4 Clinical Support from Low-Affinity GlyT1 Inhibitors and NMDAr Modulators

Numerous clinical studies with schizophrenic patients have been reported that assess the effects of (1) NMDAR glycine-site agonists (glycine, D-serine), (2) partial agonists (D-cycloserine), and (3) the low-affinity GlyT1 inhibitor sarcosine [49]. Across these studies, a generally consistent outcome was improvement in negative symptoms (Fig. 8.2). While improvement in the cognitive deficits of schizophrenia might be expected, the adjunctive trials did not include definitive tests to examine this domain. Since these studies typically involved patients that were maintained on standard antipsychotic treatment during the trials, further improvements in positive symptoms might be difficult to detect.

Several studies are particularly noteworthy. Javitt, Zukin, and co-workers reported in double-blind studies that low doses of glycine (30 mg/day), when administered with conventional antipsychotics, significantly reduced negative symptoms [50]. Subsequent studies by these and other researchers reported that adjunctive therapy with higher doses of glycine (60 g/day) led to improvements in negative symptoms [51–53] in otherwise treatment-resistant patients. In a double-blind trial, sarcosine (a low-affinity GlyT1 inhibitor) reportedly improved negative and positive symptoms and cognitive deficits when administered at 2 g/day in conjunction with conventional antipsychotics [54, 55]. The results of these studies and others have been collectively analyzed [56] and are summarized in Figure 8.3. Interestingly, the reported beneficial effects of treatments with glycine or sarcosine on negative symptoms and cognition were generally apparent within two weeks of initiation whereas conventional antipsychotics take 3–4 weeks to show improvement in positive symptoms.

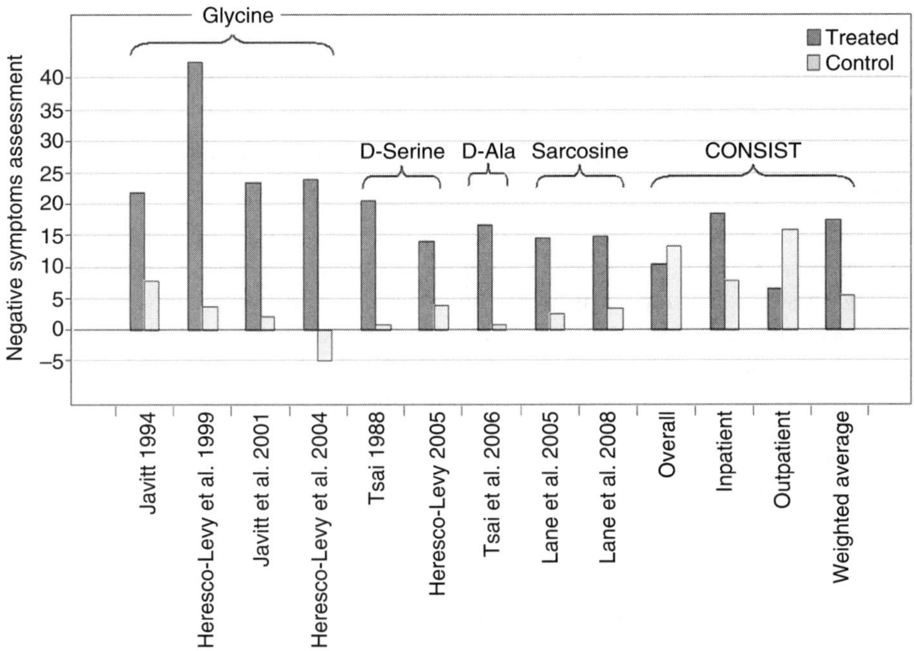


**FIGURE 8.3** Overview of several clinical studies reporting effects on negative symptoms in trials involving co-administration of NMDAR modulatory agents with conventional antipsychotics (other than clozapine); adapted from analysis by Javitt [56]. References: Glycine [50–52, 70] D-Serine [71, 72] D-Alanine [73] Sarcosine [74, 75] CONSIST [76].

### 8.4.5 Support in Nonhuman Primate Behavioral Studies

Based on the observation that NMDAR modulator ketamine produces schizophrenia-like symptoms, the reversal of ketamine-induced effects is frequently employed as a preclinical *in vivo* model to test GlyT1 inhibitors and other NMDAR modulators. Pfizer reported that administration of ketamine to rhesus monkeys induced working memory deficits that could be reversed [57] by the high-affinity, selective, GlyT1 inhibitor PF3463275 (**7**) [58]; however, the hallucinatory side effects of ketamine were not reversed by the drug. This compound was reportedly in Phase II clinical studies in 2010.

### 8.4.6 Clinical Support from High-Affinity GlyT1 Inhibitors

The strongest support for GlyT1 inhibitors as potential schizophrenia treatments to date may come from Phase II studies by Roche. In a nonpeer-reviewed disclosure, Roche reported that R-1678 (**8**) [42] improved Positive and Negative Syndrome Scale (PANSS) negative symptom factor scores in patients to a significantly greater extent than placebo after 8 weeks with co-administration of an atypical antipsychotic. Significant improvements were also reportedly seen in improvements in the personal and social performance (PSP) scale. Phase III studies were reportedly under way in 2012.

### 8.4.7 Other Clinical Studies Involving Selective, High-Affinity GlyT1 Inhibitors

Clinical studies involving Org25935/SCH900435 (**5**) (Organon/Schering/Merck) and R-1678 (**8**) (Roche) have been discussed above. Clinical studies involving several other compounds have also been described. From Johnson and Johnson, compounds R213129[59] (**9**) and R231857[60] (**10**) have been clinically evaluated. They reportedly evaluated drug exposure levels, electroencephalogram (EEG) effects, and behavioral effects due to the drug alone and in combination with scopolamine. In prior studies, scopolamine has been used to induce cognitive deficits as a model of schizophrenia to assess if potential NMDAR modulatory drugs can reverse those deficits. These compounds were reportedly administered at doses projected to achieve >50% target occupancy (based on preclinical studies); however, no consistent dose-dependent effects were found for either compound. The failure to demonstrate significant effects was attributed to potentially inadequate CNS exposure of the compounds.

Merck's compound DCCCyB (**11**) was reported as a potent ($IC_{50}$ 29 nM) selective GlyT1 inhibitor with good distributional properties in rat, rhesus, and dog [61]. It reportedly increased central glycine levels and reversed PCP-induced cognitive deficits in rat. PET imaging studies in rhesus monkey showed highest levels of distribution in pons, thalamus, and cerebellum. As of 2010, the details of clinical studies had not yet appeared in peer-reviewed publications but had been described at scientific conferences. According to these reports on DCCCyB, target occupancy of 50–70% is associated with activity in their rodent cognition model (reversal of ketamine-induced set shifting) and occupancy of >90% led to unspecified side effects in rodents. Occupancy in rhesus reached as high as 90%, with $Occ_{50}$ at about 120 nM drug concentration in plasma. In Merck's clinical studies, they reported 50% receptor occupancy of DCCCyB was achieved at plasma concentration of 98 nM and patients achieved occupancy levels as high as 80% [62].

## 8.5 SAFETY CONSIDERATIONS

The earliest reported potent and selective GlyT1 inhibitors could be described as lipophilic variations of sarcosine and are represented by NFPS/Alx5407 (**1**) and the prototypical scaffold **12**. It reportedly became apparent that such compounds could cause significant side effects in rodent such as aberrant locomotor effects, breathing deficits, convulsive behaviors, and death (at higher doses). Indeed, researchers at Allelix reportedly compared behavioral and safety effects for a series of compounds and showed that the effects could be different despite small structural changes [63].

The effects observed in rodents at escalated doses of GlyT1 inhibitors have been reported in various ways. Alx5407 has been described as inducing "akathesia-like" effects in mice [8] (the animal positions itself in the corner of a square cage), as inducing "compulsive toe walking" and ataxia in rats [40], and as "obstinate progression" [64]. The exact manifestation of the behavioral effects is likely to depend on the type of rodent and the type of cage used as well as, of course, the delivery method and the drug itself. GlyT1 knockout mice show effects that are consistent with those seen from pharmacological blockade; those effects include locomotor and respiratory deficits, and then death on the first postnatal day [29, 65].

Compounds that share some structural moieties can show differences in rodent side effect profiles. For example, Lilly reported that LY2365109 (**13**) ($IC_{50}$ 16 nM) showed faster onset and greater severity of side effects in rats than Alx540 (**1**) ($IC_{50}$ 7 nM), despite sharing some structural moieties, properties, and level of glycine increase in brain regions according to microdialysis [40]. Overall, however, the doses of LY2365109 or Alx540 that reportedly were required to show detectable glycine elevation were only slightly lower than doses that elicit locomotor side effects.

Based on the NMDAR hypofunction hypothesis, it is presumed that pharmacological blockade of GlyT1 in the forebrain region (principally prefrontal cortex [PFC] and other regions of high NMDAR-mediated glutamatergic neurotransmission) will be relevant for treatment of schizophrenia. However, GlyT1 is also expressed, and at significantly higher levels, in caudal regions like the brainstem and cerebellum. In these regions glycinergic neurotransmission prevails and NMDAR expression is relatively low. It is possible that in regions of high GlyR expression, the consequence of profound block of GlyT1 would result in detectable increases of glycine that may activate GlyRs. Using dual probe microdialysis, the Lilly group reported that glycine elevation was higher and more sustained in the cerebellum than in the PFC. Moreover, the onset and severity of the side effects reportedly correlated better with glycine levels measured in the cerebellum than in the PFC. Based on these observations, the Lilly group hypothesized that the locomotor and respiratory side effects of LY2365109 (**13**) and Alx540 (**1**) could be attributed to sustained inhibition of GlyT1 in caudal regions where elevated glycine levels activates the glycine-A (strychnine-sensitive) receptor. Effects on glycine elevation due to administration of Alx540 were different in different brain regions; glycine elevation was higher and more sustained in the cerebellum than in the PFC. The hypothesis that the side effects are associated with GlyR activation in hindbrain regions is supported by studies reporting that respiratory activity is greatly reduced in GlyT1 deficient mice but that this reduction can be normalized by application of the GlyR antagonist strychnine [66]. Additionally the Lilly team reported that the locomotor effects of LY2365109 can also be transiently reversed by co-administration of strychnine.

The concerns around these rodent side effects led to speculation that GlyT1 inhibitors could not achieve a suitable safety margin to be therapeutically useful. However, these observations were associated with the "lipophilic sarcosine" chemotype. It is now increasingly appreciated that other classes of GlyT1 inhibitors may not share these safety issues [2]. Nevertheless, it is likely that the features that contribute to the observed toxicity in rodent is more complex than just the chemotype. It is almost certainly not the case that the reported severe locomotor, respiratory, and convulsive-like effect in rodent due to Org25935 (**5**) (a "lipophilic sarcosine") will translate to human since the compound reportedly has been safely administered to monkeys, and human volunteers, and had reached Phase II clinical trials in 2010 by Merck (redesignated as SCH900435). It is known that GlyT1 inhibitors exist with different mechanistic profiles (*vide infra*) and such differences may contribute to the safety profile of each compound. Finally, it is known that expression levels of GlyT1 and regional distribution are different across species, with expression in the brainstem being much higher in mouse, rat, and monkey relative to human [40]. Such differences could influence if or how effects in rodents translate to effects in humans.

## 8.6 MECHANISTIC DIFFERENCES AMONG GlyT1 INHIBITORS

As already discussed, reported GlyT1 inhibitors exist across a range of mechanistic properties. At least three properties have been investigated: GlyT1 inhibitors can (1) bind competitively with glycine or not, (2) binding may require sodium or be sodium-independent, and (3) the effects of binding can be reversible or pseudo-irreversible (as much as 24 hours or greater). These distinctions are illustrated for the compounds in Table 8.2 which have approximately the same binding affinity to GlyT1 ($K_D$ 2–3 nM) but differ significantly in their mechanistic features.

Compounds ACPPB [25] (**2**), SB733993 [26] (**3**), and GSK931145 [26] (**4**) bind competitively with glycine, while others, such as NFPS [15] (**1**), bind noncompetitively with glycine (Table 8.3). It has been inferred from such results that the glycine-competitive compounds are glycine-orthosteric binders, while the others bind at a site that is distinct from the glycine binding site. Translocation of glycine by GlyT1 requires the co-transport of sodium (and chloride) ions. The glycine-competitive compounds SB733993 and ACPPB both require sodium for binding, whereas the glycine-noncompetitive compound NFPS does not. Interestingly, GSK931145 binding is not sodium-dependent despite being competitive with glycine. The glycine-competitive properties along with the sodium dependency may suggest that multiple, distinct ligand binding sites exist on GlyT1 some that are co-located with the glycine binding site and others that are more distant. Dissociation and functional activity rates can also vary considerably. It is noteworthy that in binding studies, NFPS dissociates relatively rapidly ($t_{1/2}$ 28 minutes [24]), and the func-

**TABLE 8.2 Representative Compounds Illustrating Different Mechanistic Properties**

| | ACPPB [25] **2** | SB733993 [26] **3** | GSK931145 [26] **4** | NFPS [15, 24] **1** |
|---|---|---|---|---|
| $K_D$ (nM) | 2 | 2 | 2 | 3 |
| Competitive binding with glycine? | Competitive | Competitive | Competitive | Noncompetitive |
| Sodium-dependent binding? | Yes | Yes | No | No |
| Dissociation rate ($t_{1/2}$) | 70 minutes | ~5 minutes | ~40 minutes | 28 minutes |

**TABLE 8.3 Representative Compounds Illustrating Ligand Competition Characteristics**

| | | Glycine | SB733993 **3** | GSK931145 **4** | SSR504734 **6** |
|---|---|---|---|---|---|
| | Glycine | | Competitive | Competitive | Competitive |
| **3** | SB733993 [26] | Competitive | | Competitive | Competitive |
| **4** | GSK931145 [26] | Competitive | Competitive | | Competitive |
| **6** | SSR504734 [37, 67] | Competitive | Competitive | Competitive | |
| **1** | NFPS/ Alx5407 [26, 67] | Noncompetitive | Uncompetitive | Uncompetitive | |
| **5** | Org25935 [26] | Noncompetitive | Uncompetitive | Uncompetitive | |

tional effects on binding reportedly are pseudo-irreversible, with recovery of GlyT1 activity taking longer than 24 hours after washout [15].

Ligand competition studies have provided additional details about mode of binding. As illustrated in Table 8.3, the nonsarcosine-based compounds SB733993 [26], GSK931145 [26], and SSR504734 all bind competitively with glycine and are mutually competitive with one another. In contrast, sarcosine-based compounds, including NFPS/Alx5407 and Org25935, bind noncompetitively with glycine and uncompetitively with SB733993 and GSK931145. Overall, available evidence may suggest that there are two classifications of binding modes, one for the sarcosine-based compounds and one for nonsarcosine-based compounds.

Similar conclusions were reached by the Abbott group to indicate that SSR504734 (**6**) was a glycine-competitive, reversible inhibitor, whereas Alx5407 (**1**) and other sarcosine-based inhibitors were glycine-noncompetitive and functionally irreversible [67].

While clear mechanistic differences are apparent, the functional consequences of those differences are not. It was discussed in Section 8.5 that the motor and respiratory effects may be due to GlyT1 inhibition in hindbrain regions due to activation of GlyR (augmentation of glycinergic neurotransmission) and, therefore, potentially distinct from the therapeutic effects that may be due to GlyT1 inhibition in forebrain regions due to NMDAR activation (augmentation of glutamatergic neurotransmission). Basal glycine concentrations within glycinergic regions are higher than within glutamatergic regions. This raises potentially important consequences for inhibitors that bind competitively with glycine or not. GlyT1 inhibitors that are insensitive to glycine concentrations would be expected to have relatively equivalent functional effects irrespective of whether the local concentration of glycine is high or low. Alternatively, inhibitors that are competitive with glycine would be expected to have a more selective effect in regions of low glycine concentration. Thus, glycine-competitive inhibitors may have greater effect on increasing glutamatergic neurotransmission (NMDAR activation) and less effect in the undesirable activation of GlyR-mediated glycinergic neurotransmission.

That hypothesis is consistent with reports that glycine-noncompetitive agents, like NFPS/Alx5407 (**1**), show profound rodent side effects, whereas comparable side effects have not so far been reported for glycine-competitive inhibitors like SSR504734 (**6**). On the basis of this reasoning, the sarcosine-based chemotypes should be avoided as schizophrenia therapeutics. However, the sarcosine-based compound Org25935/SCH900435 (**5**) was evidently safe enough to have reached Phase II clinical studies. Considered together, additional factors may play additional or even greater roles. As discussed above, NFPS/Alx5407 has a prolonged duration of functional activity. Although binding is relatively rapidly reversible ($t_{1/2}$ 28 minutes), glycine transport inhibition is maintained for >24 hours. Such long duration of activity could contribute to the rodent toxicity, although affected rodents generally fully recover much more quickly (typically 2–4 hours).

A report from Cephalon may be particularly noteworthy because it describes the magnitude of locomotor side effects for the nonsarcosine-based compound ACPPB (**2**) as being comparable to those seen with Alx5407 [64] (**1**). Those results provide evidence that neither a glycine-noncompetitive binding mode nor a sarcosine-derived chemotype may be solely responsible for the rodent side effects. The authors reported that all four compounds in Table 8.4 were active in the DBA/2 mouse PPI model. Next, they determined the rate of functional recovery of GlyT1 activity following inhibitor washout and hypoth-

**TABLE 8.4 Pharmacological Characterization of Selected GlyT1 Inhibitors [64]**

| | | $IC_{50}$ (nM) | Functional Recovery Rate; $t_{1/2}$ (minute) | Glycine Competition |
|---|---|---|---|---|
| **1** | Alx5407 | 0.9 | 294 | Mixed noncompetitive |
| **2** | ACPPB | 3.8 | 103 | Competitive |
| **14** | – | 25 | <10 | Mixed noncompetitive |
| – | Sarcosine | 39,000 | <10 | Competitive |

esized that this rate might be associated with the aberrant locomotor effects in mouse. Compound **14** reportedly had a faster rate of functional recovery compared with Alx5407 and ACPPB, yet it did not induce rodent aberrant locomotor effects.

It is now clear that GlyT1 inhibitors can differ in chemotype and several mechanistic ways including glycine competition, sodium dependency, kinetics, and possibly other characteristics that are yet to be described. However, it is unknown if or how such differences will directly impact the therapeutic potential for specific compounds with regard to efficacy, side effects, and safety margin. Addressing these questions will require systematic mechanistic comparisons of compounds in clinical trials.

## 8.7 CLINICAL DEVELOPMENT

Compounds that have reportedly reached the clinical development phase as of 2010 are shown in Table 8.5. As discussed above, the earliest compounds to reach development reportedly were Alx5407 and Org25935/SCH900435. These were sarcosine-based compounds. Next to follow was SSR504734 and all the rest followed thereafter. The compound that has advanced the farthest in clinical trials is RG1678 from Roche. It entered Phase III in 2010 and reportedly was evaluated as an adjunctive therapy (co-administered with an existing atypical antipsychotic) for the treatment of the negative symptoms of schizophrenia. Merck has evaluated Org25935/SCH900435 in three concurrent Phase II trials: (1) as an adjunct therapy for negative symptoms of schizophrenia, (2) as monotherapy for negative symptoms of schizophrenia, and (3) as a treatment for alcohol dependence. Preclinical support for the alcohol dependence indication comes from reported findings that the compound could block ethanol-induced increases in dopamine release in rat nucleus accumbens [68]

**TABLE 8.5 Compounds Reaching Clinical Development and Status as of 2012**

| Phase Reached | Sponsor | | Drug | Status |
|---|---|---|---|---|
| 1 | Amgen | | AMG747 | |
| 1 | GSK | | GSK1018921 | |
| 1 | J&J | **1** | Alx5407 | |
| 1 | J&J | **10** | R231857 | |
| 1 | J&J | **9** | R213129 | |
| 2 | Merck | **5** | Org25935/SCH900435 | Completed |
| 1 | Merck | **11** | DCCCyB | |
| 2 | Pfizer | **7** | PF3463275 | |
| 3 | Roche | **8** | RG1678 | Ongoing |
| 1 | Sanofi-Aventis | | SSR103800 | |
| 1 | Sanofi-Aventis | **6** | SSR504734 | |

and was active in a rat model involving reduction of ethanol intake and ethanol preference [69]. Similar to Roche, Pfizer has evaluated PF3463275 as an adjunct therapy for negative symptoms. Other companies continue to report on preclinical progress on new GlyT1 inhibitors. Thus, the field is likely to continue to expand.

## 8.8 SUMMARY

The first reported high-affinity GlyT1 inhibitors began to emerge in 1997. The early chemotypes associated with GlyT1 inhibition were sarcosine based and contained a lipophilic group on the nitrogen. Although these compounds appeared to be highly selective, they reportedly induced serious side effects in rodents, including aberrant locomotor behaviors, labored breathing, convulsive-like behaviors, and even death. As this target was explored by increasing numbers of academic and pharmaceutical groups numerous, different chemotypes were identified that are distinct from the early sarcosine-based compounds and from each other. These various GlyT1 inhibitors reportedly display a range of mechanistic properties and vary in at least three potentially important ways: they can be (1) competitive with glycine or not, (2) have sodium-dependent binding or not, and (3) the kinetics (dissociation) and duration of functional effects of binding can range from being fast (<30 minutes) to slow (<24 hours). The connection between these various properties and potential effects on the therapeutic potential (efficacy, side effects, safety margin) for any particular compound remains largely unknown. For example, the side effects seen in rodents have so far not been shown to be specifically associated with any particular chemotype or mechanistic class. Several early compounds had reached Phase I clinical development but were eventually withdrawn for reasons that remain undisclosed. An additional challenge to the development of GlyT1 inhibitors is that, as a new target, no preclinical models that have clinical validation exist. All reported rodent models of psychosis to date are generally based on $D_2$ mechanisms.

Despite these challenges, the field is expanding and progress is accelerating. There is increasing evidence that the side effects in rodents may be due to GlyT1 inhibition in regions of glycinergic neurotransmission in the hindbrain regions. More specifically, increased glycine levels in these regions may lead to overactivation of inhibitory Glycine-A receptors. The therapeutic target for schizophrenia is assumed to be GlyT1 in the forebrain regions including PFC, where inhibition of GlyT1 leads to increased activation of NMDAR. The evolving neurochemical understanding suggests that the desired effects of NMDAR activation may be differentiable from the undesired effects of Glycine-A receptor activation due to their different localization, different basal glycine concentrations, and different expression levels in humans compared with rodents and other species. Progress is also being made in developing clinical translational methodologies. For example, the functional effects of GlyT1 inhibitors have been reported in rodents using fMRI, and several PET imaging agents have been clinically studied and will allow assessment of transporter occupancy levels. In addition, dose-dependent increases in glycine concentration have been reported in the CSF of primates and humans. Finally, evidence of continued progress in Phase III and Phase III studies provides encouraging support that the uncertainties in this challenging area can be addressed.

## REFERENCES

1. van Os, J., Kapur, S. (2009). Schizophrenia. *Lancet*, *374*, 635–645.
2. Lindsley, C. (2010). Up from the ashes. The importance of not condemning a mechanism based on a single chemotype. *ACS Chem Neurosci*, *1*, 165–166.
3. Wolkenberg, S.E., Sur, C. (2010). Recent progress in the discovery of non-sarcosine based GlyT1 inhibitors. *Curr Top Med Chem (Sharjah, United Arab Emirates)*, *10*, 170–186.
4. Eulenburg, V., Gomeza, J. (2010). Neurotransmitter transporters expressed in glial cells as regulators of synapse function. *Brain Res Rev*, *63*, 103–112.
5. Javitt, D.C. (2009). Glycine transport inhibitors for the treatment of schizophrenia: symptom and disease modification. *Curr Opin Drug Discov Devel*, *12*, 468–478.
6. Yang, C.R., Svensson, K.A. (2008). Allosteric modulation of NMDA receptor via elevation of brain glycine and serine: the therapeutic potentials for schizophrenia. *Pharmacol Ther*, *120*, 317–332.
7. Bridges Thomas, M., Williams, R., Lindsley Craig, W. (2008). Design of potent GlyT1 inhibitors: in vitro and in vivo profiles. *Curr Opin Mol Ther*, *10*, 591–601.
8. Harsing, L.G.J., Juranyi, Z., Gacsalyi, I., Tapolcsanyi, P., Czompa, A., Matyus, P. (2006). Glycine transporter type-1 and its inhibitors. *Curr Med Chem*, *13*, 1017–1044.
9. Seeman, P. (2006). Targeting the dopamine D2 receptor in schizophrenia. *Expert Opin Ther Targets*, *10*, 515–531.
10. Lewis, D.A., Moghaddam, B. (2006). Cognitive dysfunction in schizophrenia: convergence of gamma-aminobutyric acid and glutamate alterations. *Arch Neurol*, *63*, 1372–1376.
11. Javitt, D.C., Zukin, S.R. (1991). Recent advances in the phencyclidine model of schizophrenia. *Am J Psychiatry*, *148*, 1301–1308.
12. Johnson, J.W., Ascher, P. (1987). Glycine potentiates the NMDA response in cultured mouse brain neurons. *Nature*, *325*, 529–531.
13. Kuryatov, A., Laube, B., Bertz, H., Kuhse, J. (1994). Mutational analysis of the glycine-binding site of the NMDA receptor: structural similarity with bacterial amino acid-binding proteins. *Neuron*, *12*, 1291–1300.
14. Bergeron, R., Meyer, T.M., Coyle, J.T., Greene, R.W. (1998). Modulation of N-methyl-D-aspartate receptor function by glycine transport. *Proc Natl Acad Sci U S A*, *95*, 15730–15374.
15. Vandenberg, R.J., Aubrey, K.R. (2001). Glycine transport inhibitors as potential antipsychotic drugs. *Expert Opin Ther Targets*, *5*, 507–518.

16. Chen, L., Muhlhauser, M., Yang, C.R. (2003). Glycine transporter-1 blockade potentiates NMDA-mediated responses in rat prefrontal cortical neurons in vitro and in vivo. *J Neurophysiol*, *89*, 691–703.
17. Danysz, W., Parsons, C.G. (1998). Glycine and N-methyl-D-aspartate receptors: physiological significance and possible therapeutic applications. *Pharmacol Rev*, *50*, 597–664.
18. Cubelos, B., Gimenez, C., Zafra, F. (2005). Localization of the GLYT1 glycine transporter at glutamatergic synapses in the rat brain. *Cereb Cortex*, *15*, 448–459.
19. Adams, R.H., Sato, K., Shimada, S., Tohyama, M., Pueschel, A.W., Betz, H. (1995). Gene structure and glial expression of the glycine transporter GlyT1 in embryonic and adult rodents. *J Neurosci*, *15*, 2524–2532.
20. Sato, K., Zhang, J.H., Saika, T., Sato, M., Tada, K., Tohyama, M. (1991). Localization of glycine receptor alpha 1-subunit mRNA-containing neurons in the rat brain: an analysis using in situ hybridization histochemistry. *Neuroscience*, *43*, 381–395.
21. Araki, T., Yamano, M., Murakami, T., Wanaka, A., Betz, H., Tohyama, M. (1988). Localization of glycine receptors in the rat central nervous system: an immunocytochemical analysis using monoclonal antibody. *Neuroscience*, *25*, 613–624.
22. Zarbin, M.A., Wamsley, J.K., Kuhar, M.J. (1981). Glycine receptor: light microscopic autoradiographic localization with [3H]strychnine. *J Neurosci*, *1*, 532–547.
23. Frostholm, A., Rotter, A. (1985). Glycine receptor distribution in mouse CNS: autoradiographic localization of [3H]strychnine binding sites. *Brain Res Bull*, *15*, 473–486.
24. Mallorga, P.J., Williams, J.B., Jacobson, M., Marques, R., Chaudhary, A., Conn, P.J., Pettibone, D.J., Sur, C. (2003). Pharmacology and expression analysis of glycine transporter GlyT1 with [3H]-(N-[3-(4'-fluorophenyl)-3-(4'phenylphenoxy)propyl]) sarcosine. *Neuropharmacology*, *45*, 585–593.
25. Zeng, Z., O'Brien, J.A., Lemaire, W., O'Malley, S.S., Miller, P.J., Zhao, Z., Wallace, M.A., Raab, C., Lindsley, C.W., Sur, C., Williams, D.L. (2008). A novel radioligand for glycine transporter 1: characterization and use in autoradiographic and in vivo brain occupancy studies. *Nucl Med Biol*, *35*, 315–325.
26. Herdon, H.J., Roberts, J.C., Coulton, S., Porter, R.A. (2010). Pharmacological characterisation of the GlyT-1 glycine transporter using two novel radioligands. *Neuropharmacology*, *59*, 558–565.
27. Dohi, T., Morita, K., Kitayama, T., Motoyama, N., Morioka, N. (2009). Glycine transporter inhibitors as a novel drug discovery strategy for neuropathic pain. *Pharmacol Ther*, *123*, 54–79.
28. Hermanns, H., Muth-Selbach, U., Williams, R., Krug, S., Lipfert, P., Werdehausen, R., Braun, S., Bauer, I. (2008). Differential effects of spinally applied glycine transporter inhibitors on nociception in a rat model of neuropathic pain. *Neurosci Lett*, *445*, 214–219.
29. Tsai, G., Ralph-Williams, R.J., Martina, M., Bergeron, R., Berger-Sweeney, J., Dunham, K.S., Jiang, Z., Caine, S.B., Coyle, J.T. (2004). Gene knockout of glycine transporter 1: Characterization of the behavioral phenotype. *Proc Natl Acad Sci U S A*, *101*, 8485–8490.
30. Yee, B.K., Balic, E., Singer, P., Schwerdel, C., Grampp, T., Gabernet, L., Knuesel, I., Benke, D., Feldon, J., Mohler, H., Boison, D. (2006). Disruption of glycine trans-

porter 1 restricted to forebrain neurons is associated with a procognitive and antipsychotic phenotypic profile. *J Neurosci*, *26*, 3169–3181.

31. Gabernet, L., Pauly-Evers, M., Schwerdel, C., Lentz, M., Bluethmann, H., Vogt, K., Alberati, D., Mohler, H., Boison, D. (2005). Enhancement of the NMDA receptor function by reduction of glycine transporter-1 expression. *Neurosci Lett*, *373*, 79–84.
32. Gomeza, J., Armsen, W., Betz, H., Eulenburg, V. (2006). Lessons from the knocked-out glycine transporters. *Handb Exp Pharmacol*, *175*, 457–483.
33. Moehler, H., Rudolph, U., Boison, D., Singer, P., Feldon, J., Yee, B.K. (2008). Regulation of cognition and symptoms of psychosis: Focus on GABAA receptors and glycine transporter 1. *Pharmacol Biochem Behav*, *90*, 58–64.
34. Singer, P., Feldon, J., Yee, B.K. (2009). Interactions between the glycine transporter 1 (GlyT1) inhibitor SSR504734 and psychoactive drugs in mouse motor behaviour. *Eur Neuropsychopharmacol*, *19*, 571–580.
35. Boulay, D., Pichat, P., Dargazanli, G., Estenne-Bouhtou, G., Terranova, J.P., Rogacki, N., Stemmelin, J., Coste, A., Lanneau, C., Desvignes, C., Cohen, C., Alonso, R., Vige, X., Biton, B., Steinberg, R., Sevrin, M., Oury-Donat, F., George, P., Bergis, O., Griebel, G., Avenet, P., Scatton, B. (2008). Characterization of SSR103800, a selective inhibitor of the glycine transporter-1 in models predictive of therapeutic activity in schizophrenia. *Pharmacol Biochem Behav*, *91*, 47–58.
36. Sur, C., Kinney, G.G. (2007). Glycine transporter 1 inhibitors and modulation of NMDA receptor-mediated excitatory neurotransmission. *Curr Drug Targets*, *8*, 643–649.
37. Depoortere, R., Dargazanli, G., Estenne-Bouhtou, G., Coste, A., Lanneau, C., Desvignes, C., Poncelet, M., Heaulme, M., Santucci, V., Decobert, M., Cudennec, A., Voltz, C., Boulay, D., Terranova, J.P., Stemmelin, J., Roger, P., Marabout, B., Sevrin, M., Vige, X., Biton, B., Steinberg, R., Francon, D., Alonso, R., Avenet, P., Oury-Donat, F., Perrault, G., Griebel, G., George, P., Soubrie, P., Scatton, B. (2005). Neurochemical, electrophysiological and pharmacological profiles of the selective inhibitor of the glycine transporter-1 SSR504734, a potential new type of antipsychotic. *Neuropsychopharmacology*, *30*, 1963–1985.
38. Leonetti, M., Desvignes, C., Bougault, I., Souilhac, J., Oury-Donat, F., Steinberg, R. (2006). 2-Chloro-N-[(S)-phenyl [(2S)-piperidin-2-yl] methyl]-3-trifluoromethyl benzamide, monohydrochloride, an inhibitor of the glycine transporter type 1, increases evoked-dopamine release in the rat nucleus accumbens in vivo via an enhanced glutamatergic neurotransmission. *Neuroscience*, *137*, 555–564.
39. Singer, P., Feldon, J., Yee, B.K. (2009). *Psychopharmacology*, *202*, 371–384.
40. Perry, K.W., Falcone, J.F., Fell, M.J., Ryder, J.W., Yu, H., Love, P.L., Katner, J., Gordon, K.D., Wade, M.R., Man, T., Nomikos, G.G., Phebus, L.A., Cauvin, A.J., Johnson, K.W., Jones, C.K., Hoffmann, B.J., Sandusky, G.E., Walter, M.W., Porter, W.J., Yang, L., Merchant, K.M., Shannon, H.E., Svensson, K.A. (2008). Neurochemical and behavioral profiling of the selective GlyT1 inhibitors ALX5407 and LY2365109 indicate a preferential action in caudal vs. cortical brain areas. *Neuropharmacology*, *55*, 743–754.
41. Lindsley, C.W., Zhao, Z., Leister, W.H., O'Brien, J., Lemaire, W., Williams, D.L., Jr, Chen, T., Chang, R.S.L., Burno, M., Jacobson, M.A., Sur, C., Kinney, G.G., Pettibone, D.J., Tiller, P.R., Smith, S., Tsou, N.N., Duggan, M.E., Conn, P.J., Hartman, G.D.

(2006). Design, synthesis, and in vivo efficacy of glycine transporter-1 (GlyT1) inhibitors derived from a series of [4-phenyl-1-(propylsulfonyl)piperidin-4-yl] methyl benzamides. *ChemMedChem*, *1*, 807–811.

42. Pinard, E., Alberati, D., Borroni, E., Fischer, H., Hainzl, D., Jolidon, S., Moreau, J., Narquizian, R., Nettekoven, M., Norcross, R.D., Stalder, H., Thomas, A.W. (2008). Discovery of benzoylpiperazines as a novel class of potent and selective GlyT1 inhibitors. *Bioorg Med Chem Lett*, *18*, 5134–5139.

43. Smith, G., Ruhland, T., Mikkelsen, G., Andersen, K., Christoffersen Claus, T., Alifrangis Lene, H., Mork, A., Wren Stephen, P., Harris, N., Wyman Barry, M., Brandt, G. (2004). The synthesis and SAR of 2-arylsulfanyl-phenyl piperazinyl acetic acids as glyT-1 inhibitors. *Bioorg Med Chem Lett*, *14*, 4027–4030.

44. Andrews, N., Ge, J., Walker, G., Schipper, J., Marston, H.M. (2007). Effect of the selective glycine re-uptake (GlyT-1) inhibitor Org 25935 on glycine levels in CSF and dialysates. *Eur Neuropsychopharmacol*, *17*, S497.

45. Gozzi, A., Herdon, H., Schwarz, A., Bertani, S., Crestan, V., Turrini, G., Bifone, A. (2008). Pharmacological stimulation of NMDA receptors via co-agonist site suppresses fMRI response to phencyclidine in the rat. *Psychopharmacology*, *201*, 273–284.

46. Kaufman, M.J., Prescot, A.P., Ongur, D., Evins, A.E., Barros, T.L., Medeiros, C.L., Covell, J., Wang, L., Fava, M., Renshaw, P.F. (2009). Oral glycine administration increases brain glycine/creatine ratios in men: a proton magnetic resonance spectroscopy study. *Psychiatry Res Neuroimaging*, *173*, 143–149.

47. Gambarota, G., Mekle, R., Xin, L., Hergt, M., van der Zwaag, W., Krueger, G., Gruetter, R. (2009). In vivo measurement of glycine with short echo-time 1H MRS in human brain at 7 T. *Magn Reson Mater Phys*, *22*, 1–4.

48. McGuire, P., Howes, O.D., Stone, J., Fusar-Poli, P. (2008). Functional neuroimaging in schizophrenia: diagnosis and drug discovery. *Trends Pharmacol Sci*, *29*, 91–98.

49. Shim, S.S., Hammonds, M.D., Kee, B.S. (2008). Potentiation of the NMDA receptor in the treatment of schizophrenia: focused on the glycine site. *Eur Arch Psychiatry Clin Neurosci*, *258*, 16–27.

50. Javitt, D.C., Zylberman, I., Zukin, S.R., Heresco-Levy, U., Lindenmayer, J.P. (1994). Amelioration of negative symptoms in schizophrenia by glycine. *Am J Psychiatry*, *151*, 1234–1236.

51. Heresco-Levy, U., Javitt, D.C., Ermilov, M., Mordel, C., Silipo, G., Lichtenstein, M. (1999). Efficacy of high-dose glycine in the treatment of enduring negative symptoms of schizophrenia. *Arch Gen Psychiatry*, *56*, 29–36.

52. Heresco-Levy, U., Ermilov, M., Lichtenberg, P., Bar, G., Javitt, D.C. (2004). High-dose glycine added to olanzapine and risperidone for the treatment of schizophrenia. *Biol Psychiatry*, *55*, 165–171.

53. Heresco-Levy, U., Javitt, D.C., Ermilov, M., Mordel, C., Horowitz, A., Kelly, D. (1996). Double-blind, placebo-controlled, crossover trial of glycine adjuvant therapy for treatment-resistant schizophrenia. *Br J Psychiatry*, *169*, 610–617.

54. Tsai, G., Lane, H., Young, P.J., Lane, N., Chong, M. (2004). Glycine transporter 1 inhibitor, N-methylglycine (sarcosine) added to antipsychotics for the treatment of schizophrenia. *Biol Psychiatry*, *155*, 452–456.

55. Lane, H., Huang, C., Wu, P., Liu, Y., Chang, Y., Lin, P., Chen, P., Tsai, G. (2006). Glycine transporter I inhibitor, N-methylglycine (sarcosine), added to clozapine for the treatment of schizophrenia. *Biol Psychiatry*, *60*, 645–649.

56. Javitt, D.C. (2008). Glycine transport inhibitors and the treatment of schizophrenia. *Biol Psychiatry*, *63*, 6–8.

57. Roberts, B.M., Shaffer, C.L., Seymour, P.A., Schmidt, C.J., Williams, G.V., Castner, S.A. (2010). Glycine transporter inhibition reverses ketamine-induced working memory deficits. *NeuroReport*, *21*, 390–394.

58. Lowe, J.A., Hou, X., Schmidt, C., David Tingley, F.,III, McHardy, S., Kalman, M., DeNinno, S., Sanner, M., Ward, K., Lebel, L., Tunucci, D., Valentine, J. (2009). The discovery of a structurally novel class of inhibitors of the type 1 glycine transporter. *Bioorg Med Chem Lett*, *19*, 2974–2976.

59. Liem-Moolenaar, M., Zoethout, R.W.M., de Boer, P., Schmidt, M., de Kam, M.L., Cohen, A.F., Franson, K.L., van Gerven, J.M.A. (2010). The effects of the glycine reuptake inhibitor R213129 on the central nervous system and on scopolamine-induced impairments in psychomotor and cognitive function in healthy subjects. *J Psychopharmacol*, *24*, 1671–1679.

60. Liem-Moolenaar, M., Zoethout, R.W.M., de Boer, P., Schmidt, M., de Kam, M.L., Cohen, A.F., Franson, K.L., van Gerven, J.M.A. (2010). The effects of a glycine reuptake inhibitor R231857 on the central nervous system and on scopolamine-induced impairments in cognitive and psychomotor function in healthy subjects. *J Psychopharmacol*, *24*, 1681–1687.

61. Blackaby, W.P., Lewis, R.T., Thomson, J.L., Jennings, A.S.R., Goodacre, S.C., Street, L.J., MacLeod, A.M., Pike, A., Wood, S., Thomas, S., Brown, T.A., Smith, A., Pillai, G., Almond, S., Guscott, M.R., Burns, H.D., Eng, W., Ryan, C., Cook, J., Hamill, T.G. (2010). Identification of an orally bioavailable, potent, and selective inhibitor of GlyT1. *ACS Med Chem Lett*, *1*, 350–354.

62. Williams, D.L.J., Jennings, A., Lewis, R., Street, L., Patel, S., Wisnoski, D., Wolkenberg, S., Lindsley, C., Zhao, Z., Krause, S.M., Ryan, C., Michener, M., Zeng, Z., Miller, M., Riffel, K., O'Malley, S.S., Sanabria, S., Eng, W., Gibson, R.E., Sur, C., Cook, J., Hargreaves, H., Burns, H.D., Hamill, T.G. (2008). A novel glycine transporter 1 PET tracer: from discovery to clinic. *Abstr Soc Neurosci*, 88515.

63. Egle, I., Delaney, W., Wang, Z., Shumacher, R., Hopper, A.T., Tehim, A., Maddarod, S. (2002). Wo Patent WO2002066456.

64. Kopec, K., Flood, D.G., Gasior, M., McKenna, B.A.W., Zuvich, E., Schreiber, J., Salvino, J.M., Durkin, J.T., Ator, M.A., Marino, M.J. (2010). Glycine transporter inhibitors with reduced residence time increase prepulse inhibition without inducing hyperlocomotion in DBA/2 mice. *Biochem Pharmacol*, *80*, 1407–1417.

65. Gomeza, J., Ohno, K., Huelsmann, S., Armsen, W., Eulenburg, V., Richter, D.W., Laube, B., Betz, H. (2003). Deletion of the mouse glycine transporter 2 results in a hyperekplexia phenotype and postnatal lethality. *Neuron*, *40*, 797–806.

66. Gomeza, J., Huelsmann, S., Ohno, K., Eulenburg, V., Szoeke, K., Richter, D., Betz, H. (2003). Inactivation of the glycine transporter 1 gene discloses vital role of glial glycine uptake in glycinergic inhibition. *Neuron*, *40*, 785–796.

67. Mezler, M., Hornberger, W., Mueller, R., Amberg, W., Schmidt, M., Braje, W., Ochse, M., Schoemaker, H., Behl, B. (2008). Inhibitors of GlyT1 affect glycine transport via discrete binding sites. *Mol Pharmacol*, *74*, 1705–1715.

68. Lidoe, H.H., Stomberg, R., Fagerberg, A., Ericson, M., Soederpalm, B. (2009). The glycine reuptake inhibitor Org 25935 interacts with basal and ethanol-induced dopamine release in rat nucleus accumbens. *Alcohol Clin Exp Res*, *33*, 1151–1157.

69. Molander, A., Lidoe, H.H., Loef, E., Ericson, M., Soederpalm, B. (2007). The glycine reuptake inhibitor Org 25935 decreases ethanol intake and preference in male Wistar rats. *Alcohol Alcohol*, *42*, 11–18.

70. Javitt, D.C., Silipo, G., Cienfuegos, A., Shelley, A., Bark, N., Park, M., Lindenmayer, J., Suckow, R., Zukin, S.R. (2001). Adjunctive high-dose glycine in the treatment of schizophrenia. *Int J Neuropsychopharmacol*, *4*, 385–391.

71. Tsai, G., Yang, P., Chung, L., Lange, N., Coyle, J.T. (1998). D-serine added to antipsychotics for the treatment of schizophrenia. *Biol Psychiatry*, *44*, 1081–1089.

72. Heresco-Levy, U., Javitt, D.C., Ebstein, R., Vass, A., Lichtenberg, P., Bar, G., Catinari, S., Ermilov, M. (2005). D-serine efficacy as add-on pharmacotherapy to risperidone and olanzapine for treatment-refractory schizophrenia. *Biol Psychiatry*, *57*, 577–585.

73. Tsai, G.E., Yang, P., Chang, Y., Chong, M. (2006). D-alanine added to antipsychotics for the treatment of schizophrenia. *Biol Psychiatry*, *59*, 230–234.

74. Lane, H., Chang, Y., Liu, Y., Chiu, C., Tsai, G.E. (2005). Sarcosine or D-serine add-on treatment for acute exacerbation of schizophrenia: a randomized, double-blind, placebo-controlled study. *Arch Gen Psychiatry*, *62*, 1196–2004.

75. Lane, H., Liu, Y., Huang, C., Chang, Y., Liau, C., Perng, C., Tsai, G.E. (2008). Sarcosine (N-methylglycine) treatment for acute schizophrenia: a randomized, double-blind study. *Biol Psychiatry*, *63*, 9–12.

76. Buchanan Robert, W., Javitt Daniel, C., Marder Stephen, R., Schooler Nina, R., Gold James, M., McMahon Robert, P., Heresco-Levy, U., Carpenter William, T. (2007). Cognitive and Negative Symptoms in Schizophrenia Trial (CONSIST): the efficacy of glutamatergic agents for negative symptoms and cognitive impairments. *Am J Psychiatry*, *164*, 1593–15602.

# 9

# COMBINED DOPAMINE $D_2$ AND 5-HYDROXYTRYPTAMINE $(5\text{-HT})_{1A}$ RECEPTOR STRATEGIES FOR THE TREATMENT OF SCHIZOPHRENIA: A PHARMACOLOGICAL AND CHEMICAL PERSPECTIVE

ANDREW C. MCCREARY, ROELOF W. FEENSTRA, AND CAITLIN A. JONES

## 9.1 INTRODUCTION

In its simplest form the dopamine hypothesis of schizophrenia predicts an overactive dopaminergic system in schizophrenia (see Chapter 2). Certainly dopamine $D_2$ receptor antagonists such as haloperidol and chlorpromazine display efficacy for the treatment of the positive symptoms of schizophrenia (auditory and visual hallucinations, delusions, conceptual disorganization, thought disorder, and some motor disturbances). Schizophrenia symptomatology is rather more complex, however, than just the expression of positive symptoms. Patients may present with additional, or a combination, of different symptom domains including negative symptoms (affective blunting, social withdrawal, anhedonia, avolition, and poverty of thought and speech), cognitive impairments such as working memory abnormalities, deficits of cognitive processing, and attention and affective disorders (depression and anxiety,

*Targets and Emerging Therapies for Schizophrenia*, First Edition.
Edited by Jeffrey S. Albert and Michael W. Wood.

which leads to blunted quality of life prognosis, suicidality, and increased relapse [1–5]).

## 9.2 THERAPEUTIC STRATEGIES FOR THE TREATMENT OF SCHIZOPHRENIA

True pharmacological management of schizophrenia was initiated in the late 1950s with the use of dopamine $D_2$ receptor antagonists such as haloperidol and chlorpromazine, which attenuate the putative hyperdopaminergic state expected to be seen in the disease [6, 7], thereby treating the positive symptoms. Apart from their limited therapeutic efficacy for the gamut of schizophrenic symptoms, dopamine antagonists have known neurological or motor side effects (or extrapyramidal side effects [EPS]) such as tardive dyskinesia dystonia, akathisia, and parkinsonism, which are treatment limiting and occur when approximately 80% of striatal $D_2$ receptor sites are occupied [8, 9]. Another common feature of dopamine antagonist administration is hyperprolactinemia, which results in a variety of hormonal disturbances [10–12]. Therefore, based on the limited therapeutic efficacy combined with adverse side effects, so-called atypical antipsychotics were developed as an alternative to the typical antipsychotics.

Atypical antipsychotics not only treat the positive symptoms but also have some, but limited, efficacy for the treatment of negative and partly cognitive aspects of schizophrenia [13]. The "richer" pharmacological activity of these agents at multi-receptor targets is hypothesised to mediate their actions in treating a range of symptom domains, whilst reducing their propensity to induce EPS or hyperprolactinemia [13, 14]. Atypical antipsychotics can, however, cause a multitude of other side effects including weight gain, insulin intolerance, dyslipidemia, and cardiac sequalae such as arrhythmia, blood pressure increases, and hyperprolactinemia (certain compounds), moreover the gold-standard drug, clozapine, has an identified risk of agranulocytosis [15–19].

A commonality of many atypical antipsychotics is their pharmacological actions at multiple serotonin (5-hydroxytryptamine; 5-HT) receptors including $5\text{-HT}_{2A}$, $5\text{-HT}_{2C}$, $5\text{-HT}_6$, and $5\text{-HT}_7$ receptors. Each of these targets are expected to convey particular effects either on the side effect profile and/or on the treatment of different symptom domains such as EPS reduction, negative symptom treatment, or effects in the cognitive or even positive symptom domains ([13, 20] see also Sections 4.2 and 4.3, respectively for further discussion). One of the 5-HT receptors that has recently gained recognition as a potential target warranting further attention is the $5\text{-HT}_{1A}$ receptor subtype (for recent pharmacological review see Reference [20]).

The pharmacological function of $5\text{-HT}_{1A}$ receptors has been extensively reviewed elsewhere [21]. Briefly, however, the $5\text{-HT}_{1A}$ receptor is a classical G-protein-linked receptor possessing high affinity for the endogenous ligand 5-HT. It was the first of the serotonergic receptors to be sequenced and is negatively coupled to adenylate cyclase [21]. The receptors are extensively distributed in limbic regions, such as hippocampus, lateral septum, cortical areas, hypothalamus, and the mid-brain raphe nuclei, and function both as a somatodendritic autoreceptor controlling feedback inhibition and as a postsynaptic receptor [21, 22]. The differential populations of receptors confer very different pharmacological actions with relevance to schizophrenia. Agonist actions at somatodendritic autoreceptors are thought to confer primary procognitive actions [22], while postsynaptic actions may attenuate cognitive processes via glutamatergic modulation of septo-hippocampal processes [22]. Together, these data have led to the suggestion that partial 5-$HT_{1A}$ receptor agonists might have utility for the treatment of cognition (for reviews see References [20, 22, 23]).

The antipsychotics risperidone, olanzapine, and haloperidol have limited affinity at 5-$HT_{1A}$ receptors [24, 25]. A variety of other clinically relevant and development candidates including ziprasidone, clozapine, nemonapride, S16924, bifeprunox, F-15063, SLV313, SSR181507, and aripiprazole have demonstrated (partial) agonist effects *in vitro* [20, 24–36] (Table 9.1).

## 9.3 COMBINED 5-$HT_{1A}$ AND $D_2$ RECEPTOR LIGANDS: CHEMICAL CONSIDERATIONS

The chemical structures of the receptor's endogenous ligands dopamine (DA) and serotonin (5-hydroxytryptamine [5-HT]), respectively, are depicted in Figure 9.1.

These small molecules have some common features: both possess the $NH_3^+$ moiety, a hydroxy group, and a phenyl ring. The first one, the $NH_3^+$ moiety, interacts with a negatively charged aspartic acid residue in the receptor, forming an electrostatic bond that contributes to the binding considerably. The hydroxy groups (may) form hydrogen bridges with, for example, serine, threonine, and tyrosine amino acid residues. The aromatic phenyl parts of the molecules may interact ($\pi$–$\pi$ interaction) with aromatic receptor residues (e.g., tryptophan, phenylalanine, tyrosine) or with positively charged residues (cation–$\pi$ interactions). Hydrophobic interactions are expected from nonpolar parts of both ligand and receptor.

A number of chemical entities (selected examples shown in Fig. 9.2) that have demonstrated simultaneous affinity for both dopamine $D_2$ and 5-$HT_{1A}$ receptors have been synthesized.

As can be seen from Figure 9.2, all molecules possess one or two phenyl rings within roughly the same distance to the basic nitrogen (circled). Although the depicted structures are quite different, it is possible to position the phenyl and the basic nitrogen (protonated under physiological conditions) in such a way that they match a common basic pharmacophore. Then the ligand may become permissive for binding. For both receptors the basic pharmacophores are depicted in Figure 9.3.

**TABLE 9.1** ***In Vitro*** **Affinities and Efficacies of Antipsychotics at DA $D_2$ and 5-$HT_{1A}$ Receptors**

| | $D_2$ | | | | 5-$HT_{1A}$ | | |
|---|---|---|---|---|---|---|---|
| | Affinity | Efficacy | | | Affinity | Efficacy | |
| | | [35S]-GTPγS Activation | | | | [35S]-GTPγS Activation | |
| Drugs | $pK_i$ | $pEC_{50}$ | $E_{max}$ | $pK_b$ | $pK_i$ | $pEC_{50}$ | $E_{max}$ |
| Haloperidol | 9.01 ± 0.01 | NC | 0.7 ± 2.3 | 9.12 ± 0.10 | 5.77 ± 0.04 | NC | –11.6 ± 2.2 |
| Clozapine | 6.83 ± 0.05 | NC | –4.0 ± 6.5 | 7.35 ± 0.10 | 6.31 ± 0.06 | NC | 7.5 ± 2.3 |
| Nemonapride | 9.92 ± 0.03 | NT | NT | NT | 8.35 ± 0.03 | 6.94 ± 0.09 | 25.7 ± 2.9 |
| Aripiprazole | 8.59 ± 0.15 | 8.56 ± 0.25 | 25.6 ± 1.2 | 9.36 ± 0.19 | 7.42 ± 0.13 | 6.43 ± 0.09 | 15.0 ± 0.6 |
| S16924 | 7.60 ± 0.01 | NR | NR | 7.47 ± 0.04 | 8.40 ± 0.01 | 8.00 ± 0.04 | 54.1 ± 11.3 |
| Bifeprunox | 8.83 ± 0.05 | 8.97 ± 0.12 | 26.6 ± 2.7 | 8.98 ± 0.33 | 7.19 ± 0.14 | 6.37 ± 0.11 | 35.9 ± 2.0 |
| F15063 | 9.38 ± 0.05 | NC | 0.00 | 8.29 ± 0.11 | 8.24 ± 0.07 | 7.47 ± 0.11 | 36.0 ± 4.0 |
| SLV313 | 8.58 ± 0.06 | NC | 8.0 ± 7.2 | 9.60 ± 0.13 | 8.64 ± 0.01 | 8.16 ± 0.03 | 19.0 ± 2.8 |
| SSR181507 | 8.41 ± 0.05 | 8.08 ± 0.15 | 17.5 ± 0.9 | 8.16 ± 0.29 | 8.53 ± 0.10 | 6.99 ± 0.27 | 35.9 ± 2.0 |

NC, value not calculated; NT, compound not tested; NR, value not reported.

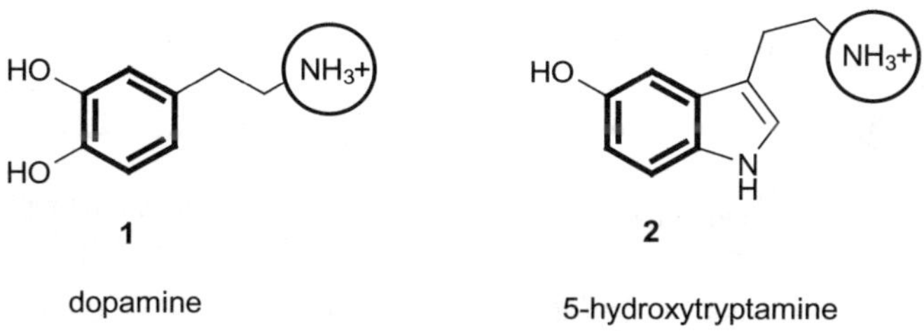


**FIGURE 9.1** Structures of dopamine and 5-hydroxytryptamine.

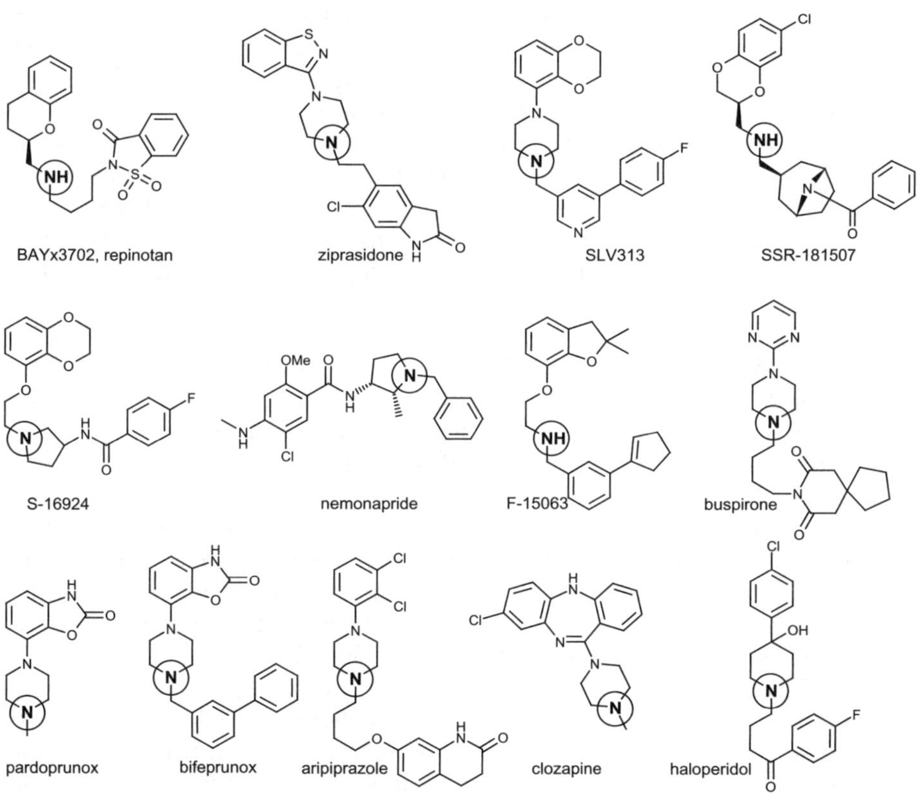


**FIGURE 9.2** Depiction of a range of molecules possessing dopamine $D_2$ receptor and/or 5-$HT_{1A}$ receptor effects. Ziprasidone, aripiprazole, SLV313, SSR181507, S16924, nemonapride, F-15063, and bifeprunox are putative atypical antipsychotics. Haloperidol is a classical antipsychotic ($D_2$ antagonist), and repinotan and buspirone have 5-$HT_{1A}$ agonist actions.

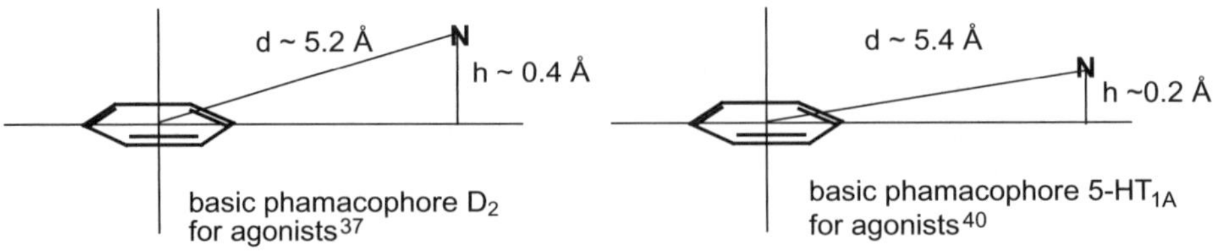


**FIGURE 9.3** Basic pharmacophores for the $D_2$ (left) and 5-$HT_{1A}$ receptors (right).

Pharmacophores for $D_2$ agonists have been proposed by Wilcox [37] while 5-$HT_{1A}$ agonist pharmacophores were developed by Hibert [38, 39] (for a recent reviews see Reference [40]). As can be seen the position of the nitrogen lies above the plane of the aromatic part for both pharmacophores, but the geometry (d and h) is different. For antagonists, the values of d and h might shift, with agonists being considerably higher, for example 5-$HT_{1A}$ antagonists d ~5.6 Å and h ~1.6 Å. The pharmacophores (Fig. 9.3) only describe the relative positions of the positively charged protonated nitrogen, which interacts strongly with the negatively charged aspartate of the receptor, and the position of the aromatic ring, but not the hydrogen bonding and hydrophobic interactions and the steric requirements that should be met. In the case of DA binding to its receptor, hydrogen-bonding interactions to three receptor serine residues and hydrophobic interaction with a receptor valine residue were proposed [41].

The molecular shape can be very different for the molecules depicted in Figure 9.2. When considering the structures of clozapine, haloperidol, and nemonapride, for example, it is not directly evident how they might all bind to the dopamine $D_2$ receptor. On preliminary inspection the molecules seem rather different in shape (Fig. 9.2), but three-dimensionally it appears possible to accommodate the three compounds into one DA $D_2$ pharmacophore [42, 43]. Interestingly, in this alignment, the phenyl of sulpiride, a close analog of nemonapride, is superimposed on haloperidol's phenyl adjacent to the carbonyl moiety and not on the phenyl connected to the piperidine portion. Other ways of generating $D_2$ pharmacophores have been described by Cottrell [43].

SLV313, SSR181507, nemonapride, and F-15063 bind potently to both DA $D_2$ and 5-$HT_{1A}$ receptors. These compounds are apparently able to adopt conformations that suit both pharmacophores, therefore yielding enough free enthalpy-driven interactions to bind to the receptors. In contrast, haloperidol only binds potently to the DA $D_2$ receptor, indicating that the molecule cannot conduct conformational alterations fitting the 5-$HT_{1A}$ receptor pharmacophore (pKi for 5-$HT_{1A}$ = 5.8).

As the chemical structure of a ligand determines the binding, it also influences the degree of agonism (i.e., the intrinsic activity, varying from 0% [full antagonist] to 100% [full agonist]). Structure–activity comparisons have been carried out, for example, for bifeprunox and SLV313 (Fig. 9.2) with regard to their intrinsic activity on DA $D_2$ and 5-HT receptors [44]. It appears that modification of the phenylpiperazine (head) part of the molecule dictates the degree of $D_2$ receptor agonism. For example, bifeprunox and pardoprunox share the benzoxazolonepiperazine head portion and both possess partial agonist properties at dopamine $D_2$ receptors (see Fig. 9.2; cf. References [44, 45]), while SLV313 contains a benzdioxyanepiperazine leading to full $D_2$ receptor antagonism. Conversely, modification of the biarylmethyl moiety (tail portion) of the molecule modulates the degree of agonism at the 5-$HT_{1A}$ receptor. The biphenylmethyl tail portion in bifeprunox induces partial agonism, whereas the 3-(4-fluoro-phenyl)pyridyl-5-yl-methyl portion in SLV313 induces full agonism at the 5-$HT_{1A}$ receptor.

Thus, within the series studied, and independent of the arylpiperazine head portion, the 3-(4-fluorophenyl) pyridyl-5-yl-methyl moiety induces full 5-$HT_{1A}$ receptor agonism [44]. Furthermore, independent of the biaryl methyl moiety, the benzdioxanepiperazine induces full $D_2$ receptor antagonism [44]. Together, such data demonstrate that molecules can be optimally designed to obtain the desired degree of 5-$HT_{1A}$ receptor agonism and $D_2$ receptor (ant)agonism.

## 9.4 EVIDENCE FOR THE UTILITY OF 5-$HT_{1A}$ RECEPTOR AGONISTS IN THE TREATMENT OF SCHIZOPHRENIA

Postmortem radioligand binding studies have assessed 5-$HT_{1A}$ receptor density in the schizophrenic brain. From such studies, mixed results have been noted in different brain areas, leading to contradictory findings. For example, in the prefrontal cortex (PFC), hippocampus, and medial and temporal lobes (including the amygdala), no changes, increases, or slight decreases in 5-$HT_{1A}$ receptor density were reported [46–49]. However, these data are confounded by the mixed-treatment status of patients (including patients receiving benzodiazepine treatment) and the inclusion of schizoaffective patients. Therefore, although these data are not conclusive, they do suggest that 5-$HT_{1A}$ receptor changes are apparent in the schizophrenic brain. Coupled with additional evidence (Section 13.5), a role of 5-$HT_{1A}$ receptors in the pathogenesis of schizophrenia is strongly implicated [20, 22, 50].

While probably an oversimplified hypothesis (for review see Reference [51]), it is thought that there is a "hypofrontal" phenomenon seen at the level of the medial PFC in schizophrenia [22]. Given the role of this brain area in the decision process, working memory, and attentional processing [52], this pathology might result in the expression of cognitive deficits, and some negative symptoms [53]. This suggests that normalization of "hypofrontality" per se represents a potential treatment strategy for negative or positive symptoms of schizophrenia. One such vehicle by which this could be mediated is by agonist actions at 5-$HT_{1A}$ receptors [20, 24]. The atypical antipsychotics, in contrast to typical antipsychotics, have demonstrated ability to augment DA and acetylcholine levels in the mPFCx by 5-$HT_{1A}$ receptor-dependent mechanisms [54–61], which are expected to predict their utility in treating negative and cognitive symptoms. Interestingly, SSR181507 and SLV313 display an increase in synaptic DA and acetylcholine in the mPFCx, which may play important roles in the mediation of mnemonic and cognitive processes [24, 62].

Mesolimbic dopaminergic projections originating from the ventral tegmental area (VTA) are important in the hyperactive dopaminergic system resulting in positive symptoms, while a hypoactive system is proposed for mesocortical DA tone [63–66]. The VTA receives serotonergic efferents from the dorsal raphe nucleus (DRN), which are under negative feedback control by somatodendritic 5-$HT_{1A}$ receptors [67–69]. The firing of dopaminergic neurons in the VTA is also modulated by pyramidal cell afferents from the mPFCx as projections from the mPFCx to the VTA caused 5-$HT_{1A}$ receptor-dependent excitation of 75% of neurons [61, 70]. This indicates that effects on 5-$HT_{1A}$ receptors can modulate pyramidal cell function, leading either to direct (pyramidal) or to indirect (via $\gamma$-aminobutyric acid [GABA] interneurons synapsing on pyramidal neurons) changes in the VTA. Furthermore, *in vivo* microdialysis studies following reverse microdialysis administration of repinotan into the mPFCx augmented local DA efflux in the VTA [61]. These effects were absent in homozygous 5-$HT_{1A}$ receptor knockout mice where DA augmentation following antipsychotics was also absent [61]. Taken together, these data support a pivotal role of mPFCx 5-$HT_{1A}$ receptors in modulating mesocorticolimbic dopaminergic neurotransmission and reinforce the potential importance of 5-$HT_{1A}$ receptors in the modulation of the neurocircuitry impacted in schizophrenia.

## 9.5 THE THERAPEUTIC EFFICACY OF COMBINED 5-$HT_{1A}$ RECEPTOR (PARTIAL) AGONISTS AND $D_2$ RECEPTOR (PARTIAL) ANTAGONISTS AGAINST SCHIZOPHRENIA

The hypothesis therefore suggests that 5-$HT_{1A}$-dependent enhancement of dopaminergic and cholinergic function will translate into efficacy in negative and cognitive domains. This is partly supported clinically by combined treatment with the 5-$HT_{1A}$ receptor (partial) agonist buspirone or tandospirone with antipsychotics, and the observation that certain types of cognitive performance in schizophrenic patients are improved [71–74]. However, data showing the improvement of negative symptoms have been less convincing; beneficial effects of tandospirone and buspirone were not seen in double-blind placebo-controlled studies [71–75], although open-label data were positive [76]. In animal models of the cognitive deficits of schizophrenia, the mixed dopamine $D_2$ receptor (partial) (ant)agonists and 5-$HT_{1A}$ receptor (partial) (ant)agonists SSR181507, aripiprazole, SLV313, and F-15063 improved cognitive flexibility [29, 77, 78], and SLV313 and bifeprunox have both been reported to reduce novel object recognition deficits induced by MK-801 and PCP [79]. Moreover, the five-choice-serial reaction time task showed that either systemic or intra-PFC administration of the 5-$HT_{1A}$ receptor agonist 8-OH-DPAT improved attentional processing [80]. Aripiprazole, SSR181507, and F-15063 also improve negative-symptom-like behavior in the social interaction test [78, 81, 82]. Thus, there is compelling evidence that 5-$HT_{1A}$ receptor agonism could help in modulating negative, cognitive, and attentional processes that might be relevant in the treatment of schizophrenia (see Table 9.2).

The ability of dopamine $D_2$ receptor antagonists to induce treatment-limiting EPS has been well documented. Although atypical antipsychotics remain the drugs of choice in the treatment of schizophrenia symptoms, other relevant avenues have been evaluated due to concerns regarding the side effects of atypical antipsychotics, for example, olanzapine and the induction of metabolic syndrome. The combination of $D_2$ receptor antagonism (or partial agonism) with 5-$HT_{1A}$ (partial receptor) receptor agonism suggests an extension of the therapeutic window over $D_2$ receptor antagonism alone. DA receptor partial agonists have received much attention in recent years as potential therapeutic targets for schizophrenia as they have reportedly displayed improved treatment efficacy with fewer and less severe side effects when compared with full $D_2$ receptor antagonists [83]. It is thought that this improved efficacy stems from the more modulatory nature or "dopamine stabilizing" properties of the compounds in conditions of both high and low tone [83]. During periods of low dopaminergic tone or in areas with a high $D_2$ receptor reserve, a partial agonist will act as full dopaminergic agonist and thus stuimulate activity. Conversely under high tone conditions they will act as full inhibitory antagonists. In conditions of normotensive tone, partial agonists will remain inert.

The role of the 5-$HT_{1A}$ receptor in ameliorating dopamine $D_2$ receptor-mediated catalepsy has been demonstrated in rodents (Table 9.2). Administration of the 5-$HT_{1A}$ receptor antagonist WAY100635 prior to bifeprunox, SLV313, and F-15063 unmasked catalepsy [84, 85]. Moreover, the 5-$HT_{1A}$ agonist effects of these compounds reduced haloperidol-mediated catalepsy [84, 85]. The mesolimbic (vs. mesostriatal) selectivity of combined $D_2$ receptor antagonists and 5-$HT_{1A}$ agonists is also supported by data suggesting that depolarization blockade of identified VTA dopaminergic neurons (vs. substantia nigra zona compacta DA neurons) is seen following chronic administration of SLV313 [24]. The contribution of 5-$HT_{1A}$ receptors in mediating this effect is suggested [67], but the population of receptors mediating the effect needs to be elucidated.

One prospective limitation of combined $D_2$ receptor antagonism and 5-$HT_{1A}$ receptor agonism lies not only with the ability of 5-$HT_{1A}$ agonists to induce components of the 5-HT syndrome, but also with the ability to disrupt sensorimotor gating (or prepulse inhibition [PPI]). SLV313, SSR181507, and bifeprunox were indeed found to disrupt PPI [86, 87]. Furthermore, in antagonist studies with WAY100635, this disruption was transformed into a reversal of PPI deficits [86, 87]. However, if one is to consider that PPI (in the rat)

**TABLE 9.2 The Effect of Drugs in Preclinical Models Predictive of Positive Symptoms, EPS, and Hyperprolactinemia**

| | | | Behavioral Model | | | | | | | |
|---|---|---|---|---|---|---|---|---|---|---|
| | | | Apomorphine-Induced | | *d*-Amph-Induced | Conditioned Avoidance Response | Catalepsy | | Prolactin | |
| | | | ED$_{50}$ (95% CI) | | | | | | | |
| Drug | Dose Range | Route | Climbing | PPI Disruption | Hyperactivity | | CLP Test | Bar Test | | $E_{max}$ |
| Haloperidol | 0.01–10 | s.c. | 0.09 (0.05–0.17) | 0.63 | 0.09 (0.04–0.17) | 0.07 (0.03–0.16) | 0.3 (0.16–0.55) | 0.59 (0.28–1.3) | 0.22 (0.06–0.8) | 82.8 ± 5.4 |
| Clozapine | 0.01–40 | i.p./s.c. | 8.7 (3.1–25) | 40 | 1.6 (0.65–3.7) | 1.4 (0.37–4.7) | 28 (12–66) | >40 | 20 | 41.5 ± 6.9 |
| Aripiprazole | 0.01–40 | i.p. | 2.2 (0.39–12) | 0.04 | 6.2 (2.6–15) | 3.2 (1.1–9.1) | >40 | >40 | 0.66 (0.04–10) | 31.6 ± 9.0 |
| S16924 | 0.01–80 | s.c. | 0.17 (0.08–0.4) | NT | 2.4 (1.6–3.7) | 1.4 (0.8–2.3) | >80 | NT | 2.5[a] | 51.7 ± 7.7 |
| Bifeprunox | 0.01–40 | i.p. | 0.03 (0.01–0.07) | 0.04 | 0.32 (0.06–1.8) | 0.03 (0.01–0.05) | >40 | >40 | >40 | 12.6 ± 1.4 |
| F15063 | 0.1–40 | i.p. | 0.3 (0.14–0.63) | 16 | 0.23 (0.15–0.31) | 0.33 (0.19–0.55) | >40 | >40 | 0.63[a] | 91.6 ± 9.6 |
| SLV313 | 0.04–40 | i.p./s.c. | 0.04 (0.01–0.16) | >10 | 0.28 (0.13–0.59) | 0.25 (0.12–0.52) | >40 | >40 | 0.12 (0.04–0.37) | 86.1 ± 11.9 |
| SSR181507 | 0.16–40 | i.p./s.c. | 3.6 (1.5–8.7) | >10 | 3.2 (1.1–9.0) | 0.58 (0.19–1.8) | >40 | >40 | 4.9 (0.81–29.8) | 23.0 ± 4.1 |

models the positive symptoms (or even cognitive symptoms of schizophrenia), then 5-$HT_{1A}$ receptor agonism might be considered detrimental to the treatment of the disease [20]. However, no empirical data from clinical studies support this assumption in healthy volunteers or schizophrenic patients. Moreover, buspirone and tandospirone might be expected to worsen clinical parameters of schizophrenia, while the contrary is the case. Therefore, there appears no emphatic evidence for this hypothesis. 5-$HT_{1A}$ receptor-mediated syndrome has been seen following SLV313 in contrast to SSR181507 [24, 88]. This has led to the suggestion that compounds that mediate 5-$HT_{1A}$ syndrome behaviors in rats (or mice) are expected to mediate this phenomenon in humans. To the best of the authors' knowledge, no translational data are yet available supporting this hypothesis.

## 9.6 EFFECTS ON COMORBID AFFECTIVE DISORDERS

One of the many aspects of schizophrenia deserving of better clinical management is the treatment of the anxiety and depressive symptoms, which are common in schizophrenics, and of key prognostic relevance [1, 2, 4, 5, 13, 89]. The role of 5-$HT_{1A}$ receptors in the modulation of anxiety and depressive symptoms is well known [90, 91]. Therefore compounds possessing 5-$HT_{1A}$ receptor agonist effects are expected to offer significant advantages in the clinical management of anxiolytic and antidepressant clinical management potential [20, 22, 92, 93]. Recent preclinical evidence supports this notion. Bifeprunox, SSR181507, and SLV313 all demonstrate anxiolytic-like and antidepressive-like properties [88, 94].

## 9.7 CONCLUSIONS

In general conclusion, there is a body of preclinical and clinical evidence supporting a role for the utility of 5-$HT_{1A}$ receptor (partial) agonists combined with $D_2$ receptor antagonist or partial agonists for treating the full range of the clinical manifestations of schizophrenia. However, while 5-$HT_{1A}$ receptor agonism does not impact $D_2$ receptor antagonist-induced hyperprolactinemia, the reduction of other side effects is observed. However, with careful chemical modification, it is possible to switch from a more antagonist profile to a partial agonist nature, thereby reducing prolactin increase while maintaining antipsychotic efficacy. The employment of partial DA receptor agonists appears to create a stabilization of the dopaminergic system, for example abrogating prolactin increases and EPS. The addition of a 5-$HT_{1A}$ agonist moiety assists in reducing side effects such as EPS and may reduce additional symptom sequalae of schizophrenia. Together, such properties may effectively increase the therapeutic window for the treatment of schizophrenia, rendering this an important area for research toward novel antipsychotic medications.

## REFERENCES

1. Andreasen, N. (1995). Symptoms, signs, and diagnosis of schizophrenia. *Lancet*, *346*, 477–481.
2. Meltzer, H. (1998). Suicide in schizophrenia: risk factors and clozapine treatment. *J Clin Psychiatry*, *59*(Suppl 3), 15–20.
3. Meltzer, H. (1999). The role of serotonin in antipsychotic drug action. *Neuropsychopharmacology*, *21*, 106S–115S.
4. Möller, H. (2005). Occurrence and treatment of depressive comorbidity/cosyndromality in schizophrenic psychoses: conceptual and treatment issues. *World J Biol Psychiatry*, *6*, 247–263.
5. Siris, S.G. (2000). Depression in schizophrenia: perspective in the era of "atypical" antipsychotic agents. *Am J Psychiatry*, *157*, 1379–1389.
6. Granger, B., Albu, S. (2005). The haloperidol story. *Ann Clin Psychiatry*, *17*, 137–140.
7. López-Muñoz, F., Alamo, C., Cuenca, E., Shen, W., Clervoy, P., Rubio, G. (2005). History of the discovery and clinical introduction of chlorpromazine. *Ann Clin Psychiatry*, *17*, 113–135.
8. Seeman, P., Lee, T., Chau-Wong, M., Wong, K. (1976). Antipsychotic drug doses and neuroleptic/dopamine receptors. *Nature*, *261*, 717–719.
9. Seeman, P., Kapur, S. (2000). Schizophrenia: more dopamine, more D2 receptors. *Proc Natl Acad Sci U S A*, *97*, 7673–7675.
10. Langer, G., Sachar, E. (1977). Dopaminergic factors in human prolactin regulation: effects of neuroleptics and dopamine. *Psychoneuroendocrinology*, *2*, 373–378.
11. Halbreich, U., Kinon, B., Gilmore, J., Kahn, L. (2003). Elevated prolactin levels in patients with schizophrenia: mechanisms and related adverse effects. *Psychoneuroendocrinology*, *28*(Suppl 1), 53–67.
12. Kinon, B., Gilmore, J., Liu, H., Halbreich, U. (2003). Hyperprolactinemia in response to antipsychotic drugs: characterization across comparative clinical trials. *Psychoneuroendocrinology*, *28*(Suppl 2), 69–82.
13. Meltzer, H.Y., Park, S., Kessler, R. (1999). Cognition, schizophrenia, and the atypical antipsychotic drugs. *Proc Natl Acad Sci U S A*, *96*, 13591–13593.
14. Meltzer, H., Li, Z., Kaneda, Y., Ichikawa, J. (2003). Serotonin receptors: their key role in drugs to treat schizophrenia. *Prog Neuropsychopharmacol Biol Psychiatry*, *27*, 1159–1172.
15. Meltzer, H. (1994). An overview of the mechanism of action of clozapine. *J Clin Psychiatry*, *55*(Suppl B), 47–52.
16. Allison, D., Mentore, J., Heo, M., Chandler, L., Cappelleri, J., Infante, M., Weiden, P. (1999). Antipsychotic-induced weight gain: a comprehensive research synthesis. *Am J Psychiatry*, *156*, 1686–1696.
17. Kasper, S., Hale, A., Azorin, J., Möller, H. (1999). Benefit-risk evaluation of olanzapine, risperidone and sertindole in the treatment of schizophrenia. *Eur Arch Psychiatry Clin Neurosci*, *249*, 1–14.
18. Haddad, P. (2005). Weight change with atypical antipsychotics in the treatment of schizophrenia. *J Psychopharmacol*, *19*, 16–27.

19. Haupt, D. (2006). Differential metabolic effects of antipsychotic treatments. *Eur Neuropsychopharmacol*, *16*(Suppl 3), S149–S155.

20. Jones, C.A., McCreary, A.C. (2008). Serotonergic approaches in the development of novel antipsychotics. *Neuropharmacology*, *55*, 1056–1065.

21. Barnes, N.M., Sharp, T. (1999). A review of central 5-HT receptors and their function. *Neuropharmacology*, *38*, 1083–1152.

22. Millan, M.J. (2000). Improving the treatment of schizophrenia: focus on serotonin (5-HT)1A receptors. *J Pharmacol Exp Ther*, *295*, 853–861.

23. King, M., Marsden, C., Fone, K. (2008). A role for the 5-HT(1A), 5-HT4 and 5-HT6 receptors in learning and memory. *Trends Pharmacol Sci*, *29*, 482–492.

24. McCreary, A.C., Glennon, J.C., Ashby, C.R., Jr, Meltzer, H.Y., Li, Z., Reinders, J.-H., Hesselink, M.B., Long, S.K., Herremans, A.H., van Stuivenberg, H., Feenstra, R.W., Kruse, C.G. (2007). SLV313 (1-(2,3-dihydro-benzo[lsqb]1,4[rsqb]dioxin-5-yl)-4-[lsqb]5-(4-fluoro-phenyl)-pyridin-3-ylmethyl[rsqb]-piperazine monohydrochloride): a novel dopamine D2 receptor antagonist and 5-HT1A receptor agonist potential antipsychotic drug. *Neuropsychopharmacology*, *32*, 78–94.

25. Newman-Tancredi, A., Assié, M., Leduc, N., Ormière, A., Danty, N., Cosi, C. (2005). Novel antipsychotics activate recombinant human and native rat serotonin 5-HT1A receptors: affinity, efficacy and potential implications for treatment of schizophrenia. *Int J Neuropsychopharmacol*, *8*, 341–356.

26. Cosi, C., Carilla-Durand, E., Assie, M.B., Ormiere, A.M., Maraval, M., Leduc, N., Newman-Tancredi, A. (2006). Partial agonist properties of the antipsychotics SSR181507, aripiprazole and bifeprunox at dopamine D2 receptors: G protein activation and prolactin release. *Eur J Pharmacol*, *535*, 135–144.

27. Newman-Tancredi, A., Assie, M.B., Martel, J.C., Cosi, C., Slot, L.B., Palmier, C., Rauly-Lestienne, I., Colpaert, F., Vacher, B., Cussac, D. (2007). F15063, a potential antipsychotic with D2//D3 antagonist, 5-HT1A agonist and D4 partial agonist properties: (I) in vitro receptor affinity and efficacy profile. *Br J Pharmacol*, *151*, 237–252.

28. Newman-Tancredi, A., Chaput, C., Verriele, L., Millan, M.J. (1996). Clozapine is a partial agonist at cloned, human serotonin 5-HT1A receptors. *Neuropharmacology*, *35*, 119–121.

29. Newman-Tancredi, A., Cussac, D., Depoortere, R. (2007). Neuropharmacological profile of bifeprunox: merits and limitations in comparison with other third-generation antipsychotics. *Curr Opin Investig Drugs*, *8*, 539–554.

30. Newman-Tancredi, A., Gavaudan, S., Conte, C., Chaput, C., Touzard, M., Verriele, L., Audinot, V., Millan, M.J. (1998). Agonist and antagonist actions of antipsychotic agents at 5-HT1A receptors: a []GTP[gamma]S binding study. *Eur J Pharmacol*, *355*, 245–256.

31. Millan, M.J., Schreiber, R., Dekeyne, A., Rivet, J.-M., Bervoets, K., Mavridis, M., Sebban, C., Maurel-Remy, S., Newman-Tancredi, A., Spedding, M., Muller, O., Lavielle, G., Brocco, M.S. (1998). 16924 ((R)-2-{1-[2-(2,3-dihydro-benzo[1,4] dioxin-5-yloxy)-ethyl]-pyrrolidin-3yl}-1-(4-fluoro-phenyl)-ethanone), a novel, potential antipsychotic with marked serotonin (5-HT)1A agonist properties: II. Functional profile in comparison to clozapine and haloperidol. *J Pharmacol Exp Ther*, *286*, 1356–1373.

32. Mason, S., Reynolds, G. (1992). Clozapine has submicromolar affinity for 5-HT1A receptors in human brain tissue. *Eur J Pharmacol*, *221*, 397–398.

33. Burris, K.D., Molski, T.F., Xu, C., Ryan, E., Tottori, K., Kikuchi, T., Yocca, F.D., Molinoff, P.B. (2002). Aripiprazole, a novel antipsychotic, is a high-affinity partial agonist at human dopamine D2 receptors. *J Pharmacol Exp Ther*, *302*, 381–389.

34. Tadori, Y., Miwa, T., Tottori, K., Burris, K., Stark, A., Mori, T., Kikuchi, T. (2005). Aripiprazole's low intrinsic activities at human dopamine D2L and D2S receptors render it a unique antipsychotic. *Eur J Pharmacol*, *515*, 10–19.

35. Jordan, S., Koprivica, V., Chen, R., Tottori, K., Kikuchi, T., Altar, C.A. (2002). The antipsychotic aripiprazole is a potent, partial agonist at the human 5-HT1A receptor. *Eur J Pharmacol*, *441*, 137–140.

36. Shapiro, D.A., Renock, S., Arrington, E., Chiodo, L.A., Liu, L.-X., Sibley, D.R., Roth, B.L., Mailman, R. (2003). Aripiprazole, a novel atypical antipsychotic drug with a unique and robust pharmacology. *Neuropsychopharmacology*, *28*, 1400–1411.

37. Wilcox, R.E., Huang, W.-H., Brusniak, M.-Y..K., Wilcox, D.M., Pearlman, R.S., Teeter, M.M., DuRand, C.J., Wiens, B.L., Neve, K.A. (2000). CoMFA-based prediction of agonist activities at recombinant wild type versus serine to alanine point mutated D2 dopamine receptors. *J Med Chem*, *43*, 3005–3019.

38. Hibert, M.F., Gittos, M.W., Middlemiss, D.N., Mir, A.K., Fozard, J.R. (1988). Graphics computer-aided receptor mapping as a predictive tool for drug design: development of potent, selective, and stereospecific ligands for the 5-HT1A receptor. *J Med Chem*, *31*, 1087–1093.

39. Hibert, M.F., McDermontt, I., Middlemiss, D.N., Mir, A.K., Fozard, J.R. (1989). Radioligand binding study of a series of 5-HT1A receptor agonists and definition of a steric model of this site. *Eur J Med Chem*, *24*, 31–37.

40. Bojarski, A.J. (2006). Pharmacophore models for metabotropic 5-HT receptor ligands. *Curr Top Med Chem*, *6*, 2005–2026.

41. Xhaard, H., Rantanen, V.-V., Nyrönen, T., Johnson, M.S. (2006). Molecular evolution of adrenoceptors and dopamine receptors: implications for the binding of catecholamines. *J Med Chem*, *49*, 1706–1719.

42. Atlamazoglou, V., Thireou, T., Eliopoulos, E. (2007). Using a pharmacophore presentation concept to elucidate molecular similarity of dopamine antagonists. *J Comput Aided Mol Des*, *21*, 239–241.

43. Cottrell, S.J., Gillet, V.J., Taylor, R., Wilton, D.J. (2004). Generation of multiple pharmacophore hypotheses using multiobjective optimisation techniques. *J Comput Aided Mol Des*, *18*, 665–682.

44. Feenstra, R.W., van den Hoogenband, A., Stroomer, C.N.J., van Stuivenberg, H.H., Tulp, M.T.M., Long, S.K., van der Heyden, J.A.M., Kruse, C.G. (2006). SAR study of 1-aryl-4-(phenylarylmethyl)piperazines as ligands for both dopamine D2 and serotonin 5-HT1A receptors showing varying degrees of (ant)agonism. Selection of a potential atypical antipsychotic. *Chem Pharm Bull (Tokyo)*, *54*, 1326–1330.

45. Glennon, J., Van Scharrenburg, G., Ronken, E., Hesselink, M., Reinders, J., Van Der Neut, M., Long, S., Feenstra, R., McCreary, A. (2006). In vitro characterization of SLV308 (7-[4-methyl-1-piperazinyl]-2(3H)-benzoxazolone, monohydrochloride): a novel partial dopamine D2 and D3 receptor agonist and serotonin 5-HT1A receptor agonist. *Synapse*, *60*, 599–608.

46. Hashimoto, T., Nishino, N., Nakai, H., Tanaka, C. (1991). Increase in serotonin 5-HT1A receptors in prefrontal and temporal cortices of brains from patients with chronic schizophrenia. *Life Sci*, *48*, 355–363.
47. Burnet, P., Eastwood, S., Harrison, P. (1996). 5-HT1A and 5-HT2A receptor mRNAs and binding site densities are differentially altered in schizophrenia. *Neuropsychopharmacology*, *15*, 442–455.
48. Tauscher, J., Kapur, S., Verhoeff, N.P.L.G., Hussey, D.F., Daskalakis, Z.J., Tauscher-Wisniewski, S., Wilson, A.A., Houle, S., Kasper, S., Zipursky, R.B. (2002). Brain serotonin 5-HT1A receptor binding in schizophrenia measured by positron emission tomography and [11C]WAY-100635. *Arch Gen Psychiatry*, *59*, 514–520.
49. Yasuno, F., Suhara, T., Ichimiya, T., Takano, A., Ando, T., Okubo, Y. (2004). Decreased 5-HT1A receptor binding in amygdala of schizophrenia. *Biol Psychiatry*, *55*, 439–444.
50. Bantick, R.A., Deakin, J.F.W., Grasby, P. (2001). The 5-HT1A receptor in schizophrenia: a promising target for novel atypical neuroleptics? *J Psychopharmacol*, *15*, 37–46.
51. Glahn, D., Ragland, J., Abramoff, A., Barrett, J., Laird, A., Bearden, C., Velligan, D. (2005). Beyond hypofrontality: a quantitative meta-analysis of functional neuroimaging studies of working memory in schizophrenia. *Hum Brain Mapp*, *25*, 60–69.
52. Goldman-Rakic, P. (1998). The cortical dopamine system: role in memory and cognition. *Adv Pharmacol*, *42*, 707–711.
53. Weinberger, D., Lipska, B. (1995). Cortical maldevelopment, anti-psychotic drugs, and schizophrenia: a search for common ground. *Schizophr Res*, *16*, 87–110.
54. Ichikawa, J., Dai, J., Meltzer, H. (2002). 5-HT(1A) and 5-HT(2A) receptors minimally contribute to clozapine-induced acetylcholine release in rat medial prefrontal cortex. *Brain Res*, *939*, 34–42.
55. Ichikawa, J., Dai, J., O'Laughlin, I., Fowler, W., Meltzer, H. (2002). Atypical, but not typical, antipsychotic drugs increase cortical acetylcholine release without an effect in the nucleus accumbens or striatum. *Neuropsychopharmacology*, *26*, 325–339.
56. Ichikawa, J., Ishii, H., Bonaccorso, S., Fowler, W., O'Laughlin, I., Meltzer, H. (2001). 5-HT(2A) and D(2) receptor blockade increases cortical DA release via 5-HT(1A) receptor activation: a possible mechanism of atypical antipsychotic-induced cortical dopamine release. *J Neurochem*, *76*, 1521–1531.
57. Li, Z., Ichikawa, J., Dai, J., Meltzer, H. (2004). Aripiprazole, a novel antipsychotic drug, preferentially increases dopamine release in the prefrontal cortex and hippocampus in rat brain. *Eur J Pharmacol*, *493*, 75–83.
58. Pehek, E., Meltzer, H., Yamamoto, B. (1993). The atypical antipsychotic drug amperozide enhances rat cortical and striatal dopamine efflux. *Eur J Pharmacol*, *240*, 107–109.
59. Nomikos, G., Iurlo, M., Andersson, J., Kimura, K., Svensson, T. (1994). Systemic administration of amperozide, a new atypical antipsychotic drug, preferentially increases dopamine release in the rat medial prefrontal cortex. *Psychopharmacology*, *115*, 147–156.
60. Rollema, H., Lu, Y., Schmidt, A., Zorn, S. (1997). Clozapine increases dopamine release in prefrontal cortex by 5-HT1A receptor activation. *Eur J Pharmacol*, *338*, R3–R5.

61. Diaz-Mataix, L., Scorza, M.C., Bortolozzi, A., Toth, M., Celada, P., Artigas, F. (2005). Involvement of 5-HT1A receptors in prefrontal cortex in the modulation of dopaminergic activity: role in atypical antipsychotic action. *J Neurosci*, *25*, 10831–10843.
62. Claustre, Y., Peretti, D.D., Brun, P., Gueudet, C., Allouard, N., Alonso, R., Lourdelet, J., Oblin, A., Damoiseau, G., Francon, D., Suaud-Chagny, M.-F., Steinberg, R., Sevrin, M., Schoemaker, H., George, P., Soubrie, P., Scatton, B. (2003). SSR181507, a dopamine D2 receptor antagonist and 5-HT1A receptor agonist. I: neurochemical and electrophysiological profile. *Neuropsychopharmacology*, *28*, 2064–2076.
63. Abi-Dargham, A., Rodenhiser, J., Printz, D., Zea-Ponce, Y., Gil, R., Kegeles, L.S., Weiss, R., Cooper, T.B., Mann, J.J., van Heertum, R.L., Gorman, J.M., Laruelle, M. (2000). Increased baseline occupancy of D2 receptors by dopamine in schizophrenia. *Proc Natl Acad Sci U S A*, *97*, 8104–8109.
64. Laruelle, M., Abi-Dargham, A., van Dyc, C.H., Gil, R., D'Souza, C.D., Erdos, J., McCance, E., Rosenblatt, W., Fingado, C., Zoghbi, S.S., Baldwin, R.M., Seibyl, J.P., Krystal, J.H., Charney, D.S., Innis, R.B. (1996). Single photon emission computerized tomography imaging of amphetamine-induced dopamine release in drug-free schizophrenic subjects. *Proc Natl Acad Sci U S A*, *93*, 9235–9240.
65. Carlsson, A. (1988). The current staus of the the dopamine hypothesis of schizophrenia. *Neuropsychopharmacology*, *1*, 179–186.
66. Weinberger, D.R., Aloia, M.S., Goldberg, T.E., Berman, K.F. (1994). The frontal lobes and schizophrenia. *J Neuropsychiatry Clin Neurosci*, *6*, 419–427.
67. Nakamura, K., Suzuki, K., McCreary, A., Ashby, C.J. (2006). The acute and chronic administration of (+/–)-8-hydroxy-2-(Di-n-propylamino)tetralin significantly alters the activity of spontaneously active midbrain dopamine neurons in rats: an in vivo electrophysiological study. *Synapse*, *59*, 359–367.
68. Lejeune, F., Millan, M.J. (1998). Induction of burst firing in ventral tegmental area dopaminergic neurons by activation of serotonin (5-HT)1A receptors: WAY 100,635-reversible actions of the highly selective ligands, flesinoxan and S 15535. *Synapse*, *30*, 172–180.
69. Arborelius, L., Chergui, K., Murase, S., Nomikos, G., Höök, B., Chouvet, G., Hacksell, U., Svensson, T. (1993). The 5-HT1A receptor selective ligands, (R)-8-OH-DPAT and (S)-UH-301, differentially affect the activity of midbrain dopamine neurons. *Naunyn Schmiedebergs Arch Pharmacol*, *347*, 353–362.
70. Santana, N., Bortolozzi, A., Serrats, J., Mengod, G., Artigas, F. (2004). Expression of serotonin1A and serotonin2A receptors in pyramidal and GABAergic neurons of the rat prefrontal cortex. *Cereb Cortex*, *14*, 1100–1109.
71. Sumiyoshi, T., Matsui, M., Nohara, S., Yamashita, I., Kurachi, M., Sumiyoshi, C., Jayathilake, K., Meltzer, H.Y. (2001). Enhancement of cognitive performance in schizophrenia by addition of tandospirone to neuroleptic treatment. *Am J Psychiatry*, *158*, 1722–1725.
72. Sumiyoshi, T., Matsui, M., Yamashita, I., Nohara, S., Kurachi, M., Uehara, T., Sumiyoshi, S., Sumiyoshi, C., Meltzer, H. (2001). The effect of tandospirone, a serotonin1A agonist, on memory function in schizophrenia. *Biol Psychiatry*, *49*, 861–868.
73. Sumiyoshi, T., Matsui, M., Yamashita, I., Nohara, S., Uehara, T., Kurachi, M., Meltzer, H. (2000). Effect of adjunctive treatment with serotonin-1A agonist tandospirone on memory functions in schizophrenia. *J Clin Psychopharmacol*, *20*, 386–388.

74. Sumiyoshi, T., Park, S., Jayathilake, K., Roy, A., Ertugrul, A., Meltzer, H. (2007). Effect of buspirone, a serotonin1A partial agonist, on cognitive function in schizophrenia: a randomized, double-blind, placebo-controlled study. *Schizophr Res*, *95*, 158–168.

75. Goff, D., Midha, K., Brotman, A., McCormick, S., Waites, M., Amico, E. (1991). An open trial of buspirone added to neuroleptics in schizophrenic patients. *J Clin Psychopharmacol*, *11*, 193–197.

76. Sirota, P., Epstein, B., Benatov, R., Sousnostzky, M., Kindler, S. (2001). An open study of buspirone augmentation of neuroleptics in patients with schizophrenia. *J Clin Psychopharmacol*, *21*, 454–455.

77. Bardin, L., Kleven, M.S., Barret-Grevoz, C., Depoortère, R., Newman-Tancredi, A. (2006). Antipsychotic-like vs cataleptogenic actions in mice of novel antipsychotics having D2 antagonist and 5-HT1A agonist properties. *Neuropsychopharmacology*, *31*, 1869–1879.

78. Depoortère, R., Auclair, A.L., Bardin, L., Slot, L.B., Kleven, M.S., Colpaert, F., Vacher, B., Newman-Tancredi, A. (2007). F15063, a compound with D2//D3 antagonist, 5-HT1A agonist and D4 partial agonist properties: (III) activity in models of cognition and negative symptoms. *Br J Pharmacol*, *151*, 266–277.

79. Neill, J., Grayson, B., Idris, N., Arnt, J. (2008). Bifeprunox and aripiprazole improve PCP-induced object recognition and deficits in rats: potential role for 5-HT1A receptor agonism in ameliorating cognitive deficit symptoms in schizophrenia. *Fundam Clin Pharmacol*, *22*, 119–131.

80. Winstanley, C., Chudasama, Y., Dalley, J., Theobald, D., Glennon, J., Robbins, T. (2003). Intra-prefrontal 8-OH-DPAT and M100907 improve visuospatial attention and decrease impulsivity on the five-choice serial reaction time task in rats. *Psychopharmacology*, *167*, 304–314.

81. Bruins Slot, L.A., Kleven, M.S., Newman-Tancredi, A. (2005). Effects of novel antipsychotics with mixed D2 antagonist/5-HT1A agonist properties on PCP-induced social interaction deficits in the rat. *Neuropharmacology*, *49*, 996–1006.

82. Boulay, D., Depoortere, R., Louis, C., Perrault, G., Griebel, G., Soubrie, P. (2004). SSR181507, a putative atypical antipsychotic with dopamine D2 antagonist and 5-HT1A agonist activities: improvement of social interaction deficits induced by phencyclidine in rats. *Neuropharmacology*, *46*, 1121–1129.

83. Tamminga, C., Carlsson, A. (2002). Partial dopamine agonists and dopaminergic stabilizers, in the treatment of psychosis. *Curr Drug Targets CNS Neurol Disord*, *1*, 141–147.

84. Bardin, L., Auclair, A., Kleven, M., Prinssen, E., Koek, W., Newman-Tancredi, A., Depoortère, R. (2007). Pharmacological profiles in rats of novel antipsychotics with combined dopamine D2/serotonin 5-HT1A activity: comparison with typical and atypical conventional antipsychotics. *Behav Pharmacol*, *18*, 103–118.

85. Kleven, M., Barret-Grévoz, C., Bruins Slot, L., Newman-Tancredi, A. (2005). Novel antipsychotic agents with 5-HT(1A) agonist properties: role of 5-HT(1A) receptor activation in attenuation of catalepsy induction in rats. *Neuropharmacology*, *49*, 135–143.

86. Auclair, A., Galinier, A., Besnard, J., Newman-Tancredi, A., Depoortère, R. (2007). Putative antipsychotics with pronounced agonism at serotonin 5-HT1A and partial

agonist activity at dopamine D2 receptors disrupt basal PPI of the startle reflex in rats. *Psychopharmacology*, *193*, 45–54.

87. Auclair, A.L., Kleven, M.S., Besnard, J., Depoortère, R., Newman-Tancredi, A. (2006). Actions of novel antipsychotic agents on apomorphine-induced PPI disruption: influence of combined serotonin 5-HT1A receptor activation and dopamine D2 receptor blockade. *Neuropsychopharmacology*, *31*, 1900–1909.
88. Depoortère, R., Boulay, D., Perrault, G., Bergis, O., Decobert, M., Francon, D., Jung, M., Simiand, J., Soubrie, P., Scatton, B. (2003). SSR181507, a dopamine D2 receptor antagonist and 5-HT1A receptor agonist. II: behavioral profile predictive of an atypical antipsychotic activity. *Neuropsychopharmacology*, *28*, 1889–1902.
89. Keck, P.J., Strakowski, S., McElroy, S. (2000). The efficacy of atypical antipsychotics in the treatment of depressive symptoms, hostility, and suicidality in patients with schizophrenia. *J Clin Psychiatry*, *61*(Suppl 3), 4–9.
90. Blier, P., Ward, N.M. (2003). Is there a role for 5-HT1A agonists in the treatment of depression? *Biol Psychiatry*, *53*, 193–203.
91. Schreiber, R., De Vry, J. (1993). 5-HT1A receptor ligands in animal models of anxiety, impulsivity and depression: multiple mechanisms of action? *Prog Neuropsychopharmacol Bioll Psychiatry*, *17*, 87–104.
92. Roy, A., Thompson, R., Kennedy, S. (1983). Depression in chronic schizophrenia. *Br J Psychiatry*, *142*, 465–470.
93. Birchwood, M., Mason, R., MacMillan, F., Healy, J. (1993). Depression, demoralization and control over psychotic illness: a comparison of depressed and non-depressed patients with a chronic psychosis. *Psychol Med*, *23*, 387–395.
94. McCreary, A.C., Glennon, J., Tuinstra, T., Herremans, A.H.J., Van der Heyden, J.A.M., Feenstra, R., Long, S.K., Kruse, C.G. (2002). SLV313: a novel antipsychotic with additional antidepressant and anxiolytic-like actions. *European Neuropsychopharmacology*, *12*, 274.

# 10

# 5-$HT_{2C}$ AND 5-$HT_6$ RECEPTOR TARGETED EMERGING APPROACHES IN SCHIZOPHRENIA

SHARON ROSENZWEIG-LIPSON, JOHN DUNLOP, LEE E. SCHECHTER, THOMAS A. COMERY, JONATHAN GROSS, AND KAREN L. MARQUIS

Schizophrenia is a disorder with multiple symptom domains including positive, negative, cognitive, and depressive. Although existing agents treat positive symptoms of schizophrenia relatively well, it comes at a price with respect to side effects related to extrapyramidal side effects (EPS) and weight gain/diabetogenesis. Over the last several decades, predominant interest in serotonergic targets with respect to schizophrenia has centered around 5-$HT_{2A}$ antagonism/inverse agonism and indeed second-generation antipsychotics (SGAs) that combine 5-$HT_{2A}$ antagonism with $D_2$ antagonism reduce the EPS liability associated with first-generation antipsychotics (FGAs). More recently, interest in the therapeutic potential of compounds with agonist or antagonist activities at 5-$HT_{2C}$ and 5-$HT_6$ receptors to address unmet medical needs across the symptom domains of schizophrenia has emerged. Interest in these receptors stems, in part, from the activities of many psychiatric drugs at these receptors. 5-$HT_{2C}$ agonists or antagonists (Table 10.1) have been suggested as treatments for multiple symptom domains including positive, negative, cognitive, and depressive symptoms without the adverse events or tolerability issues associated with existing agents. Attention around 5-$HT_6$ antagonists (Table 10.2) has focused primarily on adjunctive treatment with SGAs to treat the cognitive symptoms of schizophrenia. The current chapter will review the state of knowledge with respect to these receptors and the potential of compounds

*Targets and Emerging Therapies for Schizophrenia*, First Edition.
Edited by Jeffrey S. Albert and Michael W. Wood.

**TABLE 10.1 5-$HT_2$C Agonist and Antagonist Compounds**

| Compound | Mechanism | Structure |
|---|---|---|
| Vabicaserin | 5-$HT_{2C}$ agonist | 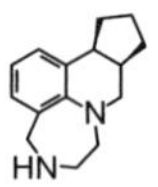 |
| Lorcaserin | 5-$HT_{2C}$ agonist | 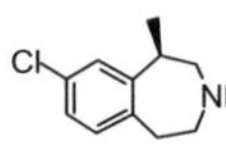 |
| CP-809,101 | 5-$HT_{2C}$ agonist | 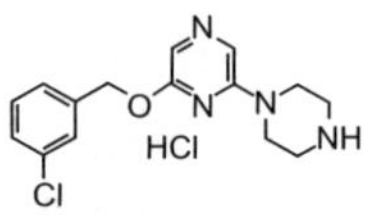 |
| WAY-163909 | 5-$HT_{2C}$ agonist | 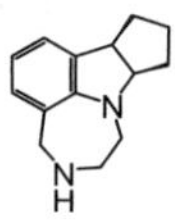 |
| Ro-60-0175 | 5-$HT_{2C}$ agonist | 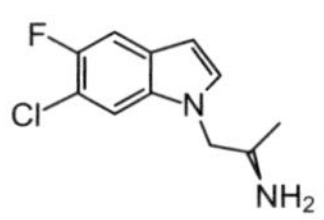 |
| SB-206553 | 5-$HT2_{2C/2B}$ antagonist | 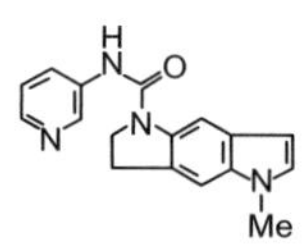 |
| SB-242084 | 5-$HT_{2C}$ antagonist | 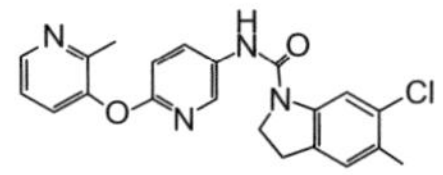 |
| SB-243213 | 5-$HT_{2C}$ antagonist | 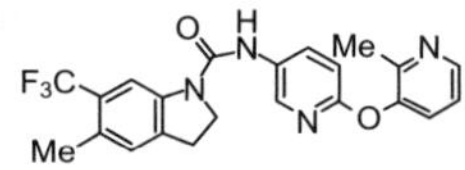 |
| SB-228357 | 5-$HT_{2C/2B}$ antagonist | 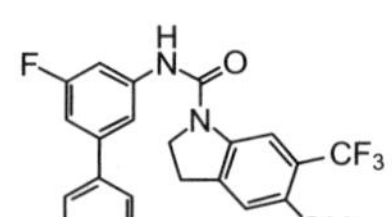 |

acting at these receptors for treating the multiple symptom domains of schizophrenia.

## 10.1 5-$HT_{2C}$

### 10.1.1 Receptor Localization

The 5-$HT_{2C}$ receptor is a member of the seven transmembrane spanning G-protein-coupled receptor (GPCR) superfamily and is classified within the

**TABLE 10.2 5-HT$_6$ Agonist and Antagonist Compounds**

| Compound | Mechanism | Structure |
|---|---|---|
| WAY-181187 | 5-HT$_6$ agonist | 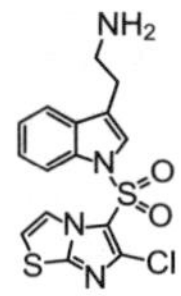 |
| WAY-208466 | 5-HT$_6$ agonist | 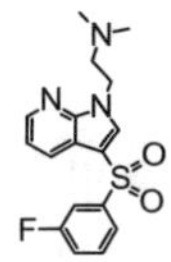 |
| Ro-04-6790 | 5-HT$_6$ antagonist | 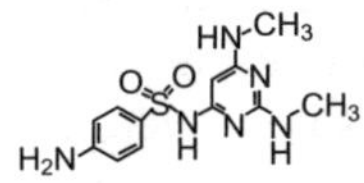 |
| SB-271046 | 5-HT$_6$ antagonist | 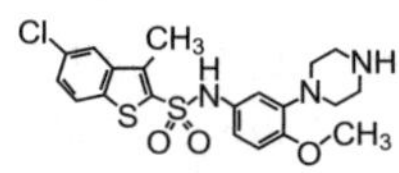 |
| SB-357134 | 5-HT$_6$ antagonist | 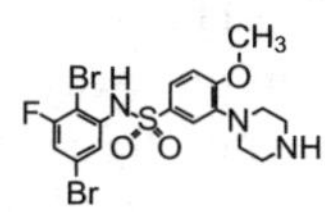 |
| SB-399885 | 5-HT$_6$ antagonist | 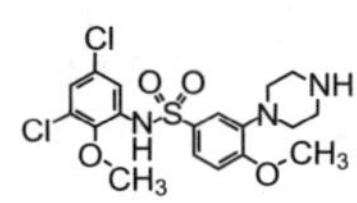 |
| Ro-4368554 | 5-HT$_6$ antagonist | 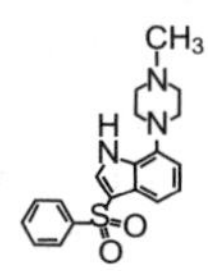 |
| BGC 20-761 | 5-HT$_6$ antagonist | 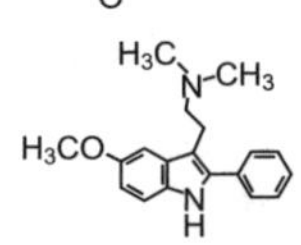 |
| GSK-74257 | 5-HT$_6$ Antagonist | 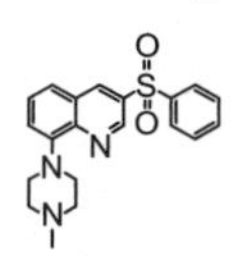 |
| GSK-773812 | 5-HT$_6$ Antagonist | 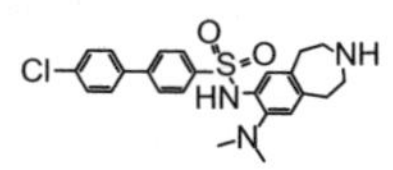 |
| PRX-07034 | 5-HT$_6$ Antagonist | 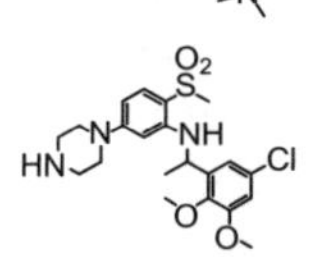 |

5-HT2 subfamily of 14 serotonin receptor subtypes based on sequence homology to the 5-$HT_{2A}$ and 5-$HT_{2B}$ receptors, and their common signal transduction pathway, via activation of the G-proteins Gq and G12/13. Receptor localization studies have revealed predominant central nervous system localization with widespread expression of the 5-$HT_{2C}$ receptor subtype throughout the brain, suggestive of an important role in central nervous system (CNS) function. More specifically, localization of the receptor to the limbic system, frontal cortex, and hippocampus [1–2] are of particular relevance to the potential involvement of this receptor subtype in schizophrenia.

### 10.1.2 Multiple Signaling Pathways and Agonist Trafficking

Like many GPCRs, the 5-$HT_{2C}$ receptor is coupled to multiple signal transduction pathways leading to engagement of a number of intracellular signaling molecules. This is particularly diverse for the 5-$HT_{2C}$ receptor including signal transduction via activation of Gq/11, G12/13 and Gi G-proteins, activation of phospholipases A, C, and D, and signaling via inositol second messengers, arachidonic acid and elevations in intracellular calcium levels [3]. In addition, the capacity for 5-$HT_{2C}$ receptor agonists to differentially activate distinct signal transduction pathways coupled to receptor activation has been demonstrated [4]. For example, 3-trifluoromethylphenylpiperazine has been shown to preferentially activate phospholipase C-mediated phosphoinositide hydrolysis while lysergic acid diethylamide favored the phospholipase $A_2$ ($PLA_2$) coupled release of arachidonic acid (AA). This property of so-called agonist-directed trafficking of receptor stimulus [5] has been proposed as a means of accounting for the ability of an agonist to selectively stimulate a subset of signal pathways coupled to a single receptor subtype. Although this receptor property has been clearly demonstrated *in vitro*, the extent to which preferential activation of one signal transduction pathway over another might impact drug activity *in vivo* is not understood.

### 10.1.3 RNA Editing

A further degree of complexity of 5-$HT_{2C}$ receptor functional activity is governed by RNA editing in the coding region of the receptor, resulting in a possible 32 mRNA variants and 24 protein isoforms [6]. The resultant receptor isoforms differ in the many aspects of receptor signaling including constitutive activation, magnitude and potency of responses to receptor agonists, and receptor desensitization. Basal activity or constitutive receptor activation is most pronounced in the unedited INI variant, is intermediate in partially edited receptor isoforms, and is lowest in the fully edited isoform VGV [7, 8]. The existence of RNA-edited 5-$HT_{2C}$ receptor isoforms also presents a different window of drug-induced activation of the receptor depending on the particular isoform expressed. Morever, a number of antipsychotic drugs have been shown to exhibit inverse agonist activity at the constitutively active INI isoform, resulting in diminished basal activity [7, 9, 10]. Indeed, the *in vitro* functional profile of antipsychotic drugs such as olanzapine and aripiprazole at the cloned $5\text{-HT}_{2C}$ receptor expressed in cell lines appears to be highly dependent on the isoform expressed [11]. In addition, the ability of agonists to differentially activate different signal transduction pathways as described above is influenced by the editing state of the receptor [12].

### 10.1.4 RNA Editing and Schizophrenia

Of the possible 24 $5\text{-HT}_{2C}$ receptor isoforms, the fully edited (VSV, VGV isoforms), unedited (INI), and partially edited (VNI, VSI, VNV) are highly represented in rat and human brain. With respect to RNA editing of the $5\text{-HT}_{2C}$ receptor and schizophrenia, a limited number of studies have been documented and have not provided strong evidence in favor of altered editing in the disease state. In two independent studies, no changes in the relative distribution of the INI, VNV, and VSV isoforms of the receptor were observed between controls and schizophrenics [13, 14]. In contrast, in a small study of five patients and controls, an increase in the expression of the INI isoform in the frontal cortex of schizophrenics was observed [15], although the small sample size precludes a definitive conclusion from this study. Clearly, additional studies are required to resolve this important question since, as discussed previously, there are functional consequences associated with different isoform expression; for example, an increase in the expression of the INI isoform would be associated with increased basal receptor activity, increased sensitivity to serotonin, and a potential for inverse agonist activity of antipsychotic drugs.

### 10.1.5 $5\text{-HT}_{2C}$ Genetic Polymorphisms and Schizophrenia

In addition to RNA-edited variants of the $5\text{-HT}_{2C}$ receptor, a number of genetic polymorphisms in the promoter and coding region of the $5\text{-HT}_{2C}$ receptor gene have been identified. These include a single nucleotide polymorphism (SNP) in the coding region (68 G/C; cys/ser substitution) and three SNPs in the promoter region close to the transcription initiation site [16]. Unlike the RNA-edited isoforms, there is no definitive functional consequences of these SNPs, although two of the SNPs in the promoter region have been shown to result in decreased promoter activity [17], possibly leading to decreased receptor expression. These SNPs have been studied extensively in the context of antipsychotic drug-induced side effect liability, in particular weight gain [18], extrapyramidal side effects (EPS), and tardive dyskinesia [16, 19, 20]. C-G-Cys23 is particularly relevant in pharmacogenetics since $5\text{-HT}_{2C}$ receptor antagonism has been implicated in antipsychotic drug-induced weight gain, and $5\text{-HT}_{2C}$ receptor agonists reduce food intake and weight gain [21–23]. An important role for the $5\text{-HT}_{2C}$ receptor subtype in appetite regulation and obesity is further supported by the phenotype of $5\text{-HT}_{2C}$ receptor knockout mice; these animals are insensitive to the hypohagic activity of the 5-$HT_{2C}$ receptor agonist mCPP, are obese and hyperphagic, and have elevated insulin and leptin levels and impaired glucose utilization [24–26]. Association studies of 5-$HT_{2C}$ receptor polymorphisms and antipsychotic drug-induced weight gain have provided mixed results [18], although more than one study has now suggested a significant association with the –759 C/T promoter polymorphism, with the presence of the T allele being associated with less antipsychotic drug-induced weight gain [3, 27–39]. In contrast, studies with clozapine [30, 31] and olanzapine [32] have not revealed an association with the 5-$HT_{2C}$ receptor polymorphisms and their antipsychotic drug efficacy. Since both these agents exhibit 5-$HT_{2C}$ receptor antagonist activity, this latter observation is of particular relevance in the context of the antipsychotic-like activity of selective 5-$HT_{2C}$ receptor agonists, discussed in the next section. Lastly, recent evidence supports an association between the presence of the 23Ser variant and a higher incidence of EPS and tardive dyskinesia [19, 33, 34]. As discussed in Section 10.2.3, 5-$HT_{2C}$ receptor antagonist activity, although not predicted preclinically to offer antipsychotic-like activity, might be beneficial in the context of these antipsychotic drug-induced side effects.

## 10.2 5-$HT_{2C}$ ANTAGONISM VERSUS AGONISM

### 10.2.1 Current Antipsychotics: 5-$HT_{2C}$ Inverse Agonists/Antagonists

All clinically effective antipsychotics share in common the ability to antagonize dopamine (DA) $D_2$ receptors. Most of the SGAs, those agents with reduced potential to induce extrapyramidal motor symptom (EPS) side effects, also produce 5-$HT_{2A}$ receptor antagonism [35]. In addition, many SGAs, including the gold standard clozapine, show antagonist effects at 5-$HT_{2C}$ receptors both *in vitro* and *in vivo* [36]. Over the last few years both 5-$HT_{2C}$ agonists and antagonists have been suggested as treatments for schizophrenia, leading to much confusion regarding how to target this receptor. In order to evaluate fully the potential utility of 5-$HT_{2C}$ agonists versus antagonists for the treatment of schizophrenia, it is important to review the neurochemical, electrophysiological, and behavioral data.

### 10.2.2 5-$HT_{2C}$ Antagonists: Neurochemistry and Electrophysiology

5-$HT_{2C}$ antagonism is reported to enhance DA neurotransmission in the prefrontal cortex [37], suggesting that this mechanism might contribute to improvements in negative symptoms and possibly cognition. In preclinical studies, a similar enhancement in DA neurotransmission has also been observed in the nucleus accumbens following treatment with some, but not all, 5-$HT_{2C}$ antagonists. In this regard, SB-206553 [38], but not SB-243213 [39], elevates nucleus accumbens DA, a region putatively associated with the positive symptoms of schizophrenia. While the increase in frontal cortex DA produced by a $5\text{-HT}_{2C}$ antagonist may be valuable, increases in nucleus accumbens DA may be a liability for a $5\text{-HT}_{2C}$ antagonist. Although this profile is similar to that of SGAs, the blockade of DA $D_2$ receptors postsynaptically by antipsychotics mitigates against this increase in DA in the nucleus accumbens. However, a selective $5\text{-HT}_{2C}$ receptor antagonist may exacerbate positive symptoms of schizophrenia by virtue of elevating subcortical DA neurotransmission. In contrast, electrophysiological studies have shown that chronic administration of both SB-200646A and SB-243213 decreases the number of spontaneously active DA neurons in the ventral tegmental area (VTA) but not in the substantia nigra (SN), which is indicative of an atypical antipsychotic-like profile [40, 41]. Interestingly, SB-243213, but not SB-200646A, shows an acute decrease in the number of spontaneously active DA neurons in the VTA; however, these effects are not dose-dependent [40] and are not accompanied by decreases in nucleus accumbens DA [39].

### 10.2.3 $5\text{-HT}_{2C}$ Antagonists: Behavior

Despite these neurochemical and electrophysiological findings, selective $5\text{-HT}_{2C}$ antagonists fail to demonstrate antipsychotic-like efficacy in preclinical models [42, 43]. However, $5\text{-HT}_{2C}$ antagonism may have beneficial effects in offsetting the EPS of antipsychotics. To this end, the $5\text{-HT}_{2C}$ antagonist SB-228357 attenuates haloperidol-induced catalepsy in rats [44]. Additionally, it has been suggested that in models of tardive dyskinesia, $5\text{-HT}_{2C}$ receptors become hypersensitive [45] and that $5\text{-HT}_{2C}$ antagonists may be effective in reducing the vacuous movements in a tardive dyskinesia model [45]. These results, coupled with the association of the $5\text{-HT}_{2C}$ receptor polymorphisms with EPS and TD [19, 20, 34], suggest that $5\text{-HT}_{2C}$ antagonists may be valuable treatments for EPS and TD.

### 10.2.4 $5\text{-HT}_{2C}$ Agonists: Neurochemistry and Electrophysiology

The electrophysiological and neurochemical evidence for reported selective $5\text{-HT}_{2C}$ receptor agonists is more consistent and supports the idea that these compounds produce antipsychotic-like properties with low potential for EPS side effects. Along these lines, acute or chronic administration of $5\text{-HT}_{2C}$ agonists such as RO 60-00175, WAY-163909, and vabicaserin significantly diminish the number of spontaneously active DA neurons of the VTA without significantly affecting the number of spontaneously active DA neurons in the SN [42, 46–48]. Similarly, acute or chronic administration of these $5\text{-HT}_{2C}$ agonists selectively reduce DA levels in the nucleus accumbens relative to striatum [23, 42, 46–48]. The decrease in VTA DA cell firing relative to SN DA cell firing, coupled with a decrease in nucleus accumbens DA, is similar to the effects of clozapine following chronic administration [39, 42]. That these compounds produce these effects both acutely and chronically may reflect a more rapid onset of activity. The selective effects of 5-$HT_{2C}$ receptor agonists on the mesolimbic DA pathway suggests that 5-$HT_{2C}$ receptor agonists should have antipsychotic efficacy without the EPS associated with typical antipsychotics.

### 10.2.5 5-$HT_{2C}$ Agonists: Behavior

The behavioral profile of 5-$HT_{2C}$ agonists provides even more compelling data supporting the use of 5-$HT_{2C}$ agonists in the treatment of schizophrenia. In this regard, CP-809,101, WAY-163909, and vabicaserin inhibit conditioned avoidance responding in rats, block apomorphine-induced climbing but not apomorphine-induced stereotypy in mice, and reverse phencyclidine (PCP) and amphetamine-induced locomotor activity, suggesting antipsychotic potential [42, 46–49]. Moreover, many of these effects are antagonized by pretreatment with 5-$HT_{2C}$ antagonists. Despite the potential for 5-$HT_{2C}$ antagonists to offset or reverse EPS or TD effects of antipsychotics [45, 50], 5-$HT_{2C}$ agonists do not induce catalepsy, suggesting low potential for extrapyramidal motor symptom side effects [42, 46–49]. These antipsychotic-like effects in the absence of catalepsy are consistent with the mesolimbic selectivity observed neurochemically and electrophysiologically. In contrast with the effects of 5-$HT_{2C}$ agonists in animal models predictive of antipsychotic-like activity, selective 5-$HT_{2C}$ antagonists fail to demonstrate antipsychotic-like efficacy in these models [42, 43].

Interestingly, 5-$HT_{2C}$ agonists also affect prepulse inhibition (PPI) of acoustic startle. CP-809,101 is reported to attenuate an apomorphine-induced deficit, while WAY-163909 and vabicaserin affect deficits induced by MK-801 or 2,5-dimethoxy-4-iodoamphetamine DOI and enhance PPI in DBA2N mice [42, 48, 49]. Thus, stimulation of 5-$HT_{2C}$ receptors can affect processes involved in sensorimotor gating, a pre-attentive process that is abnormal in schizophrenia [49, 51]. These data suggest the potential for 5-$HT_{2C}$ agonists to influence cognitive-related processes. Additionally, both WAY-163909 and vabicaserin elevate levels of medial prefrontal cortex acetylcholine that is consistent with potential procognitive activity [52] . Indeed, both CP-801,101 and vabicaserin improve performance in a novel object recognition assay [42, 51]. Similar effects have not been demonstrated for 5-$HT_{2C}$ receptor antagonists.

Recent studies have also suggested that 5-$HT_{2C}$ agonists may be effective in treating impulsivity. In this regard, both Ro-60-0175 and WAY-163909 decrease premature responses in a long intertrial interval variation of the five-choice serial reaction time task [49, 51]. Conversely, the 5-$HT_{2C}$ antagonist SB-242084 enhanced premature responding, suggestive of increased impulsivity [53, 54], effects likely mediated via by the nucleus accumbens [53, 55].

The role that 5-$HT_{2C}$ receptor activity plays in either the efficacy or the side effect liabilities of the current antipsychotics is not fully known. Recently, the 5-$HT_{2C}$ receptor has been implicated in the weight gain liability associated with several antipsychotic medications [56] while 5-$HT_{2C}$ agonism induces reduction in feeding behavior and decreases weight gain [57]. Taken together with the antipsychotic-like effects of 5-$HT_{2C}$ agonists, these studies suggest that 5-$HT_{2C}$ agonists may produce antipsychotic activity in the absence of the weight gain and diabetogenesis associated with atypical antipsychotics that are also 5-$HT_{2C}$ receptor antagonists.

These studies suggest the potential for selective 5-$HT_{2C}$ receptor agonists to address positive and cognitive symptoms of schizophrenia. Additional evidence suggests the potential to treat mood disorder symptoms [58]. These effects, coupled with the reduced risk for extrapyramidal side effects and weight gain, suggest that selective 5-$HT_{2C}$ receptor agonists represent a potential treatment approach for schizophrenia.

## 10.3 5-$HT_6$

### 10.3.1 Receptor Identification and Localization

The rodent 5-$HT_6$ receptor was first cloned and reported by Monsma and coworkers [59], and subsequently the human 5-$HT_6$ receptor was cloned and determined to be 89% homologous to the rat sequence [60]. Structural evaluations defined minor differences between the rat and human such as a short third intracellular loop (50 and 57 amino acids in the rat and human, respectively) and a long carboxy tail that is similar to that reported for other GPCRs positively coupled to adenylate cyclase. Whereas there have not been any subtypes reported for the 5-$HT_6$ receptor, a truncated splice variant of the receptor occurring prior to the first intron was identified [61] but does not appear to have any functional significance to date. This alternatively spliced variant of the 5-$HT_6$ receptor was not detected in rat or mouse whole brain cDNA by polymerase chain reaction (PCR) due to the lack of a consensus 5′ donor site. Co-expression of the variant 5-$HT_6$ transcript, which only yields the first three transmembrane domains and the full-length 5-$HT_6$ receptor in the human brain, was observed in caudate and SN but not in the hippocampus, cortex, cerebellum, and thalamus. Whether the splice variant plays a role in disease states has yet to be determined.

*In situ* hybridization and northern blot studies revealed an exclusive distribution of 5-$HT_6$ mRNA in the rat CNS with the highest density found in the olfactory tubercle, followed by the frontal and entorhinal cortices, dorsal hippocampus (i.e., dentate gyrus and CA1, CA2, and CA3 regions), nucleus accumbens, and striatum [62]. Lower levels were observed in the hypothalamus, amygdala, SN, and several diencephalic nuclei. These findings have been corroborated by immunolocalization studies and radioligand binding using [$^{125}$I]SB-258585 showing a similar distribution of 5-$HT_6$ receptor protein in the rat CNS [62]. Additionally, destruction of 5-HT cell bodies in the raphe nuclei were not found to alter 5-$HT_6$ Mrna, suggesting that 5-$HT_6$ receptors are not autoreceptors on 5-HT perikarya and are not upregulated in postsynaptic areas following degeneration [63–65]. This is consistent with the previous suggestions that in the striatum the 5-$HT_6$ receptor is postsynaptic and may be localized on interneurons [66]. This was further substantiated by studies evaluating the neurochemical effects of 5-$HT_6$ agonists and antagonists that suggest that the 5-HT6 receptor is localized on GABAergic interneurons [67].

### 10.3.2 Receptor Signaling

Cloning of the rat 5-$HT_6$ receptor [59] identified a new subfamily of G-coupled 5-HT receptors linked to the stimulation of adenylyl cyclase activity. Interesting it has been revealed that the 5-$HT_6$ receptor also directly couples to Fyn, which is a member of the Src kinase family [68]. Thus, in addition to coupling to G$\alpha$s, the 5-$HT_6$ receptor can have a G-protein-independent signaling system that can directly interact with Fyn and accordingly directly activate ERK1/2 [69]. Although ERK1/2 cascade can also be activated indirectly through PKA, the data raise intriguing possibilities regarding alternative signaling pathways. The physiological significance of this has yet to be revealed but raises interesting possibilities as *fyn*$^-$ mutant mice demonstrate impaired LTP, impaired spatial memory, and fearfulness [70, 71].

### 10.3.3 5-$HT_6$ Receptors in Schizophrenia

The pharmacology of the 5-$HT_6$ receptor subtype has received considerable attention due to the high affinity for the receptor of a wide range of drugs used in psychiatry and its exclusive localization to the CNS [72]. Studies on selective 5-$HT_6$ receptor ligands have suggested their potential use in the treatment of learning and memory disorders, depression, and schizophrenia. In particular, the high affinity for this receptor exhibited by both FGAs and SGAs has led to speculation that the 5-$HT_6$ receptor represents a therapeutic target for schizophrenia [72]. Several other lines of evidence have implicated the 5-$HT_6$ receptor in the control of cholinergic transmission, leading to the proposal that the receptor might be a target for restoring cognitive function.

### 10.3.4 5-$HT_6$ Genetic Polymorphisms and Schizophrenia

The interest in the role that 5-HT6 receptors play in the action of antipsychotics stimulated a genetic association analysis. While one study reported an increased expression of the 267T allele in schizophrenic patients [69], several other studies failed to find such an association with this silent polymorphism [73] or with a trinucleotide repeat $(GCC)_{2/3}$, upstream of the translation start site [74–77]. The T/C 267 genotype has been reported to be associated with the response to atypical antipsychotic treatment in some [78], but not all studies [79, 80].

Beyond genetic polymorphisms, others have investigated expression levels of the 5-$HT_6$ receptors as it might be altered in the disease or by drug treatment. Repeated treatment with glutamatergic antagonists decreased striatal, but not hippocampal, 5-$HT_6$ mRNA in rats [81], suggesting that glutamatergic regulators of serotonin release could impact expression of the receptor. 5-$HT_6$ receptor mRNA was reported to be decreased in the hippocampal, but not in dorsolateral prefrontal cortical tissue from postmortem schizophrenic brain, while no effect was seen following antipsychotic treatment, suggesting that the effect on receptor expression was due to the disease [82]. These data contrast with an earlier report showing decreased 5-$HT_6$ mRNA in the hippocampus, but not in the cortex, in rats treated with clozapine, but not haloperidol [83]. Autoradiographic studies confirmed the lack of change in 5-$HT_6$ receptor density in the prefrontal cortex from schizophrenic patients, as well as the lack of effect of chronic antipsychotic treatment [84], thereby suggesting that altered receptor density does not play a role in the disease or drug action, at least in this brain region.

## 10.4 NEUROCHEMISTRY

Multiple studies have investigated the neurochemical effects of 5-$HT_6$ antagonists. Consistent with observations from behavioral studies suggesting a role of the cholinergic neurotransmitter system in the behavioral effects following treatment with a 5-$HT_6$ antagonist, *in vitro* and *in vivo* neurochemical studies have reported an increase in release of acetylcholine in the cortex [85], hippocampus [86–88], and striatum [89]. In addition, studies have reported that 5-$HT_6$ antagonism increases extracellular concentration of glutamate (and in one study aspartate) in the cortex *in vitro* [86] and *in vivo* [86], as well as in the hippocampus *in vivo* [90, 91]. Taken together, these increases in neurotransmitters such as glutamate and acetylcholine in brain regions associated with cognition are consistent with potential pro-cognitive effects of 5-$HT_6$ antagonists.

Given the fact that several antipsychotics have affinity for 5-$HT_6$ receptors, there has been much interest in defining the role of monoamines in the actions of selective antagonists. Despite the observation that a 5-$HT_6$ antagonist decreases the number of spontaneously active DA neurons in VTA following acute, but not chronic treatment [90], whereas DA neurons in the SN compacta were less active following chronic, but not acute 5-$HT_6$ antagonism, there has been little consistent evidence of an effect on extracellular DA level changes in nucleus accumbens or striatum brain regions [92]. Only one report indicated that a 5-$HT_6$ antagonist treatment increased DA levels in the medial prefrontal cortex, the projection target of the mesocortical dopaminergic pathway [86, 90, 91]. In contrast, another study reported no significant effect of a 5-$HT_6$ antagonist in this brain region, but a significant increase in DA levels in the hippocampus [93].

5-$HT_6$ antagonist treatment appears to influence DA when combined with other agents. The combination of 5-$HT_6$ antagonist with the FGA haloperidol and the SGA risperidone, neither of which possesses significant 5-$HT_6$ affinity

[94], yielded a potentiated increase in DA in the medial prefrontal cortex and hippocampus, while the combination with haloperidol increased levels in the hippocampus only. These increases in DA in the hippocampus and medial prefrontal cortex produced by the combination of 5-HT$_6$ antagonists and antipsychotics suggest that co-administration of these compounds may lead to improvements in the cognitive and negative symptoms of schizophrenia beyond what an FGA or SGA can do alone.

## 10.5 COGNITION

The cognitive deficits observed in schizophrenia are considered the strongest indicator of patient rehabilitation and are very poorly treated by existing antipsychotic medications. 5-HT$_6$ antagonist treatment improves performance in a number of cognitive tasks that evaluate episodic memory and problem solving, consistent with their ability to enhance cholinergic and glutamatergic neurotransmitter activity.

Prior to the development of selective pharmacological tools with good blood–brain barrier penetration, repeated intracerebroventricular injection with antisense oligonucleotides was shown to improve hippocampus-dependent spatial memory in the Morris water maze task, with no significant effect on acquisition of the task [94]. The early lead Ro-04-6790 had similar effects in the same study, as did other 5-HT$_6$ antagonists developed later [95]. In some studies, the effects were observed only during probe trials to assess memory, while in others improved acquisition was reported, especially in aged subjects [96].

In other tasks, where delays between events are imposed to induce natural forgetting, 5-HT$_6$ antagonists have shown mixed results. Both improvements [88, 97, 98] and no significant effects [99, 100] have been reported in the novel object recognition task. In contrast, several 5-HT$_6$ antagonists have been reported to reverse the cognitive impairing effects of the nonselective muscarinic antagonist scopolamine in a number of tasks, including autoshaping [101, 102], novel object recognition [103], social recognition [88, 101, 102], and passive avoidance [101], but not contextual fear conditioning [98]. Interestingly, despite the clear evidence of the effect of 5-HT$_6$ antagonists on glutamate neurotransmission, relatively few studies have explored the ability of these compounds to reverse glutamatergic NMDA antagonist-induced cognitive deficits. The 5-HT$_6$ antagonists SB-357134 and SB-399885 reversed MK-801 impaired autoshaping [104] and MK-801 precluded the expression of the cognitive improving effects of Ro-04-6790 on novel object recognition [103]. Additionally, 5-HT$_6$ antagonists blocked scopolamine impaired fear potentiated startle, a model of emotional memory [99], but did not normalize the reduction in social interaction induced by the NMDA antagonist PCP [105].

The attention set shift task in rodents was developed to be analogous to the human Wisconsin Card Sorting Task on which schizophrenic patients perform poorly. This task requires the subject to shift attention within (intradimensional, ID) and between stimulus dimensions (odors vs. digging media in rodents) in order to receive a reward. This task requires the subject to shift attention within (intradimensional, ID; e.g., between different odors in rodents) and between stimulus dimensions (extradimensional, ED; e.g., odor vs. digging media in rodents). 5-$HT_6$ antagonists abolish the ID/ED shift [106] in normal animals and reversed the impairment induced by withdrawal from chronic treatment with the NMDA antagonist PCP [107].

Interestingly, there are data to suggest that 5-$HT_6$ agonists may also have cognitive benefits. In this regard, 5-$HT_6$ agonists have been suggested to improve cognition in a 4-hour delay NOR paradigm and enhance ED shift in an attentional set-shifting assay [108].

## 10.6 SYNAPTIC PLASTICITY

The mechanisms and pathways involved in 5-$HT_6$ antagonist effects on learning and memory are poorly understood. A single study [109] has investigated the effect of 5-$HT_6$ antagonists on polysialated neural cell adhesion molecules (PSA NCAM) based on prior evidence that synaptic remodeling is accompanied by a transient increase in this marker [110]. In this study chronic administration of two different 5-$HT_6$ antagonists increased the frequency of PSA-NCAM immunopositive cells in the infragranular zone of the hippocampal dentate gyrus, as well as regions of the medial temporal cortex including piriform, perirhinal, and entorhinal cortex, which gives rise to perforant pathway input to the hippocampus. Moreover, the effect of a single day's training on a water maze task (five trials) to increase dentate PSA-NCAM immunopositive cells 12 hours post training was further enhanced in rats treated with the 5-$HT_6$ antagonists. PSA-NCAM expression was also observed in newly born cells in the dentate; however, chronic 5-$HT_6$ antagonism did not increase the frequency of BrdU immunopositive cells found in this brain region. The mechanism by which 5-$HT_6$ antagonism increases PSA-NCAM is unclear but may be related to effects on cholinergic neurotransmission as the cholinergic projection of the septohippocampal pathway is enriched in PSA-NCAM expression and is influenced by training on cognitive tasks [111, 112].

## 10.7 SENSORY GATING

In addition to cognitive deficits, schizophrenics show deficits in sensory processing. These deficits can be assessed in models such as PPI. In this model, a small nonstartle-eliciting stimulus presented immediately prior to a startle-eliciting stimulus can dampen the motor reflex response. Early representative

5-HT$_6$ antagonists failed to reverse various pharmacologically induced PPI deficits [113]; however, it has been suggested that this lack of effect may have been due to poor brain penetration. The 5-HT$_6$ antagonists with improved brain exposure have been reported to reverse both direct (apomorphine) [114, 115] and indirect (d-amphetamine) [105] DA agonists, but not disruptions due to the NMDA antagonist PCP [106] or the muscarinic antagonist scopolamine [106].

## 10.8 SUMMARY

Despite decades of research, effective treatments for the multiple symptom domains of schizophrenia remain elusive. It is critical that novel therapeutics address the cognitive, negative, and depressive symptoms in order to have true benefit to patients with schizophrenia. Recent advances in understanding the potential of therapeutics targeting 5-HT$_{2C}$ or 5-HT$_6$ receptors provide compelling preclinical support that these mechanisms have the potential to address these critical unmet needs either as stand-alone therapies or as adjuncts to SGAs. 5-HT$_{2C}$ agonists have the potential to have a broad spectrum of activity (positive, negative, cognitive, depressive) without the tolerability issues associated with FGAs or SGAs. 5-HT$_{2C}$ antagonists have the potential to mitigate against some of the adverse events of antipsychotics. 5-HT$_6$ antagonists, as adjunctive therapies, have the potential to address the cognitive impairments associated with schizophrenia. These are clearly exciting times in the development of novel treatments for schizophrenia. The therapeutic potential of compounds that act as 5-HT$_{2C}$ agonists or antagonists and 5-HT$_6$ antagonists across the spectrum of unmet needs in schizophrenia is quite high. Clinical trials to characterize the potential of these compounds will be critical in determining the true value of these mechanisms.

## REFERENCES

1. Hoffman, B., Mezey, E. (1989). Distribution of serotonin 5-HT$_{1C}$ receptor mRNA in adult rat brain. *FEBS Letters*, *247*(2), 453–462.
2. Abramowski, D., et al. (1995). Localization of the 5-hydroxytryptamine $_{2c}$ receptor protein in human and rat brain using specific antisera. *Neuropharmacology*, *24*(12), 1635–1645.
3. Miller, K.J. (2005). Serotonin 5-HT2C receptor agonists: potential for the treatment of obesity. *Molecular Interventions*, *5*(5), 282–291.
4. Berg, K.A., et al. (1998). Effector pathway-dependent relative efficacy at serotonin type 2A and 2C receptors: evidence for agonist-directed trafficking of receptor stimulus. *Molecular Pharmacology*, *54*(1), 94–104.
5. Kenakin, T. (1995). Agonist-receptor efficacy II: agonist trafficking of receptor signals. *Trends in Pharmacological Sciences*, *16*(7), 232–238.

6. Niswender, C.M., Sanders-Bush, E., Emeson, R.B. (1998). Identification and characterization of RNA editing events within the 5-HT2C receptor. *Annals of the New York Academy of Sciences*, *861*, 38–48.
7. Niswender, C.M., et al. (1999). RNA editing of the human serotonin 5-hydroxytryptamine 2C receptor silences constitutive activity. *The Journal of Biological Chemistry*, *274*(14), 9472–9478.
8. Herrick-Davis, K., Grinde, E., Niswender, C.M. (1999). Serotonin 5-HT2C receptor RNA editing alters receptor basal activity: implications for serotonergic signal transduction. *Journal of Neurochemistry*, *73*(4), 1711–1717.
9. Herrick-Davis, K., Grinde, E., Teitler, M. (2000). Inverse agonist activity of atypical antipsychotic drugs at human 5-hydroxytryptamine2c receptors. *The Journal of Pharmacology and Experimental Therapeutics*, *295*(1), 226–232.
10. Rauser, L., et al. (2001). Inverse agonist actions of typical and atypical antipsychotic drugs at the human 5-hydroxytryptamine(2C) receptor. *The Journal of Pharmacology and Experimental Therapeutics*, *299*(1), 83–89.
11. Zhang, J.Y., et al. (2006). Distinct functional profiles of aripiprazole and olanzapine at RNA edited human 5-HT2C receptor isoforms. *Biochemical Pharmacology*, *71*(4), 521–529.
12. Berg, K.A., et al. (2008). A conservative, single-amino acid substitution in the second cytoplasmic domain of the human serotonin2c receptor alters both ligand-dependent and -independent receptor signaling. *The Journal of Pharmacology and Experimental Therapeutics*, *324*(3), 1084–1092.
13. Niswender, C.M., et al. (2001). RNA editing of the human serotonin 5-HT2C receptor. alterations in suicide and implications for serotonergic pharmacotherapy. *Neuropsychopharmacology*, *24*(5), 478–491.
14. Dracheva, S., et al. (2003). RNA editing and alternative splicing of human serotonin 2C receptor in schizophrenia. *Journal of Neurochemistry*, *87*(6), 1402–1412.
15. Sodhi, M.S., et al. (2001). RNA editing of the 5-HT(2C) receptor is reduced in schizophrenia. *Molecular Psychiatry*, *6*(4), 373–379.
16. Reynolds, G.P., Templeman, L.A., Zhang, Z.J. (2005). The role of 5-HT2C receptor polymorphisms in the pharmacogenetics of antipsychotic drug treatment. *Progress in Neuro-Psychopharmacology & Biological Psychiatry*, *29*(6), 1021–1028.
17. Hill, M.J., Reynolds, G.P. (2007). 5-HT2C receptor gene polymorphisms associated with antipsychotic drug action alter promoter activity. *Brain Research*, *1149*, 14–17.
18. Muller, D., Kennedy, J.L. (2006). Genetics of antipsychotic treatment emergent weight gain in schizophrenia. *Pharmacogenomics*, *7*(6), 863–887.
19. Gunes, A., et al. (2008). Further evidence for the association between 5-HT2C receptor gene polymorphisms and extrapyramidal side effects in male schizophrenic patients. *European Journal of Clinical Pharmacology*, *64*(5), 477–482.
20. Zhang, Z., Zhang, X., Sha, W. (2002). Association of a polymorphism in the promoter region of the serotonin 5-HT2C receptor gene with tardive dyskinesia in patients with schizophrenia. *Molecular Psychiatry*, *7*(7), 670–671.
21. Clifton, P., Lee, M., Dourish, C. (2000). Similarities in the action of Ro 60-0175, a 5-HT2c receptor agonist and d-fenfluramine on feeding patterns in the rat. *Psychopharmacology (Berl)*, *152*(3), 256–267.

22. Rosenzweig-Lipson, S., et al. (2006). Antiobesity-like effects of the 5-HT2C receptor agonist WAY-161503. *Brain Research*, *1073–1074*, 240–251.

23. Dunlop, J., et al. (2005). WAY-163909 [(7bR, 10aR)-1,2,3,4,8,9,10,10a-octahydro-7bH-cyclopenta-[b][1,4]diazepino[6,7,1hi]indole], a novel 5-hydroxytryptamine 2C receptor-selective agonist with anorectic activity. *The Journal of Pharmacology and Experimental Therapeutics*, *313*(2), 862–869.

24. Tecott, L., et al. (1995). Eating disorder and epilepsy in mice lacking 5-HT2c serotonin receptors. *Nature*, *374*(6522), 542–546.

25. Heisler, L.K., Chu, H.M., Tecott, L.H. (1998). Epilepsy and obesity in serotonin 5-HT2C receptor mutant mice. *Annals of the New York Academy of Sciences*, *861*, 74–78.

26. Nonogaki, K., et al. (1998). Leptin-independent hyperphagia and type 2 diabetes in mice with a mutated serotonin 5-HT2C receptor gene. *Nature Medicine*, *4*(10), 1152–1156.

27. Templeman, L., et al. (2005). Polymorphisms of the 5HT2C receptor and leptin genes are associated with antipsychotic drug-induced weight gain in Caucasian subjects with a first-episode psychosis. *Pharmacogenetics and Genomics*, *15*, 195–200.

28. Ellingrod, V., Perry, P., Ringold, J. (2005). Weight gain associated with the –759C/T polymorphism of the 5HT2C receptor and olanzapine. *American Journal of Medical Genetics. Part B, Neuropsychiatric Genetics*, *134*, 76–78.

29. Reynolds, G., Zhang, Z., Zhang, X. (2002). Association of antipsychotic drug-induced weight gain with a 5-HT2C receptor gene polymorphism. *Lancet*, *359*, 2086–2087.

30. Masellis, M., et al. (1998). Serotonin subtype 2 receptor genes and clinical response to clozapine in schizophrenia patients. *Neuropsychopharmacology*, *19*(2), 123–132.

31. Rietschel, M., et al. (1997). Efficacy and side-effects of clozapine not associated with variation in the 5-HT2C receptor. *Neuroreport*, *8*(8), 1999–2003.

32. Ellingrod, V., et al. (2002). 5HT2A and 5HT2C receptor polymorphisms and predicting clinical response to olanzapine in schizophrenia. *Journal of Clinical Psychopharmacology*, *22*(6), 622–624.

33. Segman, R., Heresco-Levy, U., Finkel, B. (2000). Association between the serotonin 2C receptor gene and tardive dyskinesia in chronic schizophrenia: additive contribution of 5-HT2Cser and DRD3gly alleles to susceptibility. *Psychopharmacology (Berl)*, *152*(4), 408–413.

34. Gunes, A., Scordo, M., Jaanson, P. (2007). Serotonin and dopamine receptor gene polymorphisms and the risk of extrapyramidal side effects in perphenazine-treated schizophrenic patients. *Psychopharmacology (Berl)*, *190*, 479–484.

35. Miyamoto, S., et al. (2005). Treatments for schizophrenia: a critical review of pharmacology and mechanisms of action of antipsychotic drugs. *Molecular Psychiatry*, *10*(1), 79–104.

36. Wood, M.D., et al. (2006). Pharmacological profile of antipsychotics at monoamine receptors: atypicality beyond 5-HT2A receptor blockade. *CNS & Neurological Disorders Drug Targets*, *5*(4), 445–452.

37. Gobert, A., et al. (2000). Serotonin(2C) receptors tonically suppress the activity of mesocortical dopaminergic and adrenergic, but not serotonergic, pathways: a combined dialysis and electrophysiological analysis in the rat. *Synapse (New York, N.Y.)*, *36*(3), 205–221.

38. Di Matteo, V., et al. (1998). Selective blockade of serotonin2C/2B receptors enhances dopamine release in the rat nucleus accumbens. *Neuropharmacology*, *37*(2), 265–272.

39. Shilliam, C.S., Dawson, L.A. (2005). The effect of clozapine on extracellular dopamine levels in the shell subregion of the rat nucleus accumbens is reversed following chronic administration: comparison with a selective 5-HT2C receptor antagonist. *Neuropsychopharmacology*, *30*(2), 372–380.

40. Blackburn, T.P., et al. (2002). Effect of acute and chronic administration of the selective 5-HT2C receptor antagonist SB-243213 on midbrain dopamine neurons in the rat: an in vivo extracellular single cell study. *Synapse (New York, N.Y.)*, *46*(3), 129–139.

41. Blackburn, T.P., Suzuki, K., Ashby, C.R. Jr. (2006). The acute and chronic administration of the 5-HT(2B/2C) receptor antagonist SB-200646A significantly alters the activity of spontaneously active midbrain dopamine neurons in the rat: an in vivo extracellular single cell study. *Synapse (New York, N.Y.)*, *59*(8), 502–512.

42. Marquis, K.L., et al. (2007). WAY-163909 [(7bR,10aR)-1,2,3,4,8,9,10,10a-Octahydro-7bH-cyclopenta-[b][1,4]diazepino[6,7,1hi]indole]: a novel 5-hydroxytryptamine 2C receptor-selective agonist with preclinical antipsychotic-like activity. *The Journal of Pharmacology and Experimental Therapeutics*, *320*(1), 486–496.

43. Di Giovanni, G., et al. (1999). Selective blockade of serotonin-2C/2B receptors enhances mesolimbic and mesostriatal dopaminergic function: a combined in vivo electrophysiological and microdialysis study. *Neuroscience*, *91*(2), 587–597.

44. Reavill, C., et al. (1999). Attenuation of haloperidol-induced catalepsy by a 5-HT2C receptor antagonist. *British Journal of Pharmacology*, *126*(3), 572–574.

45. Ikram, H., Samad, N., Haleem, D.J. (2007). Neurochemical and behavioral effects of m-CPP in a rat model of tardive dyskinesia. *Pakistan Journal of Pharmaceutical Sciences*, *20*(3), 188–195.

46. Di Matteo, V., et al. (1999). SB 242084, a selective serotonin2C receptor antagonist, increases dopaminergic transmission in the mesolimbic system. *Neuropharmacology*, *38*(8), 1195–1205.

47. Di Giovanni, G., et al. (2000). Preferential modulation of mesolimbic vs. nigrostriatal dopaminergic function by serotonin(2C/2B) receptor agonists: a combined in vivo electrophysiological and microdialysis study. *Synapse (New York, N.Y.)*, *35*(1), 53–61.

48. Marquis, K.L., et al. *SCA-136: a novel 5-HT$_{2C}$ receptor agonist possessing atypical antipsychotic-like effects in preclinical models*. Program No. 93.4, Neuroscience Meeting Planner. Atlanta, GA: Society for Neuroscience, 2006.

49. Siuciak, J.A., et al. (2007). CP-809,101, a selective 5-HT(2C) agonist, shows activity in animal models of antipsychotic activity. *Neuropharmacology*, *52*(2), 279–290.

50. Kostrzewa, R.M., et al. (2007). Modeling tardive dyskinesia: predictive 5-HT2C receptor antagonist treatment. *Neurotoxicity Research*, *11*(1), 41–50.
51. Rosenzweig-Lipson, S., et al. *Vabicaserin: effects of a novel 5-HT2C agonist on prefrontal cortical neurotransmission, cognition and sensorimotor gating*. ECNP abstract, 2007.
52. Ellenbroek, B.A. (2004). Pre-attentive processing and schizophrenia: animal studies. *Psychopharmacology (Berl)*, *174*(1), 65–74.
53. Fletcher, P., et al. (2007). Opposing effects of 5-HT2A and 5-HT2C receptor antagonists in the rat and mouse on premature responding in the five-choice serial reaction time test. *Psychopharmacology (Berl)*, *195*(2), 223–234.
54. Navarra, R., et al. (2008). The 5-HT2C receptor agonist WAY-163909 decreases impulsivity in the 5-choice serial reaction time test. *Behavioural Brain Research*, *188*(2), 412–415.
55. Winstanley, C.A., et al. (2004). 5-HT 2A and 5-HT 2C receptor antagonists have opposing effects on a measure of impulsivity: interactions with global 5-HT depletion. *Psychopharmacology (Berl)*, *176*(3), 376–385.
56. Robinson, E.S.J., et al. (2007). Opposing roles for 5-HT2A and 5-HT2C receptors in the nucleus accumbens on inhibitory response control in the 5-choice serial reaction time task. *Neuropsychopharmacology*, *33*(10), 2398–2406.
57. Chagnon, Y.C. (2006). Susceptibility genes for the side effect of antipsychotics on body weight and obesity. *Current Drug Targets*, *7*(12), 1681–1695.
58. Rosenzweig-Lipson, S., et al. (2007). Antidepressant-like effects of the novel, selective, 5-HT(2C) receptor agonist WAY-163909 in rodents. *Psychopharmacology (Berl)*, *192*(2), 159–170.
59. Monsma, F.J. Jr., et al. (1993). Cloning and expression of a novel serotonin receptor with high affinity for tricyclic psychotropic drugs. *Molecular Pharmacology*, *43*(3), 320–327.
60. Kohen, R., et al. (1996). Cloning, characterization, and chromosomal localization of a human 5-HT6 serotonin receptor. *Journal of Neurochemistry*, *66*(1), 47–56.
61. Olsen, M.A., et al. (1999). Identification of a human 5-HT6 receptor variant produced by alternative splicing. *Brain Research. Molecular Brain Research*, *64*(2), 255–263.
62. Gerard, C., et al. (1997). Immuno-localization of serotonin 5-HT6 receptor-like material in the rat central nervous system. *Brain Research*, *746*(1–2), 207–219.
63. Hamon, M., et al. (1999). Antibodies and antisense oligonucleotide for probing the distribution and putative functions of central 5-HT6 receptors. *Neuropsychopharmacology*, *21*(2 Suppl), 68S–76S.
64. Gerard, C., et al. (1996). Quantitative RT-PCR distribution of serotonin 5-HT6 receptor mRNA in the central nervous system of control or 5,7-dihydroxytryptamine-treated rats. *Synapse (New York, N.Y.)*, *23*(3), 164–173.
65. Roberts, J.C., et al. (2002). The distribution of 5-HT6 receptors in rat brain: an autoradiographic binding study using the radiolabelled 5-HT6 receptor antagonist [125I]SB-258585. *Brain Research*, *934*, 49–57.
66. Ward, R.P., Dorsa, D.M. (1996). Colocalization of serotonin receptor subtypes 5-HT2A, 5-HT2C, and 5-HT6 with neuropeptides in rat striatum. *The Journal of Comparative Neurology*, *370*(3), 405–414.

67. Schechter, L.E., et al. (2008). Neuropharmacological profile of novel and selective 5-HT6 receptor agonists: WAY-181187 and WAY-208466. *Neuropsychopharmacology*, *33*(6), 1323–1335.
68. Bentley, J.C., et al. (1999). Investigation of stretching behaviour induced by the selective 5-HT6 receptor antagonist, Ro 04-6790, in rats. *British Journal of Pharmacology*, *126*(7), 1537–1542.
69. Yun, H.-M., et al. (2007). The novel cellular mechanism of human 5-HT6 receptor through an interaction with Fyn. *The Journal of Biological Chemistry*, *282*(8), 5496–5505.
70. Grant, S.G., et al. (1992). Impaired long-term potentiation, spatial learning, and hippocampal development in fyn mutant mice. *Science*, *258*(5090), 1903–1910.
71. Miyakawa, T., et al. (1994). Increased fearfulness of Fyn tyrosine kinase deficient mice. *Brain Research Molecular Brain Research*, *27*(1), 179–182.
72. Roth, B.L., et al. (1994). Binding of typical and atypical antipsychotic agents to 5-hydroxytryptamine-6 and 5-hydroxytryptamine-7 receptors. *The Journal of Pharmacology and Experimental Therapeutics*, *268*(3), 1403–1410.
73. Tsai, S.J., et al. (1999). Association study of serotonin-6 receptor variant (C267T) with schizophrenia and aggressive behavior. *Neuroscience Letters*, *271*(2), 135–137.
74. Shinkai, T., et al. (1999). Association study of the 5-HT6 receptor gene in schizophrenia. *American Journal of Medical Genetics. Part A*, *88*(2), 120–122.
75. Chiu, H.J., et al. (2001). Serotonin 6 receptor polymorphism in schizophrenia: frequency, age at onset and cognitive function. *Neuropsychobiology*, *43*(3), 113–116.
76. Vogt, I.R., et al. (2000). Investigation of the human serotonin 6 [5-HT6] receptor gene in bipolar affective disorder and schizophrenia. *American Journal of Medical Genetics. Part A*, *96*(2), 217–221.
77. Zhang, M.L., et al. (2003). [Associations between six functional genes and schizophrenia]. *Zhonghua Yi Xue Yi Chuan Xue Za Zhi*, *20*(1), 69–71.
78. Ohmori, O., et al. (2001). Novel polymorphism in the 5′-upstream region of the human 5-HT6 receptor gene and schizophrenia. *Neuroscience Letters*, *310*(1), 17–20.
79. Lane, H.Y., et al. (2006). Risperidone-related weight gain: genetic and nongenetic predictors. *Journal of Clinical Psychopharmacology*, *26*(2), 128–134.
80. Yu, Y.W., et al. (1999). Serotonin-6 receptor variant (C267T) and clinical response to clozapine. *Neuroreport*, *10*(6), 1231–1233.
81. Masellis, M., et al. (2001). Lack of association between the T-->C 267 serotonin 5-HT6 receptor gene (HTR6) polymorphism and prediction of response to clozapine in schizophrenia. *Schizophrenia Research*, *47*(1), 49–58.
82. Healy, D.J., Meador-Woodruff, J.H. (1999). Ionotropic glutamate receptor modulation of 5-HT6 and 5-HT7 mRNA expression in rat brain. *Neuropsychopharmacology*, *21*(3), 341–351.
83. East, S.Z., et al. (2002). An RT-PCR study of 5-HT(6) and 5-HT(7) receptor mRNAs in the hippocampal formation and prefrontal cortex in schizophrenia. *Schizophrenia Research*, *57*(1), 15–26.

84. Frederick, J.A., Meador-Woodruff, J.H. (1999). Effects of clozapine and haloperidol on 5-HT6 receptor mRNA levels in rat brain. *Schizophrenia Research*, *38*(1), 7–12.

85. East, S.Z., et al. (2002). 5-HT6 receptor binding sites in schizophrenia and following antipsychotic drug administration: autoradiographic studies with [125I]SB-258585. *Synapse (New York, N.Y.)*, *45*(3), 191–199.

86. Marcos, B., et al. (2006). Lack of localization of 5-HT6 receptors on cholinergic neurons: implication of multiple neurotransmitter systems in 5-HT6 receptor-mediated acetylcholine release. *The European Journal of Neuroscience*, *24*(5), 1299–1306.

87. Riemer, C., et al. (2003). Influence of the 5-HT6 receptor on acetylcholine release in the cortex: pharmacological characterization of 4-(2-bromo-6-pyrrolidin-1-ylpyridine-4-sulfonyl)phenylamine, a potent and selective 5-HT6 receptor antagonist. *Journal of Medicinal Chemistry*, *46*(7), 1273–1276.

88. Hirst, W.D., et al. (2006). SB-399885 is a potent, selective 5-HT6 receptor antagonist with cognitive enhancing properties in aged rat water maze and novel object recognition models. *European Journal of Pharmacology*, *553*(1–3), 109–119.

89. Shirazi-Southall, S., Rodriguez, D.E., Nomikos, G.G. (2002). Effects of typical and atypical antipsychotics and receptor selective compounds on acetylcholine efflux in the hippocampus of the rat. *Neuropsychopharmacology*, *26*(5), 583–594.

90. Dawson, L.A., Nguyen, H.Q., Li, P. (2001). The 5-HT(6) receptor antagonist SB-271046 selectively enhances excitatory neurotransmission in the rat frontal cortex and hippocampus. *Neuropsychopharmacology*, *25*(5), 662–668.

91. Dawson, L.A., Nguyen, H.Q., Li, P. (2000). In vivo effects of the 5-HT(6) antagonist SB-271046 on striatal and frontal cortex extracellular concentrations of noradrenaline, dopamine, 5-HT, glutamate and aspartate. *British Journal of Pharmacology*, *130*(1), 23–26.

92. Minabe, Y., et al. (2004). Effect of the acute and chronic administration of the selective 5-HT6 receptor antagonist SB-271046 on the activity of midbrain dopamine neurons in rats: an in vivo electrophysiological study. *Synapse (New York, N.Y.)*, *52*(1), 20–28.

93. Lacroix, L.P., et al. (2004). 5-HT6 receptor antagonist SB-271046 enhances extracellular levels of monoamines in the rat medial prefrontal cortex. *Synapse (New York, N.Y.)*, *51*(2), 158–164.

94. Li, Z., et al. (2007). 5-HT6 receptor antagonist SB-399885 potentiates haloperidol and risperidone-induced dopamine efflux in the medial prefrontal cortex or hippocampus. *Brain Research*, *1134*(1), 70–78.

95. Woolley, M.L., et al. (2001). A role for 5-ht6 receptors in retention of spatial learning in the Morris water maze. *Neuropharmacology*, *41*(2), 210–219.

96. Rogers, D.C., Hagan, J.J. (2001). 5-HT6 receptor antagonists enhance retention of a water maze task in the rat. *Psychopharmacology (Berl)*, *158*(2), 114–119.

97. Stean, T.O., et al. (2002). Pharmacological profile of SB-357134: a potent, selective, brain penetrant, and orally active 5-HT(6) receptor antagonist. *Pharmacology, Biochemistry, and Behavior*, *71*(4), 645–654.

98. Foley, A.G., et al. (2004). The 5-HT(6) receptor antagonist SB-271046 reverses scopolamine-disrupted consolidation of a passive avoidance task and ameliorates spatial task deficits in aged rats. *Neuropsychopharmacology*, *29*(1), 93–100.

99. King, M.V., et al. (2004). 5-HT6 receptor antagonists reverse delay-dependent deficits in novel object discrimination by enhancing consolidation—an effect sensitive to NMDA receptor antagonism. *Neuropharmacology*, *47*(2), 195–204.

100. Mitchell, E.S., et al. (2006). BGC20-761, a novel tryptamine analog, enhances memory consolidation and reverses scopolamine-induced memory deficit in social and visuospatial memory tasks through a 5-HT6 receptor-mediated mechanism. *Neuropharmacology*, *50*(4), 412–420.

101. Woolley, M.L., et al. (2003). Reversal of a cholinergic-induced deficit in a rodent model of recognition memory by the selective 5-HT6 receptor antagonist, Ro 04-6790. *Psychopharmacology (Berl)*, *170*(4), 358–367.

102. Lieben, C.K., et al. (2005). The selective 5-HT6 receptor antagonist Ro4368554 restores memory performance in cholinergic and serotonergic models of memory deficiency in the rat. *Neuropsychopharmacology*, *30*(12), 2169–2179.

103. Perez-Garcia, G., Meneses, A. (2005). Oral administration of the 5-HT6 receptor antagonists SB-357134 and SB-399885 improves memory formation in an autoshaping learning task. *Pharmacology, Biochemistry, and Behavior*, *81*(3), 673–682.

104. Lindner, M.D., et al. (2003). An assessment of the effects of serotonin 6 (5-HT6) receptor antagonists in rodent models of learning. *The Journal of Pharmacology and Experimental Therapeutics*, *307*(2), 682–691.

105. Mitchell, E.S., Neumaier, J.F. (2008). 5-HT6 receptor antagonist reversal of emotional learning and prepulse inhibition deficits induced by apomorphine or scopolamine. *Pharmacology, Biochemistry, and Behavior*, *88*(3), 291–298.

106. Pouzet, B., Didriksen, M., Arnt, J. (2002). Effects of the 5-HT(6) receptor antagonist, SB-271046, in animal models for schizophrenia. *Pharmacology, Biochemistry, and Behavior*, *71*(4), 635–643.

107. Hatcher, P.D., et al. (2005). 5-HT6 receptor antagonists improve performance in an attentional set shifting task in rats. *Psychopharmacology (Berl)*, *181*(2), 253–259.

108. King, M.V., Marsden, C.A., Fone, K.C.F. (2008). A role for the 5-HT1A, 5-HT4 and 5-HT6 receptors in learning and memory. *Trends in Pharmacological Sciences*, *29*(9), 482–492.

109. Rodefer, J.S., et al. (2008). Reversal of subchronic PCP-induced deficits in attentional set shifting in rats by sertindole and a 5-HT(6) receptor antagonist: comparison among antipsychotics. *Neuropsychopharmacology*, *33*(11), 2657–2666.

110. Foley, A.G., et al. (2008). The selective 5-HT6 receptor antagonists SB-271046 and SB-399885 potentiate NCAM PSA immunolabeling of dentate granule cells, but not neurogenesis, in the hippocampal formation of mature Wistar rats. *Neuropharmacology*, *54*(8), 1166–1174.

111. Murphy, K.J., O'Connell, A.W., Regan, C.M. (1996). Repetitive and transient increases in hippocampal neural cell adhesion molecule polysialylation state following multitrial spatial training. *Journal of Neurochemistry*, *67*(3), 1268–1274.

112. Foley, A.G., et al. (2003). Consolidation of memory for odour-reward association requires transient polysialylation of the neural cell adhesion molecule in the rat hippocampal dentate gyrus. *Journal of Neuroscience Research*, *74*(4), 570–576.
113. Foley, A.G., et al. (2003). Distribution of polysialylated neural cell adhesion molecule in rat septal nuclei and septohippocampal pathway: transient increase of polysialylated interneurons in the subtriangular septal zone during memory consolidation. *Journal of Neuroscience Research*, *74*(6), 807–817.
114. Leng, A., et al. (2003). Effect of the 5-HT6 receptor antagonists Ro04-6790 and Ro65-7199 on latent inhibition and prepulse inhibition in the rat: comparison to clozapine. *Pharmacology, Biochemistry, and Behavior*, *75*(2), 281–288.
115. Ouagazzal, A., et al. (2001). Effect of LSD on prepulse inhibition and spontaneous behavior in the rat. A pharmacological analysis and comparison between two rat strains. *Neuropsychopharmacology*, *25*(4), 565–575.

# 11

# THE CHOLINERGIC HYPOTHESIS: AN INTRODUCTION TO THE HYPOTHESIS AND A SHORT HISTORY

JOSEPH I. FRIEDMAN, ISABELLA KANELLOPOULOU, AND VLADAN NOVAKOVIC

## 11.1 INTRODUCTION

Over the last several years psychiatric research has been engaged in a search for new drugs with novel mechanisms of action to improve symptom domains of schizophrenia, such as cognitive impairments, which are poorly addressed by current treatments. It has been particularly challenging to develop drugs that act on targets other than dopamine because recognition of the involvement of other neurotransmitter systems in the pathophysiology of schizophrenia has lagged behind. Although acetylcholine (ACh) has long been recognized as playing an important role in cognition, and its involvement in the cognitive symptoms of Alzheimer's disease has been solidly established, it has only been recently that disruption of normal cholinergic transmission has been recognized as part of the pathophysiology of schizophrenia. Indeed, interest in cholinergic system involvement in the pathophysiology of schizophrenia was reawakened with the demonstration of the cholinergic effects of second-generation antipsychotics and the reported superior cognitive effects of second-generation antipsychotics in schizophrenia. The hypothesis that central nervous system (CNS) cholinergic system disruptions are involved in the pathology of schizophrenia and possibly related to the cognitive impairments

*Targets and Emerging Therapies for Schizophrenia*, First Edition.
Edited by Jeffrey S. Albert and Michael W. Wood.

of schizophrenia is now supported by a growing understanding of the involvement of more specific ACh receptor subtypes in normal cognitive processes, and observations that more subtle cholinergic disruptions at the receptor level are a part of the pathophysiology underlying schizophrenia.

## 11.2 ORGANIZATION OF THE CENTRAL CHOLINERGIC SYSTEM

### 11.2.1 Cholinergic Projections

In order to better approach potential points of intervention in the cholinergic system to target the cognitive impairments of schizophrenia, it is important to first understand the organization of the cholinergic system in the brain.

The cholinergic system in the brain is distributed in a variety of different nuclei. Two groups of cholinergic nuclei, the basal forebrain and pedunculopontine groups, both have extensive projections to the cortex and thalamus (see Fig. 11.1). The basal forebrain cholinergic group innervates the entire cerebral cortex, including the hippocampus and amygdale, and these projections are considered essential for normal cognitive functioning. The basal forebrain cholinergic group includes the nucleus basalis of Meynert (NbM), the medial septal, and the vertical and horizontal limbs of the diagonal band. Among the basal forebrain nuclei, the NbM has the highest content of cholinergic fibers (90%). The septal nuclei have 10% cholinergic fibers, the vertical nucleus of Broca's diagonal band has 70%, and the horizontal nucleus of the diagonal band has only 1%. The NbM is not a discrete, well-circumscribed structure, but consists of groups of large neurons scattered in the substantia innominata beneath and impinging into the lenticular nucleus. Anteriorly, cells of the NbM intermingle with cells of the diagonal band of Broca, and the two structures are difficult to differentiate. The largest bulk of the nucleus is situated beneath the anterior globus pallidus, dorsolateral to the optic tract and ventromedial to the anterior commissure. The NbM has rich afferent and efferent projections. Its input arises primarily from the limbic system and related structures and its output projects to most of the neocortex. The NbM receives afferents from the orbitofrontal cortex, temporal lobe, pre-pyriform regions, entorhinal cortex, medial inferotemporal cortex, and anterior insula. Subcortical afferent input arises from the hypothalamus, septal nuclei, nucleus accumbens, amygdala, and peripendicular nucleus of the midbrain. Efferent projections of the NbM project to all areas of the neocortex and the amygdala. The degree of cholinergic innervation in the cortex is very high in layer I, less intense in the middle layers, and intense in layers IV and V. The efferent projections are topographically ordered so that the anteromedial division of the NbM connects with the frontoparietal operculum and the amygdala; the intermediate division projects to dorsal frontal and parietal regions as well as inferotemporal and peristriate cortex; and the posterior division provides efferents to the superior temporal cortex and adjacent regions. The other

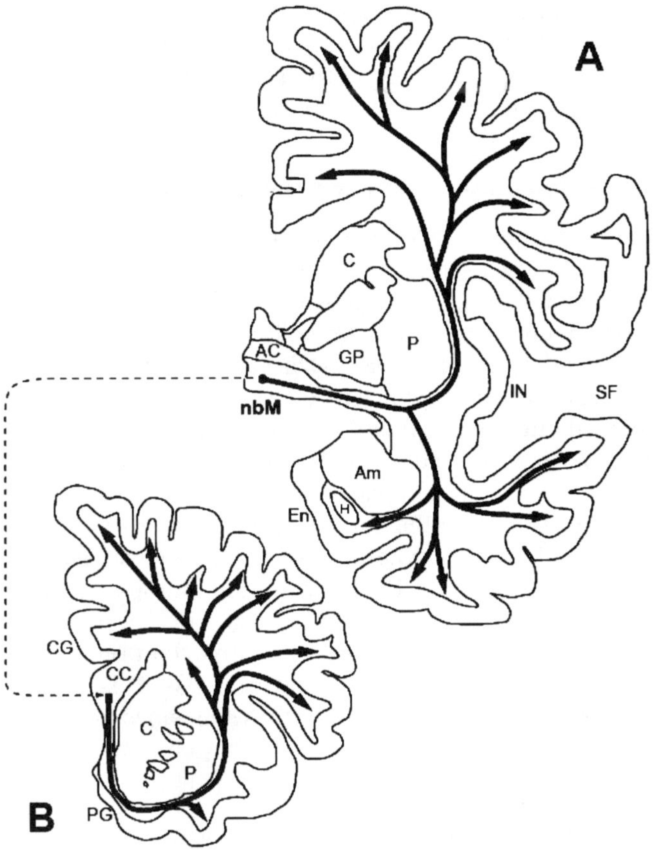


**FIGURE 11.1** Coronal view of the lateral and medial cholinergic projections from the basal forebrain group. (A) is more caudal and (B) is more rostral. Both medial and lateral pathways emanate from the nucleus basalis of Meynert (nbM).The medial pathway (B) gives off fibers to the cingulate gyrus (CG) and medial prefrontal cortex. The lateral pathway (A) courses within the frontal lobe white matter and gives off fibers to the dorsolateral prefrontal cortex.Two major componets of the lateral pathway course through external capsule and claustrum projecting to the frontoparietal cortex (dorsally) and temporal lobe (ventrally). In addition, discrete AchE-rich fiber bundles project to temporal, parietal, and occipital cotical areas. The minor subset of the basal cholinergic group—medial septal nuclei (MSN), and vertical limb of the diagonal bandof Broca (VDB) are not shown. The pontomesencephalic (PM) cholinergic group that carries input to brainstem bioaminergic nuclei (e.g., VTA, SN, Raphe) is not shown. Ac, anterior commissure; nbM, nucleus basalis of Meynert; GP, globus pallidus; P, putamen; C, caudate; CC, corpus callosum; IN, insular cortex; SF, Sylvian fissure; En, enthorhinal cortex; H, hipocampus; AM, amygdala; CG, cingulate gyrus; PG, parolfactory gyrus; V, ventricule.

medial forebrain nuclei have different efferent connections: the medial septal nucleus projects to the hippocampus, the vertical nucleus of the diagonal band projects both to the hippocampus and to the hypothalamus, and the horizontal nucleus of the diagonal band projects to the olfactory bulb.

### 11.2.2 Acetylcholine Biosynthesis and Degradation

ACh is synthesized from acetyl-CoA and choline by the enzyme choline acetyltransferase (ChAT). This enzyme is located almost exclusively in the cytoplasm of cholinergic fibers. The acetyl-CoA derives from pyruvate generated by the glucose metabolism in the mitochondria. The choline derives from dietary sources and from phosphatidylcholine. Furthemore, choline can be supplied from ACh hydrolysis, which is released into the synaptic cleft. Choline is then reimported into the cholinergic neuron through the choline transporter. The amount of ACh produced in cholinergic neurons is determined by the concentration of the choline in these neurons.

ACh is stored in vesicles at the nerve terminals. In response to action potentials, ACh is released into the synaptic cleft via exocytosis, which is facilitated by membrane calcium channels. Botulinum toxin inhibits the function of these channels, and consequently, the release of ACh.

ACh is hydrolyzed by esterases. The most important ones are acetylcholinesterase (AChE) and butyrylesterase (BuChE). AChE is located extracellularly in the synaptic complex. Blockade of these enzymes increases the half-life of Ach in the synapse.

### 11.2.3 Acetylcholine Receptors

Cholinergic transmission is mediated by two families of receptors, the ligand-gated ion channels, which comprise the nicotinic receptor family, and the G-protein-mediated muscarinic receptor family.

Nicotinic acetylcholine receptors (nAChRs) are ligand-gated cationic channels wherein the movement of $Na^+$ and $Ca^{2+}$ results in membrane depolarization and neuronal excitation. Diverse nACh receptor types are formed as pentamers from different combinations of genetically distinct subunits which confer distinctive functional and structural properties to the nACh receptor types that they form (reviewed by Lukas et al; [1]). The 16 nACh receptor subunits identified to date are defined using a Greek letter, with nine alpha subunit ($\alpha$1–$\alpha$9), four beta subunits ($\beta$1–$\beta$4), one gamma ($\gamma$), delta ($\delta$), and epsilon ($\varepsilon$) subunit (Reviewed by Lukas et al; [1]). Various combinations of $\alpha$ and $\beta$ subunits form two primary subtypes of neuronal nAChRs: (1) those containing a combination of $\alpha$ and $\beta$ subunits, and (2) those containing only $\alpha$ subunits. nAChRs mediate pre- and postsynaptic excitation and presynaptic control of neurotransmitter release. Neurotransmitters mediated by presynaptic nAChRs include ACh [2], norepinephrine [3], dopamine [4], serotonin [5], glutamate [6], and GABA [7]. The subtypes of nAChR expressed most highly in the brain are α4β2 subunit-containing receptors and α7 subunit-containing receptors [8], with both subtypes being richly expressed in the hippocampus.

Muscarinic acetylcholine receptors (mAChRs) are widely expressed throughout the CNS, of which five subtypes have been identified: $M_1$, $M_2$, $M_3$, $M_4$, $M_5$. mAChRs are G-protein coupled and can be divided into two distinct classes based on the type of G-protein with which they couple (reviewed by Langmead [9]). The group comprising $M_1$, $M_3$, and $M_5$ subtypes are coupled via $G_{q/11}$ proteins that activate phospholipase-C and increase intracellular calcium. $M_2$ and $M_4$ subtypes are coupled via $G_{i/o}$ proteins and inhibit adenylate cyclase and reduce intracellular concentrations of cAMP. The predominant mAChR subtype in the CNS is the $M_1$ subtype, which is located in the cortex, hippocampus, striatum, and thalamus, where it is found postsynaptically [10]. $M_2$ mAChRs are located predominantly in the brainstem and thalamus, though also in the cortex, hippocampus, and striatum, where they reside on cholinergic synaptic terminals [11] and are thought to control ACh release [12]. $M_3$ and $M_5$ mAChRs are expressed at much lower levels than $M_1$ or $M_2$ mAChRs in the CNS; nevertheless, $M_3$ mAChRs are found in the cortex and hippocampus [10], whereas $M_5$ mAChRs have a very discrete localization in the substantia nigra [10]. $M_4$ mAChRs are found in many brain regions including the cortex and hippocampus but are most prominent in the striatum [10], where they are thought to play a role in controlling dopamine release and locomotor activity.

## 11.3 THE RELATIONSHIP BETWEEN CENTRAL CHOLINERGIC NEUROTRANSMISSION AND COGNITION

### 11.3.1 Lesion Studies

The relationship between memory and ACh has been well established in animal lesion models and behavioral pharmacology investigations. The correlation between lesions in septo-hippocampal and NbM-cortical cholinergic pathways and subsequent memory deficits indicates the involvement of these pathways in memory processes [13]. Lesions of the septohippocampal pathway decrease performance in the delayed nonmatch to position paradigm in rats [14, 15], whereas lesions of the NbM produces deficits in passive avoidance conditioned responses, radial arm maze, and water maze performance [16, 17]. Taken together, these findings demonstrate that the septohippocampal pathway is associated with working memory processes through hippocampal storage of intermediate-term memory [18–20] and that the NbM-cortical pathway is involved in reference memory through long-term information storage in the neocortex [21, 22]. The memory deficits caused by the above lesions are ameliorated by administration of AChE inhibitors, such as physostigmine [23], which increase synaptic levels of ACh.

### 11.3.2 Pharmacological Manipulations of Acetylcholine

Further insight into the importance of ACh in memory and learning comes from pharmacological studies of behavior. Administration of either of the muscarininc receptor antagonists, scopolamine, or atropine induces memory dysfunction in rats, primates, and humans [24–26]. This drug-induced impairment is subsequently reversed after displacement of the blocking agent [27] and can be overcome by the use of AChE inhibitors. AChE inhibitor drugs act by preventing the breakdown of ACh in the synaptic cleft. The administration of the AChE inhibitor physostigmine to both young and aged monkeys produces an overall improvement of mnemonic processes in both groups [28]. Tacrine and donepezil, two AChE inhibitors, can reverse the deficits induced by scopolamine in T-maze and passive avoidance tests in rats [29, 30] and induced deficits in memory in monkeys [31]. This supports the notion that memory function can be improved by increasing synaptic ACh, and specifically by AChE inhibition.

A role for ACh in the processes of attention has also been demonstrated in rats. Performance on the five-choice serial reaction task is impaired following basal forebrain lesions [32]. Furthermore, both the systemic administration of physostigmine and the transplant of cholinergic embryonic cells into the brains of rats with basal forebrain lesions improve the visual attentional impairments [33]. The role of ACh in attentional processes has also been described in monkeys. Continuous intraventricular injections of scopolamine during a continuous performance task requiring localization of briefly presented visual stimuli results in a decrease in the number of responses. This effect becomes more apparent when the stimulus presentation is shortened, and toward the end of the testing session [34].

### 11.3.3 Pharmacological Manipulations of the Muscarinic Acetylcholine Receptor

mAChRs in the hippocampus are relevant to learning and memory. Moreover, memory consolidation in the rat appears to involve participation of both $M_1$ and $M_4$ hippocampal receptors [35]. However, a more defined role for the $M_1$ receptor subtype in memory processes has been demonstrated by the $M_1$ mAChR knockout mouse phenotype, which suggests a role for these receptors in the induction of long-term potentiation, learning, and working memory [36, 37]. The $M_4$ mAChR subtype appears to exert control over midbrain dopamine release. For example, $M_4$ knockout mice display a twofold increase in dopamine efflux and dopamine metabolites in the nucleus accumbens compared with wild-type mice [38].

### 11.3.4 Pharmacological Manipulations of the nAChR Nicotinic Acetylcholine Receptor

Nicotine and other nAChR agonists can improve performance on cognitive tasks, while nicotinic antagonists can impair performance [39, 40]. The principal nicotinic receptor subtypes that have been characterized with regard to cognitive function are the low-affinity α7 and the high-affinity α4β2 nAChRs. α7 knockout mice have significant impairment in attentional processes [41], whereas the partial α7 nAChR agonist GTS 21 significantly improves learning and memory [42]. In addition, the α4β2 nAChR agonist RJR2403 significantly improves working memory functions in rats [43].

## 11.4 ALTERATIONS OF CENTRAL CHOLINERGIC FUNCTIONS IN SCHIZOPHRENIA

### 11.4.1 Changes in Choline Acetyl Transferase

Post mortem investigations have demonstrated that the obvious neuropathology of the cholinergic system in Alzheimer's disease is absent from the brains of schizophrenic patients. Specifically, the size and number of cells in the NbM of schizophrenic patients is not significantly different from that of normal controls [44]. Moreover, the activity of ChAT, a marker of cholinergic function, is not significantly reduced in the parietal cortex of schizophrenic patients compared with normal elderly controls [45]. Despite these findings, more subtle alterations in cholinergic pathways in the brain of schizophrenic patients may make significant contributions to the cognitive impairments of schizophrenia. For example, although the activity of ChAT in the parietal cortex of schizophrenic patients is not significantly reduced in comparison to normal elderly controls [45], its relative activity may nevertheless contribute to the cognitive dysfunction of schizophrenia. Indeed, ChAT activity in the parietal cortex significantly correlates with the severity of cognitive impairment in schizophrenic patients [45].

### 11.4.2 Muscarinic Receptor Changes

At the receptor level, numerous observations implicate the involvement of the muscarinic cholinergic system in schizophrenia. For example, investigations of *in vivo* mAChR availability using [123I]IQNB (Idoquinuclidinyl benzialte) SPECT (single photon emission computed tomography) have demonstrated decreased mAChR binding in the frontal, temporal and occipital cortex and, caudate, putamen and thalamus of un-medicated schizophrenic patients [46]. Interestingly, the level of $M_1$ receptor protein has been found to also be decreased in Brodmann's area 9 in schizophrenic patients [47], an area specifically linked to some of the cognitive impairments of schizophrenia. Moreover, these findings also have relevance in light of involvement of the $M_1$ subtype in memory processes found to be impaired in schizophrenic patients. Indeed, the $M_1$ receptor subtype is the most abundant of the mAChRs in forebrain and hippocampus [10, 48], brain regions both crucial to normal cognitive functions.

### 11.4.3 Nicotinic Receptor Changes

Other receptor alterations of the cholinergic system found in schizophrenia include reduced numbers of low affinity (containing the $\alpha7$ subunit) nAChRs in the hippocampus [49], prefrontal cortex and corpus callosum [50], and reduced numbers of high affinity (containing $\alpha4\beta2$ subunits) nAChRs in the hippocampus, cortex, striatum and thalamus [51]. Consistent with these findings is the observation that nicotine administration normalizes two psychophysiological deficits found in schizophrenia; the auditory sensory gating deficit [52] and abnormal smooth pursuit eye movement [53].

## 11.5 CHOLINERGICALLY BASED PHARMACOLOGICAL STRATEGIES FOR COGNITIVE ENHANCEMENT IN SCHIZOPHRENIA

### 11.5.1 Early Studies of Augmenting Central Cholinergic Function in Schizophrenia

The data already presented provide a sufficient basis for testing various strategies to augment central cholinergic function for the purposes of enhancing the cognitive functions of patients with schizophrenia. Moreover, these data provide several potential points of intervention to achieve this goal. Potential cholinergically based strategies include increasing concentration of ACh at the synapse (e.g., AChE inhibitors), directly agonizing mAChRs involved in cognition, and directly agonizing nAChRs involved in cognition (see Table 11.1).

The earliest suggestion that increased central cholinergic activity might improve symptoms of schizophrenia was published in 1957 in a report that the cholinomimetic arecoline produced a brief period of lucidity in patients with

**TABLE 11.1 Cholinergically Based Targets for Pharmacological Treatment of Cognitive Impairments in Schizophrenia**

| Target | | Action | Result |
|---|---|---|---|
| Acetylcholinesterase | | Inhibitor | Prolonged activity of acetylcholine at both nicotinic and muscarinic receptor types. |
| Muscarinic receptor | $M_1$ subtype | Agonist | G-protein-mediated activation of phospholipase-C and mobilization of intracellular calcium |
| | $M_4$ subtype | Agonist | G-protein-mediated inhibition of adenylate cyclase and reduction of intracellular cAMP |
| Nicotinic receptor | $\alpha7$ containing | Agonist | Stabilize the open state of the cationic channels |
| | $\alpha4\beta2$ containing | Agonist | Stabilize the open state of the cationic channels |

catatonic schizophrenia [54]. Similarly, oxotremorine, another central muscarinic agonist, was reported to produce a lucid interval in chronic schizophrenic patients [55]. However, neither arecoline nor oxotremorine produced more than brief periods of remission. Longer remission in chronic schizophrenic patients, refractory to traditional antipsychotics, was reported following the combination of antipsychotics and the reversible AChE inhibitor, physostigmine [56]. However, patients seemed to develop tolerance to this combination and a few days later, they returned to the same level of psychopathology as prior to the physostigmine administration. In addition, physostigmine has been shown to be effective in preventing and reversing methylphenidate-induced symptoms of psychosis in schizophrenic patients [57].

Interestingly, increases in ACh in the synapse may be one mechanism by which second generation antipsychotics exert their putative pro-cognitive effects in schizophrenic patients. Although less well known than their dopaminergic and serotonergic effects, second-generation antipsychotic drugs significantly increase ACh release in the medial prefrontal cortex, whereas the first-generation antipsychotics do not [58]. This important distinction could explain, in part, the limited differences in cognitive effects between first- and second-generation antipsychotics.

### 11.5.2 Cholinesterase Inhibitors

Presently, most drugs used in the treatment of Alzheimer's disease are AChE inhibitors. The inhibition of AChE increases the duration of time ACh remains active at the synapse. This strategy has been proven useful in Alzheimer's disease by improving cognition and disruptive behavior associated with this disorder. Subsequent to the earlier studies of cholinomimetics in schizophrenia, newer AChE inhibitors have been developed with improved pharmacokinetic and side effect profiles.

The AChE inhibitors approved for the treatment of Alzheimer's disease including donepezil, rivastigmine, and galantamine [59–62] have all been tested as adjunctive treatment for the cognitive impairments of schizophrenia. To date, a total of 26 clinical trials have been published describing the effects of these three AChE inhibitors on cognitive performance in patients with schizophrenia (see Table 11.2).

Donepezil has been the most frequently studied with a total of 15 published trials involving a total of 540 subjects (see Table 11.2). While the majority of these trials evaluated donepezil's effects on neurocognition, two assessed symptom severity effects only [63, 64]. Four studies reported statistically significant pro-cognitive effects of donepezil; however, three of these were open label designed [65–67]. The single positive double-blind study reported significant improvement in delayed recall with 5 mg of daily donepezil augmentation of first- and second-generation antipsychotics [68]. However, in this crossover designed study, the group randomized to donepezil first had better baseline delayed recall performance, and it is unclear if this discrepancy between groups

**TABLE 11.2 Review of Acetylcholinesterase Inhibitor Augmentation Trials to Treat the Cognitive Impairments of Schizophrenia**

| Sample Size | Cholinesterase Inhibitor | Dose (mg) | Antipsychotic Treatment | Trial Design | Outcome | Comment | Reference |
|---|---|---|---|---|---|---|---|
| 30 | Donepezil | 10 | Second-generation antipsychotics | 12-week, double-blind, placebo-controlled, parallel | • Improvement in negative symptoms with donepezil.<br>• No differences between the donepezil and placebo groups on any neurocognitive assessments. | 15/15 subjects completed the trial.<br>Mostly chronic outpatient subjects aged 22–44.<br>Baseline cognitive deficit at least 20 on MMSE. | [77] |
| 251 | Donepezil | 5–10 | Second-generation antipsychotics | 12-week, double-blind, placebo-controlled, parallel | • Placebo treated subjects showed greater neurocognitive improvement.<br>• No change in PANSS symptom severity rating with donepezil. | 98/121 donepezil treated-subjects and 97/124 placebo-treated subjects completed the study. | [69] |
| 28 | Donepezil | 5–10 | Second-generation antipsychotics | 12-week, open label | • Improvement in several cognitive domains with donepezil. | Concurrent use of anticholinergic medication and benzodiazepines was allowed. | [65] |
| | | | | | • No improvements in Positive and Negative Syndrome Scale (PANSS) symptom severity rating with donepezil. | 13/28 subjects completed the trial. | |
| 26 | Donepezil | 5–10 | Second-generation antipsychotics | 12 week, double-blind, placebo-controlled, parallel | • No improvement in neurocognition with donepezil.<br>• No improvement in social cognition with donepezil.<br>• No improvement in positive or negative symptoms with donepezil. | 22/26 subjects completed the trial. | [70] |

| | | | | | | | |
|---|---|---|---|---|---|---|---|
| 13 | Donepezil | 5–10 | Second-generation antipsychotics | 24-week double-blind, placebo-controlled, crossover | • Improvement in PANSS symptom severity ratings with donepezil. treatment. | 12 weeks placebo, 12 weeks donepezil treatment. | [63] |
| 21 | Donepezil | 5–10 | Ziprasidone | 4-month double-blind, placebo-controlled, parallel | • Placebo-treated patients improved on immediate verbal recall and planning efficiency. | 11/21 subjects completed the study (7 donepezil, 4 placebo). | [71] |
| 24 | Donepezil | 5 | Haloperidol | 12-week double-blind, placebo-controlled, parallel | • Donepezil treatment associated with trend level improvement in Mini Mental Status Examination. | | [72] |
| 24 | Donepezil | 5 | First- and second-generation antipsychotics, and combinations thereof. | 24-week double-blind, placebo-controlled, crossover | • Donepezil associated with nonsignificant improvement in PANSS symptom severity.<br>• Donepezil associated with modestly significant improvement in delayed recall. | 8 weeks of active treatment, 8 weeks washout between treatments.<br>15/22 subjects completed the protocol.<br>Significant placebo effects on PANSS symptom severity and delayed recall.<br>Group randomized to donepezil first had better baseline recall performance. | [68] |

(*Continued*)

**TABLE 11.2 (*Continued*)**

| Sample Size | Cholinesterase Inhibitor | Dose (mg) | Antipsychotic Treatment | Trial Design | Outcome | Comment | Reference |
|---|---|---|---|---|---|---|---|
| 40 | Donepezil | 5–10 | First- and second-generation antipsychotics | 8-week double-blind, placebo-controlled, parallel | • No improvement in symptomatology with donepezil.<br>• No improvement in neuorcognition with donepezil. | 32/40 subjects completed the study.<br>Significantly lower IQ in the donepezil-treated group. | [73] |
| 8 | Donepezil | 5–10 | Clozapine | 18-week open label, placebo-controlled, crossover | • No improvement in PANSS symptom severity with donepezil. | 8 weeks of treatment with a 2-week washout period.<br>6/8 subjects completed the study. | [64] |
| 12 | Donepezil | 5–10 | First-generation antipsychotics | 12-week double-blind, placebo-controlled, crossover | • No improvement in neurocognition with donepezil.<br>• No improvement in PANSS symptom severity with donepezil. | | [74] |
| 6 | Donepezil | 5–10 | Second-generation antipsychotics | 12-week double-blind, placebo-controlled, crossover | • No improvement in verbal fluency with donepezil.<br>• Donepezil treatment associated with greater task related activation of left prefrontal and cingulate cortex and deactivation of left superior temporal gyrus | 2-week washout period between treatments. | [75] |

| | | | | | | | |
|---|---|---|---|---|---|---|---|
| 6 | Donepezil | 5 | First- and second-generation antipsychotics | 4-week open label | • Significant improvement in MMSE.<br>• No improvement in Alzheimer's Disease Assessment Scale-cognitive.<br>• No significant improvement in PANSS symptom severity. | Subjects aged 54–76 with comorbid dementia (MMSE≤24).<br>Some subjects receiving anticholinergic medication. | [66] |
| 15 | Donepezil | 5–10 | Olanzapine | 6 weeks open label | • Donepezil produced modest improvement in P50 suppression,<br>• Donepezil produced significant improvement in Grooved Pegboard. | 14/15 subjects completed the trial. | [67] |
| 36 | Donepezil | 5–10 | Risperidone | 12-week double-blind, placebo-controlled, parallel | • No improvement in neurocognition with donepezil.<br>• No improvement in PANSS symptom severity with donepezil. | 34/36 subjects completed the study. | [76] |
| 21 | Galantamine | 4–8 | NA | Double-blind, placebo-controlled | • No main effects of galantamine on neurocognition. | Smoking status affected neurocognition. | [85] |
| 20 | Galantamine | 32 | Second-generation antipsychotics | 8-week double-blind, placebo-controlled, parallel | • Galantamine worsened neurocognitive performance.<br>• Galantamine had no effect on symptom severity. | 18/20 subjects completed the study.<br>All subjects were nonsmokers. | [86] |

(*Continued*)

**TABLE 11.2 (*Continued*)**

| Sample Size | Cholinesterase Inhibitor | Dose (mg) | Antipsychotic Treatment | Trial Design | Outcome | Comment | Reference |
|---|---|---|---|---|---|---|---|
| 86 | Galantamine | 5–24 | Second-generation antipsychotic and low-dose first-generation antipsychotic | 12-week double-blind, placebo-controlled, parallel | • Galantamine significantly improved processing speed., modestly improved verbal memory.<br>• Galantamine associated with worse performance on test of distractibility. | 73/86 subjects completed the study. | [83] |
| 24 | Galantamine | 8–16 | First-generation antipsychotics | 12-week double-blind, placebo-controlled, parallel | • No effect of galantamine on neurocognition. | Subjects had MMSE scores between 18 and 24. | [87] |
| 17 | Galantamine | 8–24 | Risperidone | 8-week double-blind, placebo-controlled, parallel | • Galantamine treatment produced significant improvement in overall neurocognitivwe performance.<br>• Galantamine did not affect symptom severity. | 14/17 subjects completed the trial. | [84] |
| 12 | Galantamine | 8–24 | Second-generation antipsychotic | 12-week open label | • No effect of galantamine on neurocognition. | 9 patients received galantamine and 3 received no treatment. | [88] |
| 5 | Galantamine | 16 | Clozapine | 8-week open label | • Neurocognitive improvement in some cases. | Group means not analyzed, individual data presented. | [89] |
| 24 | Rivastigmine | 3–9 | First- and second-generation antipsychotics | 3-month open label crossover design | • No improvement in neurocognition with rivastigmine.<br>• No improvement in symptom severity with rivastigmine. | 20/24 subjects completed the study.<br>4 subjects were taking anticholinergic medication. | [82] |

| | | | | | | | |
|---|---|---|---|---|---|---|---|
| 21 | Rivastigmine | 24 | Second-generation antipsychotics | 24-week double-blind, placebo-controlled, parallel | • No improvement in neurocognition with rivastigmine. | 9/21 subjects completed the study | [80] |
| 36 | Rivastigmine | 12 | Second-generation antipsychotics | 12-week double-blind, placebo-controlled, parallel | • No improvement in neurocognition with rivastigmine.<br>• No improvement in symptom severity with rivastigmine.<br>• Rivastigmine produced enhanced task-related visual cortex activation. | 21/36 subjects completed the study. | [81] |
| 13 | Rivastigmine | 9 | First- and second-generation antipsychotics | 12-week open label | • Rivastigmine produced significant neurocognitive improvement.<br>• Rivastigmine produced significant improvement in Activities of Daily Living<br>• Rivastigmine produced significant improvement in symptom severity.- | All subjects were above age 65.<br>All subjects had comorbid dementia (MMSE ≤ 24). | [78] |
| 16 | Rivastigmine | 3–12 | Second-generation antipsychotics | 12-month open label | • Rivastigmine produced a significant improvement in a quality of life measure.<br>• Rivastigmine produced a significant improvement in neurocognition. | 10/16 subjects completed the study. | [79] |

MMSE, Mini Mental Status Examination.

was accounted for in the statistical analyses. Moreover, the majority of these trials failed to show a significant pro-cognitive effect of donepezil [69–77]. In sum, the preponderance of evidence does not support a cognitive enhancing effect of donepezil in patients with schizophrenia.

The results from trials using rivastigmine as adjunctive treatment for cognitive enhancement in patients with schizophrenia have been equally disappointing. To date, a total of five trials reporting on a total of 110 subjects have been published (see Table 11.2). Two of these trials demonstrated significant pro-cognitive effects of rivastigmine [78, 79]; however, both were open label designed. The only two double-blind, placebo-controlled trials conducted to date [80, 81] both showed no cognitive enhancing effect of rivastigmine relative to placebo, as was the same for an additional open label trial [82].

Relative to donepezil and rivastigmine, the data on galantamine is somewhat more supportive of a modest pro-cognitive effect in patients with schizophrenia. A total of seven studies reporting on 185 subjects have been published (see Table 11.2). Two of these trials reported significant beneficial effects of galantamine on neurocognition and both were double blind designed [83, 84]. Moreover, the pattern of cognitive improvement was similar between these studies. The Schubert study [84] demonstrated significant improvements in verbal memory performance, which overlaps with the improvement in verbal memory observed in the Buchannan study [83], the largest in the series of galantamine trials (i.e., 86 subjects). However, it should be noted that the significance of the verbal memory effect of galantamine in the Buchanan study [83] was lost after correction for multiple comparisons. In contrast with these findings, three double-blind, placebo-controlled trials failed to replicate the pro-cognitive effects of galantamine in schizophrenic patients [85–87], as did two small open label trials [88, 89]. Overall, these data are more supportive of a cognitive enhancing effect than that for donepezil or rivastigmine, but nonetheless they are only modestly positive and generally inconsistent.

### 11.5.3 Actions Other Than Inhibition of Acetylcholinesterase May Explain Galantamine's Efficacy

Although modest, galantamine appears to be more effective as a cognitive enhancer in schizophrenia relative to the other AChE inhibitors studied. However, this conclusion is speculative and based on the comparison of data from different studies. Unfortunately, there have been no head to head comparisons of AChE inhibitors in schizophrenic patients on their cognitive enhancing effects. However, there is a substantial amount of pharmacological comparison data between AChE inhibitors generated from animal studies.

Interestingly, the AChE inhibitory activity of galantamine is relatively weak, and on a mg/kg basis, is less than that of donepezil [90]. So what is to explain this possible gain in efficacy over other AChE inhibitors such as donepezil? Indeed, galantamine has pharmacological properties that set it apart from other AChE inhibitors and may explain its possible increased efficacy in schizophrenia. There is evidence that, in addition to its AChE inhibitory effects, galantamine binds to a site distinct from the ACh binding site to allosterically potentiate both α4β2 and α7 nAChRs [91, 92]. Thus, while other AChE inhibitors simply increase cholinergic neurotransmission at both mAChRs and nAChRs through increases in ACh, galantamine additionally potentiates nAChR response to endogenous ACh. Moreover, through its action as an allosteric modulator of nAChRs, galantamine may, consequently, facilitate increased dopaminergic firing through potentiation of nAChR function in the Ventral Tegmental Area (VTA), thereby increasing dopamine output in the prefrontal cortex [93]. In contrast to galantamine, donepezil does not activate dopamine cell firing. In fact, higher doses of donepezil produces a significant attenuation of firing rate of dopaminergic cells in the VTA [93].

## 11.6 CONCLUSIONS AND THERAPEUTIC IMPLICATIONS

The data presented provide a solid rationale for enhancement of central cholinergic activity as a means to enhance the cognitive functions of schizophrenic patients. However, a strategy based on raising ACh levels at the synapse with AChE inhibitors has not proven effective to date. The exception to this statement is tentatively galantamine, which seems to have modestly greater procognitive effects relative to other AChE inhibitors based on currently available clinical trials data. Doses of AChE inhibitors evaluated in the studies reviewed were within the recommended therapeutic range for Alzheimer's disease. Perhaps this is insufficient to produce increased muscarinic or nicotinic receptor activation to levels necessary to improve the cognitive functions of schizophrenic patients. Thus, it is possible that supratherapeutic doses of the AChE inhibitors donepezil and rivastigmine would produce significant cognitive effects. However, given the nonselective activation of mAChR and nAChR subtypes produced by AChE inhibitors, unwanted side effects such as gastrointestinal (GI) distress and muscle cramps mediated by mAChRs and nAChRs would be a limiting factor.

The modestly increased cognitive effects of galantamine in schizophrenic patients implies that more selective and greater activation of α4β2 and α7 subunit containing nAChRs could be a more effective strategy for cognitive enhancement in schizophrenic patients. This is particularly true in light of the data demonstrating relationships between these nAChR subtypes and cognitive functions. There are compounds that act directly on nicotinic receptors currently being evaluated which will be discussed in proceeding chapters. Moreover, direct acting muscarinic activation strategies are also in development and will be discussed in the next chapters. These more selective mAChR and nAChR agonists, which are targeted as those ACh receptor subtypes that are critical to cognitive functions, hold promise to be more effective cognitive enhancers than AChE inhibitors.

## REFERENCES


1. Lukas, R.J., Changeux, J.P., Le Novère, N., Albuquerque, E.X., Balfour, D.J., Berg, D.K., Bertrand, D., Chiappinelli, V.A., Clarke, P.B., Collins, A.C., Dani, J.A., Grady, S.R., Kellar, K.J., Lindstrom, J.M., Marks, M.J., Quik, M., Taylor, P.W., Wonnacott, S. (1999). International Union of Pharmacology. XX. Current status of the nomenclature for nicotinic acetylcholine receptors and their subunits. *Pharmacol Rev*, *51*(2), 397–401.
2. Wilkie, G.I., Hutson, P.H., Stephens, M.W., Whiting, P., Wonnacott, S. (1993). Hippocampal nicotinic autoreceptors modulate acetylcholine release. *Biochem Soc Trans*, *21*(2), 429–431.
3. Clarke, P.B., Reuben, M. (1996). Release of [3H]-noradrenaline from rat hippocampal synaptosomes by nicotine: mediation by different nicotinic receptor subtypes from striatal [3H]-dopamine release. *Br J Pharmacol*, *117*(4), 595–606.
4. Rapier, C., Lunt, G.G., Wonnacott, S. (1990). Nicotinic modulation of [3H]dopamine release from striatal synaptosomes: pharmacological characterisation. *J Neurochem*, *54*(3), 937–945.
5. Takahashi, H., Takada, Y., Nagai, N., Urano, T., Takada, A. (1998). Nicotine increases stress-induced serotonin release by stimulating nicotinic acetylcholine receptor in rat striatum. *Synapse*, *28*(3), 212–219.
6. Wang, B.W., Liao, W.N., Chang, C.T., Wang, S.J. (2006). Facilitation of glutamate release by nicotine involves the activation of a Ca2+/calmodulin signaling pathway in rat prefrontal cortex nerve terminals. *Synapse*, *59*(8), 491–501.
7. Yang, X., Criswell, H.E., Breese, G.R. (1996). Nicotine-induced inhibition in medial septum involves activation of presynaptic nicotinic cholinergic receptors on gamma-aminobutyric acid-containing neurons. *J Pharmacol Exp Ther*, *276*(2), 482–489.
8. Perry, D.C., Xiao, Y., Nguyen, H.N., Musachio, J.L., Davila-Garcia, M.I., Kellar, K.J. (2002). Measuring nicotinic receptors with characteristics of α4ß2, α3ß2, and α3ß4 subtypes in rat tissues by autoradiography. *J Neurochem*, *82*, 468–481.
9. Langmead, C.J., Watson, J., Reavill, C. (2008). Muscarinic acetylcholine receptors as CNS drug targets. *Pharmacol Ther*, *117*(2), 232–243.
10. Levey, A.I., Kitt, C.A., Simonds, W.F., Price, D.L., Brann, M.R. (1991). Identification and localization of muscarinic acetylcholine receptor proteins in brain with subtype-specific antibodies. *J Neurosci*, *11*(10), 3218–3226.
11. Rouse, S.T., Thomas, T.M., Levey, A.I. (1991). Muscarinic acetylcholine receptor subtype, m2l: diverse functional implications of differential synaptic localization. *Life Sci*, *60*(13–14), 1031–1038.
12. Raiteri, M., Marchi, M., Paudice, P. (1990). Presynaptic muscarinic receptors in the central nervous system. *Ann N Y Acad Sci*, *604*, 113–129.
13. Miyamoto, M., Kato, J., Narumi, S., Nagaoka, A. (1987). Characteristics in memory impairment following lesioning of the basal forebrain and septal nucleus in rats. *Brain Res*, *419*, 19–31.
14. Aggleton, J., Keith, A., Rawlins, J., Hunt, P., Sahgal, A. (1992). Removal of the hippocampus and transection of the fornix produce comparable deficits on delyed non-match to position by rats. *Behav Brain Res*, *52*, 61–71.

15. McAlonan, G., Wilkinson, L., Robbins, T., Everitt, B. (1995). The effects of AMPA-induced lesions of the septohippocampal cholinergic projection on aversive conditioning to explicit and contextual cues and spatial learning in the water maze. *Eur J Neurosci*, *7*, 281–292.
16. Page, K., Everitt, B., Robbins, T., Marston, H., Wilkinson, L. (1991). Dissociable effects on spatial maze and passive avoidance acquisition and retention following AMPA- and ibotenic acid-induced excitotoxic lesions of the basal forebrain in rats: differential dependence on cholinergic neuronal loss. *Neuroscience*, *43*, 457–472.
17. Winkler, J., Suhr, S., Gage, F., Thal, L., Fisher, L. (1995). Essential role of neocortical acetylcholine in spatial memory. *Nature*, *375*, 484–487.
18. Brito, G., Davis, B., Stopp, L., Stanton, M. (1983). Memory and the septohippocampal cholinergic system in the rat. *Psychopharmacology (Berl)*, *81*, 315–320.
19. Eichenbaum, H., Otto, T., Cohen, N. (1994). Two functional components of the hippocampal memory system. *Behav Brain Sci*, *17*, 449–518.
20. Fadda, F., Melis, F., Stancampiano, R. (1996). Increased hippocampal acetylcholine release during a working memory task. *Eur J Pharmacol*, *307*, R1–R2.
21. Dunnett, S. (1985). Comparative effects of cholinergic drugs and lesions of the nucleus basalis or fimbria-fornix on delayed-matching in rats. *Psychopharmacology (Berl)*, *87*, 357–363.
22. Meek, W., Chuch, R., Wenk, G., Olton, D. (1987). Nucleus basalis magnocellularis and medial septal area lesions differentially impair temporal memory. *J Neurosci*, *7*, 3505–3511.
23. Mandel, R., Chen, A., Connor, D., Thal, L. (1989). Continuous physostigmine infusion in rats with excitotoxic lesions of the nucleus basalis magnocellularis: effects on performance in the water maze task and cortical cholinergic markers. *J Pharmacol Exp Ther*, *251*, 612–619.
24. Blozovski, D., Cudennec, A., Garrigou, D. (1977). Deficits in passive avoidance learning following atropine in the developing rat. *Psychopharmacology (Berl)*, *54*, 139–144.
25. Aigner, T., Mishkin, M. (1986). The effects of physostigmine and scopolamine on recognition memory in monkeys. *Behav Neural Biol*, *45*, 81–87.
26. Drachman, D. (1977). Memory and cognitive function in man. Does the cholinergic system have a specific role? *Neurology*, *27*, 783–790.
27. Dawson, G., Heyes, C., Iversen, S. (1992). Pharmacological mechanisms and animal models of cognition. *Behav Pharmacol*, *3*, 285–297.
28. Bartus, R., Uehara, Y. (1979). Physostigmine and recent memory: effects in young and aged nonhuman primates. *Science*, *206*, 1085–1087.
29. Nielsen, J., Mena, A., Williams, I., Nocerini, M., Liston, D. (1989). Correlation of brain levels of 9-amino-1,2,3,4-tetrahydroacridine (THA) with neurochemical and behavioral changes. *Eur J Pharmacol*, *173*, 53–64.
30. Wanibuchi, F., Nishida, T., Yamashita, H., Hidaka, K., Koshiya, K., Tsukamoto, S., Usuda, S. (1994). Characterization of a novel muscarinic receptor agonist, YM796: comparison with cholinesterase inhibitors in in vivo pharmacological studies. *Eur J Pharmacol*, *265*(3), 151–158.
31. Rupniak, N., Spencer, T., Field, M. (1997). Enhanced performance of spatial and visual memory tasks by the selective acetylcholinesterase inhibitor E2020 in rhesus monkeys. *Psychopharmacology (Berl)*, *131*, 406–410.

32. Robbins, T., Everitt, B., Marston, H., Wilkinson, J., Jones, G., Page, K. (1989). Comparative effects of ibotenic acid and quisqualic acid-induced lesions of the substantia innominata on attentional function in the rat: further implications for the role of the cholinergic neurons of the nucleus basalis in cognitive processes. *Behav Brain Res*, *35*, 221–240.
33. Muir, J., Dunnett, S., Robbins, T., Everitt, B. (1992). Attentional functions of the forebrain cholinergic systems: effects of intraventricular hemicholinium, physostigmine, basal cortical lesions and intracortical grafts on a multiple choice serial reaction time task. *Exp Brain Res*, *89*, 611–622.
34. Callahan, M., Kinsora, J., Harbaugh, R., Reeder, T., Davis, R. (1993). Continuous icv infusion of scopolamine impairs sustained attention of rhesus monkeys. *Neurobiol Aging*, *14*, 147–151.
35. Ferreira, A.R., Fürstenau, L., Blanco, C., Kornisiuk, E., Sánchez, G., Daroit, D., Castro e Silva, M., Cerveñansky, C., Jerusalinsky, D., Quillfeldt, J.A. (2003). Role of hippocampal M1 and M4 muscarinic receptor subtypes in memory consolidation in the rat. *Pharmacol Biochem Behav*, *74*(2), 411–415.
36. Anagnostaras, S.G., Murphy, G.G., Hamilton, S.E., Mitchell, S.L., Rahnama, N.P., Nathanson, N.M., Silva, A.J. (2003). Selective cognitive dysfunction in acetylcholine M1 muscarinic receptor mutant mice. *Nat Neurosci*, *6*(1), 51–58.
37. Shinoe, T., Matsui, M., Taketo, M.M., Manabe, T. (2005). Modulation of synaptic plasticity by physiological activation of M1 muscarinic acetylcholine receptors in the mouse hippocampus. *J Neurosci*, *25*(48), 11194–11200.
38. Tzavara, E.T., Bymaster, F.P., Davis, R.J., Wade, M.R., Perry, K.W., Wess, J., McKinzie, D.L., Felder, C., Nomikos, G.G. (2004). M4 muscarinic receptors regulate the dynamics of cholinergic and dopaminergic neurotransmission: relevance to the pathophysiology and treatment of related CNS pathologies. *FASEB J*, *18*(12), 1410–1412.
39. Levin, E.D., Simon, B.B. (1998). Nicotinic acetylcholine involvement in cognitive function in animals. *Psychopharmacology (Berl)*, *138*, 217–230.
40. Levin, E., Christopher, N. (2002). Persistence of the nicotinic agonist RJR2403 induced working memory improvement in rats. *Drug Dev Res*, *55*, 97–103.
41. Young, J.W., Finlayson, K., Spratt, C., Marston, H.M., Crawford, N., Kelly, J.S., Sharkey, J. (2004). Nicotine improves sustained attention in mice: evidence for involvement of the alpha7 nicotinic acetylcholine receptor. *Neuropsychopharmacology*, *29*(5), 891–900.
42. Arendash, G.W., Sengstock, G.J., Sanberg, P.R., Kem, W.R. (1995). Improved learning and memory in aged rats with chronic administration of the nicotinic receptor agonist GTS-21. *Brain Res*, *674*(2), 252–259.
43. Lippiello, P.M., Bencherif, M., Gray, J.A., Peters, S., Grigoryan, G., Hodges, H., Collins, A.C. (1996). RJR-2403: a nicotinic agonist with CNS selectivity II. In vivo characterization. *J Pharmacol Exp Ther*, *279*(3), 1422–1429.
44. El-Mallack, R., Kirch, D., Shelton, R., Fan, K., Pezeshkpour, G., Kanhouwa, Wyatt, R., Kleinman, J. (1991). The NbM, senile plaques, and intellectual impairment in schizophrenia. *J Neuropsychiatry Clin Neurosci*, *3*, 383–386.
45. Powchik, P., Davidson, M., Haroutunian, V., Gabriel, S.M., Purohit, D.P., Perl, D.P., Harvey, P.D., Davis, K.L. (1998). Postmortem studies in schizophrenia. *Schizophr Bull*, *24*(3), 325–341.

46. Raedler, T.J., Knable, M.B., Jones, D.W., Urbina, R.A., Gorey, J.G., Lee, K.S., Egan, M.F., Coppola, R., Weinberger, D.R. (2003). In vivo determination of muscarinic acetylcholine receptor availability in schizophrenia. *Am J Psychiatry*, *160*(1), 118–127.

47. Dean, B., McLeod, M., Keriakous, D., McKenzie, J., Scarr, E. (2002). Decreased muscarinic1 receptors in the dorsolateral prefrontal cortex of subjects with schizophrenia. *Mol Psychiatry*, *7*(10), 1083–1091.

48. Wei, J., Walton, E.A., Milici, A., Buccafusco, J.J. (1994). M1-M5 muscarinic receptor distribution in rat CNS by RT-PCR and HPLC. *J Neurochem*, *63*(3), 815–821.

49. Freedman, R., Hall, M., Adler, L.E., Leonard, S. (1995). Evidence in postmortem brain tissue for decreased numbers of hippocampal nicotinic receptors in schizophrenia. *Biol Psychiatry*, *38*, 22–33.

50. Severance, E.G., Yolken, R.H. (2008). Novel α7 nicotinic receptor isoforms and deficient cholinergic transcription in schizophrenia. *Genes Brain Behav*, *7*, 37–45.

51. Breese, C.R., Lee, M.J., Adams, C.E., Sullivan, B., Logel, J., Gillen, K.M., Marks, M.J., Collins, A.C., Leonard, S. (2000). Abnormal regulation of high affinity nicotinic receptors in subjects with schizophrenia. *Neuropsychopharmacology*, *23*(4), 351–364.

52. Adler, L.E., Hoffer, L.D., Wiser, A., Freedman, R. (1993). Normalization of auditory physiology by cigarette smoking in schizophrenic patients. *Am J Psychiatry*, *150*, 1856–1861.

53. Olincy, A., Ross, R.G., Young, D.A., Roath, M., Freedman, R. (1998). Improvement in smooth pursuit eye movements after cigarette smoking in schizophrenic patients. *Neuropsychopharmacology*, *18*, 175–185.

54. Fulcher, J.H., Gallagher, W.J., Pfeiffer, C.C. (1957). Comparative lucid intervals after amobarbital, CO2 and arecoline in the chronic schizophrenic. *AMA Arch Neurol Psychiatry*, *75*, 392–395.

55. Collard, J., Lecoq, R., Damaret, A. (1965). Un essaie de therapeutic pathogenique de la schizophrenic par un acetylcholinic: L' oxotremorine. *Acta Biol Belg*, *65*, 122–127.

56. Modestn, J., Schwartz, R.B., Hunger, J. (1973). Zur Frage Beeinflussung schizophrener symptoms durch physostigmine. *Pharmakopsychiatr Neuropsychopharmakol*, *6*, 300–304.

57. Janowski, D.S., EL-Yousef, M.D., Davis, J.M. (1973). Antagonistic effects of physostigmine and methylphenidate in man. *Am J Psychiatry*, *130*, 1370.

58. Ichikawa, J., Dai, J., O'Laughlin, A., Fowler, W.L., Meltzer, H.Y. (2002). Atypical, but not typical, antipsychotic drugs increase cortical acetylcholine release without an effect in the nucleus accumbens or striatum. *Neuropsychopharmacology*, *26*(3), 325–339.

59. Rogers, S.L., Doody, R.S., Mohs, R.C., Friedhoff, L.T. (1998). Donepezil improves cognition and global function in Alzheimer disease: a 15-week, double-blind, placebo-controlled study. Donepezil Study Group. *Arch Intern Med*, *158*, 1021–1031.

60. Rogers, S.L., Farlow, M.R., Doody, R.S., Mohs, R., Friedhoff, L.T. (1998). A 24-week, double blind, placebo-controlled trial of donepezil in patients with Alzheimer's disease: Donepezil Study Group. *Neurology*, *50*, 136–145.

61. Rosler, M., Anand, R., Cicin-Sain, A., Gauthier, S., Agid, Y., Dal-Bianco, P., Stahelin, H.B., Hartman, R., Gharabawi, M. (1999). Efficacy and safety of rivastigmine in patients with Alzheimer's disease: international randomised controlled trial. *BMJ*, *318*(7184), 633–638.

62. Tariot, P.N., Solomon, P.R., Morris, J.C., Kershaw, P., Lilienfeld, S., Ding, C. (2000). A 5-month, randomized, placebo-controlled trial of galantamine in AD. The Galantamine USA-10 Study Group. *Neurology*, *54*(12), 2269–2276.

63. Risch, S.C., Horner, M.D., McGurk, S.R., Palecko, S., Markowitz, J.S., Nahas, Z., DeVane, C.L. (2007). Double-blind donepezil-placebo crossover augmentation study of atypical antipsychotics in chronic, stable schizophrenia: a pilot study. *Schizophr Res*, *93*(1–3), b131–b135.

64. Stryjer, R., Strous, R., Bar, F., Shaked, G., Shiloh, R., Rozencwaig, S., Grupper, D., Buchman, N., Kotler, M., Rabey, J.M., Weizman, A. (2004). Donepezil augmentation of clozapine monotherapy in schizophrenia patients: a double blind cross-over study. *Hum Psychopharmacol*, *19*(5), 343–346.

65. Chung, Y.C., Lee, C.R., Park, T.W., Yang, K.H., Kim, K.W. (2007). Effect of donepezil added to atypical antipsychotics on cognition in patients with schizophrenia: an open-label trial. *World J Biol Psychiatry*, *10*, 1–7.

66. Stryjer, R., Strous, R.D., Bar, F., Werber, E., Shaked, G., Buhiri, Y., Kotler, M., Weizman, A., Rabey, J.M. (2003). Beneficial effect of donepezil augmentation for the management of comorbid schizophrenia and dementia. *Clin Neuropharmacol*, *26*(1), 12–17.

67. Buchanan, R.W., Summerfelt, A., Tek, C., Gold, J. (2003). An open-labeled trial of adjunctive donepezil for cognitive impairments in patients with schizophrenia. *Schizophr Res*, *59*(1), 29–33.

68. Erickson, S.K., Schwarzkopf, S.B., Palumbo, D., Badgley-Fleeman, J., Smirnow, A.M., Light, G.A. (2005). Efficacy and tolerability of low-dose donepezil in schizophrenia. *Clin Neuropharmacol*, *28*(4), 179–184.

69. Keefe, R.S., Malhotra, A.K., Meltzer, H.Y., Kane, J.M., Buchanan, R.W., Murthy, A., Sovel, M., Li, C., Goldman, R. (2008). Efficacy and safety of donepezil in patients with schizophrenia or schizoaffective disorder: significant placebo/practice effects in a 12-week, randomized, double-blind, placebo-controlled trial. *Neuropsychopharmacology*, *33*(6), 1217–1228.

70. Kohler, C.G., Martin, E.A., Kujawski, E., Bilker, W., Gur, R.E., Gur, R.C. (2007). No effect of donepezil on neurocognition and social cognition in young persons with stable schizophrenia. *Cognit Neuropsychiatry*, *12*(5), 12–21.

71. Fagerlund, B., Søholm, B., Fink-Jensen, A., Lublin, H., Glenthøj, B.Y. (2007). Effects of donepezil adjunctive treatment to ziprasidone on cognitive deficits in schizophrenia: a double-blind, placebo-controlled study. *Clin Neuropharmacol*, *30*(1), 3–12.

72. Lee, B.J., Lee, J.G., Kim, Y.H. (2007). A 12-week, double-blind, placebo-controlled trial of donepezil as an adjunct to haloperidol for treating cognitive impairments in patients with chronic schizophrenia. *J Psychopharmacol*, *21*(4), 421–427.

73. Freudenreich, O., Herz, L., Deckersbach, T., Evins, A.E., Henderson, D.C., Cather, C., Goff, D.C. (2005). Added donepezil for stable schizophrenia: a double-blind, placebo-controlled trial. *Psychopharmacology (Berl)*, *181*(2), 358–363.

74. Tuğal, O., Yazici, K.M., Anil Yağcioğlu, A.E., Göğüş, A. (2004). A double-blind, placebo controlled, cross-over trial of adjunctive donepezil for cognitive impairment in schizophrenia. *Int J Neuropsychopharmacol*, *7*(2), 117–123.

75. Nahas, Z., George, M.S., Horner, M.D., Markowitz, J.S., Li, X., Lorberbaum, J.P., Owens, S.D., McGurk, S., DeVane, L., Risch, S.C. (2003). Augmenting atypical antipsychotics with a cognitive enhancer (donepezil) improves regional brain activity in schizophrenia patients: a pilot double-blind placebo controlled BOLD fMRI study. *Neurocase*, *9*(3), 274–282.

76. Friedman, J.I., Adler, D.N., Howanitz, E., Harvey, P.D., Brenner, G., Temporini, H., White, L., Parrella, M., Davis, K.L. (2002). A double blind placebo controlled trial of donepezil adjunctive treatment to risperidone for the cognitive impairment of schizophrenia. *Biol Psychiatry*, *51*(5), 349–357.

77. Shahin Akhondzadeh, S., Gerami, M., Noroozian, M., Karamghadiri, N., Ghoreishi, A., Abbasi, S.-H., Ali Rezazadeh, S. (2008). A 12-week, double-blind, placebo-controlled trial of donepezil adjunctive treatment to risperidone in chronic and stable schizophrenia. *Prog Neuropsychopharmacol Biol Psychiatry*, *32*, 1810–1815.

78. Mendelsohn, E., Rosenthal, M., Bohiri, Y., Werber, E., Kotler, M., Strous, R.D. (2004). Rivastigmine augmentation in the management of chronic schizophrenia with comorbid dementia: an open-label study investigating effects on cognition, behaviour and activities of daily living. *Int Clin Psychopharmacol*, *19*(6), 319–324.

79. Lenzi, A., Maltinti, E., Poggi, E., Fabrizio, L., Coli, E. (2003). Effects of rivastigmine on cognitive function and quality of life in patients with schizophrenia. *Clin Neuropharmacol*, *26*(6), 317–321.

80. Sharma, T., Reed, C., Aasen, I., Kumari, V. (2006). Cognitive effects of adjunctive 24-weeks rivastigmine treatment to antipsychotics in schizophrenia: a randomized, placebo-controlled, double-blind investigation. *Schizophr Res*, *85*(1–3), 73–83.

81. Kumari, V., Aasen, I., Ffytche, D., Williams, S.C., Sharma, T. (2006). Neural correlates of adjunctive rivastigmine treatment to antipsychotics in schizophrenia: a randomized, placebo-controlled, double-blind fMRI study. *Neuroimage*, *29*(2), 545–556.

82. Chouinard, S., Stip, E., Poulin, J., Melun, J.P., Godbout, R., Guillem, F., Cohen, H. (2007). Rivastigmine treatment as an add-on to antipsychotics in patients with schizophrenia and cognitive deficits. *Curr Med Res Opin*, *23*(3), 575–583.

83. Buchanan, R.W., Conley, R.R., Dickinson, D., Ball, M.P., Feldman, S., Gold, J.M., McMahon, R.P. (2008). Galantamine for the treatment of cognitive impairments in people with schizophrenia. *Am J Psychiatry*, *165*(1), 82–89.

84. Schubert, M.H., Young, K.A., Hicks, P.B. (2006). Galantamine improves cognition in schizophrenic patients stabilized on risperidone. *Biol Psychiatry*, *60*(6), 530–533.

85. Sacco, K.A., Creeden, C., Reutenauer, E.L., George, T.P. (2008). Effects of galantamine on cognitive deficits in smokers and non-smokers with schizophrenia. *Schizophr Res*, *103*(1–3), 326–327.

86. Dyer, M.A., Freudenreich, O., Culhane, M.A., Pachas, G.N., Deckersbach, T., Murphy, E., Goff, D.C., Evins, A.E. (2008). High-dose galantamine augmentation inferior to placebo on attention, inhibitory control and working memory performance in nonsmokers with schizophrenia. *Schizophr Res*, *102*(1–3), 88–95.

87. Lee, S.W., Lee, J.G., Lee, B.J., Kim, Y.H. (2007). A 12-week, double-blind, placebo-controlled trial of galantamine adjunctive treatment to conventional antipsychotics

for the cognitive impairments in chronic schizophrenia. *Int Clin Psychopharmacol*, *22*(2), 63–68.

88. Norén, U., Björner, A., Sonesson, O., Eriksson, L. (2006). Galantamine added to antipsychotic treatment in chronic schizophrenia: cognitive improvement? *Schizophr Res*, *85*(1–3), 302–304.
89. Bora, E., Veznedaroğlu, B., Kayahan, B. (2005). The effect of galantamine added to clozapine on cognition of five patients with schizophrenia. *Clin Neuropharmacol*, *28*(3), 139–141.
90. Geerts, H., Guillaumat, P.O., Grantham, C., Bode, W., Anciaux, K., Sachak, S. (2005). Brain levels and acetylcholinesterase inhibition with galantamine and donepezil in rats, mice, and rabbits. *Brain Res*, *1033*(2), 186–193.
91. Samochocki, M., Zerlin, M., Jostock, R., Groot Kormelink, P.J., Luyten, W.H., Albuquerque, E.X., Maelicke, A. (2000). Galantamine is an allosterically potentiating ligand of the human alpha4/beta2 nAChR. *Acta Neurol Scand Suppl*, *176*, 68–73.
92. Texidó, L., Ros, E., Martín-Satué, M., López, S., Aleu, J., Marsal, J., Solsona, C. (2005). Effect of galantamine on the human alpha7 neuronal nicotinic acetylcholine receptor, the Torpedo nicotinic acetylcholine receptor and spontaneous cholinergic synaptic activity. *Br J Pharmacol*, *145*(5), 672–678.
93. Schilström, B., Ivanov, V.B., Wiker, C., Svensson, T.H. (2007). Galantamine enhances dopaminergic neurotransmission in vivo via allosteric potentiation of nicotinic acetylcholine receptors. *Neuropsychopharmacology*, *32*, 43–53.

# 12

# α7 NICOTINIC ACETYLCHOLINE RECEPTORS IN THE TREATMENT OF SCHIZOPHRENIA

Mihály Hajós and Bruce N. Rogers

## 12.1 STRUCTURE AND FUNCTIONAL PROPERTIES OF α7 nAChRs

The nicotinic acetylcholine receptors (nAChRs) are a well-defined subset of acetylcholine-sensitive receptors, named for their activation by the alkaloid nicotine [1, 2]. The structural makeup of nAChRs consists of five transmembrane subunits which form an ion channel that becomes permeable to cations such as $Na^{+}$, $K^{+}$, and $Ca^{2+}$ upon agonist-induced activation. There are currently 17 distinct nAChR subunits known, which can be assembled into nAChR pentamers, potentially providing a large variation of different nAChRs [3]. These subunits, however, display preferential arrangements in native pentameric receptors, showing region-specific expressions and assemblies. Individual subunits have been classified based on their genetic encoding, and distinguished into muscle-type and neuronal-type subunits. The nAChRs are broadly distributed throughout the body, including the central and peripheral nervous system, skeletal muscles, endocrine cells, as well as nonexcitable endothelial, epithelial, and immune cells. The first structurally characterized nAChRs were the receptors located at the neuromuscular junction, transmitting signals from motor neurons to skeletal muscles. The subunits of native neuronal nAChRs include two subfamilies: groups of alpha (α2–α10) and beta (β2–β4) subunits

*Targets and Emerging Therapies for Schizophrenia*, First Edition.
Edited by Jeffrey S. Albert and Michael W. Wood.

[4]. Combinations of different alpha and beta subunits give rise to a variety of heteromeric nAChRs. Among the best known and most characterized are the α3β4 nAChRs (expressed at mammalian ganglionic synapses and within the hippocampus) and the α4β2 nAChRs (expressed in most brain regions and representing the high-affinity nicotinic agonist binding sites in the brain) [5]. Although the true diversity of the heteromeric nAChRs is unknown with respect to their different subunit compositions and exact stoichiometry, there is evidence for the existence of a number of native heteromeric receptors, including the α3β2, α3β4, α3β2β4, and α6α4β2β3 nAChRs [6]. In addition to heteromeric nAChRs, there are homomeric nAChRs that are composed from the same subunits, including the homomeric α7 nAChRs. In recent years, α7 nAChRs have attracted substantial interest since they are considered a potential target in the treatment of schizophrenia, particularly for the cognitive symptoms of schizophrenia [7], and potentially for other cognitive disorders such as Alzheimer's disease and attention deficit/hyperactivity disorder (ADHD).

The pentameric α7 nAChR consists of five α7 subunits, and each subunit provides an orthosteric binding site for its endogenous ligand, acetylcholine [8]. The orthosteric binding site of the α7 subunits has a low affinity for ACh and nicotine, and therefore activation of the receptor requires a micromolar concentration of ACh (the apparent binding affinity for ACh is 55 μM, and the apparent affinity of activation is 155 μM) [9]. Agonist-induced activation of α7 nAChRs generates a conformational change of subunit protein, shifting the receptor functional state from a resting state to an activated state, according to the now canonical concept introduced by Monod, Wyman, and Changeux [10]. In the functionally active state, the channel becomes permeable to cations, and in particular calcium ($Ca^{+2}$), leading to a cation influx. In the presence of agonist, the α7 nAChRs undergo further conformational change to a desensitized closed state, when these receptors are no longer permeable to cation influx, and thus cannot be activated by agonists. Subsequently, receptors from the desensitized state shift to a resting state when they can once again be activated by agonists [11]. In the case of the α7 nAChR, the onset of activation and desensitization is very rapid, and consequently this fast receptor desensitization could present significant pharmacological challenges in the development of agonists for this receptor [12].

The rapid onset of α7 nAChR activation renders them suitable to transmit fast synaptic activity, and one might thus expect that α7 nAChRs are located within the direct synaptic connections between neurons. The exact subcellular synaptic arrangements of α7 nAChRs have not been fully revealed, but it is believed that α7 nAChRs are relatively far from ACh release sites of varicosities on cholinergic axons. It is postulated that since α7 nAChRs are found at both presynaptic and postsynaptic sites, ACh could modulate neurotransmission by various pre- and postsynaptic mechanisms [13].

Although fast excitatory transmissions via α7 nAChRs have been demonstrated [14], the current thinking is that α7 nAChRs function mostly as presynaptic receptors in the brain [15], in line with the notion that "presynaptic nACh receptors might be the exclusive or predominant role of nACh receptors in the CNS" [6]. Since expression of the α7 nAChR subunit mRNAs has been demonstrated in brain cholinergic neurons [16], it has been suggested that α7 nAChRs can play a presynaptic autoreceptor role. Furthermore, α7 nAChRs have been also identified at axon terminals of noncholinergic neurons functioning as heteroreceptors, including glutamatergic, γ-aminobutyric acid (GABA)ergic, dopaminergic, noradrenergic, and serotonergic neurons, and shown to facilitate transmitter release [17, 18]. Therefore, each and every neurotransmitter associated with schizophrenia could be theoretically modulated via α7 nAChRs.

Distribution of α7 nAChRs in the brain have been mapped with selective radioligand antagonists such as the alkaloid [$^{3}$H]-methyllycaconitine and the snake toxin [$^{125}$I] alpha-bungarotoxin [19–21]. The α7 nAChRs are expressed in high density in many forebrain and brainstem regions, including the hippocampus, cortex, amygdala, hypothalamus, dorsal tegmental nucleus of the pons, and colliculi [19]. The high level expression of α7 nAChRs within the limbic circuitry, including the hippocampus and prefrontal cortical areas, is in line with their involvement in various cognitive functions (see below). Interestingly, little overlap was observed in the distribution of high-affinity heteromeric—and low-affinity α7 nAChRs in the rat brain. In regions where both low- and high-affinity nAChRs are expressed (cortex and hippocampus), their respective distributions are reciprocally restricted to subregions. Expression and distribution of α7 nAChRs show changes during brain maturation, indicating possible contributions to the development of functional neuronal connections [21].

## 12.2 LINKAGE OF α7 NACHRS TO SCHIZOPHRENIA

It is recognized that schizophrenia is a genetically predisposed disease, and twin studies show unequivocally that schizophrenia is predominantly a genetic disorder, with estimates of heritability of risk of around 80% [22]. However, like other complex disorders, schizophrenia is characterized by the contribution of multiple risk genes, which could contribute in combination with epigenetic and environmental processes to the development of the disease [23]. Therefore, schizophrenia does not show simple patterns of inheritance, and simple major gene effects in the disease are unlikely but rather implicated genes will each account for only a small increment in risk [24]. Among a number of genetic linkage sites, the α7 nAChR subunit gene *CHRNA7* has been implicated in schizophrenia by considerable, although partially circumstantial, evidence. Thus, a genetic linkage of the 15q13-15 region of chromosome 15 containing *CHRNA7* has been established to impaired auditory gating (P50), a presumed indicator of dysfunctional sensory processing in schizophrenia [25–28]. The original observation made by Freedman and colleagues on association between the region of chromosome 15 that contains *CHRNA7* (15q13-14), auditory gating deficits, and schizophrenia has been confirmed in most of the subsequent studies. For further details on polymorphisms in *CHRNA7* gene and schizophrenia, see the comprehensive review published by Stitzel [29].

In addition to genetic observation, a potential link between schizophrenia and α7 nAChRs is further supported by postmortem pathological studies. Thus, expression of α7 nAChRs, measured as immunoreactivity or binding site densities, is reduced in schizophrenia in several brain areas closely associated with schizophrenia, including hippocampus [30], thalamic reticular nucleus [31], and cingulated cortex [32]. The association between the *CHRNA7* gene and impaired P50 auditory gating provided a very attractive endophenotype not only for genetic research in schizophrenia but also for antipsychotic drug discovery [33–35]. Auditory gating can be evaluated in experimental pharmacological studies and applied as a translational biomarker. Limited human studies suggest that nicotine's mechanism of action in cognition may be via the α7 nAChR [36].

Although the biological connection of α7 nAChRs to schizophrenia is prominent, an association between *CHRNA7* gene alterations and other psychiatric disorders has been also revealed. In bipolar disorder, alteration in ratio between the *CHRNA7* gene and its partial duplication that constitutes the α7-like nicotinic receptor gene (CHRFAM7A), or its polymorphism has been reported [37–39]. Furthermore, an association between genetic variations in the α7 nAChR with delusional symptoms in Alzheimer's disease has been recently disclosed [40]. Taken together, these findings indicate that alteration in *CHRNA7* gene or its α7 nAChR expression might contribute to psychotic or delusional symptoms in various psychiatric disorders, and not specifically linked to development of schizophrenia.

## 12.3 ACTIVATION OF α7 nACHRS BY AGONISTS

### 12.3.1 Endogenous Agonists

Activation of α7 nAChRs by their endogenous agonists has been studied in great detail, with research describing molecular-level interactions between agonists and receptor binding sites of the receptor [8, 9, 13]. In addition to the well-established endogenous agonist acetylcholine, choline, a precursor and a metabolite of Ach, has been also considered an endogenous, relatively selective agonist of α7 nAChRs (Fig. 12.1) [41]. Acetylcholine and choline have similar kinetic properties of activation and desensitization on α7 nAChRs [42].

### 12.3.2 Overview of the Chemistry of α7 nAChR Agonists

Interest in the development of an agonist of the α7 nAChR in medicinal chemistry has greatly expanded over the past decade, with a focus on the

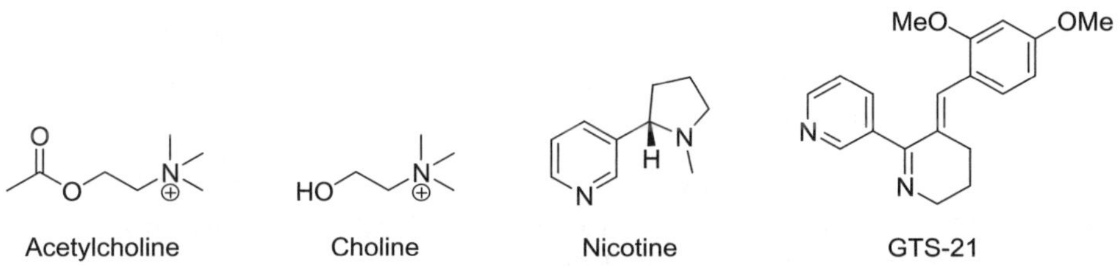


**FIGURE 12.1** Structures of the endogenous nAChR ligands acetyl choline and choline; the natural ligand nicotine, and the partial agonist GTS-21.

identification of novel and selective chemical entities, and the area has been extensively reviewed [43–53]. For the purpose of this section we will focus on those ligands that have been most extensively characterized in the primary literature, and thus have served as tools to significantly advance the overall field. Many of the ligands described in the primary literature as α7 nAChR agonists are derived from the quinuclidine scaffold and include such structures as spirooxazolidinone [54], quinuclidine carbamates [55, 56], amides [57], and ethers [58]. Several other templates have appeared, expanding the field, and these include additional azabicyclic amine templates, and the significant departure from the quinuclidine template with the anabaseine analog GTS-21 (DMXBA).

The endogenous ligand of the α7 nAChR, acetylcholine, and its natural ligand, nicotine, are both small molecular weight molecules that are highly efficient activators of the receptor. The inherent challenge with these two natural ligands is in their lack of selectivity for the α7 nAChR over other nAChRs, and thus they have limited utility in developing an understanding of the α7 nAChR subtype. Among the earliest reported non-nicotine ligands for the α7 nAChR is the anabasine analog GTS-21 (DMXBA) [59, 60]. GTS-21 is reported as a functionally selective partial agonist of the α7 nAChR. The compound does, however, show potent binding activity to the α4β2 nAChR, on the order of 100-fold greater potency than its α7 binding [61]. The compound has been extensively characterized *in vitro* and *in vivo* and is also one of a handful of compounds that have advanced to clinical studies (these studies are discussed elsewhere in this chapter).

The most heavily investigated class of ligands for the α7 nAChR are the quinuclidine amine-based compounds. One of the earliest entries in this area was from the group at AstraZeneca, with the spirooxazolidinones (Fig. 12.2) [54]. Initially characterized by AR-R17779, this class has been evolved by several groups to a selective *in vivo* active series of compounds. AR-R17779 was the first entry from AstraZeneca and was reported to be a full agonist at the α7 nAChR and highly selective over other subtypes [54]. Although a great small molecule tool, the challenges that this initial compound provided were that it also activated the 5-$HT_3$ receptors and had limited brain penetration. The spirooxazolidinones have been further refined at both AstraZeneca and

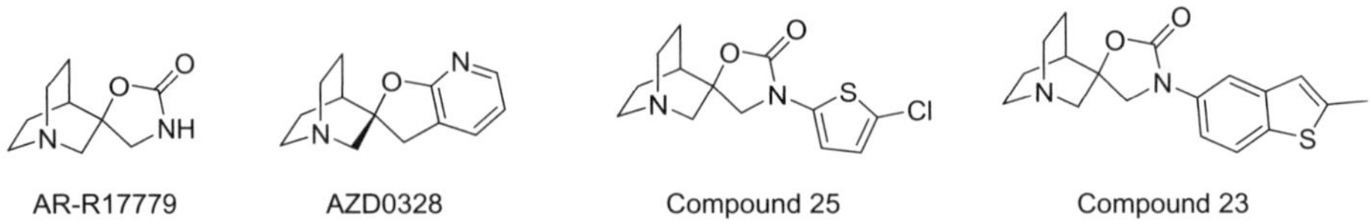


**FIGURE 12.2** Structures of spirooxazolidinones α7 nAChR agonist ligands AR-R17779, AZD0328, Compound **25** and Compound **23**.

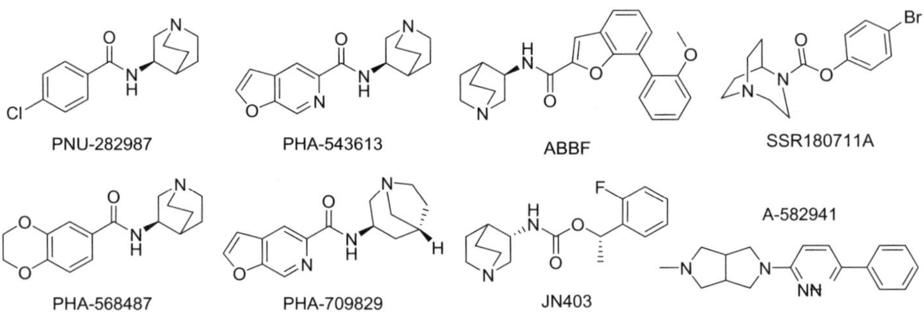


**FIGURE 12.3** Structures of α7 nAChR agonist ligands PNU-282987, PHA-543613, ABBF, SSR180711A, PHA-568487, PHA-709829, JN403, and A-582941.

the Mitsubishi Corporation. AZD0328 has been extensively characterized by the group at AstraZeneca [62, 63]. This potent α7 nAChR agonist (Ki = 3 nM) is described as a selective partial agonist with adequate pharmacokinetic (PK) characteristics to progress to human studies. AZD0328 also demonstrates *in vivo* activity when dosed in a variety of models including mouse novel object recognition, reversal of short-term memory deficits in fimbria/fornix-lesioned rats, and improvement in working memory in rhesus monkey spatial delayed response performance. Researchers at Mitsubishi reported that the potent spirooxazolidinone (compound **25**) ($K_i$ = 9 nM) significantly improves MK-801-induced auditory gating deficits, but was an inhibitor of CYP2D6 [64]. Further refinement of this class of compounds has resulted in compounds with high binding affinity ($K_i$ = 3 nM) at the α7 nAChR, no CYP2D6 activity, and in the case of compound **25**, active *in vivo*, demonstrating improved cognition in several rodent models [65].

Many of the recent ligands disclosed in the literature come from the quinuclidine scaffold (Fig. 12.3), and include such structures as quinuclidine carbamates [55, 56] amides, and ethers [58]. The most extensively characterized ligands in this area are the quiniclidine amides and carbamates. An early key compound to emerge in the literature was the quinuclidine benzamide PNU-282987 by researchers at Pharmacia/Pfizer [66]. PNU-282987 is a potent and selective α7 nAChR agonist ($K_i$ = 29 nM), with full efficacy relative to nicotine in functional assays. A key issue that emerged with this compound was its significant activity at the hERG channel. The compound has been extensively characterized *in vitro* and *in vivo* and served as an excellent tool to guide research efforts, including the restoration of P50 gating deficits in rodent [67]. The group at Pharmacia/Pfizer has also more recently described a series of compounds that progressed to clinical studies that had similar profiles to PNU-282987 with significantly improved hERG profiles, ADME properties and adequate safety profiles to advance into clinical studies (PHA-543613 and PHA-568487) [68–70]. Recently, the potent quinuclidine amide ABBF was reported by Bayer as a full agonist at α7 nAChRs ($pEC_{50} = 5.5$), with weak antagonist activity at other nAChRs [71]. Like the amide series from the Pharmacia group, ABBF shows antagonism at the 5-$HT_3$ receptor. ABBF shows *in vivo* activity when dosed orally (0.3 and 1.0 mg/kg) in a variety of models including rat social recognition, mouse novel object recognition, and rat water maze. Novartis also recently disclosed an entry in the quinuclidine area with JN403 [72]. The *in vitro* properties of this compound demonstrate that it is a potent and selective α7 nAChR (pKD = 6.7) and is a partial agonist relative to Ach in *Xenepus oocytes*. The *in vivo* characteristics have also recently been reported, and this compound demonstrates good PK characteristics with rapid brain penetration and activity in rat social exploration, mouse sensory gating (DBA/2), and two models of permanent pain [73]. Several other companies including Memory (MEM-3454), En-Vivo (EVP-6124), Targacept (TC-5619), and others have compounds that likely come from this class, but the exact structures have yet to be disclosed.

Reports in the primary literature describing additional structural diversity in the amine portion of α7 nAChR ligands have also appeared. Within the nAChR field, alternative azabicyclic amines are prevalent among ligands for other subtypes of receptors. Three alternate amines that have recently appeared for the α7 nAChR where significant characterization in the literature exists include the diazabicyclononanes such as SSR180711A [74, 75], the octahydropyrrolo[3,4-c]pyrrole, A-582949 [76], and the (3R,5R)-1-azabicyclo-[3.2.1]oct-3-yl-carboxamide, PHA-709829 [77]. The selective partial agonist SSR180711A is a 1,4-diazabicyclo[3.2.2]nonane carbamate derivative ($K_i = 50$ nM, $EC_{50} = 800$ nM) active in novel object recognition, Morris water maze, and an MK-801-induced memory deficit model. Researchers at Abbott have recently described a novel biaryl diamine α7 nAChR agonist, A-582941 [76]. This compound shows potent affinity for the human α7 nAChR ($K_i = 16.7$ nM) and is stated to be a partial agonist with acceptable PK and central nervous system (CNS) distribution properties. In addition, A-582941 enhanced cognitive performance in behavioral assays including the monkey delayed matching-to-sample, rat social recognition, and mouse inhibitory avoidance, and it normalized sensory gating deficits induced by the nAChR antagonist methyllycaconitine in rats [78]. PHA-709829, N-[(3R,5R)-1-azabicyclo[3.2.1]oct-3-yl]furo[2,3-c]pyridine-5-carboxamide is a novel α7 nAChR agonist that shows potent and selective α7 nAChR *in vitro* activity ($K_i = 3$ nM, $EC_{50} = 46$ nM), excellent brain penetration, good rat oral bioavailability, and an improved human ether-à-go-go-related gene (hERG) profile relative to PNU-282987. This compound also demonstrates robust dose-related *in vivo* efficacy in a rat auditory sensory gating model. As is demonstrated from the ligands that are fairly well characterized in the primary literature, the diversity of α7 nAChR ligands has expanded greatly in the past decade. Numerous ligands that are potent and selective for the α7 nAChR exist, and a clear understanding of the *in vivo* pharmacology and absorption, distribution, metabolism, and excretion (ADME) properties has led to the initiation of clinical studies with a variety of agonists for this receptor.

## 12.4 ACTIVATION OF α7 nAChRs BY POSITIVE ALLOSTERIC MODULATORS

Interest continues to grow in the use of positive allosteric modulators (PAMs) of the α7 nAChRs, and recent reviews cite their therapeutic potential in the treatment of cognition [51, 79–82]. The obvious inherent benefit of a PAM is in the fact that it increases the probability of channel opening while potentially decreasing the inherent agonist potential for receptor desensitization.

### 12.4.1 Endogenous Modulators

In physiological conditions, endogenous modulators could theoretically adjust agonist-induced receptor activation of α7 nAChRs. For example, it has been demonstrated that activity of the $GABA_A$ receptor is modulated by endogenous neurosteroids acting at different allosteric sites of the pentameric receptors [83]. 5-Hydroxyindole (5-HI), a metabolite of tryptophan, has been recognized as a low-potency α7 nAChR PAM at both human recombinant and rat naïve receptors [84, 85]. Using rat brain hippocampal slices, it was demonstrated that 5-HI facilitates GABAergic neurotransmission via excitation of the α7 nAChR at the presence of the endogenous agonist Ach [84]. Furthermore, facilitation of α7 nAChR-mediated glutamate release from mouse cortical synaptosomes by 5-HI has been also reported [86]. Additional endogenous substances have been shown to act as PAMs at α7 nAChRs, although a potential physiological role for any of these ligands is unknown at the present [80].

### 12.4.2 Overview of the Chemistry of α7 nAChR Positive Allosteric Modulators

Interest in the development of allosteric modulators of the α7 nAChR in medicinal chemistry has begun to expand over recent years, with a focus on the identification of novel chemical entities (Fig. 12.4). For the purpose of this section we will focus on those ligands that have been most extensively characterized in the primary literature and thus have served as tools to significantly advance the overall field. These compounds represent a new class of ligands

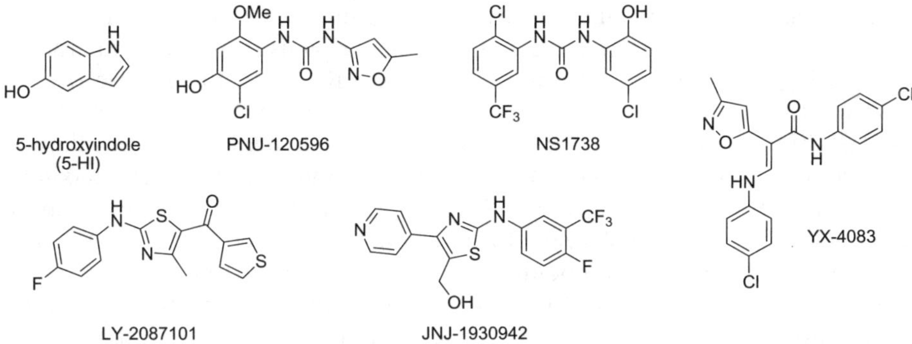


**FIGURE 12.4** Structures of α7 nAChR positive allosteric modulators (PAMs) 5-hydroxyindole, PNU-120596, NS1738, LY-2087101, JNJ-1930942, and YX-4083.

that activate the α7 nAChR and thus provide a potential mechanism to treat the cognitive deficits in schizophrenia.

Much of the early work to demonstrate the benefit of an allosteric modulator was accomplished utilizing 5-hydroxyindole as a modulator of the α7 nAChR [84]. The recent disclosure of the selective α7 nAChR positive allosteric modulator PNU-120596 provided a selective tool for further exploration of this mechanism [87]. PNU-120596 increases agonist-evoked $Ca^{+2}$ flux mediated by an engineered variant of the human α7 nAChR and enhances the acetylcholine-evoked inward currents in hippocampal interneurons. This compound also suppresses desensitization when tested *in vitro* and shows robust *in vivo* activity in an amphetamine-induced P50 gating deficit model (0.1–3 mg/kg, i.v.). The structure–activity relationship (SAR) of this series has more recently been discussed, and although a narrow SAR is observed, compounds with improved potency, physiochemical properties, and PK were identified and tested *in vivo* [88, 89]. More recently, a biaryl urea series has appeared in the literature from the group at NeuroSearch and is exemplified by NS1738 [90]. This compound is also reported to enhance the potency as well as the efficacy of an agonist but does not appear to affect desensitization to the extent that PNU-120596 does. Although the compound has only modest brain penetration, it was able to reverse a (-)-scopolamine-induced deficit in acquisition of a water-maze learning task in rats, and improved performance in rat social recognition *in vivo*.

A very interesting connection that a group at the University of California-Irvine recently made was between the $GABA_A$ receptor and the α7 nAChR based on sequence homology [91]. In a screening effort looking at a library of modulators of $GABA_A$, the group identified a class of compounds exemplified by XY4083 [92]. XY4083 evokes a positive modulation of agonist induced currents, which were demonstrated to retain the kinetic and desensitization properties of the α7 nAChR. This compound was also shown to reverse sensory gating deficits in rodents and improve working memory *in vivo*. Eli Lilly and JNJ have recently reported a series of thiazole derivatives that were identified through high-throughput screening as α7 nAChR PAMs. In the case of LY-2087101, the compound appears to be selective for the brain forms of the nAChR, but not specifically for the α7 nAChR subtype. Further profiling of these compounds demonstrated that they indeed enhance potency and maximal efficacy at both the α7 and α4β2 nAChRs [93]. More recently, the group at JNJ disclosed JNJ-1930942, also a thizalo, and it was stated to be selective for the α7 nAChR [94]. This compound increases the peek current amplitude and like PNU-120596 appears to slow desensitization kinetics and affects auditory evoked potential (AEPs) in DBA/2 mice. It is interesting to note that subtle differences in this class appear to have profound effects on selectivity for the neuronal nAChR subtypes.

### 12.4.3 Receptor Pharmacology. Type I and II Positive Allosteric Modulators

As the literature on PAMs for the α7 nAChR emerges, it is growing clear that there are at least two modes of action of these modulators [95], (Fig. 12.5). Studies with the homomeric α7 nAChRs indicate that such ligand interactions can be well described by an allosteric model [82] and that PAMs can affect energy transitions by (1) predominantly influencing the peak current response (type I profile) or (2) by increasing both peak current responses and the desensitization profile of an agonist response (type II profile) [80].

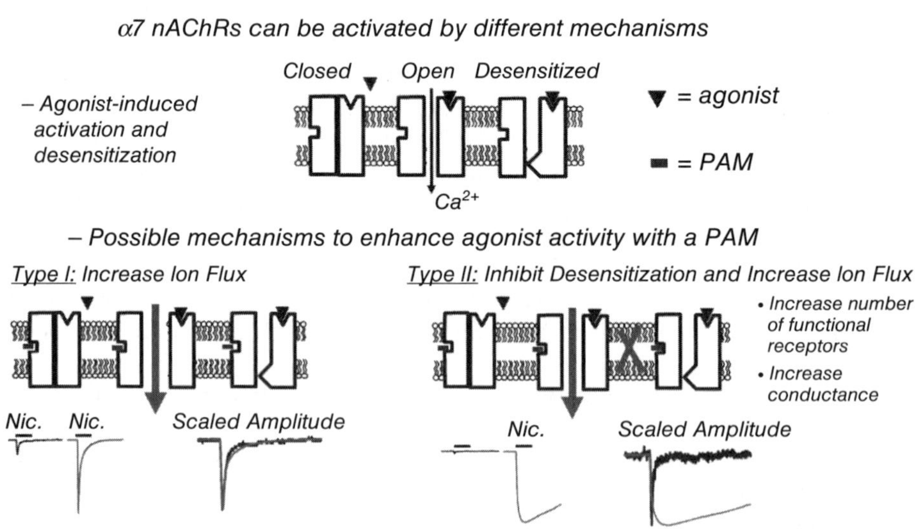


**FIGURE 12.5** Type I and type II mechanisms of positive allosteric potentiation. Nic, nicotine.

The recent literature, as described above, discloses a chemically diverse group of molecules capable of differentially modifying nAChR properties without interacting at the ligand binding site. Compounds that clearly appear to fit into the type I mechanism including 5-HI, XY-4083, and NS1738 have little to no effect on desensitization kinetics *in vitro*. Compounds that fit into the type II mechanism including PNU-120596, LY-2087101, and JNJ-1930942 all affect the desensitization kinetics, but to differing degrees, with PNU-120596 producing the most profound effect *in vitro*. It is interesting to note that although there are at least two possible mechanisms acting, both produce similar effects *in vivo*.

## 12.5 PHARMACOLOGICAL EFFECTS OF α7 nACh RECEPTOR AGONISTS AND PAMs: RELEVANCE FOR TREATMENT OF SCHIZOPHRENIA

### 12.5.1 Activation of α7 Receptors: Downstream Cellular Mechanisms

Extensive projections of cholinergic neurons provide widespread innervation to the entire brain, establishing various morphological connections between cholinergic axon terminals and targeted neurons. Cholinergic axon terminals establish proper synaptic connections or "classical synapses" in the cortex [96], although volume transmission (i.e., diffusion to receptors from distal release sites) as a nonsynaptic neurotransmission is broadly assumed in cholinergic transmission [97]. Since α7 nAChRs are located at both pre- and postsynaptic sites [13], endogenous ACh could theoretically directly activate them via synapses, or provide indirect activation via transmitter spillover from synapses or diffuse volume transmission [8]. Although rapid, direct nicotinic synaptic transmission has been demonstrated in rat hippocampus [14, 98], the sparse and diffuse nature of cholinergic axons makes detection or studying of this type of postsynaptic response methodologically very challenging.

Since α7 nAChRs are ligand-gated ion channels permeable to cations, activation of the channel results in direct depolarization of neuronal membrane potential. This depolarization might in turn change the neuron's responsiveness to synaptic input, alter its firing rate and/or firing pattern, and thus lead to modulation of axonal transmitter release (Fig. 12.6). However, α7 nAChRs are highly permeable to $Ca^{2+}$, and a subsequent increase in intracellular $Ca^{2+}$ has been considered the most significant response to activation of α7 nAChRs [99]. Enhanced neurotransmitter release could be just one consequence of increased intracellular $Ca^{+2}$, as it might also initiate a series of downstream intracellular processes, influencing a broad range of cellular functions ranging from synaptic plasticity to gene expression. Using the expression of the neuronal immediate-early gene c-fos as an indicator for neuronal activity, it has been shown that the selective α7 nAChR agonists PNU-282987 and SSR180711 induce dose-dependent c-fos expression in the limbic forebrain similar to

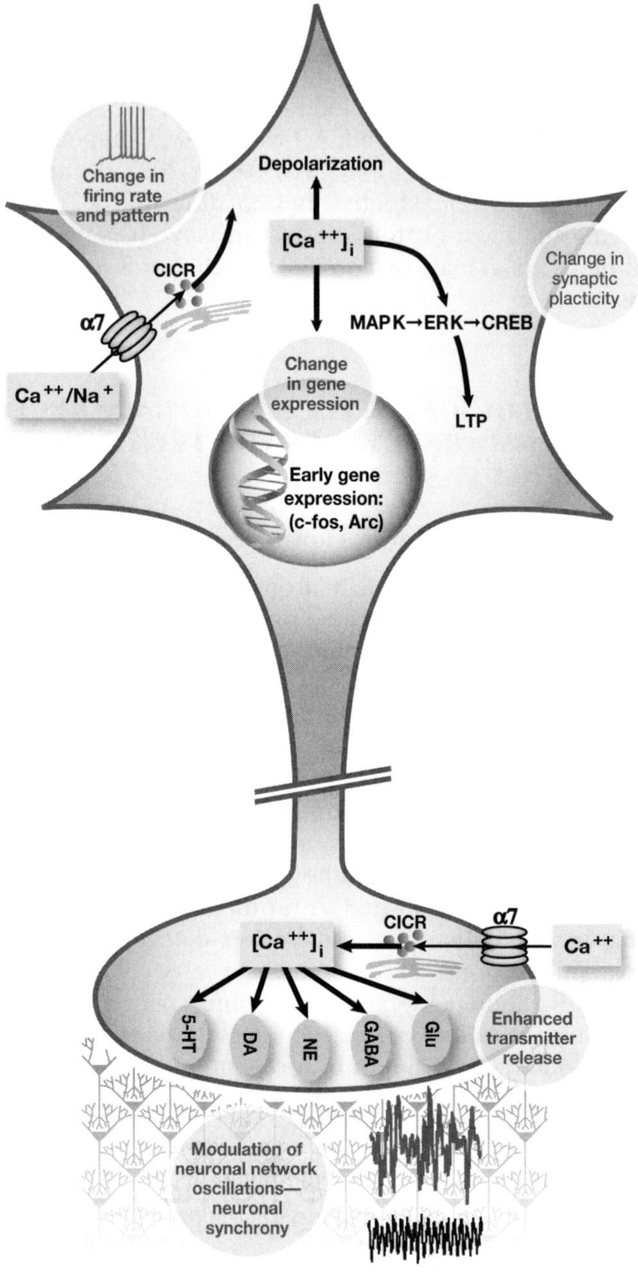
Change in
firing rate
and pattern
Depolarization
[Ca ++]i
CICR
α7
Ca ++/Na +
Change in
synaptic
placticity
MAPK→ERK→CREB
Change
in gene
expression
LTP
Early gene
expression:
(c-fos, Arc)
CICR
α7
[Ca ++]i
Ca ++
5-HT
DA
NE
GABA
Glu
Enhanced
transmitter
release
Modulation of
neuronal network
oscillations—
neuronal
synchrony

**FIGURE 12.6** Summary of subsequent cellular processes in response to activation of α7 nAChRs at the soma and axon terminals. Agonists binding to the pentameric α7 nAChRs (α7) induce a conformational change of subunit protein, making the channel permeable to cations, including calcium ($Ca^{++}$). Cation influx leads to membrane depolarization, and elicits calcium-induced calcium release (CICR) from intracellular stores. Increased intracellular $Ca^{++}$ levels, by activating the cascades of calcium-sensitive mitogen-activated protein kinase (MAPK) and extracellular-signal regulated kinase 1/2 (ERK) phosphorylation, and cAMP response element-binding protein (CREB) cascade, can lead to long-term synaptic plasticity (LTP). Higher intracellular $Ca^{++}$ levels also initiate expression of the neuronal immediate-early gene c-fos (c-fos) and activity-regulated cytoskeleton-associated protein (Arc). Facilitation of neurotransmitter release is also linked to an increase of intracellular calcium in response to receptor activation. Calcium influx via α7nAChR channels, together with calcium release from intracellular stores, triggers release of various neurotransmitters, including glutamate (Glu), γ-aminobutyric acid (GABA), norepinephrine (NE), dopamine (DA), and serotonin (5-HT). Via presynaptic regulation of release of several neurotransmitters, broadly distributed α7nAChRs are well positioned to modulate neuronal network activity, such as network oscillations and neuronal synchrony.

conventional antipsychotics [100]. Induction of two cellular markers, the activity-regulated cytoskeleton-associated protein (Arc) and c-fos, by the α7 nAChR agonist A-582941 was more pronounced in juvenile than in adult rats in limbic forebrain regions associated with working memory and attention [101]. This study indicates that the juvenile forebrain is more responsive to α7 nAChR stimulation that the adult brain [101].

Among various calcium-regulated second-messenger signaling pathways, the calcium-sensitive mitogen-activated protein kinase (MAPK) cascade has been studied as a potential mechanism involved in the pro-cognitive activity of α7 nAChRs. The selective α7 nAChR agonist A-582941 increased extracellular signal regulated kinase 1/2 (ERK 1/2) phosphorylation and cAMP response element-binding protein (CREB) phosphorylation in mouse cingulate cortex and hippocampus [78]. These responses were observed after acute administration of A-582941 at a dose range that was also efficacious in producing precognitive behavioral effects in animal models such as monkey delayed matching-to-sample, rat social recognition, and mouse inhibitory avoidance models [78]. Based on these observations, it has been suggested that α7 nAChR-mediated increases in intracellular calcium activate calcium-dependent MAPK–ERK signal transduction, a pathway known to regulate various cellular functions, including synaptic plasticity events such as long-term potentiation (LTP) [102].

Facilitation of neurotransmitter release, the best established neuromodulatory role of α7 nAChRs, is also linked to an increase of intracellular calcium in response to receptor activation. Calcium influx via α7 nAChR channels can trigger calcium release from intracellular stores (calcium-induced calcium release [CICR]) and subsequently triggering neurotransmitter release from the terminals [103]. Furthermore, calcium influx, together with the simultaneous influx of $Na^+$, produces membrane depolarization that might lead to the activation of voltage-gated calcium channels (VGCCs), thus ensuring effective transmitter release [99]. Since α7 nAChRs expressed by a large variety of neurons as presynaptic (or preterminal) receptors, they are well positioned to modulate neuronal network activity, such as network oscillations and neuronal synchrony (see Section 12.5.3).

### 12.5.2 Auditory Gating: Preclinical and Clinical Findings

Since auditory gating deficits are considered an endophenotype for schizophrenia, and the P50 gating deficit has been linked to the α7nAChR gene (*CHRNA7*), considerable clinical and preclinical research has been initiated in this field. Acoustic stimulation elicits a number of AEPs with various latencies that can be detected by human scalp EEG recordings. In a healthy individual, if the same acoustic stimulation is repeated within sufficiently short intervals, (typically at 0.5 seconds), the AEPs to the second stimuli are significantly attenuated. This phenomenon is known as auditory gating, and was first demonstrated by examining AEPs, which occur with 50-millisecond latency as a positive deflection (positive potential at 50 milliseconds = P50 gating). Schizophrenic patients, their first-degree relatives, and subjects with schizotypal personality disorder show impaired auditory gating and exhibit identical responses to the first and second stimuli (for review see References[7, 104, 105]) Although a recent meta-analysis of 20 studies on P50 auditory gating revealed a robust deficiency in schizophrenic patients in this neurophysiological measure, the relationship between abnormal sensory gating and clinical symptoms of schizophrenia is not fully understood [106]. In addition, impaired auditory gating has been described in other psychiatric and neurological diseases, including bipolar disorder and Alzheimer's disease [107]. Based on the association between the polymorphism in the α7 nAChR gene and auditory gating, and the clinical observations that nicotine transiently improves auditory gating in schizophrenics [108, 109], it has been proposed that activation of α7 nAChRs would improve sensory processing and thus provide benefit for impaired cognitive function and perhaps positive and/or negative symptoms in schizophrenic patients as well [110]. It has also been suggested that the high prevalence of heavy smoking among patients with schizophrenia (>80%) may be a form of self-medication [108].

Sensory gating processes resembling those in humans have been demonstrated in experimental animals using clinically equivalent acoustic stimulation paradigms. A large body of evidence clearly demonstrates that abnormal information processing in schizophrenia could be reproduced in these preclinical models using pharmacological, genetic, or environmental manipulations (Fig. 12.7). Thus, pharmacologically disrupted auditory gating in rodents can be induced by direct or indirect dopamine receptor agonists (amphetamine, apo-

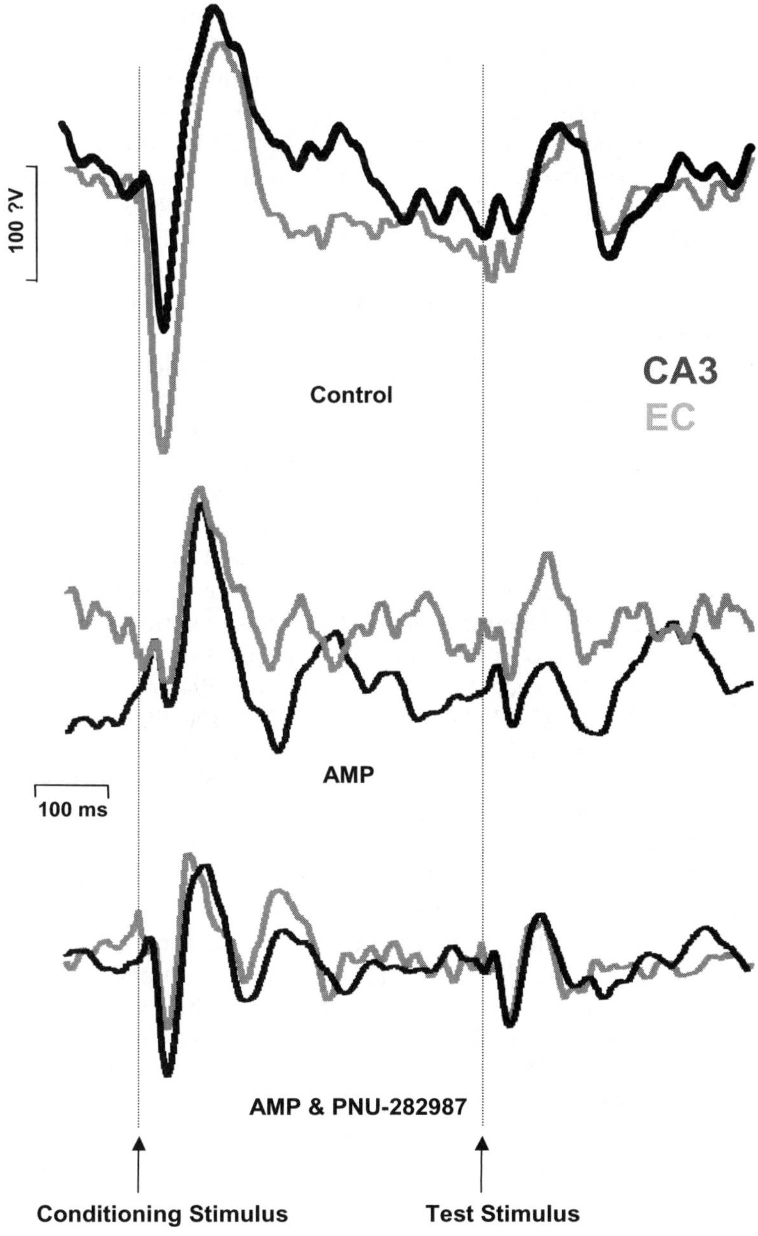


**FIGURE 12.7** Simultaneously recorded auditory evoked potentials to conditioning and test acoustical stimuli (arrows) in the hippocampus CA3 region (CA3) and entorhinal cortex of an anesthetized rat. Evoked potentials (marked with asterisks) show auditory gating (Control); administration of amphetamine disrupts auditory gating in both regions (AMP). Amphetamine-induced gating deficit is reversed by the selective α7 nAChR agonist PNU-282987, 1 mg/kg, i.v. (AMP and PNU-282987).

morphine, or cocaine), NMDA receptor antagonists (PCP, ketamine, or MK-801) or cannabinoid-1 receptor agonists [111–115]. Most of these compounds are also known to disrupt sensory gating in humans and/or elicit psychosis [107, 116, 117]. Furthermore, social isolation [118] and early maternal deprivation [119] also impair sensory gating in adult rats, providing an excellent alternative to pharmacologically based animal models. The inbred mouse strain DBA/2, which have a relatively reduced α7 nAChR expression, as well as the C3H α7 nAChRs null mutant heterozygous mice (with approximately a 60% reduction in α7nAChR expression) both show significantly reduced auditory gating [120]. The methodology of animal modeling in auditory gating has been extensively reviewed in recent years [33, 111, 113, 114].

Systemic administration of nicotine has been shown to normalize or improve gating deficits in various animal models of auditory gating deficits, including DBA/2 mice, fornix-lesioned rats, and amphetamine or cocaine-induced gating deficit (for review see Reference [33]). These findings are in line with the clinical findings showing that nicotine transiently improves or normalizes the P50 auditory gating deficit in schizophrenic patients. The effectiveness of many agonists and PAMs of α7 nAChRs have been tested in animal models, and confirmed that selective activation of α7 nAChRs is sufficient to improve auditory gating deficits. It has been shown that the auditory gating deficit of DBA/2 mice is improved by the α7 nAChR partial agonist, GTS-21 (DMXBA), full agonists of α7 nAChRs, such as PHA-543613, A-582941, and JN403 [68, 72, 76], as well as PAMs of α7 nAChRs, including PNU-120596 and XY4083 [92]. In addition, α7 nAChR agonists showed activity in auditory gating deficits induced by social isolation or central administration of the α7 nAChR antagonist MLA [118]. Dopamine hyperfunction in schizophrenic patients has been demonstrated by neuroimaging findings [121], validating the choice of amphetamine as a pharmacological tool for modeling disrupted auditory gating of schizophrenic patients [122]. Enhanced dopaminergic neurotransmission by pharmacological manipulation leads to impaired auditory gating in humans [116, 117] and in animals [111, 112, 123]. Using the amphetamine-induced gating deficit model in rats, several azabicyclic α7 nAChRs agonists have been evaluated. The amphetamine-induced gating deficit was reversed by PNU-282987 [57, 67], PHA-543613 [68], PHA-568487 [124], and PHA-709829 [77], as well as the PAM PNU-120569 [87]. Since PAMs of α7 nAChRs showed activity in auditory gating assays (as well as in a cognitive animal test), it can be inferred that α7 nAChRs are tonically activated by their endogenous ligand(s) and therefore that their allosteric potentiation results in a measurable pharmacological effect.

Considering the fast desensitizing characteristics of α7 nAChRs, activity of α7 nAChR agonists has been tested after repeated administration. It has been demonstrated that PHA-543613, PHA-709829, and PHA-568487 were active after repeated administration (twice daily for 6 days) in the amphetamine-induced gating deficit model [77, 124, 125]. Similarly, A-582941 was found to be active after subsequent daily, 5-day repeated administration in DBA/2 mice as well [76]. Furthermore, the efficacy of α7 nAChR agonists could be maintained even in the presence of chronic nicotine exposure, as demonstrated by the fact that PHA-543613 restores amphetamine-induced auditory gating deficits in rats after chronic nicotine treatment (i.e., 14 days, implanted minipump) [125].

Although the effectiveness of α7 nAChR activation has been shown unequivocally in various gating deficits, there are a growing number of observations demonstrating that other nicotinic receptors, particularly α4β2 nAChRs, might impact auditory gating mechanisms as well. Involvement of α4β2 nAChRs has been shown in the effect of nicotine on auditory gating in DBA/2 mice [126]. The nAChR agonist ABT-480, as well as the selective α4β2 nAChR full agonists 5-I A-85380 and TC-2403, and the partial agonist varenicline all improve gating deficit in DBA/2 mice [127, 128]. It has also been shown that varenicline reverses amphetamine-induced gating deficits in rats, similarly to selective α7 nAChR agonists [129]. Therefore, non α7 nAChR agonists might also be efficacious in schizophrenia, regardless of probable genetic connection between α7 nAChRs and the disease. Ultimately, clinical studies will determine whether these compounds can impact auditory gating mechanisms in schizophrenic patients and, subsequently, improve perception and cognitive functions.

There is a considerable ongoing effort to understand neuronal network activities underlying sensory evoked potentials, including analysis of event-related network oscillations at various frequencies [130–132] The time-frequency analysis of event related or induced oscillations can ultimately shed light on processes involved in sensory gating deficits in schizophrenic patents. In fact, recent findings indicate that lower frequency band oscillations (theta-alpha-band) contribute to paired-click paradigm auditory gating, and it is significantly different between control and schizophrenic subjects, representing a better neurophysiological measure than traditional P50 gating [131]. In addition, the heritability of theta-alpha-band gating is at least 4-fold higher than the P50 heritability estimate, suggesting that this marker is well suited for genetic studies of the gating deficit in schizophrenia. Recent findings on α7 nAChR partial agonists in schizophrenic patients showed improvement in P50 auditory gating and some measures of schizophrenia symptoms. It is therefore now possible to evaluate the effects of relatively selective nicotinic compounds on event-related neuronal network activities in patients. These findings could initiate further preclinical studies modeling abnormal oscillations using *in vivo* models, *in vitro* preparations, as well as computational modeling [133].

### 12.5.3 Effects on Neuronal Network Oscillations

There is a growing interest in the pathophysiology of oscillatory activity of cortical neuronal networks in schizophrenia. To study neuronal network oscillations, naturally arising brain rhythms are recorded that occur while the brain performs specific sensory, cognitive, or motor operations. These oscillations reflect synchrony in neuronal activity and synchronous brain activity within and between brain regions. Gamma-band (30–200 Hz) measures have been of particular interest in schizophrenia as they are linked to the concept of perceptual feature binding and interbrain-area synchronization [134]. Deficits in gamma generation have been observed in sensory discrimination tasks in schizophrenia patients, although deficits also appear at slower (0.5–12 Hz) frequencies [135]. In addition, abnormal steady-state visually- or auditory-evoked oscillations have been reported in schizophrenic patients, indicating a reduction in generating or maintaining oscillations in neural networks [136, 137]. Taken together, these studies suggest that schizophrenia involves abnormal oscillations and synchrony of neuronal networks that are related to cognitive dysfunctions and presumably positive symptoms of the disorder. For further discussion on this topic, see recent reviews [33, 107, 138, 139].

As neuronal synchrony and network oscillation share many common processes in humans and animals, pharmacological studies of network oscillations could disclose some pathophysiological processes that are associated with schizophrenia, and provide a unique opportunity to evaluate novel therapeutic targets. Growing preclinical literature and computational modeling of oscillatory brain activity during perception and cognitive operations can support this effort. Current theories on the generation of neuronal network oscillations attribute a central role to interconnected, inhibitory GABA neurons, suggesting that morphologically and neurochemically distinct subsets of GABA neurons contribute differently to theta- and gamma-frequency oscillations [140, 141]. Importantly, recent postmortem studies provide consistent evidence to support abnormalities of GABA functioning in schizophrenic brains, and augmentation of efficacy of GABA neurotransmission has been suggested as a therapeutic strategy [139].

Since α7 nAChRs predominantly facilitate GABA-mediated inhibitory neurotransmission, it is of great interest to learn whether these receptors can modulate neuronal network oscillations at various frequency bands in the cortex or hippocampus. Among the neurochemically diverse $GABA_A$ interneurons, cholecystokinin (CCK)-containing interneurons have been identified as expressing α7 nAChRs [142]. CCK-positive cells receive synaptic input from various and distant circuitries, and their activity is modulated by cholinergic afferents [140, 143]. In contrast to the well-defined role of muscarinic cholinergic receptors [144], less is known about the potential involvement of nicotinic receptors in neuronal network oscillation. However, recent findings indicate that activity of α7 nAChRs can modulate oscillatory activity. Using *in vitro* rat hippocampal slice preparations, it has been demonstrated that tetanic stimulation-induced gamma oscillation is enhanced by α7 nAChRs [145]. The selective α7nAChR agonist PNU-282987 has been tested on hippocampal oscillation in anesthetized rats. Although PNU-282987 does not elicit hippocampal oscillatory activity in anesthetized rats, it can significantly enhance amphetamine-induced theta and gamma oscillations [67, 146]. Similarly, recording brainstem stimulation-induced hippocampal theta oscillation, it has been found that PNU-282987 significantly enhances total power of oscillation at theta frequency [147]. PNU-282987 also augmented elicited theta frequency (at a frequency range above 6.5 Hz) [148], indicating that although muscarinic acetylcholine receptors appear to promote the power but not the frequency of theta, α7 nAChRs may play some role in the control of frequency as well. Based on these observations, it seems clear that activation of α7 nAChRs is capable of enhancing ongoing hippocampal oscillations that could, in turn, contribute to the known mnemonic effects of α7 nAChR agonists [148]. In the above experiments, the action of α7 nAChRs on oscillatory activitry could be attributed to modulation of GABA neurotransmission. However, α7 nAChRs might modulate oscillation via regulating glutamate neurotransmission at presynaptic sites as well. Recording from hypoglossal motoneurons in rat brainstem slices, it was demonstrated that persistent activation of α7 nAChRs could evoke sustained oscillations in the theta frequency range via release of endogenous glutamate [149]. Whether activation of α7 nChRs could adjust pathological oscillations in schizophrenic patents and concomitantly improve cognitive functions could be determined in future clinical trials, which could also help to validate the relevance of oscillatory abnormalities in cortical networks in the pathophysiology of schizophrenia.

### 12.5.4 Behavioral Precognitive Effects

In order to elucidate the physiological roles of neurotransmitter receptors, behavioral, electrophysiological, and neurochemical studies of genetically modified mice have been an important alternative to pharmacological research. The first studies on knockout (KO) mice lacking α7 nAChRs showed remarkably normal behavior, including normal sensory-motor gating, affective, and cognitive functions [150]. However, more recent studies on homozygous and heterozygous KO mice have revealed an impairment in attentional performance in the five-choice serial reaction time task [151, 152], spatial discrimination [153], and Morris water maze [154]. In order to overcome potential adaptive or compensatory changes in neurotransmission in α7 KO mice, alternative methods have been used to interfere with α7 nAChR expression and function. Thus, using an antisense oligonucleotide targeted toward the rat α7 nAChR, it has been shown that rats exhibited a significant decrease in α7 nAChR densities in the hippocampus and cortex, and an impaired acquisition of Morris water maze performance [155]. Furthermore, increasing neuronal α7 receptor functions by α7 nAChR receptor gene delivery into mouse hippocampal neurons using neuron-selective recombinant adeno-associated virus vectors resulted in functional receptor expression and improved spatial memory-related performance [156]. These findings demonstrate a connection between functional α7 nAChRs and various domains of cognition, including attention, spatial learning, and working/episodic memory.

As an increasing number of selective α7 nAChR agonists have been developed, their behavioral effects have been studied in a broad range of assays. In line with observations in genetically modified mice, improvement in several cognitive functions has been reported after administration of α7 nAChR agonists or PAMs. In rodent cognitive models, α7 nAChR agonists were active in social recognition tests (i.e., A-582941 [76], AR-R 17779 [157], ABBF [71], and JN403 [158]) novel object recognition (i.e., SSR180711 [75], ABBF [157], and PHA-543613 [68]), in radial arm or Y maze (i.e., AR-R 17779 [159], A-582941 [160], SSR180711 [161], and PNU-282987 [162]), and Morris water maze (i.e., ABBF [157], GTS-21 [59], and SSR180711 [75]), as well as in delayed matching-to-sample test in primates (i.e., A-582941 [78] and GTS-21 [61]). Similarly, α7 nAChR PAMs demonstrate cognitive enhancing effects, including NS1738 (in social recognition test and Morris water maze [90]) and YX4083 (in eight-arm radial maze [92]). Furthermore, agonists and PAMs of α7 nAChRs have been shown to reverse impaired cognitive functions induced by scopolamine [61, 156, 159], the NMDA receptor antagonists, MK-801, and PCP [160, 163], and aging-related decline of cognition [164, 165].

The exact synaptic or cellular mechanisms involved in cognitive effects of α7 nAChRs ligands are not fully explored. Since long-term modulations of synaptic activity, such as LTP, are considered probable correlates of learning and memory [166, 167], it is of a significance that activation of α7 nAChR agonists facilitate LTP in both *in vitro* and *in vivo* preparations [168–170]. For instance, AZD0328, a potent and selective α7 neuronal nicotinic receptor agonist, has been shown to restore LTP induction in fimbria/fornix-transectioned rats in response to theta burst stimulation [170]. At these same doses, AZD0328 also improved cognitive performance in a working memory task of fimbria/fornix-lesioned rats; therefore, the agonist-induced restoration of hippocampal plasticity has been considered the putative underlying mechanism of its mnemonic action [171]. In addition, activation of α7 nAChRs has been shown to enhance hippocampal theta oscillation [146, 147], a neuronal network activity considered a natural, endogenous stimulus for inducing LTP [172]. In line with the recognized functional importance of acetylcholine in learning and memory [144], a considerable amount of preclinical data demonstrate pro-cognitive effects of α7nAChR agonists, although there are only very limited data on their cognitive effects in humans as outlined in the next section.

## 12.6 THERAPEUTIC PROMISES AND UNCERTAINTIES ABOUT α7 nAChR LIGANDS IN TREATMENT OF SCHIZOPHRENIA: FUTURE DIRECTIONS

With the possible exception of clozapine, most of the antipsychotics currently used in clinical practice do not normalize gating deficits. It has been reported that clozapine significantly improves P50 auditory gating, which might be associated with parallel improvement in clinical symptoms [173–175]. Recently, tropisetron, which is a potent α7 nAChR partial agonist and a 5-$HT_3$ antagonist, has been shown to improve the gating deficit in schizophrenic patients [176]. Interestingly, ondansetron, a selective 5-$HT_3$ antagonist also improves P50 gating in schizophrenia patients treated with typical antipsychotics [177]. Since 5-$HT_3$ receptors modulate acetylcholine release, it is speculated that ondansetron could indirectly activate α7 nAChRs via release of acetylcholine and thereby improve gating [177]. A similar, indirect activation of α7 nAChRs has been proposed as a possible underlying mechanism of clozapine-induced normalization of P50 gating in schizophrenics [173]. Whether cognitive symptoms or subsets of cognitive, negative, or positive symptoms of schizophrenia would recover in parallel with improving auditory gating following α7 nAChR stimulation is still an open, intriguing question.

### 12.6.1 Proof-of-Concept Studies on GTS-21

Numerous companies have stated that they are currently in clinical trials with α7 nAChR agonists including AZD-0328 [178], EVP-6124 [179], MEM-3454, PHA-543613, PHA-568487, and SSR180711. Although some of the preliminary results have been presented at meetings and indeed demonstrate a modest improvement in certain cognitive domains, GTS-21 (DMXBA) is the only compound where clinical results have been published. The partial nAChR agonist DMBX-A showed statistically significant enhancement of attention, working memory, and episodic secondary memory in healthy male subjects [180]. In the study reported by Olincy and co-workers, the primary objective was to determine if DMBX-A improves cognition in nonsmoking patients currently taking antipsychotics [181], as measured by the effect on P50 AEP inhibition. In this initial study, significant improvement was found on the Repeatable Battery for the Assessment of Neuropsychology on the total scale score, particularly for the lower GTS-21 dose compared with placebo. In this study, the effects seen were greater than that of nicotine. The study also demonstrated a significant improvement in P50 inhibition.

The results of the Phase I trial with GTS-21 were deemed significantly robust to prompt a larger Phase II trial of 31 patients with schizophrenia treated for a 4-week period (75 mg BID or 150 mg BID, orally) [182]. Patients in this study were evaluated using the MATRICS Consensus Cognitive Battery to assess cognitive effects, the Scale for the Assessment of Negative Symptoms (SANS), and the Brief Psychiatric Rating Scale (BPRS) to assess clinical effects. In this trial, the investigators did not find a significant improvement in the primary cognition measure (MATRICS), but patients dosed at the high dose did see an improvement in the negative symptoms as measured by the SANS. The study was, however, complicated by a significant practice effect in the test battery. Although these results fall short of the original hypothesis of the study, they are encouraging, particularly given the limitations of the GTS-21 compound that was used to test the nicotinic strategy. Therefore, the clinical utility of α7 nAChR agonists or partial agonists in schizophrenia pharmacotherapy, particularly for cognitive dysfunction, has yet to be fully determined.

### 12.6.2 Potential Adverse Effects of α7 nAChR Ligands

As compounds containing α7 nAChR activity enter clinical trials, a more complete understanding of the potential challenges of this class will emerge. The safety concerns that nicotine itself raises range from abuse liability, cardiovascular, seizure liability, cytotoxicity, and the risk of a bell-shaped dose response curve [45]. Specifically for α7, the rapid desensitization profile of the receptor could contribute to a tachyphylaxis potential. In many ways, this could serve as a protection mechanism to ensure that a significant increase in calcium flux does not result in a cytotoxicity [183]; likewise, this may provide a rationale for increased interest in PAMs of nAChRs to ensure that minimization of the desensitization profile is considered.

Cardiovascular safety assessments of compounds will be critical for the success of agents in this class. Nicotine, a nonselective nAChR agonist, is linked to cardiovascular changes [184], and the expectation is that selective agents will reduce cardiovascular safety issues. To date, a primary issue of interest has been ensuring that sufficient hERG selectivity is attained [185]. Many compounds reported to date contain very potent hERG blocking effects, including PNU-282987, while many others have shown adequate selectivity against this ion channel [68]. More recently, Pfizer has disclosed that the clinical development of two compounds in the class, PHA-543613 and PHA-568487, have been discontinued from development due to a low incidence (5%) of asymptomatic cardiac arrhythmia in healthy volunteers (asymptomatic ventricular tachycardia and asymptomatic nonsustained ventricular tachycardia) [70]. Although it is unclear at this point if this finding is related to the target or the class of compounds, work should be done to fully elucidate the nature of these findings in the future. As the data from patients emerge from the clinical trial of agents that are partial and full agonists of the α7 nAChR, a full understanding of the potential safety concerns will emerge.

## 12.7 CONCLUSIONS

Significant progress has been made over the past decade in the area of the α7 nAChR research as evidenced by the many compounds now making their way into the clinical setting. Emerging evidence from meetings and initial publications suggests that compounds containing α7 activity do affect the P50 gating deficits and may improve cognitive deficits. As compounds are dosed in greater numbers of patients and for longer periods, a clear understanding of the safety and efficacy of these agents will emerge. It is a very exciting time in the field, and as the mechanism is better understood in patients, a clear answer will emerge on the full therapeutic utility of this important receptor family.

## REFERENCES


1. Arneric, S.P., Brioni, J.D., eds. (1999). *Neuronal Nicotinic Receptors: Pharmacology and Therapeutic Opportunities*, 1st ed. New York: Wiley-Liss.
2. Clementi, F., Fornasari, D., Gotti, C., eds. (2000). *Neuronal Nicotinic Receptors*, 1st ed. New York: Springer.
3. Lukas, R.J., Changeux, J.-P., Le Novère, N., Albuquerque, E.X., Balfour, D.J.K., Berg, D.K., Bertrand, D., Chiappinelli, V.A., Clarke, P.B.S., Collins, A.C., Dani, J.A., Grady, S.R., Kellar, K.J., Lindstrom, J.M., Marks, M.J., Quik, M., Taylor, P.W., Wonnacott, S. (1999). International Union of Pharmacology. XX. Current status of the nomenclature for nicotinic acetylcholine receptors and their subunits. *Pharmacol Rev*, *51*, 397–401.
4. Weiland, S., Bertrand, D., Leonard, S. (2000). Neuronal nicotinic acetylcholine receptors: from the gene to the disease. *Behav Brain Res*, *113*, 43–56.
5. Skok, M.V., Voitenko, L.P., Voitenko, S.V., Lykhmus, E.Y., Kalashnik, E.N., Litvin, T.I., Tzartos, S.J., Skok, V.I. (1999). Alpha subunit composition of nicotinic acetylcholine receptors in the rat autonomic ganglia neurons as determined with subunit-specific anti-alpha.(181-192) peptide antibodies. *Neuroscience*, *93*, 1427–1436.
6. McGehee, D.S., Role, L.W. (1995). Physiological diversity of nicotinic acetylcholine receptors expressed by vertebrate neurons. *Annu Rev Physiol*, *57*, 521–546.
7. Freedman, R., Olincy, A., Ross, R.G., Waldo, M.C., Stevens, K.E.W., Adler, L.E., Leonard, S. (2003). The genetics of sensory gating deficits in schizophrenia. *Curr Psychiatry Rep*, *5*, 155–161.
8. Dani, J.A., Bertrand, D. (2007). Nicotinic acetylcholine receptors and nicotinic cholinergic mechanisms of the central nervous system. *Annu Rev Pharmacol Toxicol*, *47*, 699–729.
9. Corringer, P.-J., Bertrand, S., Bohler, S., Edelstein, S.J., Changeux, J.-P., Bertrand, D. (1998). Critical elements determining diversity in agonist binding and desensitization of neuronal nicotinic acetylcholine receptors. *J Neurosci*, *18*, 648–657.
10. Monod, J., Wyman, J., Changeux, J.P. (1965). On the nature of allosteric transition: a plausible model. *J Mol Biol*, *12*, 88–118.
11. Changeux, J.P., Edelstein, S.J. (1998). Allosteric receptors after 30 years. *Neuron*, *21*(5), 959–980.
12. Gay, E.A., Giniatullin, R., Skorinkin, A., Yakel, J.L. (2008). Aromatic residues at position 55 of rat alpha7 nicotinic acetylcholine receptors are critical for maintaining rapid desensitization. *J Physiol*, *586*, 1105–1115.
13. McKay, B.E., Placzek, A.N., Dani, J.A. (2007). Regulation of synaptic transmission and plasticity by neuronal nicotinic acetylcholine receptors. *Biochem Pharmacol*, *74*, 1120–1133.
14. Alkondon, M., Pereira, E.F., Albuquerque, E.X. (1998). Alpha-bungarotoxin- and methyllycaconitine-sensitive nicotinic receptors mediate fast synaptic transmission in interneurons of rat hippocampal slices. *Brain Res*, *810*, 257–263.
15. Wonnacott, S. (1997). Presynaptic nicotinic ACh receptors. *Trends Neurosci*, *20*, 92–97.

16. Azam, L., Winzer-Serhan, U., Leslie, F.M. (2003). Co-expression of α7 and β2 nicotinic acetylcholine receptor subunit mRNAs within rat brain cholinergic neurons. *Neuroscience*, *119*, 965–977.
17. Aznar, S., Kostova, V., Christiansen, S.H., Knudsen, G.M. (2005). Alpha 7 nicotinic receptor subunit is present on serotonin neurons projecting to hippocampus and septum. *Synapse*, *55*(3), 196–200.
18. Marchi, M., Risso, F., Viola, C., Cavazzani, P., Raiteri, M. (2002). Direct evidence that release-stimulating alpha7* nicotinic cholinergic receptors are localized on human and rat brain glutamatergic axon terminals. *J Neurochem*, *80*(6), 1071–1078.
19. Chen, D., Patrick, J.W. (1997). The alpha-bungarotoxin-binding nicotinic acetylcholine receptor from rat brain contains only the alpha7 subunit. *J Biol Chem*, *272*(38), 24024–24029.
20. Whiteaker, P., Davies, A.R., Marks, M.J., Blagbrough, I.S., Potter, B.V., Wolstenholme, A.J., Collins, A.C., Wonnacott, S. (1999). An autoradiographic study of the distribution of binding sites for the novel alpha7-selective nicotinic radioligand [3H]-methyllycaconitine in the mouse brain. *Eur J Neurosci*, *11*(8), 2689–2696.
21. Tribollet, E., Bertrand, D., Marguerat, A., Raggenbass, M. (2004). Comparative distribution of nicotinic receptor subtypes during development, adulthood and aging: an autoradiographic study in the rat brain. *Neuroscience*, *124*, 405–420.
22. Sullivan, P.F., Kendler, K.S., Neale, M.C. (2003). Schizophrenia as a complex trait—evidence from a meta-analysis of twin studies. *Arch Gen Psychiatry*, *60*, 1187–1192.
23. Karayiorgou, M., Gogos, J.A. (1997). Dissecting the genetic complexity of schizophrenia. *Mol Psychiatry*, *2*(3), 211–223.
24. Harrison, P.J., Weinberger, D.R. (2005). Schizophrenia genes, gene expression, and neuropathology: on the matter of their convergence. *Mol Psychiatry*, *10*, 40–68.
25. Stassen, H.H., Bridler, R., Hagele, S., Hergersberg, M., Mehmann, B., Schinzel, A., Weisbrod, M., Scharfetter, C. (2000). Schizophrenia and smoking: evidence for a common neurobiological basis? *Am J Med Genet*, *96*, 173–177.
26. Freedman, R., Coon, H., Myles-Worsley, M., Orr-Urtreger, A., Olincy, A., Davis, A., Polymeropoulous, M., Holik, J., Hopkins, J., Hoff, M., Rosenthal, J., Waldo, M.C., Reimherr, F., Wender, P., Yaw, J., Young, D.A., Breese, C.R., Adams, C., Patterson, D., Adler, L., Kruglyak, L., Leonard, S., Byerley, W. (1997). Linkage of a neurophysiological deficit in schizophrenia to a chromosome 15 locus. *Proc Natl Acad Sci U S A*, *94*, 587–592.
27. Leonard, S., Gault, J., Hopkins, J., Logel, J., Vianzon, R., Short, M., Drebing, C., Berger, R., Venn, D., Pinkhas, S., Zerbbe, G., Olincy, A., Ross, R., Adler, L., Freedman, R. (2002). Association of promoter variants in the a7 nicotinic acetylcholine receptor subunit gene with an inhibitory deficit found in schizophrenia. *Arch Gen Psychiatry*, *59*, 1085–1096.
28. Gault, J., Hopkins, J., Berger, R., Drebing, C., Logel, J., Walton, C., Short, M., Vianzon, R., Olincy, A., Ross, R.G., Adler, L.E., Freedman, R., Leonard, S. (2003). Comparison of polymorphisms in the alpha7 nicotinic receptor gene and its partial duplication in schizophrenic and control subjects. *Am J Med Genet B Neuropsychiatr Genet*, *123B*(1), 39–49.

29. Stitzel, J.A. (2008). Naturally occurring genetic variability in the nicotinic acetylcholine receptor alpha4 and alpha7 subunit genes and phenotypic diversity in humans and mice. *Front Biosci*, *13*, 477–491.

30. Freedman, R., Hall, M., Adler, L.E., Leonard, S. (1995). Evidence in postmortem brain tissue for decreased numbers of hippocampal nicotinic receptors in schizophrenia. *Biol Psychiatry*, *38*, 22–33.

31. Court, J., Spurden, D., Lloyd, S., McKeith, I., Ballard, C., Cairns, N., Kerwin, R., Perry, R., Perry, E. (1999). Neuronal nicotinic receptors in dementia with Lewy bodies and schizophrenia: a-bungarotoxin and nicotine binding in the thalamus. *J Neurochem*, *73*, 1590–1597.

32. Marutle, A., Zhang, X., Court, J., Piggott, M., Johnson, M., Perry, R., Perry, E., Nordberg, A. (2001). Laminar distribution of nicotinic receptor subtypes in cortical regions in schizophrenia. *J Chem Neuroanat*, *22*, 115–126.

33. Hajós, M. (2006). Targeting information-processing deficit in schizophrenia: a novel approach to psychotherapeutic drug discovery. *Trends Pharmacol Sci*, *27*, 391–398.

34. Thaker, G. (2008). Psychosis endophenotypes in schizophrenia and bipolar disorder. *Schizophr Bull*, *34*, 720–721.

35. Hong, L.E., Summerfelt, A., Mitchell, B.D., McMahon, R.P., Wonodi, I., Buchanan, R.W., Thaker, G.K. (2008). Sensory gating endophenotype based on its neural oscillatory pattern and heritability estimate. *Arch Gen Psychiatry*, *65*, 1008–1016.

36. Ripoll, N., Bronnec, M., Bourin, M. (2004). Nicotinic receptors and schizophrenia. *Curr Med Res Opin*, *20*, 1057–1074.

37. Freedman, R., Adams, C.E., Leonard, S. (2000). The alpha7-nicotinic acetylcholine receptor and the pathology of hippocampal interneurons in schizophrenia. *J Chem Neuroanat*, *20*, 299–306.

38. Hong, C.J., Lai, I.C., Liou, L.L., Tsai, S.J. (2004). Association study of the human partially duplicated alpha7 nicotinic acetylcholine receptor genetic variant with bipolar disorder. *Neurosci Lett*, *355*, 69–72.

39. De Luca, V., Likhodi, O., Van Tol, H.H., Kennedy, J.L., Wong, A.H. (2006). Regulation of alpha7-nicotinic receptor subunit and alpha7-like gene expression in the prefrontal cortex of patients with bipolar disorder and schizophrenia. *Acta Psychiatr Scand*, *114*, 211–215.

40. Carson, R., Craig, D., Hart, D., Todd, S., McGuinness, B., Johnston, J.A., O'Neill, F.A., Ritchie, C.W., Passmore, A.P. (2008). Genetic variation in the alpha7 nicotinic acetylcholine receptor is associated with delusional symptoms in Alzheimer's disease. *Neuromolecular Med*, *10*, 377–384.

41. Alkondon, M., Pereira, E.F., Cortes, W.S., Maelicke, A., Albuquerque, E.X. (1997). Choline is a selective agonist of alpha7 nicotinic acetylcholine receptors in the rat brain neurons. *Eur J Neurosci*, *9*, 2734–2742.

42. Mike, A., Castro, N.G., Albuquerque, E.X. (2000). Choline and acetylcholine have similar kinetic properties of activation and desensitization on the alpha7 nicotinic receptors in rat hippocampal neurons. *Brain Res*, *882*, 155–168.

43. Lightfoot, A.P., Kew, J.N.C., Skidmore, J. (2008). 3 α7 nicotinic acetylcholine receptor agonists and positive allosteric modulators. *Prog Med Chem*, *46*, 131–171.

44. Cincotta, S.L., Yorek, M.S., Moschak, T.M., Lewis, S.R., Rodefer, J.S. (2008). Selective nicotinic acetylcholine receptor agonists: potential therapies for neuropsychiatric disorders with cognitive dysfunction. *Curr Opin Investig Drugs*, *9*, 47–57.
45. Chiamulera, C., Fumagalli, G. (2007). Nicotinic receptors and the treatment of attentional and cognitive deficits in neuropsychiatric disorders: focus on the .alpha.7 nicotinic acetylcholine receptor as a promising drug target for schizophrenia. *CNS Agents Med Chem*, *7*, 269–288.
46. Mazurov, A., Hauser, T., Miller, C.H. (2006). Selective .alpha.7 nicotinic acetylcholine receptor ligands. *Curr Med Chem*, *13*, 1567–1584.
47. Jensen, A.A., Frolund, B., Liljefors, T., Krogsgaard-Larsen, P. (2005). Neuronal nicotinic acetylcholine receptors: structural revelations, target identifications, and therapeutic inspirations. *J Med Chem*, *48*, 4705–4745.
48. Hashimoto, K., Koike, K., Shimizu, E., Iyo, M. (2005). α7 nicotinic receptor agonists as potential therapeutic drugs for schizophrenia. *Curr Med Chem*, *5*, 171–184.
49. Breining, S.R., Mazurov, A.A., Miller, C.H. (2005). Neuronal nicotinic acetylcholine receptor modulators: recent advances and therapeutic potential. *Annu Rep Med Chem*, *40*, 3.
50. Bunnelle, W.H., Dart, M.J., Schrimpf, M.R. (2004). Design of ligands for the nicotinic acetylcholine receptors: the quest for selectivity. *Curr Med Chem*, *4*, 299–334.
51. Romanelli, M.N., Gualtieri, F. (2003). Cholinergic nicotinic receptors: competitive ligands, allosteric modulators, and their potential applications. *Med Res Rev*, *23*, 393–426.
52. Astles, P.C., Baker, S.R., Boot, J.R., Broad, L.M., Dell, C.P., Keenan, M. (2002). Recent progress in the development of subtype selective nicotinic acetylcholine receptor ligands. *Curr Drug Target CNS Neurol Disord*, *1*, 337–348.
53. Schmitt, J.D. (2000). Exploring the nature of molecular recognition in nicotinic acetylcholine receptors. *Curr Med Chem*, *7*, 749–800.
54. Mullen, G., Napier, J., Balestra, M., DeCory, T., Hale, G., Macor, J., Mack, R., Loch, J., Wu, E., Kover, A., Verhoest, P., Sampognaro, A., Phillips, E., Zhu, Y., Murray, R., Griffith, R., Blosser, J., Gurley, D., Machulskis, A., Zongrone, J., Rosen, A., Gordon, J. (2000). (-)-Spiro[1-azabi-cyclo [2.2.2]octane-3,5'-oxazolidin-2'-one], a conformationally restrict-ed analog of acetylcholine, is a highly selective full agonist at the α7 nicotinic acetylcholine receptor. *J Med Chem*, *43*, 4045–4050.
55. Macor, J., Wu, E. (1997) Azabicyclic esters of carbamic acids useful in therapy. PCT Int. Appl. WO9730998.
56. Guendisch, D., Andrae, M., Munoz, L., Tilotta, M.C. (2004). Synthesis and evaluation of phenylcarbamate derivatives as ligands for nicotinic acetylcholine receptors. *Bioorg Med Chem*, *12*, 4953–4962.
57. Bodnar, A.L., Cortes-Burgos, L.A., Cook, K.K., Dinh, D.M., Groppi, V.E., Hajós, M., Higdon, N.R., Hoffmann, W.E., Hurst, R.S., Myers, J.K., Rogers, B.N., Wall, T.M., Wolfe, M.L., Wong, E. (2005). Discovery and structure-activity relationship of quinuclidine benzamides as agonists of alpha7 nicotinic acetylcholine receptors. *J Med Chem*, *48*, 905.
58. Tatsumi, R., Seio, K., Fujio, M., Katayama, J., Horikawa, T., Hashimoto, K., Tanaka, H. (2004). (+)-3-[2-(Benzo[b]thiophen-2-yl)-2-oxoethyl]-1-azabicyclo[2.2.2]octane

as potent agonists for the alpha7 nicotinic acetylcholine receptor. *Bioorg Med Chem Lett*, *14*, 3781.

59. Meyer, E.M., Tay, E.T., Papke, R.L., Meyers, C., Huang, G.-L., de Fiebre, C.M. (1997). 3-[2,4-Dimethoxybenzylidene]anabaseine (DMXB) selectively activates rat alpha 7 receptors and improves memory-related behaviors in a mecamylamine-sensitive manner. *Brain Res*, *768*, 49–56.
60. de Fiebre, C.M., Meyer, E.M., Henry, J.C., Muraskin, S.I., Kem, W.R., Papke, R.L. (1995). Characterization of a series of anabaseine-derived compounds reveals that the 3-(4)-dimethylaminocinnamylidine derivative is a selective agonist at neuronal nicotinic alpha7/125I-bungarotoxin receptor subtypes. *Mol Pharmacol*, *47*, 164–171.
61. Briggs, C.A., Anderson, D.J., Brioni, J.D., Buccafusco, J.J., Buckley, M.J., Campbell, J.E., Decker, M.W., Donnelly-Roberts, D., Elliott, R.L., Gopalakrishnan, M., Holladay, M.W., Hui, Y.-H., Jackson, W.J., Kim, D.J.B., Marsh, K.C., O'Neill, A., Prendergast, M.A., Ryther, K.B., Sullivan, J.P., Arneric, S.P. (1997). Functional characterization of the novel neuronal nicotinic acetylcholine receptor ligand GTS-21 in vitro and in vivo. *Pharmacol Biochem Behav*, *57*, 231–241.
62. Castner, S.A., Hudzik, T., Maier, D.L., Mrzljak, L., Piser, T., Smith, J.S., Widzowski, D., Williams, G.V. (2008) A composition comprising (R)-spiro[1-azabicyclo[2.2.2] octane-3,2'(3′H)-furo[2,3 -b]pyridine (AZD0328) and its use in the treatment of Alzheimer's disease, and or cognitive dysfunction. PCT Int. Appl. WO2008115139 A1, 60.
63. Phillips, E., Mack, R., Macor, J., Semus, S. (1999) (Astra AB) Novel spiroazabicyclic heterocyclic compounds. WO9903859, 71.
64. Tatsumi, R., Fujio, M., Satoh, H., Katayama, J., Takanashi, S., Hashimoto, K., Tanaka, H. (2005). Discovery of the α7 nicotinic acetylcholine receptor agonists. (R)-3'-(5-Chlorothiophen-2-yl)spiro-1-azabicyclo[2.2.2]octane-3,5'-[1',3'] oxazolidin-2'-one as a novel, potent, selective, and orally bioavailable ligand. *J Med Chem*, *48*, 2678–2786.
65. Tatsumi, R., Fujio, M., Takanashi, S.-I., Numata, A., Katayama, J., Satoh, H., Shiigi, Y., Maeda, J.-I., Kuriyama, M., Horikawa, T., Murozono, T., Hashimoto, K., Tanaka, H. (2006). (R)-3'-(3-Methylbenzo[b]-thiophen-5-yl)spiro[1-azabicyclo[2,2,2] octane-3,5'-oxazolidin]-2'-one, a novel and potent .alpha.7 nicotinic acetylcholine receptor partial agonist displays cognitive enhancing properties. *J Med Chem*, *49*, 4374–4383.
66. Bodnar, A.L., Cortes-Burgos, L.A., Cook, K.K., Dinh, D.M., Groppi, V.E., Hajós, M., Higdon, N.R., Hoffmann, W.E., Hurst, R.S., Myers, J.K., Rogers, B.N., Wall, T.M., Wolfe, M.L., Wong, E. (2005). Discovery and SAR of quiniclidine benzamides as agonists of α7 nicotinic acetylcholine receptors. *J Med Chem*, *48*, 905–908.
67. Hajós, M., Hurst, R.S., Hoffmann, W.E., Krause, M., Wall, T.M., Higdon, N.R., Groppi, V.E. (2005). The selective .alpha.7 nicotinic acetylcholine receptor agonist PNU-282987 [N-[(3R)-1-azabicyclo[2.2.2]oct-3-yl]-4-chlorobenzamide hydrochloride] enhances GABAergic synaptic activity in brain slices and restores auditory gating deficits in anesthetized rats. *J Pharmacol Exp Ther*, *312*, 1213–1222.
68. Wishka, D.G., Walker, D.P., Yates, K.M., Reitz, S.C., Jia, S., Myers, J.K., Olson, K.L., Jacobsen, E.J., Wolfe, M.L., Groppi, V.E., Hanchar, A.J., Thornburgh, B.A., Cortes-

Burgos, L.A., Wong, E.H.F., Staton, B.A., Raub, T.J., Higdon, N.R., Wall, T.M., Hurst, R.S., Walters, R.R., Hoffmann, W.E., Hajós, M., Franklin, S., Carey, G., Gold, L.H., Cook, K.K., Sands, S.B., Zhao, S.X., Soglia, J.R., Kalgutkar, A.S., Arneric, S.P., Rogers, B.N. (2006). Discovery of N-[(3R)-1-Azabicyclo[2.2.2]oct-3-yl]furo[2,3-c] pyridine-5-carboxamide, an agonist of the .alpha.7 nicotinic acetylcholine receptor, for the potential treatment of cognitive deficits in schizophrenia: synthesis and structure-activity relationship. *J Med Chem*, *49*, 4425–4436.

69. Walker, D.P., Wishka, D.G., Piotrowski, D.W., Jia, S., Reitz, S.C., Yates, K.M., Myers, J.K., Vetman, T.N., Margolis, B.J., Jacobsen, E.J., Acker, B.A., Groppi, V.E., Wolfe, M.L., Thornburgh, B.A., Tinholt, P.M., Cortes-Burgos, L.A., Walters, R.R., Hester, M.R., Seest, E.P., Dolak, L.A., Han, F., Olson, B.A., Fitzgerald, L., Staton, B.A., Raub, T.J., Hajós, M., Hoffmann, W.E., Li, K.S., Higdon, N.R., Wall, T.M., Hurst, R.S., Wong, E.H.F., Rogers, B.N. (2006). Design, synthesis, structure-activity relationship, and in vivo activity of azabicyclic aryl amides as .alpha.7 nicotinic acetylcholine receptor agonists. *Bioorg Med Chem*, *14*, 8219–8248.
70. Rogers, B.N. (2007) Agonists of alpha 7 nAChRs for the potential treatment of cognitive deficits in schizophrenia.Nicotinic acetylcholine Receptors as Therapeutic Targets: Emerging Frontiers in Basic research and Clinical Sciences, San Diego, CA, October 31–November 2, 2007.
71. Boess, F.G., De Vry, J., Erb, C., Flessner, T., Hendrix, M., Luithle, J., Methfessel, C., Riedl, B., Schnizler, K., van der Staay, F.-J., van Kampen, M., Wiese, W.B., Koenig, G. (2007). The novel .alpha.7 nicotinic acetylcholine receptor agonist N-[(3R)-1-azabicyclo[2.2.2]oct-3-yl]-7-[2-(methoxy)phenyl]-1-benzofuran-2-carboxamide improves working and recognition memory in rodents. *J Pharmacol Exp Ther*, *321*, 716–725.
72. Feuerbach, D., Nozulak, J., Lingenhoehl, K., McAllister, K., Hoyer, D. (2007). JN403, in vitro characterization of a novel nicotinic acetylcholine receptor .alpha.7 selective agonist. *Neurosci Lett*, *416*, 61–65.
73. Feuerbach, D., Lingenhoehl, K., Olpe, H.-R., Vassout, A., Gentsch, C., Chaperon, F., Nozulak, J., Enz, A., Bilbe, G., McAllister, K., Hoyer, D. (2009). The selective nicotinic acetylcholine receptor α7 agonist JN403 is active in animal models of cognition, sensory gating, epilepsy and pain. *Neuropsychopharmacology*, *56*, 254–263.
74. Biton, B., Bergis, O.E., Galli, F., Nedelec, A., Lochead, A.W., Jegham, S., Godet, D., Lanneau, C., Santamaria, R., Chesney, F., Leonardon, J., Granger, P., Debono, M.W., Bohme, G.A., Sgard, F., Besnard, F., Graham, D., Coste, A., Oblin, A., Curet, O., Vige, X., Voltz, C., Rouquier, L., Souilhac, J., Santucci, V., Gueudet, C., Francon, D., Steinberg, R., Griebel, G., Oury-Donat, F., George, P., Avenet, P., Scatton, B. (2007). SSR180711, a novel selective .alpha.7 nicotinic receptor partial agonist: (1) binding and functional profile. *Neuropsychopharmacology*, *32*, 1–16.
75. Pichat, P., Bergis, O.E., Terranova, J.-P., Urani, A., Duarte, C., Santucci, V., Gueudet, C., Voltz, C., Steinberg, R., Stemmelin, J., Oury-Donat, F., Avenet, P., Griebel, G., Scatton, B. (2007). SSR180711, a novel selective .alpha.7 nicotinic receptor partial agonist: (II) efficacy in experimental models predictive of activity against cognitive symptoms of schizophrenia. *Neuropsychopharmacology*, *32*, 17–34.
76. Tietje, K.R., Anderson, D.J., Bitner, R.S., Blomme, E.A., Brackemeyer, P.J., Briggs, C.A., Browman, K.E., Bury, D., Curzon, P., Drescher, K.U., Frost, J.M., Fryer, R.M., Fox, G.B., Gronlien, J.H., Hakerud, M., Gubbins, E.J., Halm, S., Harris, R., Helfrich,

R.J., Kohlhaas, K.L., Law, D., Malysz, J., Marsh, K.C., Martin, R.L., Meyer, M.D., Molesky, A.L., Nikkel, A.L., Otte, S., Pan, L., Puttfarcken, P.S., Radek, R.J., Robb, H.M., Spies, E., Thorin-Hagene, K., Waring, J.F., Ween, H., Xu, H., Gopalakrishnan, M., Bunnelle, W.H. (2008). Preclinical characterization of A-582941: a novel .alpha.7 neuronal nicotinic receptor agonist with broad spectrum cognition-enhancing properties. *CNS Neurosci Ther*, *14*, 65–82.

77. Acker, B.A., Jacobsen, E.J., Rogers, B.N., Wishka, D.G., Reitz, S.C., Piotrowski, D.W., Myers, J.K., Wolfe, M.L., Groppi, V.E., Thornburgh, B.A., Tinholt, P.M., Walters, R.R., Olson, B.A., Fitzgerald, L., Staton, B.A., Raub, T.J., Krause, M., Li, K.S., Hoffmann, W.E., Hajós, M., Hurst, R.S., Walker, D.P. (2008). Discovery of N-[(3R,5R)-1-azabicyclo[3.2.1]oct-3-yl]furo[2,3-c]pyridine-5-carboxamide as an agonist of the .alpha.7 nicotinic acetylcholine receptor: in vitro and in vivo activity. *Bioorg Med Chem Lett*, *18*, 3611–3615.

78. Bitner, R.S., Bunnelle, W.H., Anderson, D.J., Briggs, C.A., Buccafusco, J., Curzon, P., Decker, M.W., Frost, J.M., Gronlien, J.H., Gubbins, E., Li, J., Malysz, J., Markosyan, S., Marsh, K., Meyer, M.D., Nikkel, A.L., Radek, R.J., Robb, H.M., Timmermann, D., Sullivan, J.P., Gopalakrishnan, M. (2007). Broad-spectrum efficacy across cognitive domains by .alpha.7 nicotinic acetylcholine receptor agonism correlates with activation of ERK1/2 and CREB phosphorylation pathways. *J Neurosci*, *27*, 10578–10587.

79. Faghih, R., Gopalakrishnan, M., Briggs, C.A. (2008). Allosteric modulators of the .alpha.7 nicotinic acetylcholine receptor. *J Med Chem*, *51*, 701–712.

80. Bertrand, D., Gopalakrishnan, M. (2007). Allosteric modulation of nicotinic acetylcholine receptors. *Biochem Pharmacol*, *74*, 1155–1163.

81. Romanelli, M.N., Gualtieri, F. (2007). The quest for the treatment of cognitive impairment.alpha.7 nicotinic and .alpha.5 GABAA receptor modulators. *Expert Opin Ther Pat*, *17*(11), 1365–1377.

82. Changeux, J.-P., Edelstein, S.J. (2001). Allosteric mechanisms in normal and pathological nicotinic acetylcholine receptors. *Curr Opin Neurobiol*, *11*, 369–377.

83. Hosie, A.M., Wilkins, M.E., da Silva, H.M., Smart, T.G. (2006). Endogenous neurosteroids regulate GABAA receptors through two discrete transmembrane sites. *Nature*, *444*, 486–489.

84. Zwart, R., De Filippi, G., Broad, L.M., McPhie, G.I., Pearson, K.H., Baldwinson, T., Sher, E. (2002). 5-Hydroxyindole potentiates human alpha 7 nicotinic receptor-mediated responses and enhances acetylcholine-induced glutamate release in cerebellar slices. *Neuropharmacology*, *43*, 374–384.

85. Mok, M.H.S., Kew, J.N. (2006). Excitation of rat hippocampal interneurons via modulation of endogenous agonist activity at the alpha7 nicotinic ACh receptor. *J Physiol*, *574*, 699–710.

86. Grilli, M., Raiteri, L., Patti, L., Parodi, M., Robino, F., Raiteri, M., Marchi, M. (2006). Modulation of the function of presynaptic alpha7 and non-alpha7 nicotinic receptors by the tryptophan metabolites, 5-hydroxyindole and kynurenate in mouse brain. *Br J Pharmacol*, *149*, 724–732.

87. Hurst, R.S., Hajós, M., Raggenbass, M., Wall, T.M., Higdon, N.R., Lawson, J.A., Rutherford-Root, K.L., Berkenpas, M.B., Hoffmann, W.E., Piotrowski, D.W., Groppi, V.E., Allaman, G., Ogier, R., Bertrand, S., Bertrand, D., Arneric, S.P. (2005).

A novel positive allosteric modulator of the 7 neuronal nicotinic acetylcholine receptor: in vitro and in vivo characterization. *J Neurosci*, *25*, 4396–4405.

88. Piotrowski, D.W., Rogers, B.N., Wilhite, D.M., Margolis, B.J., Vetman, T.N., Sarapa, D., Wishka, D.G., Yates, K.M., Acker, B.A., Jacobsen, E.J., McWhorter, W.W., Badescu, V.O., Xu, W., Walker, D.P., Myers, J.K., Berkenpas, M.B., Dinh, D.M., Hurst, R.S., Wall, T.M., Higdon, N.R., Hajós, M., Hoffmann, W.E., Lee, E.K., Groppi, V.E. (2005) Positive allosteric modulators of the alpha 7 nicotonic acetylcholine receptor. 13th RSC-SCI Medicinal Chemistry Symposium, Chembridge, UK, September 14–17, 2005.
89. Dinklo, T., Shaban, H., Thuring, J.W., Lavreysen, H., Stevens, K.E., Zheng, L., Mackie, C., Grantham, C., Vandenberk, I., Meulders, G., Peeters, L., Verachtert, H., De Prins, E., Lesage, A.S. (2011) Characterization of 2-[[4-fluoro-3-(trifluoromethyl) phenyl]amino]-4-(4-pyridinyl)-5-thiazolemethanol (JNJ-1930942), a novel positive allosteric modulator of the {alpha}7 nicotinic acetylcholine receptor. *J Pharmacol Exp Ther*, *336*(2), 560–574.
90. Timmermann, D.B., Groenlien, J.H., Kohlhaas, K.L., Nielsen, E.O., Dam, E., Joergensen, T.D., Ahring, P.K., Peters, D., Holst, D., Christensen, J.K., Malysz, J., Briggs, C.A., Gopalakrishnan, M., Olsen, G.M. (2007). An allosteric modulator of the . alpha.7 nicotinic acetylcholine receptor possessing cognition-enhancing properties in vivo. *J Pharmacol Exp Ther*, *323*, 294–307.
91. Connolly, C.N., Wafford, K.A. (2004). The Cys-loop superfamily of ligand-gated ion channels: the impact of receptor structure on function. *Biochem Soc Trans*, *32*, 529–534.
92. Ng, H.J., Whittemore, E.R., Tran, M.B., Hogenkamp, D.J., Broide, R.S., Johnstone, T.B., Zheng, L., Stevens, K.E., Gee, K.W. (2007). Nootropic .alpha.7 nicotinic receptor allosteric modulator derived from GABAA receptor modulators. *Proc Natl Acad Sci U S A*, *104*, 8059–8064.
93. Broad, L.M., Zwart, R., Pearson, K.H., Lee, M., Wallace, L., McPhie, G.I., Emkey, R., Hollinshead, S.P., Dell, C.P., Baker, S.R., Sher, E. (2006). Identification and pharmacological profile of a new class of selective nicotinic acetylcholine receptor potentiators. *J Pharmacol Exp Ther*, *318*, 1108–1117.
94. Dinklo, T., Meeus, K., Peeters, L., Lavreysen, H., van Roosbroeck, Y., Grantham, C., Vandenberk, I., Pouzet, B., Stevens, K.E., Zheng, L., Mackie, C., Macdonald, G., Lesage, A., Thuring, J. (2007). In vitro and in vivo evaluation of JNJ1930942, a novel α7 nAChR selective positive allosteric modulator. *Biochem Pharmacol*, *74*, SMA–S33.
95. Groenlien, J.H., Haakerud, M., Ween, H., Thorin-Hagene, K., Briggs, C.A., Gopalakrishnan, M., Malysz, J. (2007). Distinct profiles of .alpha.7 nAChR positive allosteric modulation revealed by structurally diverse chemotypes. *Mol Pharmacol*, *72*, 715–724.
96. Turrini, P., Casu, M.A., Wong, T.P., De Koninck, Y., Ribeiro-Da-Silva, A., Cuello, A.C. (2001). Cholinergic nerve terminals establish classical synapses in the rat cerebral cortex: synaptic pattern and age-related atrophy. *Neuroscience*, *105*, 277–285.
97. Descarries, L., Gisiger, V., Steriade, M. (1997). Diffuse transmission by acetylcholine in the CNS. *Prog Neurobiol*, *53*, 603–625.

98. Hefft, S., Hulo, S., Bertrand, D., Muller, D. (1999). Synaptic transmission at nicotinic acetylcholine receptors in rat hippocampal organotypic cultures and slices. *J Physiol*, *515*, 769–776.
99. Berg, D.K., Conroy, W.G. (2002). Nicotinic alpha 7 receptors: synaptic options and downstream signaling in neurons. *J Neurobiol*, *53*, 512–523.
100. Hansen, H.H., Timmermann, D.B., Peters, D., Walters, C., Damaj, M.I., Mikkelsen, J.D. (2007). Alpha-7 nicotinic acetylcholine receptor agonists selectively activate limbic regions of the rat forebrain: an effect similar to antipsychotics. *J Neurosci Res*, *85*, 1810–1818.
101. Thomsen, M.S., Mikkelsen, J.D., Timmermann, D.B., Peters, D., Hay-Schmidt, A., Martens, H., Hansen, H.H. (2008). The selective alpha7 nicotinic acetylcholine receptor agonist A-582941 activates immediate early genes in limbic regions of the forebrain: differential effects in the juvenile and adult rat. *Neuroscience*, *154*, 741–753.
102. Bozon, B., Kelly, A., Josselyn, S.A., Silva, A.J., Davis, S., Laroche, S. (2003). MAPK, CREB and zif268 are all required for the consolidation of recognition memory. *Philos Trans R Soc Lond B Biol Sci*, *358*, 805–814.
103. Sharma, G., Vijayaraghavan, S. (2003). Modulation of presynaptic store calcium induces release of glutamate and postsynaptic firing. *Neuron*, *38*, 929–939.
104. Adler, L.E., Olincy, A., Waldo, M., Harris, J., Griffith, J., Stevens, K., Flach, K., Nagamoto, H., Bickford, P., Leonard, S., Freedman, R. (1998). Schizophrenia, sensory gating, and nicotinic receptors. *Schizophr Bull*, *24*, 189–202.
105. Braff, D.L., Light, G.A. (2004). Preattentional and attentional cognitive deficits as targets for treating schizophrenia. *Psychopharmacology (Berl)*, *174*, 75–85.
106. Bramon, E., Rabe-Hesketh, S., Sham, P., Murray, R., Frangou, S. (2004). Meta-analysis of the P300 and P50 waveforms in schizophrenia. *Schizophr Res*, *70*, 315–329.
107. Javitt, D.C., Spencer, K.M., Thaker, G.K., Winterer, G., Hajós, M. (2008). Neurophysiological biomarkers for drug development in schizophrenia. *Nat Rev Drug Discov*, *7*, 68–83.
108. Goff, D.C., Henderson, D.C., Amico, E. (1992). Cigarette smoking in schizophrenia: relationship to psychopathology and medication side effects. *Am J Psychiatry*, *149*, 1189–1194.
109. Adler, L.E., Hoffer, L.D., Wiser, A., Freedman, R. (1993). Normalization of auditory physiology by cigarette smoking in schizophrenic patients. *Am J Psychiatry*, *150*, 1856–1861.
110. Martin, L.F., Kem, W.R., Freedman, R. (2004). Alpha-7 nicotinic receptor agonists: potential new candidates for the treatment of schizophrenia. *Psychopharmacology (Berl)*, *174*, 54–64.
111. Adler, L.E., Rose, G., Freedman, R. (1985). Neurophysiological studies of sensory gating in rats: effects of amphetamine, phencyclidine, and haloperidol. *Biol Psychiatry*, *21*, 787–798.
112. Krause, M., Hoffman, W.E., Hajós, M. (2003). Auditory sensory gating in hippocampus and reticular thalamic neurons in anesthetized rats. *Biol Psychiatry*, *53*, 244–253.

113. Ellenbroek, B.A. (2004). Pre-attentive processing and schizophrenia: animal studies. *Psychopharmacology (Berl)*, *174*, 65–74.
114. Swerdlow, N.R., Geyer, M.A., Shoemaker, J.M., Light, G.A., Braff, D.L., Stevens, K.E., Sharp, R., Breier, M., Neary, A., Auerbach, P.P. (2006). Convergence and divergence in the neurochemical regulation of prepulse inhibition of startle and N40 suppression in rats. *Neuropsychopharmacology*, *31*, 506–515.
115. Hajós, M., Hoffmann, W.E., Kocsis, B. (2008). Activation of cannabinoid-1 receptors disrupts sensory gating and neuronal oscillation: relevance to schizophrenia. *Biol Psychiatry*, *63*, 1075–1083.
116. Adler, L.E., Olincy, A., Cawthra, E., Hoffer, M., Nagamoto, H., Amass, L., Freedman, R. (2001). Reversal of diminished inhibitory sensory gating in cocaine addicts by a nicotinic cholinergic mechanism. *Neuropsychopharmacology*, *24*, 671–679.
117. Light, G.A., Malaspina, D., Geyer, G.A., Luber, B.M., Coleman, E.A., Sackheim, H.A., Braff, D.L. (1999). Amphetamine disrupts P50 suppression in normal subjects. *Biol Psychiatry*, *46*, 990–999.
118. O'Neill, H.C., Rieger, K., Kem, W.R., Stevens, K.E. (2003). DMXB, an alpha7 nicotinic agonist, normalizes auditory gating in isolation-reared rats. *Psychopharmacology (Berl)*, *169*, 332–339.
119. Ellenbroek, B.A., De Bruin, N.M.W.J., van den Kroonenburg, P.T.J.M., van Luijtelaar, E.L.J.M., Cools, A.R. (2004). The effects of early maternal deprivation on auditory information processing in adult Wistar rats. *Biol Psychiatry*, *55*, 701–707.
120. Adams, C.E., Yonchek, J.C., Zheng, L., Collins, A.C., Stevens, K.E. (2008). Altered hippocampal circuit function in C3H alpha7 null mutant heterozygous mice. *Brain Res*, *1194*, 138–145.
121. Laruelle, M., Abi-Dargham, A. (1999). Dopamine as the wind of the psychotic fire: new evidence from brain imaging studies. *J Psychopharmacol*, *13*, 358–371.
122. Snyder, S.H. (1973). Amphetamine psychosis: a "model" schizophrenia mediated by catecholamines. *Am J Psychiatry*, *130*, 61–67.
123. Stevens, K.E., Meltzer, J., Rose, G.M. (1995). Nicotinic cholinergic normalization of amphetamine-induced loss of auditory gating in freely moving rats. *Psychopharmacology (Berl)*, *119*, 163–170.
124. Hurst, R.S., Hajós-Korcsok, E., Walker, D.P., Rogers, B.N., Walters, R.R., Gorczyca, R.R., Hoffmann, W.E., Wall, T.M., Higdon, N.R., Mo, Z.-L., Hajós, M. (2007) Novel ligand of α7 nicotinic acetylcholine receptors shows dual agonist and positive allosteric modulator actions: in vitro and in vivo pharmacology. *Neuroscience Meeting Planner*, San Diego, CA 2007, *No. 574.11/J16*. Society for Neuroscience.
125. Hajós, M., Krause, M., Hoffmann, W.E., Hajós-Korcsok, E., Yu, J.H., Robinson, D.D., Wall, T.M., Higdon, N.R., Svensson, K.A., Nichols, N.F., Walters, R.R., Groppi, V.E., Arneric, S.P., Hurst, R.S. (2007) Abstract 60.9/V172007, *Abstract of Papers, 37th Society for Neuroscience*, San Diego, CA, 2007.
126. Stevens, K.E., Wear, K.D. (1997). Normalizing effects of nicotine and a novel nicotinic agonist on hippocampal auditory gating in two animal models. *Pharmacol Biochem Behav*, *57*, 869–874.
127. Wildeboer, K.M., Stevens, K.E. (2008). Stimulation of the alpha4beta2 nicotinic receptor by 5-I A-85380 improves auditory gating in DBA/2 mice. *Brain Res*, *122*, 29–36.

128. Wildeboer, K.M., Stevens, K.E. (2007) α4β2 Nicotinic receptor involvement in the auditory gating deficit in DBA/2 mice, a model of the deficit in schizophrenics, *Society for Neuroscience*, *573.12*, I17.

129. Rollema, H., Hajós, M., Seymour, P.A., Kozak, R., Majchrzak, M.J., Guanowsky, V., Horner, W.E., Chapin, D.S., Hoffmann, W.E., Johnson, D.E., McLean, S., Freeman, J., Williams, K.E. (2009). *Biochem Pharmacol*, *78*, 813–824.

130. Johannesen, J.K., Kieffaber, P.D., O'Donnell, B.F., Shekhar, A., Evans, J.D., Hetrick, W.P. (2005). Contributions of subtype and spectral frequency analyses to the study of P50 ERP amplitude and suppression in schizophrenia. *Schizophr Res*, *78*, 269–284.

131. Hong, L.E., Buchanan, R.W., Thaker, G.K., Shepard, P.D., Summerfelt, A. (2008). Beta (~16 Hz) frequency neural oscillations mediate auditory sensory gating in humans. *Psychophysiology*, *45*, 197–204.

132. Rosburg, T., Trautner, P., Fell, J., Moxon, K.A., Elger, C.E., Boutros, N.N. (2008). Sensory gating in intracranial recordings—the role of phase locking. *Neuroimage*, *44*(3), 1041–1049. [Epub ahead of print].

133. Vierling-Claassen, D., Siekmeier, P., Stufflebeam, S., Kopell, N. (2008). Modeling GABA alterations in schizophrenia: a link between impaired inhibition and altered gamma and beta range auditory entrainment. *J Neurophysiol*, *99*, 2656–2671.

134. Mima, T., Oluwatimilehin, T., Hiraoka, T., Hallett, M. (2001). Transient interhemispheric neuronal synchrony correlates with object recognition. *J Neurosci*, *21*, 3942–3948.

135. Winterer, G., Coppola, R., Goldberg, T., Egan, M., Jones, D., Sanchez, C., Weinberger, D. (2004). Prefrontal broadband noise, working memory, and genetic risk for schizophrenia. *Am J Psychiatry*, *161*, 490–500.

136. Krishnan, G.P., Vohs, J.L., Hetrick, W.P., Carroll, C.A., Shekhar, A., Bockbrader, M.A., O'Donnell, B.F. (2005). Steady state visual evoked potential abnormalities in schizophrenia. *Clin Neurophysiol*, *116*, 614–624.

137. Light, G.A., Hsu, J.L., Hsieh, M.H., Meyer-Gomes, K., Sprock, J., Swerdlow, N.R., Braff, D. (2006). Gamma band oscillations reveal neural network cortical coherence dysfunction in schizophrenia patients. *Biol Psychiatry*, *60*, 1231–1240.

138. Uhlhaas, P.J., Haenschel, C., Nikolic, D., Singer, W. (2008). The role of oscillations and synchrony in cortical networks and their putative relevance for the pathophysiology of schizophrenia. *Schizophr Bull*, *34*, 927–943.

139. Gonzalez-Burgos, G., Lewis, D.A. (2008). GABA neurons and the mechanisms of network oscillations: implications for understanding cortical dysfunction in schizophrenia. *Schizophr Bull*, *34*, 944–961.

140. Freund, T.F. (2003). Interneuron diversity series: rhythm and mood in perisomatic inhibition. *Trends Neurosci*, *26*, 489–495.

141. Buzsáki, G. (2002). Theta oscillations in the hippocampus. *Neuron*, *33*, 325–340.

142. Morales, M., Hein, K., Vogel, Z. (2008). Hippocampal interneurons co-express transcripts encoding the alpha7 nicotinic receptor subunit and the cannabinoid receptor 1. *Neuroscience*, *152*, 70–81.

143. Lawrence, J.J. (2008). Cholinergic control of GABA release: emerging parallels between neocortex and hippocampus. *Trends Neurosci*, *31*, 317–327.

144. Hasselmo, M.E. (2006). The role of acetylcholine in learning and memory. *Curr Opin Neurobiol*, *16*, 710–715.
145. Song, C., Kimura, R., Wakui, M., Ellsworth, K., Javedan, S.P., Marxer-Miller, S., Lukas, R.J., Wu, J. (2005). Role of alpha7-nicotinic acetylcholine receptors in tetanic stimulation-induced gamma oscillations in rat hippocampal slices. *Neuropharmacology*, *48*, 869–880.
146. Hoffmann, W.E., Schaeffer, E., Hajos, M. (2005). Auditory gating in rat entorhinal cortex, medial septum and hippocampus: modeling dysfunctional information processing associated with schizophrenia. *Soc Neurosci Abstr*, *1023*, 10.
147. Siok, C.J., Rogers, J.A., Kocsis, B., Hajós, M. (2006). Activation of alpha7 acetylcholine receptors augments stimulation-induced hippocampal theta oscillation. *Eur J Neurosci*, *23*, 570–574.
148. McNaughton, N., Kocsis, B., Hajós, M. (2007). Elicited hippocampal theta rhythm: a screen for anxiolytic and procognitive drugs through changes in hippocampal function? *Behav Pharmacol*, *18*, 329–346.
149. Lamanauskas, N., Nistri, A. (2006). Persistent rhythmic oscillations induced by nicotine on neonatal rat hypoglossal motoneurons in vitro. *Eur J Neurosci*, *24*, 2543–2556.
150. Paylor, R., Nguyen, M., Crawley, J.N., Patrick, J., Beaudet, A., Orr-Urtreger, A. (1998). Alpha7 nicotinic receptor subunits are not necessary for hippocampal-dependent learning or sensorimotor gating: a behavioral characterization of Acra7-deficient mice. *Learn Mem*, *5*(4–5), 302–316.
151. Hoyle, E., Genn, R.F., Fernandes, C., Stolerman, I.P. (2006). Impaired performance of alpha7 nicotinic receptor knockout mice in the five-choice serial reaction time task. *Psychopharmacology (Berl)*, *189*, 211–223.
152. Young, J.W., Crawford, N., Kelly, J.S., Kerr, L.E., Marston, H.M., Spratt, C., Finlayson, K., Sharkey, J. (2007). Impaired attention is central to the cognitive deficits observed in alpha 7 deficient mice. *Eur Neuropsychopharmacol*, *17*, 145–155.
153. Levin, E.D., Petro, A., Pollard, N., Christopher, N.C., Strauss, M., Avery, J., Nicholson, J., Rezvani, A.H. (2008). Nicotinic alpha7- or beta2-containing receptor knockout: effects on radial-arm maze learning and long-term nicotine consumption in mice. *Behav Brain Res*, *196*(2), 207–213.
154. Fernandes, C., Hoyle, E., Dempster, E., Schalkwyk, L.C., Collier, D.A. (2006). Performance deficit of alpha7 nicotinic receptor knockout mice in a delayed matching-to-place task suggests a mild impairment of working/episodic-like memory. *Genes Brain Behav*, *5*, 433–440.
155. Curzon, P., Anderson, D.J., Nikkel, A.L., Fox, G.B., Gopalakrishnan, M., Decker, M.W., Bitner, R.S. (2006). Antisense knockdown of the rat alpha7 nicotinic acetylcholine receptor produces spatial memory impairment. *Neurosci Lett*, *410*, 15–19.
156. Ren, K., Thinschmidt, J., Liu, J., Ai, L., Papke, R.L., King, M.A., Hughes, J.A., Meyer, E.M. (2007). Alpha7 nicotinic receptor gene delivery into mouse hippocampal neurons leads to functional receptor expression, improved spatial memory-related performance, and tau hyperphosphorylation. *Neuroscience*, *145*, 314–322.
157. van Kampen, M., Selbach, K., Schneider, R., Schiegel, E., Boess, F., Schreiber, R. (2004). AR-R 17779 improves social recognition in rats by activation of nicotinic alpha7 receptors. *Psychopharmacology (Berl)*, *172*, 375–383.

158. Feuerbach, D., Lingenhoehl, K., Olpe, H.R., Vassout, A., Gentsch, C., Chaperon, F., Nozulak, J., Enz, A., Bilbe, G., McAllister, K., Hoyer, D. (2008). The selective nicotinic acetylcholine receptor alpha7 agonist JN403 is active in animal models of cognition, sensory gating, epilepsy and pain. *Neuropharmacology*, *56*(1), 254–263.

159. Levin, E.D., Bettegowda, C., Blosser, J., Gordon, J. (1999). AR-R17779, and alpha7 nicotinic agonist, improves learning and memory in rats. *Behav Pharmacol*, *10*, 675–680.

160. Redrobe, J.P., Nielsen, E.O., Christensen, J.K., Peters, D., Timmermann, D.B., Olsen, G.M. (2008). Alpha7 nicotinic acetylcholine receptor activation ameliorates scopolamine-induced behavioural changes in a modified continuous Y-maze task in mice. *Eur J Pharmacol*, *602*(1), 58–65.

161. Hashimoto, K., Ishima, T., Fujita, Y., Matsuo, M., Kobashi, T., Takahagi, M., Tsukada, H., Iyo, M. (2008). Phencyclidine-induced cognitive deficits in mice are improved by subsequent subchronic administration of the novel selective alpha7 nicotinic receptor agonist SSR180711. *Biol Psychiatry*, *63*, 92–97.

162. Chan, W.K., Wong, P.T., Sheu, F.S. (2007). Frontal cortical alpha7 and alpha4beta2 nicotinic acetylcholine receptors in working and reference memory. *Neuropharmacology*, *52*, 1641–1649.

163. Levin, E.D., Rezvani, A.H. (2006). Nicotinic-antipsychotic drug interactions and cognitive function. *EXS*, *98*, 185–205.

164. Arendash, G.W., Sengstock, G.J., Sanberg, P.R., Kem, W.R. (1995). Improved learning and memory in aged rats with chronic administration of the nicotinic receptor agonist GTS-21. *Brain Res*, *674*, 252–259.

165. Marighetto, A., Valerio, S., Desmedt, A., Philippin, J.N., Trocmé-Thibierge, C., Morain, P. (2008). Comparative effects of the alpha7 nicotinic partial agonist, S 24795, and the cholinesterase inhibitor, donepezil, against aging-related deficits in declarative and working memory in mice. *Psychopharmacology (Berl)*, *197*, 499–508.

166. Lynch, G., Rex, C.S., Gall, C.M. (2007). LTP consolidation: substrates, explanatory power, and functional significance. *Neuropharmacology*, *52*, 12–23.

167. Kullmann, D.M., Lamsa, K.P. (2007). Long-term synaptic plasticity in hippocampal interneurons. *Nat Rev Neurosci*, *8*, 687–699.

168. Radcliffe, K.A., Dani, J.A. (1998). Nicotinic stimulation produces multiple forms of increased glutamatergic synaptic transmission. *J Neurosci*, *18*, 7075–7083.

169. Lagostena, L., Trocme-Thibierge, C., Morain, P., Cherubini, E. (2008). The partial alpha7 nicotine acetylcholine receptor agonist S 24795 enhances long-term potentiation at CA3-CA1 synapses in the adult mouse hippocampus. *Neuropharmacology*, *54*, 676–685.

170. Christian, E.P., Smith, J.S., Doherty, J.J., Li, C. (2007) AZD0328: Dose-dependent normalization of hippocampal long term potentiation induction deficit in the fimbria/fornix lesioned rat in vivo. Program. *Neuroscience Meeting Planner* 2007 San Diego, CA, *No. 906.9*, Society for Neuroscience.

171. Widzowski, D.V., Maier, D., McLaughlin, K., Neilson, J.K., Bock, M.J., Wang, Y., Maciag, C. (2007) AZD0328 and AZ11943872: α7 nicotinic agonists that reverse fimbria-fornix-transection-induced working memory deficits following acute or

chronic administration. *Neuroscience Meeting Planner* 2007, San Diego, CA: *Program No. 906.21*, Society for Neuroscience.

172. Huerta, P.T., Lisman, J.E. (1995). Bidirectional synaptic plasticity induced by a single burst during cholinergic theta oscillation in CA1 in vitro. *Neuron*, *15*, 1053–1063.
173. Adler, L.E., Olincy, A., Cawthra, E., McRae, K., Harris, J., Nagamoto, H., Waldo, M., Hall, M.-H., Bowles, A., Woodward, L., Ross, R., Freedman, R. (2004). Varied effects of atypical neuroleptics on P50 auditory gating in schizophrenia patients. *Am J Psychiatry*, *161*, 1822–1828.
174. Becker, J., Gomes, I., Ghisolfi, E.S., Schuch, A., Ramos, F.L., Ehlers, A.A., Nora, D.B., Lara, D.R., da Costa, J.C. (2004). Clozapine, but not typical antipsychotics, correct P50 suppression deficit in patients with schizophrenia. *Clin Neurophysiol*, *115*, 396–401.
175. Chung, C., Remington, G. (2005). Predictors and markers of clozapine response. *Psychopharmacology (Berl)*, *179*, 317–335.
176. Koike, K., Hashimot, K., Takai, N., Shimizu, E., Komatsu, N., Watanabe, H., Nakazato, M., Okamura, N., Stevens, K.E., Freedman, R. (2005). Tropisetron improves deficits in auditory P50 suppression in schizophrenia. *Schizophr Res*, *76*, 67–72.
177. Adler, L.E., Cawthra, E., Donovan, K., Harris, J., Nagamoto, H., Olincy, A., Waldo, M. (2005). Improved p50 auditory gating with ondansetron in medicated schizophrenia patients. *Am J Psychiatry*, *162*, 386–388.
178. AstraZeneca. Our Pipeline. http://www.astrazeneca-us.com/research-and-development/?itemId=1462661.
179. Envivo. Pipeline. http://www.envivopharma.com/template/5_5_1.html.
180. Kitagawa, H., Takenouchi, T., Azuma, R., Wesnes, K.A., Kramer, W.G., Clody, D.E., Burnett, A.L. (2003). Safety, pharmacokinetics, and effects on cognitive function of multiple doses of GTS-21 in healthy, male volunteers. *Neuropsychopharmacology*, *28*, 542–551.
181. Olincy, A., Harris, J.G., Johnson, L.L., Pender, V., Kongs, S., Allensworth, D., Ellis, J., Zerbe, G.O., Leonard, S., Stevens, K.E., Stevens, J.O., Martin, L., Adler, L.E., Soti, F., Kem, W.R., Freedman, R. (2006). Proof-of-concept trial of an .alpha.7 nicotinic agonist in schizophrenia. *Arch Gen Psychiatry*, *63*, 630–638.
182. Freedman, R., Olincy, A., Buchanan, R.W., Harris, J.G., Gold, J.M., Johnson, L., Allensworth, D., Guzman-Bonilla, A., Clement, B., Ball, M.P., Kutnick, J., Pender, V., Martin, L.F., Stevens, K.E., Wagner, B.D., Zerbe, G.O., Soti, F., Kem, W.R. (2008). Initial phase 2 trial of a nicotinic agonist in schizophrenia. *Am J Psychiatry*, *165*, 1040–1047.
183. Orrenius, S., Zhivotovsky, B., Nicotera, P. (2003). Calcium: regulation of cell death: the calcium-apoptosis link. *Nat Rev Mol Cell Biol*, *4*, 552–565.
184. Benowitz, N.L., Gourlay, S.G. (1997). Cardiovascular toxicity of nicotine: implications for nicotine replacement therapy. *J Am Coll Cardiol*, *29*, 1422–1431.
185. Fermini, B., Fossa, A.A. (2003). The impact of drug-induced QT interval prolongation on drug discovery and development. *Nat Rev Drug Discov*, *2*, 439–447.

# 13

# MUSCARINIC ACETYLCHOLINE RECEPTORS AS NOVEL TARGETS FOR THE DEVELOPMENT OF THERAPEUTICS FOR SCHIZOPHRENIA

CHRISTIAN C. FELDER, DAVID L. MCKINZIE,
RICHARD C. THOMPSON, AND BIN LIU

## 13.1 INTRODUCTION

Cholinergic treatment approaches for schizophrenia predate the discovery of monoamine-based typical and atypical antipsychotics such as haloperidol and clozapine, respectively. Early cholinergic agents were empirically derived from clinical experience, were nonselective for receptor subtypes, and frequently not well tolerated by the patients or control subjects, thus creating some confusion as to the relative benefit of muscarinic agonism versus antagonism. Betel nut abuse by schizophrenics revealed positive symptom relief but also induced psychotropic side effects as well as increased incidence of malignancy and liver disease [1]. The symptom relief was thought to be mediated by endogenous acetylcholine-like arecoline muscarinic agonists released by chewing of the raw betel nut pulp [2]. Acetylcholine injections to augment endogenous cholinergic tone were also used as a potential method to restore neural signaling imbalances [3]. These injections, however, resulted in the suspension of consciousness, and may have related to the restorative effect that are sometimes observed in patients following physiologic or electroshock therapy [4]. Similar

*Targets and Emerging Therapies for Schizophrenia*, First Edition.
Edited by Jeffrey S. Albert and Michael W. Wood.

**TABLE 13.1 Muscarinic Acetylcholine Receptor Modulators**

| Compound | Structure | Reference | Compound | Structure | Reference | Compound | Structure |
|---|---|---|---|---|---|---|---|
| Oxotremorine | 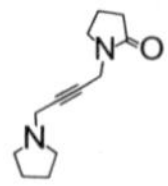 | [17] | Milameline | 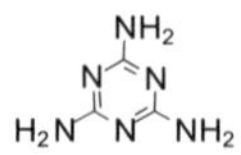 | [17] | **6** | 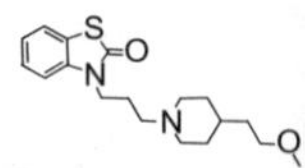 |
| Carbachol | 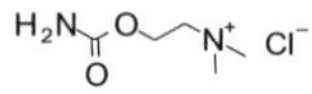 | | SCH57790 | 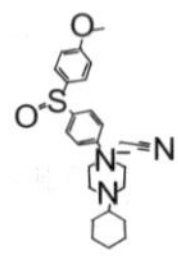 | [49] | **7** | 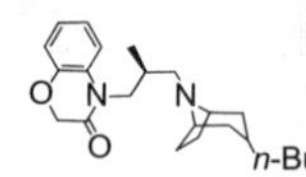 |
| Atropine (muscarinic antagonist) | 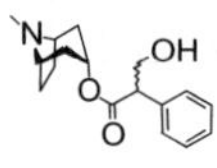 | | BIBN-99 | 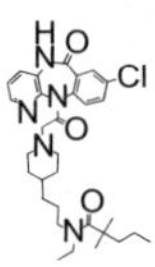 | [59, 60] | **8** | 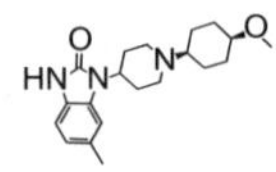 |
| Scopolamine (muscarinic antagonist) | 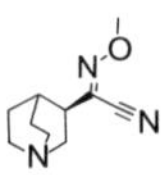 | | N-desmethyl clozapine | 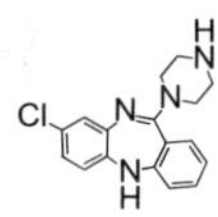 | [64, 65] | **9** | 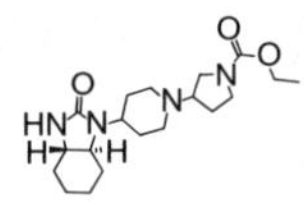 |
| Sabcomeline | 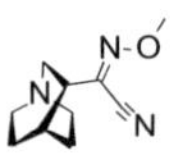 | [11, 17] | Xanomeline, **1** | 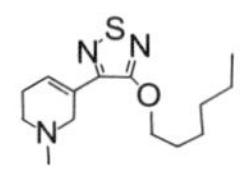 | [11, 17–18, 21, 24, 27] | **10** | 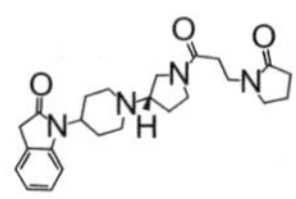 |
| Talsaclidine | 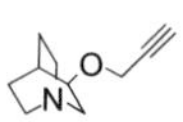 | [11] | Amidine, **2** | 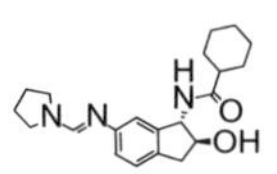 | [77] | **11** | 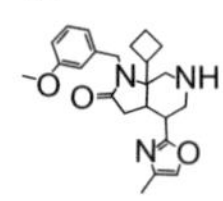 |
| BuTAC | 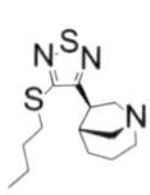 | [17, 19–20] | LY593093, **3** | 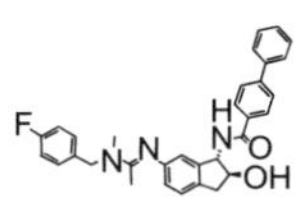 | [78–81] | **12** | 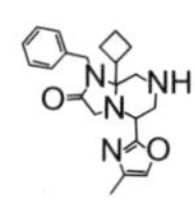 |
| RS86 | 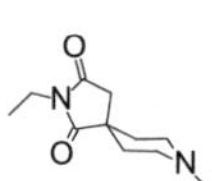 | [17] | 35AKU-21, **4** | 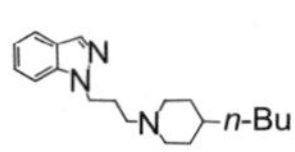 | [82] | **13** | 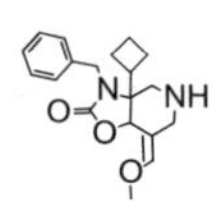 |
| Pilocarpine | 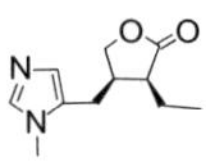 | [17] | **5** | 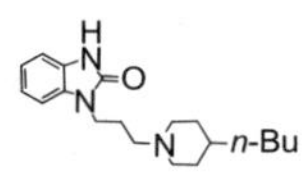 | [83] | **14** | 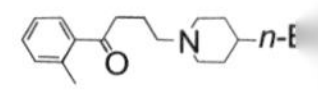 |

effects were observed with antimuscarinic-induced coma following atropine injections, a therapy reported to improve positive symptoms in subsets of schizophrenic patients [5]. Cholinesterase inhibitors, which elevate acetylcholine levels, had measurable efficacy in cognition and negative symptom measures of schizophrenia, suggesting that cholinergic agonism was preferred for treatment of these symptom domains (for a recent review see Reference [6]). However, nonselective approaches to modulation of acetylcholine tone can induce synergistic, or potentially opposing, nicotinic and muscarinic regulatory

| Reference | Compound | Structure | Reference | Compound | Structure | Reference |
|---|---|---|---|---|---|---|
| [83] | **15** | 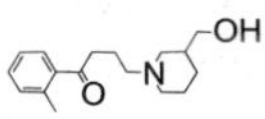 | [92] | 77-LH-28-1, **24** | 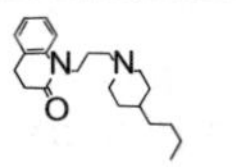 | [107, 109] |
| [84] | CDD-0304, **16** | 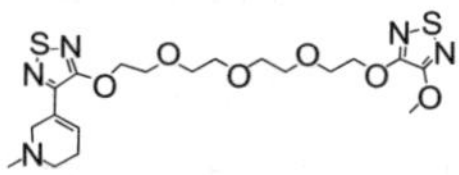 | [93–95] | LY2033298, **25** | 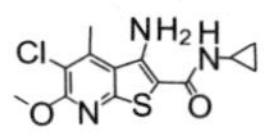 | [41] |
| [85–87] | CDD-0300, **17** | 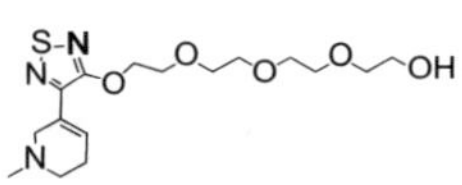 | [93–95] | 7912361, **26** | 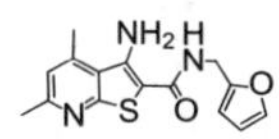 | [110] |
| [88] | **18** | 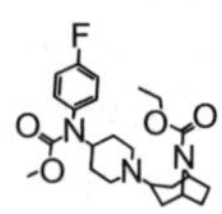 | [99] | VU100010, **27** | 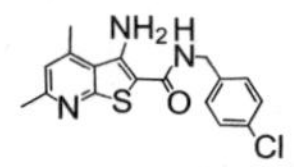 | [110] |
| [89] | **19** | 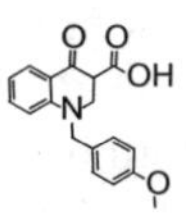 | [100, 102] | VU0152099, **28** | 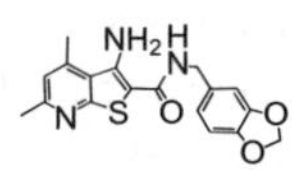 | [111] |
| [91] | **20** | 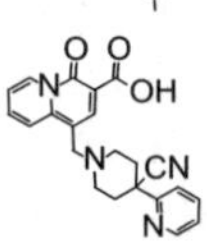 | [101] | VU0152100, **29** | 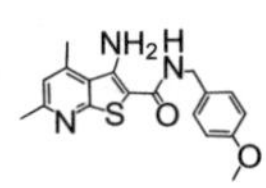 | [111] |
| [91] | VU0090157, **21** | 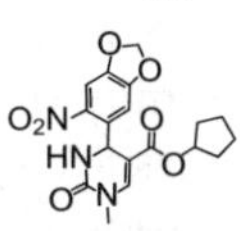 | [103] | VU0119498, **30** | 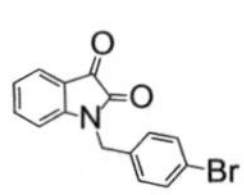 | [113] |
| [91] | VU0029767, **22** | 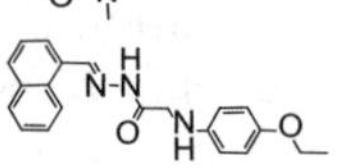 | [103] | VU0238429, **31** | 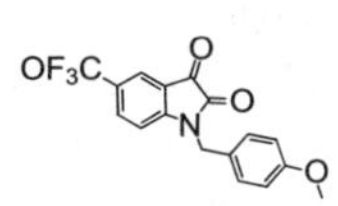 | [113] |
| [92] | TBPB, **23** | 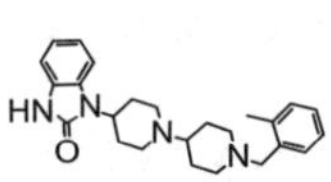 | [70] | | | |

pathways resulting in complex interactions between peripheral and central cholinergic physiology.

It was not until the 1980s that cholinergic receptor subtypes began to be identified at the molecular level, allowing selective ligands to be developed and gene deletion mice to be created. With these emerging selective tools (Table 13.1), deciphering the physiological complexity of individual nicotinic and muscarinic receptor (MRs) subtypes has become possible. Therefore, the role of the cholinergic system in the pathophysiology of schizophrenia remains controversial as to whether single or multiple muscarinic or nicotinic receptor subtypes provide better therapeutic targets and whether agonism or antagonism is the better pharmacological approach. More recent cholinergic therapeutic development efforts have focused on a deeper understanding of both muscarinic and nicotinic neurobiology and neurophysiology as well as creating selective pharmacological tools for preclinical and clinical investigations.

## 13.2 OVERVIEW OF MUSCARINIC RECEPTOR STRUCTURE, FUNCTION, AND LOCALIZATION

Acetylcholine provided the first example of a discrete biological entity that encoded complex neural signaling control [7]. This remarkable transmitter is found in virtually all living entities including mold, plants, animals, and humans. Modulation of mammalian physiology via acetylcholine was eventually discovered to be mediated by two families of acetylcholine receptor proteins that are localized to the cell membrane surface. The two receptor families include the ionotropic nicotinic ion channel receptors and the metabotropic G-protein-coupled receptor (GPCR)-type MRs, so named by their differential response to natural nicotine and muscarine alkaloids derived from tobacco and the toxic mushroom, *Amanita Muscaria*, respectively. The nicotinic receptors and their relationship to schizophrenia are discussed in a separate chapter in this volume. The MR family consists of five members numbered $M_1$–$M_5$ based on the order of their cloning [8]. $M_1$, $M_3$, and $M_5$ receptors are known for their robust coupling through Gq, and mobilization of intracellular calcium as well as their coupling to several members of the phospholipase family of lipid hydrolyzing enzymes (e.g., PLC, PLA2, PLD). $M_2$ and $M_4$ receptors are coupled to Gi and the inhibition of adenylate cyclase as well as modulation of inwardly rectifying K+ channels. Additional diverse signaling events have been linked to the MRs including tyrosine kinase activity, extracellular-signal-regulated kinases (*ERKs*)ERK1/2 activity, microtubule-associated protein *kinase* (MAPK), voltage-independent ion channels, and others [9].

Sequence alignment suggests a strong similarity of the five MR subtypes within the family and across species. The amino acid sequence similarity is 60% overall and rises to over 80% at the orthosteric binding domain (acetylcholine binding pocket) [10]. The homology is also well conserved across mammalian species, which is functionally supported by the similar species pharmacology observed for agonist and antagonist orthosteric ligands. Residues have been mapped that constitute the key determinants of orthosteric ligand binding, and these residues are conserved across the five receptor subtypes for almost all readily available orthosteric ligands. More recently, selective ligands have been developed for several of the ,MR subtypes that are detailed in the chemistry section below. In general, the selectivity is achieved at the orthosteric domain either through increasing molecular weight to create additional points of attachment or through binding at ectopic sites found beyond the traditional orthosteric binding domain. Alternatively, allosteric sites that are distinct from the orthosteric binding domain have been targeted, resulting in the development of highly receptor subtype-selective ligands. Examples of both orthosteric ligands and allosteric ligands and modulators are discussed in the chemistry section.

All five MR subtypes are broadly distributed in the central nervous system (CNS) and periphery, and are involved in the regulation of the parasympathetic nervous system, exocrine gland secretion, smooth muscle function, vascular and gastrointestinal (GI) tone, pupil constriction, nociception, arousal, sleep, and other physiologic processes [7]. In the CNS, the cholinergic system has both local interneuronal projections and projections that reach and innervate more distal brain regions. There are two major cholinergic projection complexes: one emanating from posterior pendunclopontine and lateral dorsal tegmental nuclei (ldt & ppt) and the other from the basal forebrain. The ldt and ppt complex projects to dorsal regions (e.g., thalamus, medial hebenula, and tectum), ventral regions (medullary reticular formations, cranial nerve bundles, deep cerebellar, and vestibular nuclei), and rostral areas (basal ganglia, substantia nigra, and ventral tegmentum). The forebrain bundle projects from the diagonal band of Broca, medial septum, and nucleus Baysalis of Meynart forward and upward to subcortical and cortical structures including the hippocampus, frontal/parietal/temporal cortex, and olfactory bulb. Interneurons within the striatum, olfactory tubercle, Islands of Calleja, and nucleus accumbens provide essential regional circuit control.

Therapeutic development of muscarinic ligands long preceded the cloning of the five receptor subtypes. After the genetic molecular revolution and the cloning of the five MR subtypes in the 1980s, it was discovered that muscarinic agonists (e.g., oxotremorine and carbachol) and antagonists (e.g., atropine and scopolamine) were generally nonselective across the MR family (Table 13.1). Even after the five receptor subtypes were cloned and stably expressed heterogeneously in mammalian cell lines, the purported selective ligands were discovered to be less selective than previously believed based on data generated with functional assays that allowed direct measurement of receptor subtype-signal transduction coupling events. For example, the purported $M_1$ selective ligands sabcomeline, talsaclidine, xanomeline, and others were found to have complex selectivity patterns at the ,MRs, overlapping pharmacology with other cell surface targets, and complex ligand binding site interactions [11].

A better understanding of the distribution and physiologic function of MR subtypes has contributed to the recent reemergence of interest in therapeutic development of selective muscarinic small molecule ligands. The highly homologous ligand binding sites, broad and overlapping MR subtype distribution, and lack of detailed knowledge of physiologic roles have relegated this family of receptors to the bottom of many preclinical development pipelines. Yet the knowledge of MR distribution in brain, coupled with knowledge of cholinergic neural wiring diagrams, suggests that these proteins may be promising therapeutic targets. In fact, early efforts focused on the $M_1$ receptor as a logical target based on its distribution on postsynaptic terminals in the hippocampus and prefrontal cortical areas and loss of basal forebrain cholinergic projections in Alzheimer's disease (AD) [12]. The working hypothesis suggested that replacement of MR stimulation lost with forebrain cholinergic deafferentation through $M_1$ receptor agonism would restore or at minimum delay the decline of working and short-term memory [13].

To date, the role of MRs in cognitive deficits associated with schizophrenia has received much less attention. The use of cholinesterase inhibitors in the treatment of schizophrenia was one of the earliest attempts at leveraging the cholinergic system for this disorder [6]. This approach evolved out of reverse hypothesis testing when it was observed that psychotic symptoms and attentional deficits worsened with exposure to anti-cholinergics [14]. Therefore, the resulting increase in synaptic acetylcholine following inhibition of the predominant catabolic enzyme should hypothetically enhance cholinergic tone, alleviating psychosis and improving attention. But are the domains of cognitive impairment associated with psychosis the same as those circuits regulated by MRs? Accumulating preclinical data provide support for this hypothesis [15]. For instance, $M_1$ receptor distribution is high on postsynaptic terminals in the hippocampus, cortex, and limbic areas. $M_1$ knockout mice show a deficit in cognitive operant tasks requiring vigilance and attention, two hallmark deficits associated with poorly functioning schizophrenics. Additional examples are provided below where each MR subtype is considered a potential target alone or in combination to provide symptom relief for this complex disease. Emerging evidence suggests that in some patients, MR mutations may contribute to disease etiology [16].

## 13.3 ROLE OF EACH MUSCARINIC RECEPTOR SUBTYPE AND SCHIZOPHRENIA

### 13.3.1 Mixed MR Subtypes

Many orthosteric muscarinic agonists have been reported and characterized in animal models of psychosis. In a comprehensive pharmacological evaluation, the following muscarinic agonists attenuated apomorphine-induced disruption of prepulse inhibition (PPI): xanomeline, BuTAC, oxotremorine, RS86, pilocarpine, milameline, and sabcomeline [17]. This study also demonstrated prepulse inhibition (PPI) disruption by scopolamine, which was reversed by both xanomeline and haloperidol. Efficacy of xanomeline in reversing apomorphine deficits in PPI was previously reported by Stanhope and colleagues [18]; interestingly, in their paper they also reported that xanomeline had anxiolytic efficacy in the conditioned emotional response assay. Multiple reports indicate that muscarinic agonists, such as xanomeline, PTAC, and BuTAC, block dopamine agonist-induced hyperlocomotor activity and exhibit robust efficacy in the conditioned avoidance response assay [19–20]. Although most studies were conducted in rodents, xanomeline was demonstrated to block amphetamine- and apomorphine-induced behaviors in monkeys [21]. The above pharmacological studies demonstrating reciprocal interactions between dopamine and muscarinic systems provide strong construct validity for an involvement of the muscarinic system in the pathophysiology of schizophrenia.

In an electrophysiological model of schizophrenia in which the ability of an agent to inhibit A10 versus A9 dopamine pathways is assessed, xanomeline selectively inhibited A10 dopamine neurons following both acute and 21-day chronic dosing [20]. The selectivity in inhibiting A10 (VTA), but not A9 (substantia nigra), neurons is similar to the profile of atypical antipsychotics such as olanzapine and clozapine [22] and thought to reflect reduced propensity for producing extrapyramidal motor effects. Also interesting and perhaps suggestive of a favorable onset of efficacy was the finding that xanomeline effectively inhibited A10 neurons following a single dose, whereas clozapine and olanzapine required chronic treatment before modulatory effects on cell firing were observed.

Given the known role of acetylcholine in mediating cognitive functioning, there remains much hope that muscarinic agonists will have a significant therapeutic impact on the cognitive deficits associated with schizophrenia. In direct models of cognition, a xanomeline derivative improved memory functions in aged mice [23] and facilitated spatial learning acquisition in rats [24]. Schizophrenics exhibit deficiencies in latent inhibition, and psychotomimetic agents such as amphetamine, phencyclidine, and scopolamine disrupt latent inhibition in rodents [25–26]. Scopolamine-induced disruption of latent inhibition can be reversed by atypical antipsychotics and physostigmine [14, 27]. More recently, xanomeline reversed latent inhibition deficits induced by scopolamine, amphetamine, and MK801 [28]. Although less directly tied to cognitive function, increasing dopamine efflux in the prefrontal cortex has been hypothesized to be a desirable pharmacological trait that some atypical antipsychotics exhibit, and may be related to better clinical outcomes on cognitive deficits in schizophrenic patients [29]. Similar to clozapine and olanzapine, xanomeline increased dopamine levels in the medial prefrontal cortex of rats [30].

***13.3.1.1 M1 and M4 Receptor Subtypes*** Even in schizophrenic patients that respond favorably to treatments, cognitive deficits are considered the major disability preventing schizophrenic patients from achieving productive and social lives. MRs play a role in arousal, executive function, working memory, attention, and consolidation of short and long term memory [8–9, 30–33]. The foundation of muscarinic involvement in cognition emerges from the early work in AD, where anatomical cholinergic deficits were associated with cognitive decline [34, 35]. The link to the MRs was established when nonselective muscarinic antagonists were shown to cause psychosis-like symptoms and significant cognitive impairment [36, 37]. Due to its postsynaptic localization in key brain areas regulating cognitive control, the $M_1$ receptor became the focus of therapeutic intervention. Despite little direct mechanistic evidence as well as lack of selective pharmacology and genetic models, several modestly selective muscarinic agonists advanced into clinical trials for the treatment of cognitive decline in AD [38]. $M_2$ receptors regulate acetylcholine release through their presynaptic location, making them attractive targets for antagonist therapy [39]. However, they are also highly expressed in cardiovascular tissue and therefore have proven unattractive drug targets. $M_4$ receptors are localized presynapytically as a heteroreceptor regulating the release of DA, glutamate, acetylcholine, γ-aminobutyric acid (GABA), and possibly other neurotransmitters [40], but until recently, they have been largely ignored [41]. To date, there is little evidence that $M_3$ or $M_5$ receptors are significantly involved in cognition; however, $M_5$ receptors are colocalized on DA neurons and functionally affect striatal dopamine efflux [42, 43] and may modulate cognition and other dopamine-regulated behaviors indirectly. Such findings indicate that the M5 receptor may also be a potential therapeutic target either alone or in combination with other MR subtypes for the treatment of schizophrenia.

Cognitive processes found to be most impaired in schizophrenia are attentional control regulated, in part, by the anterior cingulate cortex [44] and working memory and executive function regulated, in part, through the lateral dorsal prefrontal cortex [45]. Both of these structures express $M_1$ and $M_4$ receptors and innervate the hippocampus, a structure important for memory consolidation and encoding implicit contextual information. The hippocampus also expresses both $M_1$ and $M_4$ receptors, and deficits of $M_4$ receptors have been measured in postmortem hippocampal tissues obtained from unmedicated schizophrenics [16]. Functional changes were also noted for $M_1$ receptors in a subpopulation of "$M_1$-deficit schizophrenics [46]." The precise role of $M_1$ and $M_4$ receptors in these structures has not been fully explored. Early efforts with selective MR toxins suggested that stimulation of both $M_1$ and $M_4$ receptors in the hippocampus would improve memory tasks in rodents [47, 48]. At the cellular level, $M_1$ receptors have been shown to positively modulate N-methyl-D-aspartate (NMDA) receptor function in hippocampal slices [49], where both are localized postsynaptically. Yet follow-up studies by the same group showed that this effect was not lost in $M_1$ receptor-deficient mice [50]. The selective $M_1$ allosteric potentiator, TBPB, exhibited an antipsychotic-like profile in several behavioral and neurochemical paradigms, including potentiation of NMDA receptor currents in pyramidal neurons in the hippocampus, activation of Fos expression in rat forebrain, and reversal of amphetamine-induced hyperlocomotor activity [51]. More recently, $M_1$ selective modulators and antagonists were used to show excitatory synaptic events in the medial-prefrontal cortex (mPFC) layer V pyramidal cells that were $M_1$ receptor mediated [52, 53]. The localization in mPFC of M1 receptor-driven neural excitation is consistent with $M_1$ cortical-dependent learning in mice [15]. Therefore, $M_1$

and $M_4$ receptors may be the key subtypes to target either individually or together for therapeutic intervention, yet their role in cognitive control in various brain regions has not been fully elucidated.

***13.3.1.2 $M_2$ and $M_3$ Receptor Subtypes*** Numerous studies have demonstrated a strong presence of $M_2$ and $M_3$ receptor function in the regulation of parasympathetic control of peripheral organs tissue. For instance, an extensive loss of [$^3$H]-NMS binding is observed in heart and smooth muscle tissue of mice lacking either $M_2$ or $M_3$ receptors [54–56]. Therefore, a concern for any muscarinic agonist with appreciable $M_2$ or $M_3$ affinity is the emergence of parasympathetic side effects that preclude clinical use for schizophrenia or other diseases involving cognitive deficits. Indeed, all of the arecoline-based muscarinic agonists tested in humans and in animals have shown at least some cardiovascular signal, presumably because of a lack of MR subtype selectivity at $M_2$ and $M_3$ receptors [11].

Whereas little is known regarding a potential role of the $M_3$ receptor in schizophrenia, the $M_2$ receptor subtype is localized in key cortical and limbic structures, often exhibiting a presynaptic autoreceptor role in the regulation of acetylcholine release [57]. Therefore, $M_2$ antagonists, rather than agonists, are believed to be therapeutic targets. For instance, oral administration of the selective M2 antagonist SCH57790 elevated ACh release in rat hippocampus, cortex, and striatum [58]. These increased ACh levels were presumably linked to improved retention of passive avoidance learning in rats, reversal of scopolamine-induced passive avoidance deficits in mice, and improved working memory performance in squirrel monkeys. Similar pro-cognitive effects on spatial learning have been found in aged rats using the $M_2$ antagonist BIBN-99 [59, 60]. Regarding potential parasympathetic side effects of selective $M_2$ antagonists, reports with compounds such as SCH-57790 indicate, in animals, a margin between efficacy in cognitive models and notable cardiovascular effects [58]. It is not known whether such a tolerability window exists in clinical settings. Potential novel approaches would include $M_2$ weak partial agonists or negative allosteric modulators, which may offer a better therapeutic index.

***13.3.1.3 $M_5$ Receptor Subtype*** To date, no specific orthosteric ligands have been reported for the $M_5$ receptor. Despite the lack of pharmacological tools, the $M_5$ receptor appears to be a reasonable target for developing an antipsychotic agent. Compared with other MR subtypes in the brain, $M_5$ receptors are expressed in very low levels and are discretely localized [61]. Of particular note, the M5 receptor is the only MR subtype expressed on the dopamine cell bodies of the ventral tegmental area VTA and substantial nigra [62]. Mice lacking the $M_5$ receptor show diminished dopamine release in the nucleus accumbens and decreased stimulatory response to amphetamine [43]. Moreover, this study also demonstrated that $M_5$ knockout mice had improved latent inhibition relative to wild-type controls, suggesting a role for the $M_5$ receptor in the regulation of attention. Although explored in more depth in peripheral physiology [63], the $M_5$ receptor remains a relatively unexplored CNS target.

## 13.4 CLINICAL STUDIES

A lack of selective pharmacological tools has hampered the validation of the muscarinic agonist hypothesis for the treatment of symptoms associated with schizophrenia. A major metabolite of clozapine, N-desmethyl clozapine, has partial $M_1$ receptor agonist properties, which may provide the modest cognitive benefit observed in some patients treated with clozapine [64, 65]. Of the many arecoline-based orthosteric muscarinic agonists, xanomeline stands out as having preferential $M_1$ and $M_4$ partial agonist activity [20]; however, additional contributory pharmacology cannot be ruled out [66, 67]. More recent preclinical studies support the role of the $M_4$ receptor in regulating at least some of the psychotic behaviors in schizophrenia [68]. Xanomeline was originally studied as a potential treatment for cognitive decline in Alzheimer's patients and showed promise in psychological clinical global impression scales and cognitive scores. The improvements observed in psychotic symptoms of advanced Alzheimer's patients suggested promise as a potential antipsychotic. A small placebo-controlled clinical study was conducted with xanomeline in difficult to treat schizophrenic patients [69]. Xanomeline was dosed at 75 mg TID for 4 weeks and was well tolerated in this patient population, with nearly all subjects completing the trial. The more modest pharmacological activity at $M_2$ and $M_3$ receptors may explain the relative lack of parasympathetic side effects observed in schizophrenic and control patients compared with the AD trial with elderly patients. The primary outcome measures were Clinical Global Impression (CGI), Brief Psychiatric Rating Scale (BPRS), and Positive and Negative Syndrome Scale (PANSS). Significant improvements were observed in all measures. Xanomeline was also positive in cognitive measures indicating surprising improvements in all three major symptom domains. Although these results are preliminary, they do encourage continued exploration of the muscarinic agonist hypothesis. Promising MR-selective pharmacological tools are being developed to better understand the potential of this novel approach [40, 70].

## 13.5 MEDICINAL CHEMISTRY

Despite decades of research, the discovery of subtype-selective orthosteric ligands continues to elude medicinal chemists, both in industry and academia. This is mostly due to the fact that the orthosteric binding site (the binding site of the endogenous ligand acetylcholine) is highly conserved across all five MRs [71, 72]. Nonetheless, medicinal chemistry-based rational molecule design led to modestly selective full and partial agonists [11, 73, 74]. An emerging approach to circumvent this dilemma has been to target the allosteric binding sites, which potentially have less sequence homology across the subtypes [75, 76]. This is an attractive approach for multiple reasons: (1) the allosteric modulator has no activity on its own, but modulates the action of endogenous ACh, thus maintaining the temporal aspects of the signaling pathway; (2) the allosteric modulator has the potential to be subtype selective due to sequence heterogeneity at the allosteric sites; (3) the allosteric modulator has potential to intensify weak signaling due to disease states resulting from deficits in ACh tone. Both orthosteric and allosteric approaches are detailed in Section 13.7.

## 13.6 $M_1$ AGONISTS

Since 2000, a number of putative selective $M_1$ agonists have been reported. Previously, we reported amidines [77] such as **2** that may have some functional muscarinic subtype selectivity. Further extensive structure–activity relationship (SAR) exploration around amidines yielded a clinical candidate, LY593093 [78–81] (**3**). LY593093 is a highly functionally selective M1 agonist with diminished $M_2$ subtype activity. Moreover, it was found to be devoid of measurable $M_3$–$M_5$ activities in an *in vitro* functional assay (GTPγS binding assay $EC_{50}$: $M_1 = 144$ nM [93% efficacy] and $M_2 = 4245$ nM [27% efficacy]). This compound showed favorable pharmacokinetic properties with good rat brain exposure and good bioavailability in both rats and monkeys. It demonstrated robust efficacy over a range of doses with the minimum effective oral dose of 1 mg/kg in several rodent models of cognitive behavior including the rat eight-arm radial maze. In animal studies, no cholinergic side effects related to the activation of $M_2$ and $M_3$ receptors were observed at doses of up to 100 mg/kg. These data indicate that LY593093 is a highly selective $M_1$ agonist *in vitro* and has robust efficacy in a model of spatial learning in rat following oral dosing without apparent $M_2$/$M_3$-dependent parasympathetic effects. 35AKU-21 [82] (**4**) was reported by Acadia Pharmaceuticals as an $M_1$/$M_4$ agonist without $M_2$, $M_3$, and $M_5$ activities, whose activations produce the majority of dose-limiting side effects observed in the clinic. A selective $M_1$ and $M_4$ agonist could be effective in the treatment of cognitive impairment for both AD and schizophrenia. 35AKU-21 (**4**) was tested for ocular hypotensive effect in glaucomatous monkeys and showed a 29.2% drop in intraocular pressure change in 6 hours. After 35AKU-21, benzimidazol-2-one and benzothiazol-2-one derivatives [83], such as compounds **5** and **6**, were reported as selective $M_1$/$M_4$ agonists coupled with $D_2$ activity; however, no *in vivo* data were disclosed. Also disclosed were benzoxazinones [84], depicted by compound **7**, as selective $M_1$/$M_4$ agonists.

More recently, Glaxo disclosed benzimidazol-2-ones [85–87] such as **8**, as M1 agonists for the treatment of psychotic disorder and cognitive impairment. The reported selectivity (ratio $pEC_{50}$) for M1 receptor over $M_2$–$M_5$ receptors is 10- to 100-fold in calcium mobilization assays. Structural modification of benzimidazol-2-ones to perhydroimidazolones and perhydroindolones [88] as well as indolinones [89] led to compound **9** [88] and compound **10** [89], which were also reported for treatment of AD and schizophrenia as well as pain. Compound **9** is claimed to be a highly selective $M_1$ agonist (FLIPR $EC_{50}$: $M_1 = 5$ nM, $M3 > 40{,}000$ nM and $M_5 = 3900$ nM; GTPγS binding $EC_{50}$: $M_2 = 3700$ nM and $M_4 = 9400$ nM). The rat Freund's Complete Adjuvant (FCA)-induced heat hyperalgesia model was used as a pain model for evaluating perhydroimidazolones and perhydroindolones, but no data were disclosed. In 2009, some benzoxazole analogs [90] emerged from further modifications of benzimidazol-2-ones and were reported as selective $M_1$ agonists.

A series of compounds with more complex structures [91] exemplified as compounds **11**, **12**, and **13**, which are structurally similar to perhydroimidazolones and perhydroindolones, was reported as selective $M_1$ agonists. It is interesting to note that tissue-based assays were utilized for the evaluation of these compounds, but yet no pharmacology data were reported. Compound **13** is claimed to be a partial M1 agonist with a potency ($EC_{50}$ value) of 100 nM.

Piperidine analogs were reported as selective $M_1$ agonists that showed no significant activity at $M_2$, $M_3$, $M_4$ or $M_5$ receptors. Representative piperidine analogs are shown in Table 13.1 as compounds **14** and **15** [92].

Extensive effort has been invested in exploring structural modifications of xanomeline (**1**) in order to improve the $M_1$ and $M_4$ receptor selectivity. New findings are continuously appearing in the literature and patent forums. It was proposed that combined agonist activity at $M_1$, $M_2$, and $M_4$ receptors would be useful in the treatment of AD and schizophrenia and other cognitive impairment [93–95]. The most recent reported xanomeline analogs such as CDD0304 (**16**) and CDD0273 (**17**) were claimed to be $M_1$, $M_2$, and $M_4$ selective agonists. CDD0304 displayed functional activity at $M_1$ and $M_2$ receptors, and partial agonist at the $M_4$ receptor. It was essentially inactive at $M_3$ and $M_5$ receptors. CD0304 was also tested *in vivo* (mouse) to evaluate $M_3$-receptor mediated side effects. Only minimal side effects were observed at doses of up to 10 mg/kg (i.p). These data are consistent with a lack of efficacy of CD0304 in an *in vitro* $M_3$ receptor assay. It is interesting to note that CD0304 caused slight tremors and induced hypothermia in mouse at a dose of 10 mg/kg (i.p.). More recently an $M_1$-selective agonist series of N-substituted benzimidazolones has been described [96]. One of the examples, GSK1034702, was evaluated and shown positive in improving episodic memory in a small human nicotine withdrawal proof-of-concept clinical trial [97]. It is not clear if this compound is acting at an allosteric or orthosteric binding site on the $M_1$ receptor.

## 13.7 $M_1$ POSITIVE ALLOSTERIC MODULATORS

Due to the high degree conservation of muscarinic orthosteric binding sites and the proven challenges in developing subtype-selective ligands, targeting ligands that bind to muscarinic allosteric binding sites may be more promising for developing subtype-selective drugs. Allosteric modulators do not activate the receptors directly nor compete with endogenous ACh at the orthosteric binding site. By binding at an allosteric site, it is hypothesized that a greater structural diversity of compounds can be achieved which will promote greater subtype selectivity for the target MR. Binding of modulator at allosteric sites results in potentiation of the endogenous agonist effects. This approach has been successfully demonstrated in the development of several ligands for GPCRs, more recently mGluR 2 potentiators [98]. Previous attempts to identify and develop subtype-selective allosteric modulators were reviewed [76]. In 2005, Vertex disclosed a series of 4-aminopiperidines as muscarinic modulators for the treatment of CNS disorders (see example 18 [99]). The data indicated some of 4-aminopiperdines are selective M1 receptor modulators, but no detailed SAR was disclosed.

Merck recently reported quinolone [100] and quinolizidione [101] derivatives such as compounds **19** and **20** as $M_1$ positive allosteric modulators. Compound **19** (BQCA) was claimed to be a highly selective and efficacious positive allosteric modulator (potentiator) for the $M_1$ receptor [102]. It is an $M_1$ allosteric potentiator and does not have agonist activity at $M_1$ receptors, but compound **19** left-shifts the concentration response curve of Ach at activating $M_1$. More importantly, compound **19** does not compete for binding at the orthosteric binding site and it is not active at $M_2$, $M_3$, or $M_4$ receptors. *In vivo* studies of compound **19** indicated that it is centrally active and reverses the cognitive impairment induced by scopolamine in a contextual fear-conditioning model of episodic-like memory in mice and does not produce unwanted peripheral side effects at doses that demonstrate central responses.

In addition, several structurally diverse M1 modulators such as VU0090157 (**21**) and VU0029767 (**22**) have been reported recently by Conn, Lindsley, and colleagues at Vanderbilt University [103]. They showed that both **21** and **22** induced left-shift of ACh affinity at the $M_1$ receptor, indicating enhancement of $M_1$ activity. It is interesting to note that **21** induced similar potentiation in $M_1$ activation of phospholipase C and D (PLC and PLD), and **22** only potentiated activation of PLC but not PLD, indicating multiple, diverse modes of activity.

In addition to M1 allosteric modulators, significant progress has been made recently in identifying $M_1$ allosteric agonists. TBPB (**23**) was reported as a highly selective $M_1$ allosteric agonist without $M_2$–$M_5$ activity [70]. Data collected from binding studies of an $M_1$ receptor with a mutated orthosteric site and a competitive nonselective orthosteric mAChR antagonist demonstrated that TBPB does not bind at the muscarinic orthosteric binding site, further indicating the likely existence of allosteric binding sites [104]. TBPB showed robust effects in several preclinical antipsychotic models without producing motor or parasympathetic side effects associated with activation of central or peripheral $M_2$ and $M_3$ receptors. Although it has weak $D_2$ receptor antagonist activity ($IC_{50} = 5.1\ \mu M$), $D_2$ receptor occupancy studies indicated that the antipsychotic activity of TBPB observed in animal models was likely the result of $M_1$ activation and not the $D_2$ inhibition [70, 105, 106]. These data provide evidence that TBPB produces the antipsychotic-like effects of xanomeline in animal models through selective activation of $M_1$ receptor at the allosteric sites. Further structural exploration around TBPB did not yield significant improvement of potency and efficacy, and subtle structure changes resulted in decreasing of $M_1$ potency and agonism efficacy, indicating the challenges in development of allosteric ligands for TBPB series. The other recently reported highly selective $M_1$ agonist is 77-LH-28-1 [107] (**4**), which is an analog of previously reported selective allosteric M1 agonist, AC-42 [108]. Extensive binding and functional studies of 77-LH-28-1 with mutated M1 cell lines and orthosteric antagonists indicate its mode of action as an allosteric agonist [109].

## 13.8 $M_4$ POSITIVE ALLOSTERIC MODULATORS

Researchers at Eli Lilly have reported [41] on the identification of a functionally potent and selective muscarinic $M_4$ receptor positive allosteric modulator, LY2033298, **25**. Utilizing a FLIPR assay, a typical leftward shift of the ACh dose response curve was demonstrated upon application of increasing concentrations of LY2033298. Data analysis gave a $K_B$ of $200 \pm 40$ nM at the $hM_4$ receptor with an allosteric cooperativity factor $\alpha$ of $35 \pm 4$. No effect was observed at the human $M_1$, $M_3$, and $M_5$ receptors, and only a modest allosteric effect at the human $M_2$ receptor ($K_B = 1.0 \pm 0.3\ \mu M$, $\alpha = 3.7 \pm 0.5$) was found. These findings were confirmed in Chinese hamster ovary (CHO) cell membranes by measuring GTP$\gamma$S binding to native G proteins. LY2033298 was again found to be a potent and selective positive allosteric modulator of the $M_4$ receptor with a measured $K_B$ of $870 \pm 310$ nM and cooperativity factor $\alpha$ of $28 + 7$.

The Lilly researchers also identified a species difference between the rat and human M4 receptors. Utilizing mutational analysis, a key residue, $D^{432}$, in the extracellular loop of the M4 receptor was found to be critical for the activity of LY2033298. Comparison of the rat and human $M_4$ receptor sequences revealed two nonconserved residues in this domain, one of which corresponds to the $D^{432}$ residue of the $hM_4$ receptor. This finding correlates with a lack of observable effect upon dosing LY2033298 to rats in conditioned avoidance responding (CAR) and PPI psychosis models. However, upon co-administration of a sub-effective dose of oxotremorine, LY2033298 did attenuate CAR and reverse apomorphine-disrupted PPI in a dose-dependent manner. This finding substantiates that LY2033298 is active *in vivo* through the muscarinic mechanism as a positive allosteric modulator of the $M_4$ receptor in rodent models predictive of antipsychotic drug effects.

Researchers at Vanderbilt University applied chemoinformatics and medicinal chemistry to explore analogs of LY2033298 to aid in the identification of a series of selective and potent rM4 allosteric potentiators [110]. A total of 232 compounds were identified from commercial sources based on core similarity to LY2033298. Compound 7912361, **26**, emerged from this set and was found to be the most potent $M_4$ allosteric potentiator, having an $EC_{50}$ of 395 ± 28 nM. Subsequent chemical optimization through modification of the amide functionality of 7912361 led to the identification of VU100010, **27**, which has an $EC_{50}$ of 400 ± 100 nM and demonstrates a 47-fold leftward shift in the ACh $EC_{50}$.

These researchers further explored this structural class through a diversity-oriented synthesis approach [111]. Two compounds emerged (i.e., VU0152099, **28**, and VU0152100, **29**) as being potent (M4 $EC_{50}$ = 403 nM and 380 nM, respectively) and selective allosteric modulators. In addition, each induced a leftward shift of the ACh dose–response curve by 30-fold at 30 μM for VU0152099 and 70-fold at 10 μM for VU0152100. Although the activities of these newer derivatives were comparable to that of VU100010, VU0152100, and VU0152099 had improved physiochemical properties, which enabled their study in *in vivo* behavioral rat models. Indeed, both compounds produced robust decreases in amphetamine-induced hyperlocomotion in rats, a model predictive of antipsychotic activity, at a dose of 56.6 mg/kg (dosed i.p.). The results of Eli Lilly with LY2033298 and Vanderbilt University with VU0152099 and VU0152100 support the hypothesis that selective modulation of the $M_4$ AChR is an attractive target for treating schizophrenia.

## 13.9 $M_5$ POSITIVE ALLOSTERIC MODULATOR

An understanding of the physiological role of the central $M_5$ receptor has been hampered, as with all the MR subtypes, by a lack of subtype-selective agonists/antagonists. The use of mutant mice, deficient in the five mAChR subtypes, has provided evidence for the role of the $M_5$ AChR in various disorders including Alzheimer's disease, schizophrenia, drug addiction, and cerebrovascular diseases [112]. Recently Lindsley and co-workers from Vanderbilt University described the discovery of an $M_5$ AChR preferring the positive allosteric modulator VU0238429 [113] (**31**).

The original screening hit, VU0119498, **30**, was found to have comparable allosteric potentiator activity at $M_1$, $M_3$, and $M_5$, and lacked activity at $M_2$ and $M_4$. Efforts were undertaken to optimize the potency and selectivity of this hit for $M_5$. VU0238429 emerged as an $M_5$ preferring positive allosteric modulator of the $M_5$ AChR, having an $M_5$ $EC_{50}$ of 1.16 μM and greater than 30-fold selectivity over the receptor subtypes. Unfortunately, VU0238429 demonstrated poor systemic absorption after intraperitoneal administration, precluding its use as an *in vivo* tool. Nonetheless, VU0238429 represents the first $M_5$ subtype selective modulator reported to date.

## 13.10 FUTURE DIRECTIONS

Currently available atypical antipsychotics have reasonable therapeutic efficacy for the positive symptoms of schizophrenia. However, treatment of the cognitive deficits and negative symptoms remains as a key unmet medical challenge. Current economic pressures and health care reform initiatives will encourage payers and providers to offer generic atypical antipsychotics as the first-line treatment option. Providers will be reluctant to switch their patients on to experimental medications and will likely elect to use these novel treatment options in adjunctive treatment modalities. The challenge for pharmaceutical innovators will be to provide sufficient proof of efficacy for novel treatments to be considered as monotherapeutic or adjunctive treatment options in combination with current medications. A recent small clinical study with the mixed muscarinic agonist, xanomeline, was conducted to provide preliminary evidence that muscarinic agonism, particularly at the $M_1$ and $M_4$ subtype, might offer a new approach to either monotherapy or adjunctive therapy for treatment of symptoms associated with schizophrenia. This new approach would differ significantly from first- and second-generation typical and atypical antipsychotics, respectively, which block many receptor proteins, but the $D_2$ and 5-HT2A receptors in particular [69]. Based on positive results across multiple symptom domains, muscarinic agonism at the $M_1$ and $M_4$ receptor subtypes appear to offer promise as a potential monotherapeutic approach as well as an adjunctive treatment modality. The data are preliminary and the available pharmacological tools are imperfect to directly assess the role of each MR subtype in treating the three symptom domains of schizophrenia. Selective $M_1$ and $M_4$ molecules are beginning to emerge, however, and in the next decades these compounds will be evaluated in advanced clinical trials. Despite their neuroanatomical localization, it is unlikely that $M_2$ and $M_3$ receptors will be viable targets due to their role in cardiovascular, smooth muscle, and exocrine gland function. However, the $M_5$ receptor remains largely unexplored and might be a viable target alone or in combination with the $M_1$ and $M_4$ receptor subtypes.

## REFERENCES

1. Sullivan, R.J., Allen, J.S., Otto, C., Tiobech, J., Nero, K. (2000). Effects of chewing betel nut (Areca catechu) on the symptoms of people with schizophrenia in Palau, Micronesia. *The British Journal of Psychiatry*, *177*, 174–178.
2. Gilani, A.H., Ghayur, M.N., Saify, Z.S., Ahmed, S.P., Choudhary, M.I., Khalid, A. (2004). Presence of cholinomimetic and acetylcholinesterase inhibitory constituents in betel nut. *Life Sciences*, *75*, 2377–2389.
3. Fiamberti, A.M. (1950). Development of acetylcholine treatment of schizophrenia from the Congress of Paris (1950) to the present time. *Minerva Medica*, *49*, 3791–3793.

4. Massignan, L., Roi, G. (1948) *Researches on the therapeutic efficacy of suspension of consciousness in mental patients*, Note e Reviste di Psichiatria, Pesaro.
5. Forrer, G.R. (1954). Psychodynamic factors in atropine toxicity therapy. *The Journal of Nervous and Mental Disease*, *120*, 40–43.
6. Raedler, T.J., Bymaster, F.P., Tandon, R., Copolov, D., Dean, B. (2007). Towards a muscarinic hypothesis of schizophrenia. *Molecular Psychiatry*, *12*, 232–246.
7. Cooper, J.R., Bloom,F.E., Roth, R.H., eds. (2003). *The Biochemical Basis of Neuropharmacology*, 8th ed. Oxford: Oxford University Press.
8. Felder, C.C. (1995). Muscarinic acetylcholine receptors: signal transduction through multiple effectors. *The FASEB Journal*, *9*, 619–625.
9. Felder, C.C., Bymaster, F.P., Ward, J., DeLapp, N. (2000). Therapeutic opportunities for muscarinic receptors in the central nervous system. *Journal of Medicinal Chemistry*, *43*, 4333–4353.
10. Wess, J., Liu, J., Blin, N., Yun, J., Lerche, C., Kostenis, E. (1997). Structural basis of receptor/G protein coupling selectivity studied with muscarinic receptors as model systems. *Life Sciences*, *60*, 1007–1014.
11. Heinrich, J.N., Butera, J.A., Carrick, T., Kramer, A., Kowal, D., Lock, T., Marquis, K.L., Pausch, M.H., Popiolek, M., Sun, S.C., Tseng, E., Uveges, A.J., Mayer, S.C. (2009). Pharmacological comparison of muscarinic ligands: historical versus more recent muscarinic M1-preferring receptor agonists. *European Journal of Pharmacology*, *605*, 53–56.
12. McKinney, M., Coyle, J.T. (1991). The potential for muscarinic receptor subtype-specific pharmacotherapy for Alzheimer's disease. *Mayo Clinic Proceedings. Mayo Clinic*, *66*, 1225–1237.
13. Caccamo, A., Fisher, A., LaFerla, F.M. (2009). M1 agonists as a potential disease-modifying therapy for Alzheimer's disease. *Current Alzheimer Research*, *6*, 112–117.
14. Barak, S., Weiner, I. (2009). Towards an animal model of an antipsychotic drug-resistant cognitive impairment in schizophrenia: scopolamine induces abnormally persistent latent inhibition, which can be reversed by cognitive enhancers but not by antipsychotic drugs. *The International Journal of Neuropsychopharmacology*, *12*, 227–241.
15. Anagnostaras, S.G., Murphy, G.G., Hamilton, S.E., Mitchell, S.L., Rahnama, N.P., Nathanson, N.M., Silva, A.J. (2003). Selective cognitive dysfunction in acetylcholine M1 muscarinic receptor mutant mice. *Nature Neuroscience*, *6*, 51–58.
16. Scarr, E., Dean, B. (2008). Muscarinic receptors: do they have a role in the pathology and treatment of schizophrenia? *Journal of Neurochemistry*, *107*, 1188–1195.
17. Jones, C.K., Eberle, E.L., Shaw, D.B., McKinzie, D.L., Shannon, H.E. (2005). Pharmacologic interactions between the muscarinic cholinergic and dopaminergic systems in the modulation of prepulse inhibition in rats. *The Journal of Pharmacology and Experimental Therapeutics*, *312*, 1055–1063.
18. Stanhope, K.J., Mirza, N.R., Bickerdike, M.J., Bright, J.L., Harrington, N.R., Hesselink, M.B., Kennett, G.A., Lightowler, S., Sheardown, M.J., Syed, R., Upton, R.L., Wadsworth, G., Weiss, S.M., Wyatt, A. (2001). The muscarinic receptor agonist xanomeline has an antipsychotic-like profile in the rat. *The Journal of Pharmacology and Experimental Therapeutics*, *299*, 782–792.

19. Bymaster, F.P., Shannon, H.E., Rasmussen, K., Delapp, N.W., Mitch, C.H., Ward, J.S., Calligaro, D.O., Ludvigsen, T.S., Sheardown, M.J., Olesen, P.H., Swedberg, M.D., Sauerberg, P., Fink-Jensen, A. (1998). Unexpected antipsychotic-like activity with the muscarinic receptor ligand (5R,6R)6-(3-propylthio-1,2,5-thiadiazol-4-yl)-1-azabicyclo[3.2.1]octane. *European Journal of Pharmacology*, *356*, 109–119.

20. Shannon, H.E., Rasmussen, K., Bymaster, F.P., Hart, J.C., Peters, S.C., Swedberg, M.D., Jeppesen, L., Sheardown, M.J., Sauerberg, P., Fink-Jensen, A. (2000). Xanomeline, an M(1)/M(4) preferring muscarinic cholinergic receptor agonist, produces antipsychotic-like activity in rats and mice. *Schizophrenia Research*, *42*, 249–259.

21. Andersen, M.B., Fink-Jensen, A., Peacock, L., Gerlach, J., Bymaster, F., Lundbaek, J.A., Werge, T. (2003). The muscarinic M1/M4 receptor agonist xanomeline exhibits antipsychotic-like activity in Cebus apella monkeys. *Neuropsychopharmacology*, *28*, 1168–1175.

22. Stockton, M.E., Rasmussen, K. (1996). Electrophysiological effects of olanzapine, a novel atypical antipsychotic, on A9 and A10 dopamine neurons. *Neuropsychopharmacology*, *14*, 97–105.

23. Cui, Y., Wang, D., Si, W., Lv, W., Niu, Y., Lei, X., Hu, Y., Cao, X. (2008). Enhancement of memory function in aged mice by a novel derivative of xanomeline. *Cell Research*, *18*, 1151–1153.

24. Crile, R.S., Hart, J.C., Shaw, D.B., Bymaster, F.P., Felder, C.C., McKinzie, D.L. (2001) Characterization of the muscarinic M1-M4 receptor agonist xanomeline in radial maze acquisition, prepulse inhibition and autonomic effects. Society for Neuroscience. San Diego, CA.

25. Feldon, J., Weiner, I. (1992). From an animal model of an attentional deficit towards new insights into the pathophysiology of schizophrenia. [Review] [230 refs]. *Journal of Psychiatric Research*, *26*, 345–366.

26. Lubow, R.E., Braunstein-Bercovitz, H., Blumenthal, O., Kaplan, O., Toren, P. (2005). Latent inhibition and asymmetrical visual-spatial attention in children with ADHD. *Child Neuropsychology*, *11*, 445–457.

27. Weiner, I., Arad, M. (2009). Using the pharmacology of latent inhibition to model domains of pathology in schizophrenia and their treatment. *Behavioural Brain Research*, *204*, 369–386.

28. Barak, S., Weiner, I. (2011). The M1/M4 preferring agonist xanomeline reverses amphetamine-, MK801- and scopolamine-induced abnormalities of latent inhibition: putative efficacy against positive, negative and cognitive symptoms in schizophrenia. *International Journal of Neuropsychopharmacology 14*, 1233–1246.

29. Ichikawa, J., Dai, J., O'Laughlin, I.A., Fowler, W.L., Meltzer, H.Y. (2002). Atypical, but not typical, antipsychotic drugs increase cortical acetylcholine release without an effect in the nucleus accumbens or striatum. *Neuropsychopharmacology*, *26*, 325–339.

30. Perry, K.W., Nisenbaum, L.K., George, C.A., Shannon, H.E., Felder, C.C., Bymaster, F.P. (2001). The muscarinic agonist xanomeline increases monoamine release and immediate early gene expression in the rat prefrontal cortex. *Biological Psychiatry*, *49*, 716–725.

31. Sarter, M., Martinez, V., Kozak, R. (2009). A neurocognitive animal model dissociating between acute illness and remission periods of schizophrenia. [Review] [189 refs]. *Psychopharmacology*, *202*, 237–258.
32. Sellin, A.K., Shad, M., Tamminga, C. (2008). Muscarinic agonists for the treatment of cognition in schizophrenia. *CNS Spectrums*, *13*, 985–996.
33. Bymaster, F.P. (2001). Possible role of muscarinic receptor agonists as therapeutic agents for psychosis. In: Breier, A., Tran, P.V., Herrera, J.M., Tollefson, G.D., Bymaster, F.P., eds., *Current Issues in the Psychopharmacology of Schizophrenia*. Philadelphia: Lippincott Williams & Wilkins Healthcare, 2001, pp. 333–348.
34. Bartus, R.T. (2000). On neurodegenerative diseases, models, and treatment strategies: lessons learned and lessons forgotten a generation following the cholinergic hypothesis. [Review] [242 refs]. *Experimental Neurology*, *163*, 495–529.
35. Bartus, R.T., Dean, R.L., Beer, B. (1982). Neuropeptide effects on memory in aged monkeys. *Neurobiology of Aging*, *3*, 61–68.
36. Sunderland, T., Tariot, P., Murphy, D.L., Weingartner, H., Mueller, E.A., Cohen R.M. (1985). Scopolamine challenges in Alzheimer's disease. *Psychopharmacology*. 87, 247–249.
37. Agnoli, A., Martucci, N., Manna, V., Conti, L., Fioravanti, M. (1983). Effect of cholinergic and anticholinergic drugs on short-term memory in Alzheimer's dementia: a neuropsychological and computerized electroencephalographic study. *Clinical Neuropharmacology*, *6*, 311–323.
38. Fisher, A. (2008). Cholinergic treatments with emphasis on m1 muscarinic agonists as potential disease-modifying agents for Alzheimer's disease. *Neurotherapeutics*, *5*, 433–442.
39. Greenlee, W., Clader, J., Asberom, T., McCombie, S., Ford, J., Guzik, H., Kozlowski, J., Li, S., Liu, C., Lowe, D., Vice, S., Zhao, H., Zhou, G., Billard, W., Binch, H., Crosby, R., Duffy, R., Lachowicz, J., Coffin, V., Watkins, R., Ruperto, V., Strader, C., Taylor, L., Cox, K. (2001). Muscarinic agonists and antagonists in the treatment of Alzheimer's disease. *Farmaco*, *56*, 247–250.
40. Tzavara, E.T., Bymaster, F.P., Davis, R.J., Wade, M.R., Perry, K.W., Wess, J., McKinzie, D.L., Felder, C., Nomikos, G.G. (2004). M4 muscarinic receptors regulate the dynamics of cholinergic and dopaminergic neurotransmission: relevance to the pathophysiology and treatment of related CNS pathologies. *The FASEB Journal*, *18*, 1410–1412.
41. Chan, W.Y., McKinzie, D.L., Bose, S., Mitchell, S.N., Witkin, J.M., Thompson, R.C., Christopoulos, A., Lazareno, S., Birdsall, N.J., Bymaster, F.P., Felder, C.C. (2008). Allosteric modulation of the muscarinic M4 receptor as an approach to treating schizophrenia. *Proceedings of the National Academy of Sciences of the United States of America*, *105*, 10978–10983.
42. Zhang, W., Yamada, M., Gomeza, J., Basile, A.S., Wess, J. (2002). Multiple muscarinic acetylcholine receptor subtypes modulate striatal dopamine release, as studied with M1-M5 muscarinic receptor knock-out mice. *The Journal of Neuroscience*, *22*, 6347–6352.
43. Wang, H., Ng, K., Hayes, D., Gao, X., Forster, G., Blaha, C., Yeomans, J. (2004). Decreased amphetamine-induced locomotion and improved latent inhibition in mice mutant for the M5 muscarinic receptor gene found in the human 15q schizophrenia region. *Neuropsychopharmacology*, *29*, 2126–2139.

44. Heckers, S., Weiss, A.P., Deckersbach, T., Goff, D.C., Morecraft, R.J., Bush, G. (2004). Anterior cingulate cortex activation during cognitive interference in schizophrenia. *The American Journal of Psychiatry*, *161*, 707–715.
45. Goldman-Rakic, P.S. (1987). Circuitry of the frontal association cortex and its relevance to dementia. [Review] [55 refs]. *Archives of Gerontology and Geriatrics*, *6*, 299–309.
46. Salah-Uddin, H., Thomas, D.R., Davies, C.H., Hagan, J.J., Wood, M.D., Watson, J.M., Challiss, R.A. (2008). Pharmacological assessment of m1 muscarinic acetylcholine receptor-gq/11 protein coupling in membranes prepared from postmortem human brain tissue. *The Journal of Pharmacology and Experimental Therapeutics*, *325*, 869–874.
47. Jerusalinsky, D., Kornisiuk, E., Alfaro, P., Guillfeldt, J., Alonso, M., Rial Verde, E., Cervenansky, C., Harvey, A. (1998). Muscarinic toxin selective for m4 receptors impairs memory in the rat. *Neuroreport: An International Journal for the Rapid Communication of Research in Neuroscience*, *9*, 1407–1411.
48. Sanchez, G., Alvares Lde, O., Oberholzer, M.V., Genro, B., Quillfeldt, J., da Costa, J.C., Cervenansky, C., Jerusalinsky, D., Kornisiuk, E. (2009). M4 muscarinic receptors are involved in modulation of neurotransmission at synapses of Schaffer collaterals on CA1 hippocampal neurons in rats. *Journal of Neuroscience Research*, *87*, 691–700.
49. Rouse, S.T., Marino, M.J., Potter, L.T., Conn, P.J., Levey, A.I. (1999). Muscarinic receptor subtypes involved in hippocampal circuits. *Life Sciences*, *64*, 501–509.
50. Rouse, S.T., Hamilton, S.E., Potter, L.T., Nathanson, N.M., Conn, P.J. (2000). Muscarinic-induced modulation of potassium conductances is unchanged in mouse hippocampal pyramidal cells that lack functional M1 receptors. *Neuroscience Letters*, *278*, 61–64.
51. Jones, C.K., Brady, A.E., Davis, A.A., Xiang, Z., Bubser, M., Tantawy, M.N., Kane, A.S., Bridges, T.M., Kennedy, J.P., Bradley, S.R., Peterson, T.E., Ansari, M.S., Baldwin, R.M., Kessler, R.M., Deutch, A.Y., Lah, J.J., Levey, A.I., Lindsley, C.W., Conn, P.J. (2008). Novel selective allosteric activator of the M1 muscarinic acetylcholine receptor regulates amyloid processing and produces antipsychotic-like activity in rats. *The Journal of Neuroscience*, *28*, 10422–10433.
52. Shirey, J.K., Brady, A.E., Jones, P.J., Davis, A.A., Bridges, T.M., Kennedy, J.P., Jadhav, S.B., Menon, U.N., Xiang, Z., Watson, M.L., Christian, E.P., Doherty, J.J., Quirk, M.C., Snyder, D.H., Lah, J.J., Levey, A.I., Nicolle, M.M., Lindsley, C.W., Conn, P.J. (2009). A selective allosteric potentiator of the M1 muscarinic acetylcholine receptor increases activity of medial prefrontal cortical neurons and restores impairments in reversal learning. *The Journal of Neuroscience*, *29*, 14271–14286.
53. Lewis, L.M., Sheffler, D., Williams, R., Bridges, T.M., Kennedy, J.P., Brogan, J.T., Mulder, M.J., Williams, L., Nalywajko, N.T., Niswender, C.M., Weaver, C.D., Conn, P.J., Lindsley, C.W. (2008). Synthesis and SAR of selective muscarinic acetylcholine receptor subtype 1 (M1 mAChR) antagonists. *Bioorganic & Medicinal Chemistry Letters*, *18*, 885–890.
54. Ito, Y., Oyunzul, L., Seki, M., Fujino Oki, T., Matsui, M., Yamada, S. (2009). Quantitative analysis of the loss of muscarinic receptors in various peripheral tissues in M1-M5 receptor single knockout mice. *British Journal of Pharmacology*, *156*, 1147–1153.

55. Gautam, D., Jeon, J., Li, J.H., Han, S.J., Hamdan, F.F., Cui, Y., Lu, H., Deng, C., Gavrilova, O., Wess, J. (2008). Metabolic roles of the M3 muscarinic acetylcholine receptor studied with M3 receptor mutant mice: a review. *Journal of Receptor and Signal Transduction Research*, *28*, 93–108.

56. Stengel, P.W., Cohen, M.L. (2002). Muscarinic receptor knockout mice: role of muscarinic acetylcholine receptors M(2), M(3), and M(4) in carbamylcholine-induced gallbladder contractility. *The Journal of Pharmacology and Experimental Therapeutics*, *301*, 643–650.

57. Tzavara, E.T., Bymaster, F.P., Felder, C.C., Wade, M., Gomeza, J., Wess, J., McKinzie, D.L., Nomikos, G.G. (2003). Dysregulated hippocampal acetylcholine neurotransmission and impaired cognition in M2, M4 and M2/M4 muscarinic receptor knockout mice. *Molecular Psychiatry*, *8*, 673–679.

58. Carey, G.J., Billard, W., Binch, H. 3rd, Cohen-Williams, M., Crosby, G., Grzelak, M., Guzik, H., Kozlowski, J.A., Lowe, D.B., Pond, A.J., Tedesco, R.P., Watkins, R.W., Coffin, V.L. (2001). SCH 57790, a selective muscarinic M(2) receptor antagonist, releases acetylcholine and produces cognitive enhancement in laboratory animals. *European Journal of Pharmacology*, *431*, 189–200.

59. Rowe, W.B., O'Donnell, J.P., Pearson, D., Rose, G.M., Meaney, M.J., Quirion, R. (2003). Long-term effects of BIBN-99, a selective muscarinic M2 receptor antagonist, on improving spatial memory performance in aged cognitively impaired rats. *Behavioural Brain Research*, *145*, 171–178.

60. Tombaugh, G.C., Rowe, W.B., Chow, A.R., Michael, T.H., Rose, G.M. (2002). Theta-frequency synaptic potentiation in CA1 in vitro distinguishes cognitively impaired from unimpaired aged Fischer 344 rats. [References]. *The Journal of Neuroscience*, *22*(22), 9932–9940.

61. Yasuda, R.P., Ciesla, W., Flores, L.R., Wall, S.J., Li, M., Satkus, S.A., Weisstein, J.S., Spagnola, B.V., Wolfe, B.B. (1993). Development of antisera selective for m4 and m5 muscarinic cholinergic receptors: distribution of m4 and m5 receptors in rat brain. *Molecular Pharmacology*, *43*, 149–157.

62. Vilaro, M.T., Palacios, J.M., Mengod, G. (1990). Localization of m5 muscarinic receptor mRNA in rat brain examined by in situ hybridization histochemistry. *Neuroscience Letters*, *114*, 154–159.

63. Eglen, R.M., Nahorski, S.R. (2000). The muscarinic M(5) receptor: a silent or emerging subtype? [Review] [88 refs]. *British Journal of Pharmacology*, *130*, 13–21.

64. Li, Z., Huang, M., Ichikawa, J., Dai, J., Meltzer, H.Y. (2005). N-desmethylclozapine, a major metabolite of clozapine, increases cortical acetylcholine and dopamine release in vivo via stimulation of M1 muscarinic receptors. *Neuropsychopharmacology*, *30*, 1986–1995.

65. Sur, C., Mallorga, P.J., Wittmann, M., Jacobson, M.A., Pascarella, D., Williams, J.B., Brandish, P.E., Pettibone, D.J., Scolnick, E.M., Conn, P.J. (2003). N-desmethylclozapine, an allosteric agonist at muscarinic 1 receptor, potentiates N-methyl-D-aspartate receptor activity. *Proceedings of the National Academy of Sciences of the United States of America*, *100*, 13674–13679.

66. Watson, J., Brough, S., Coldwell, M.C., Gager, T., Ho, M., Hunter, A.J., Jerman, J., Middlemiss, D.N., Riley, G.J., Brown, A.M. (1998). Functional effects of the

muscarinic receptor agonist, xanomeline, at 5-HT1 and 5-HT2 receptors. *British Journal of Pharmacology*, *125*, 1413–1420.

67. Grant, M.K., El-Fakahany, E.E. (2005). Persistent binding and functional antagonism by xanomeline at the muscarinic M5 receptor. *The Journal of Pharmacology and Experimental Therapeutics*, *315*, 313–319.

68. Woolley, M.L., Carter, H.J., Gartlon, J.E., Watson, J.M., Dawson, L.A. (2009). Attenuation of amphetamine-induced activity by the non-selective muscarinic receptor agonist, xanomeline, is absent in muscarinic M4 receptor knockout mice and attenuated in muscarinic M1 receptor knockout mice. *European Journal of Pharmacology*, *603*, 147–149.

69. Shekhar, A., Potter, W.Z., Lightfoot, J., Lienemann, J., Dube, S., Mallinckrodt, C., Bymaster, F.P., McKinzie, D.L., Felder, C.C. (2008). Selective muscarinic receptor agonist xanomeline as a novel treatment approach for schizophrenia. *The American Journal of Psychiatry*, *165*, 1033–1039.

70. Jones, C.K., Brady, A.E., Davis, A.A., Xiang, Z., Bubser, M., Tantawy, M.N., Kane, A.S., Bridges, T.M., Kennedy, J.P., Bradley, S.R., Peterson, T.E., Ansari, M.S., Baldwin, R.M., Kessler, R.M., Deutch, A.Y., Lah, J.J., Levey, A.I., Lindsley, C.W., Conn, P.J. (2008). Novel selective allosteric activator of the M1 muscarinic acetylcholine receptor regulates amyloid processing and produces antipsychotic-like activity in rats. *The Journal of Neuroscience*, *28*, 10422–10433.

71. Lu, Z.L., Saldanha, J.W., Hulme, E.C. (2002). Seven-transmembrane receptors: crystals clarify. [Review] [79 refs]. *Trends in Pharmacological Sciences*, *23*, 140–146.

72. Hulme, E.C., Birdsall, N.J., Buckley, N.J. (1990). Muscarinic receptor subtypes. *Annual Review of Pharmacology and Toxicology*, *30*, 633–673.

73. Fisher, A., Karton, Y., Heldman, E., Gurwitz, D., Haring, R., Meshulam, H., Brandeis, R., Pittel, Z., Segall, Y., Marciano, D. (1993). Progress in medicinal chemistry of novel selective muscarinic agonists. [Review] [27 refs]. *Drug Design and Discovery*, *9*, 221–235.

74. Mazucco, R.A., Ognjenovic, M. (1993). American chemical society—225th national meeting neurological disorders 23–27 March 2003, New Orleans, LA, USA. *Current Drugs*, *6*, 407–409.

75. Birdsall, N.J., Lazareno, S. (2005). Allosterism at muscarinic receptors: ligands and mechanisms. *Mini Reviews in Medicinal Chemistry*, *5*, 523–543.

76. May, L.T., Leach, K., Sexton, P.M., Christopoulos, A. (2007). Allosteric modulation of G protein-coupled receptors. *Annual Review of Pharmacology and Toxicology*, *47*, 1–51.

77. Hollinshead, S.P., Huff, B.E., Hughes, P.F., Mendoza, J.S., Mitch, C.H., Staszak, M.A., Ward, J.S., Wilson, J.W. (1997) Preparation of indanes as antipsychotics. Patent application WO97-US997 970122. *Chem. Abstr. 127*, 176278.

78. Hansen, M.M., Border, S.S., Clayton, M.T., Heath, P.C., Kolis, S.P., Larsen, S.D., Linder, R.J., Reutzel-Edens, S.M., Smith, J.C., Tameze, S.L., Ward, J.A., Weigel L O. (2008). Development of a practical synthesis of an aminoindanol-derived M1 agonist. *Organic Process Research & Development*, *13*, 198–208.

79. Watt, M.L., Schober, D.A., Hitchcock, S., Liu, B., Chesterfield, A.K., McKinzie, D.L., Felder, C.C. (2011) Pharmacological characterization of LY593093, an M1

muscarinic acetylcholine receptor-selective partial orthosteric agonist. *Journal of Pharmacology and Experimental Therapeutics 338*, 662–632.

80. Bush, J.K., Heath, P.C. (2004) PCT Int. Appl. WO 2004018411 A1.
81. Allen, J.R., Hitchcock, S.A., Liu, B., Turner, W.W., Jamison, J.A. (2003) PCT Int. Appl. WO2003027061 A2.
82. Andersson, C.A., Frierg, B.M., Skjaerbaek, N., Spalding, T., Uldam, A.K. (2001) PCT Int. Appl. WO 2001083472 A1.
83. Kelly, N.M., Koch, K.N., Tolf, B. (2003) PCT Int. Appl. WO 2003028650 A2.
84. Skjaerbaek, N.K., Kristian, N., Friberg, B.L.M., Tolf, B.-R. (2005) Preparation of tetrahydroquinoline analogs such as benzoxazinones as muscarinic agonists useful against mental and other disorders. *U.S. Pat. Appl. Publ. 74 pp., Cont.-in-part of U.S. Ser. No. 329,455. CODEN: USXXCO.* US 2005209226 A1; 20050922; CAN 143:326374; AN 2005:1026605.
85. Copper, D.G., Forbes, I.T., Garzya, V., Jin, J., Louchart, Y., Walker, G., Wyman, P.A. (2007) PCT Int. Appl. WO 2007107565 A1; WO 2007107566 A1; WO 2007107567 A1.
86. Budzik, B., Cooper, D.G., Forbes, I.T., Jin, J., Shi, D., Smith, P.W., Walker, G. (2007) PCT Int. Appl. WO 2007036711 A1.
87. Budzik, B., Cooper, D.G., Forbes, I.T., Garzya, V., Jin, J., Shi, D., Smith, P.W., Walker, G. (2007) PCT Int. Appl. WO 2007036781 A2.
88. Cheng, Y., Mehrnaz, P., Tomaszewski, M. (2007) PCT Int. Appl. WO 2007142583.
89. Cheng, Y., Mehrnaz, P., Tomaszewski, M. (2007) PCT Int. Appl. WO 2007142585.
90. Copper, D.G., Forbes, I.T., Garzya, V., Johnson, D.J., Stevenson, G.I., Wyman, P.A. (2009) PCT Int. Appl. WO 2009037296.
91. Buffat, M., Thomas, E., Davis, R.H. (2005) PCT Int. Appl. WO 2005054242.
92. Brann, M., Messier, T., Currier, E., Duggento, K., Spalding, T., Friberg, M., Skjaerback, N. (2003) US 6, 528, 529 B1.
93. Cao, Y., Zhang, M., Wu, C., Lee, S., Wroblewski, M.E., Whipple, T., Nagy, P.I., Takacs-Novak, K., Balazs, A., Toros, S., Messer, W.S. Jr (2003). Synthesis and biological characterization of 1-methyl-1,2,5,6-tetrahydropyridyl-1,2,5-thiadiazole derivatives as muscarinic agonists for the treatment of neurological disorders. *Journal of Medicinal Chemistry*, *46*, 4273–4286.
94. Messer, W.S., Cao, Y., Tejada, F.R. (2007) PCT Int. Appl. WO 2007075297 A2.
95. Messer, W.S., Tejada, F.R. (2008) PCT Int. Appl. WO 2008118326 A1.
96. Budzik, B., Garzya, V., Shi, D., Walker, G., Wooley-Roberts, M., Pardoe, J., Lucas, A., Tehan, B., Rivero, R.A., Langmead, C.J., Watson, J., Wu, Z., Forbes, I.T., Jin, J. (2010) Novel N-substituted benzimidazolones as potent, selective, CNS-penetrant, and orally active M1 mAChR agonists. *ACS Medicinal Chemistry Letters*, *1*, 244–248.
97. Nathan, J., Watson, J., Lund, J., Peters, G.L., Dodds, C.M., Lawrence, P., Bentley, G.D., O'Neill, B.V., Robertson, J., Maruff, P., Laruelle, M., Bullmore, E.T. (2011) The potent M1 receptor allosteric agonist GSK1034702 improves episodic memory in the nicotine abstinence model of cognitive dysfunction in humans. *Neuropsychopharmacology*, *36*, S236–S237.

98. Swanson, C.J., Bures, M., Johnson, M.P., Linden, A.M., Monn, J.A., Schoepp, D.D. (2005). Metabotropic glutamate receptors as novel targets for anxiety and stress disorders. [Review] [131 refs]. *Nature Reviews Drug Discovery*, *4*, 131–144.

99. Fredrik, E., Olsson, R., Ohlsson, J. (2005) PCT Int. Appl. WO2005063254.

100. Shipe, W.D., Lindsley, C., Hallett, D.P.I.A.W. (2007) PCT Int. Appl. WO2007067489.

101. Kudul, S.D., Chang, R.K. (2009) PCT Int. Appl. WO2009051715.

102. Ray, W.J., Seager, M., Ma, L., Wittmann, M., Getty, K., Marlatt, M., Crouthamel, M-C., Wu, G., Sankaranarayananan, S., Simon, A., Burno, M., Jones, K., Graufields, V.K., Bickel, D., Posavec, D., Cook, J., Veng, L., Kuduk, S., Sur, C., Shipe, W., Lindsley, C., Kinney, G., Pascarella, D., Jacobson, M., Seabrook, G.,(2008) Allosteric potentiation of the M1 muscarinic receptors provides unprecedented selectivity and a novel therapeutic strategy for the treatment of Alzheimer's disease. *Alzheimer's and Dementia*, *4*, T761.

103. Marlo, J.E., Niswender, C.M., Days, E.L., Bridges, T.M., Xiang, Y., Rodriguez, A.L., Shirey, J.K., Brady, A.E., Nalywajko, T., Luo, Q., Austin, C.A., Williams, M.B., Kim, K., Williams, R., Orton, D., Brown, H.A., Lindsley, C.W., Weaver, C.D., Conn, P.J. (2009). Discovery and characterization of novel allosteric potentiators of M1 muscarinic receptors reveals multiple modes of activity. *Molecular Pharmacology*, *75*, 577–588.

104. Thomas, R.L., Mistry, R., Langmead, C.J., Wood, M.D., Challiss, R.A. (2008). G protein coupling and signaling pathway activation by m1 muscarinic acetylcholine receptor orthosteric and allosteric agonists. *The Journal of Pharmacology and Experimental Therapeutics*, *327*, 365–374.

105. Miller, N.R., Daniels, R.N., Bridges, T.M., Brady, A.E., Conn, P.J., Lindsley, C.W. (2008). Synthesis and SAR of analogs of the M1 allosteric agonist TBPB. Part II: amides, sulfonamides and ureas—the effect of capping the distal basic piperidine nitrogen. *Bioorganic & Medicinal Chemistry Letters*, *18*, 5443–5447.

106. Bridges, T.M., Brady, A.E., Kennedy, J.P., Daniels, R.N., Miller, N.R., Kim, K., Breininger, M.L., Gentry, P.R., Brogan, J.T., Jones, C.K., Conn, P.J., Lindsley, C.W. (2008). Synthesis and SAR of analogues of the M1 allosteric agonist TBPB. Part I: exploration of alternative benzyl and privileged structure moieties. *Bioorganic & Medicinal Chemistry Letters*, *18*, 5439–5442.

107. Langmead, C.J., Austin, N.E., Branch, C.L., Brown, J.T., Buchanan, K.A., Davies, C.H., Forbes, I.T., Fry, V.A., Hagan, J.J., Herdon, H.J., Jones, G.A., Jeggo, R., Kew, J.N., Mazzali, A., Melarange, R., Patel, N., Pardoe, J., Randall, A.D., Roberts, C., Roopun, A., Starr, K.R., Teriakidis, A., Wood, M.D., Whittington, M., Wu, Z., Watson, J. (2008). Characterization of a CNS penetrant, selective M1 muscarinic receptor agonist, 77-LH-28-1. *British Journal of Pharmacology*, *154*, 1104–1115.

108. Spalding, T.A., Trotter, C., Skjaerbaek, N., Messier, T.L., Currier, E.A., Burstein, E.S., Li, D., Hacksell, U., Brann, M.R. (2002). Discovery of an ectopic activation site on the M(1) muscarinic receptor. *Molecular Pharmacology*, *61*, 1297–1302.

109. Lebon, G., Langmead, C.J., Tehan, B.G., Hulme, E.C. (2009). Mutagenic mapping suggests a novel binding mode for selective agonists of M1 muscarinic acetylcholine receptors. *Molecular Pharmacology*, *75*, 331–341.

110. Shirey, J.K., Xiang, Z., Orton, D., Brady, A.E., Johnson, K.A., Williams, R., Ayala, J.E., Rodriguez, A.L., Wess, J., Weaver, D., Niswender, C.M., Conn, P.J. (2008). An

allosteric potentiator of M4 mAChR modulates hippocampal synaptic transmission. *Nature Chemical Biology*, *4*, 42–50.

111. Brady, A.E., Jones, C.K., Bridges, T.M., Kennedy, J.P., Thompson, A.D., Heiman, J.U., Breininger, M.L., Gentry, P.R., Yin, H., Jadhav, S.B., Shirey, J.K., Conn, P.J., Lindsley, C.W. (2008). Centrally active allosteric potentiators of the M4 muscarinic acetylcholine receptor reverse amphetamine-induced hyperlocomotor activity in rats. *The Journal of Pharmacology and Experimental Therapeutics*, *327*, 941–953.
112. Wess, J., Eglen, R.M., Gautam, D. (2007). Muscarinic acetylcholine receptors: mutant mice provide new insights for drug development. [see comment]. *Nature Reviews Drug Discovery*, *6*, 721–733.
113. Bridges, T.M., Marlo, J.E., Niswender, C.M., Jones, C.K., Jadhav, S.B., Gentry, P.R., Plumley, H.C., Weaver, C.D., Conn, P.J., Lindsley, C.W. (2009). Discovery of the first highly M5-preferring muscarinic acetylcholine receptor ligand, an M5 positive allosteric modulator derived from a series of 5-trifluoromethoxy N-benzyl isatins. *Journal of Medicinal Chemistry*, *52*, 3445–3448.

# 14

# WILL MODULATION OF NEUROPEPTIDE RECEPTORS PRODUCE THE NEXT GENERATION OF ANTIPSYCHOTIC DRUGS? A FOCUS ON THE NEUROKININ AND NEUROTENSIN SYSTEMS

LEE A. DAWSON, PAUL W. SMITH, AND JEANNETTE M. WATSON

## 14.1 INTRODUCTION

The dopaminergic and glutamatergic hypotheses have dominated and continue to dominate antipsychotic drug discovery strategies [1, 2]. The dopamine (DA) hypothesis states that hyperactivity of the mesolimbic dopaminergic pathway is associated with positive symptoms of the disease, whereas hypoactivity of the mesocortical dopaminergic pathway is associated with the negative and cognitive symptoms. Increasing evidence has also suggested that hypoactivity in the corticolimbic glutamatergic system may contribute to the complex interplay between dysfunctional aspects of these neurotransmitter systems, which could account for much of the symptomatology observed in schizophrenia [3]. Current antipsychotic drugs, whether from the "typical" (i.e., dopamine 2/3 receptor [$D_{2/3}R$] antagonist) or the newer "atypical" class (i.e., $D_{2/3}R$ antagonist + 5-$HT_2R$ antagonist), target the monoaminergic systems as a means of intervening in some of these abnormal processes and, thus, treating

*Targets and Emerging Therapies for Schizophrenia*, First Edition.
Edited by Jeffrey S. Albert and Michael W. Wood.

the various symptoms of the disease. However, even the newer atypical antipsychotic drugs display moderate efficacy in treating the positive symptoms and limited efficacy against the negative, cognitive, or other comorbid symptoms of the disease. They are also associated with tolerability issues such as extrapyramidal side effects (EPS) and associated movement disorders and metabolic disturbances (as highlighted by the recent CATIE [Clinical Antipsychotic Trials of Intervention Effectiveness]; [4]) study. Thus, pharmacologies that are able to more selectively modulate the underlying neuronal substrates of schizophrenia may have utility as efficacious and wide spectrum antipsychotic therapies with potentially improved side effect burden. The neuropeptide neuromodulator/neurotransmitter class has been suggested to be one such class. Here, we will summarize those particular neuropeptide ligands and their associated receptors that have been researched or investigated and review the literature findings reported thus far. We will focus in detail on both the neurokinin and the neurotensin systems as these are areas that have shown particular promise. We will provide an introduction to both ligands and receptors and review current preclinical understanding of their putative biological roles and, in particular, their modulatory roles in the circuitry pertinent to schizophrenia. As these are areas that have attracted significant drug development interest, a review of the available chemical strategies employed to produce selective tools and drug development candidates will be undertaken. Finally, we will summarize the available clinical information on those compounds that have progressed into patient populations, and evaluate their potential therapeutic utility.

## 14.2 BACKGROUND

Schizophrenia is a devastating chronic mental disorder that, according to the National Institute of Mental Health (NIMH), affects approximately 1% of the population. Its onset usually occurs during early adulthood and those suffering from the disease typically experience a life-long pattern of acute psychotic episodes superimposed upon chronically poor psychosocial adjustment, with only one in five of affected individuals making a full recovery. Schizophrenic symptoms are subdivided into four distinct domains, referred to as positive (e.g., delusions, hallucinations, disorganized speech and behaviour), negative (e.g., social withdrawal, avolition, blunted affect), cognitive (e.g., impaired sustained attention, executive function, and working memory), and affective (e.g., anxiety/depression, hostility/aggression, increased risk of suicide) symptoms. These occur in different combinations and to different degrees in each patient. As such, schizophrenia is a complex and highly heterogeneous disorder for which there is no common identifiable pathology and for which the etiology is poorly understood. Genetic factors appear to provide a significant contribution to the neurodevelopmental disturbances that generate the abnormalities in synaptic stabilization and connectivity that are believed to underlie the clinical disease manifestations. The condition is thought to be polygenic, and while numerous susceptibility genes have been identified, replications of these findings have frequently failed, even in the case of neuregulin-1 (NRG1), the best replicated schizophrenia susceptibility gene to date. As such, many of the treatment strategies that are being developed for schizophrenia still rely on exploiting cellular mechanisms that fit within the framework of the DA- and glutamate neurotransmitter-based theories of schizophrenia [1, 2].

Of these, DA dysfunction was the first hypothesis to be proposed on the basis that (1) established antipsychotic drugs (i.e., $D_{2/3}$ receptor antagonists or partial agonists) directly reduce dopamine $D_2$ receptor function at clinically effective exposures and (2) amphetamine, which acts to release DA, exacerbates the positive symptoms of the disease. Conceptually, hyperactivity of the mesolimbic dopaminergic pathway is believed to cause the positive symptoms of the disease, a suggestion that is strongly supported by positron emission tomography (PET) imaging studies which demonstrated that an amphetamine challenge released more DA in the striatum of patients with schizophrenia compared with healthy individuals [5]. In contrast, the negative and cognitive symptoms of the disease are believed to arise from hypoactivity of the mesocortical dopaminergic pathway.

The glutamate hypothesis of schizophrenia suggests that hypoactivity in the corticolimbic glutamatergic system underlies the disease. A recent biochemical study [6] has provided the first direct evidence of potential N-methyl-D-aspartate (NMDA) receptor hypofunction. Specifically NRG1-mediated suppression of NMDA receptor function (possibly via enhanced activation of ErbB4) was enhanced in postmortem prefrontal cortex from schizophrenic subjects relative to healthy controls. Furthermore, both phencyclidine (PCP) and ketamine, which block the NMDA subtype of ionotropic glutamate receptor, exacerbate schizophrenic symptoms and induce schizophrenic-like psychotic states and impairments in cognitive performance in healthy individuals. Dopaminergic and hypoglutamatergic deficits are not necessarily independent of one another and schizophrenic symptoms may reflect complex dysfunctional interplay between these neurotransmitter systems [7, 8]. Imaging data suggest that dopaminergic dysregulation could be secondary to synaptic dysconnectivity in the prefrontal cortex and that a deficit in glutamatergic neurotransmission leading to excessive subcortical dopaminergic activity may, in turn, exacerbate the glutamate deficit, leading to a further reduction in neuronal connectivity and plasticity. As such, pharmacological strategies that target the dysfunctions in either, or both, of these neurotransmitter systems are likely to provide significant benefit to patients with schizophrenia.

Current antipsychotic drugs, whether from the "typical" (i.e., $D_{2/3}R$ antagonists such as haloperidol, chlorpromazine, thioridazine) or the newer "atypical" class (i.e., $D_{2/3}R$ antagonist + 5-$HT_2R$ antagonist, such as clozapine, olanzapine, risperidone, ziprasidone, and aripiprazole) target the monoaminergic system as a means of intervening in some of these abnormal processes and, thus, treating the various symptoms of the disease. However, both classes of drug display only moderate efficacy in treating the positive symptoms and little, or no, efficacy against the negative and cognitive symptoms [9] of the disease. Furthermore, a number of patients with schizophrenia are resistant to both typical and atypical antipsychotics. Moreover, there is still relatively little evidence to suggest that atypical antipsychotic drugs provide a better functional outcome for patients than do typical antipsychotic drugs [10], an observation highlighted by the recent NIMH-sponsored CATIE [4] trial, which demonstrated little improvement in the efficacy of atypical over the typical antipsychotic drugs. Furthermore, both classes of antipsychotic drug produced significant side effects (typical antipsychotic drugs inducing hyperprolactinemia and EPS, whereas atypical antipsychotic drugs caused significant weight gain and metabolic disturbances) that contributed to the lack of compliance. Thus, in the CATIE trial, on average 74% of the 1493 patients enrolled in the study discontinued their treatment within 18 months mainly because of a lack of efficacy or the induction of intolerable side effects. These findings have largely been confirmed by the CUtLASS (Cost Utility of the Latest Antipsychotic Drugs in Severe Schizophrenia; [11]; [12]) study performed in the UK. Schizophrenia, thus, remains a relatively poorly treated disease, and there is an immediate need to develop more efficacious drugs with improved tolerability profiles.

The neuropeptide neuromodulator/neurotransmitter family of receptors has been suggested, due to their interaction and/or modulation of both glutamate and DA systems, to be suitable targets for potential therapeutic agents for schizophrenia and related disorders. A number of specific targets have been mooted to have potential for antipsychotic therapy and some have indeed shown some clinical proof of concept. One example is cholecystokinin (CCK), a peptide originally identified from the gut and subsequently shown to be a brain neurotransmitter primarily acting though $CCK_A$ and $CCK_B$ receptor subtypes (for review see Reference [13]). Behavioral, neurochemical, and electrophysiological studies have demonstrated the modulatory role of CCK, via both receptor subtypes, on central dopaminergic function and production of "neuroleptic-like" effects versus DA-driven behaviors (for review of preclinical observations see Reference [14]). As a consequence, this led to the speculation that CCK may play a role in the pathophysiology of schizophrenia [15, 16]. Support for this idea came from studies demonstrating reduced CCK levels in the cerebrospinal fluid (CSF) [17] and postmortem brains [18] of drug-naïve patients with schizophrenia. The hypothesis was tested in a series of clinical trials, and although 500 patients received CCK, its efficacy in the treatment of schizophrenia was equivocal (for review see Reference [19]).

The cannabanoid (CB) receptor subfamily has also received significant focus as a novel antipsychotic target. It is believed that many of the pharmacological effects of marijuana are mediated through the $CB_1$ and $CB_2$ receptors and that dysfunction of the endogenous CB system may play a role in the manifestation of at least some of the symptoms of schizophrenia (for review see Reference [20]). In support of this concept, it has been observed that the endogenous CBs anandamine and palmitoylethanolamide were increased in the CSF of patients with schizophrenia. Furthermore $CB_1$ receptor agonists have been shown to activate mesolimbic dopaminergic neurons [21], which has led to the hypothesis that antagonists of this receptor may have antipsychotic efficacy. SR141716 is a selective $CB_1$ receptor antagonist presumably developed to test this hypothesis. Its detailed pharmacology has been reported [22, 23] and it has been demonstrated to antagonize psychostimulant-induced behavior. The clinical efficacy of this molecule was examined by Meltzer and colleagues [24] in a novel trial that examined multiple novel therapeutics in schizophrenic and schizoaffective disorder patients. Despite haloperidol producing efficacy across a number of measures and a number of the novel mechanisms also showing some promising outcomes (see later), a positive signal was not attained with SR141716. Therefore, clinical support for the target has not been achieved to date.

CCK and cannabinoid receptors are obviously not the only examples of neuropeptide targets that may be useful in the treatment of schizophrenia and related disorders (e.g., the orexin/hypocretin systems [25]) but are two families that have undergone some clinical evaluation (unfortunately unsuccessfully). Two further examples that have undergone extensive preclinical evaluation and have also been evaluated in multiple clinical trials, with some success, are the neurokinin (NK)/tachykinin and neurotensin (NT) receptor subfamilies, and these will be the subject of this review, with a particular focus on the $NK_3$ receptors and a current opinion on NT receptors.

## 14.3 THE TACHYKININ/NEUROKININ FAMILY

The tachykinin peptide neurotransmitter/neuromodulator family comprises three main neuropeptides—substance P (SP), neurokinin A (NKA), and neurokinin B (NKB). Each tachykinin shares a common amino acid sequence at their carboxy terminal region and is a full agonist at each of the three family 1 (rhodopsin-like) seven transmembrane $G_q$-protein coupled neurokinin receptors; neurokinin-1 ($NK_1$), neurokinin-2 ($NK_2$), and neurokinin-3 ($NK_3$). Each tachykinin displays quite distinct rank orders of potency of activation across the three NK receptor subtypes such that SP primarily selects for $NK_1$ receptors, NKA for $NK_2$ receptors, and NKB for $NK_3$ receptors (Table 14.1). However, as can be seen from the affinities, there is potential cross reactivity within the family depending on localization and concentrations of endogenously released tachykinin.

Distribution also varies between the three receptor subtypes, which potentially underlies their diverse physiological roles. $NK_1$ receptors are expressed throughout the body, for example, in neurons, vascular endothelial cells, muscle, and a variety of immune cells [26]. The human brain distribution pattern of $NK_1$ receptors (striatum, cortex, and limbic areas such as the insula and

**TABLE 14.1 Peptide Sequences and NK Receptor Subtype Affinities (nM) of the Major Tachykinin Neuropeptides**

| | Peptide Sequence | $NK_1$ | $NK_2$ | $NK_3$ |
|---|---|---|---|---|
| Substance P | Arg-Pro-Lys-Pro-Gln-Gln-Phe-Phe-Gly-Leu- Met.$NH_2$ | **2.8** | 129 | 1292 |
| Neurokinin A | His-Lys-Thr-Asp-Ser-Phe-Val-Gly-Leu-Met.$NH_2$ | 539 | **0.8** | 647 |
| Neurokinin B | Asp-Met-His-Asp-Phe-Phe-Val-Gly-Leu-Met.$NH_2$ | 554 | 16.5 | **0.8** |

For each ligand its highest affinity for an NK receptor subtype is highlighted in bold. Data adapted from Reference [49].

cingulate cortices, hippocampus, dorsal raphe, locus coeruleus, and various nuclei of the amygdala) [27–30] is consistent with their potential role in affective disorders, and indeed ligands targeted at this receptor have been developed for the potential treatment of anxiety and depression (for review see [31]). $NK_2$ receptors are largely expressed within the periphery, in particular in the gastrointestinal (GI) tract controlling smooth muscle contraction, with very low levels in the brain. This has led to much therapeutic focus on this receptor for GI-related disorders. However, it is interesting in light of this low central nervous system (CNS) expression that antagonists of $NK_2$ receptors appear to produce efficacy in preclinical models of anxiety [32] and have shown efficacy in depression. In this regard, saredutant (SR489686, [33]), a selective $NK_2$ receptor antagonist, has been reported to have shown efficacy in two of four Phase III clinical trials in major depressive disorder (MDD) although development of this compound has recently been discontinued (Pharmaprojects 2010). In contrast, $NK_3$ receptors are localized in mammalian central, peripheral, and enteric nervous systems. In the mammalian CNS, $NK_3$ receptors are expressed within medial prefrontal cortex (mPFC), thalamus, and amygdala, while their presence in midbrain dopaminergic nuclei and a suggested role in modulating central monoaminergic systems has led to the proposition that $NK_3$ receptors may be a potential therapeutic intervention point for the treatment of psychotic disorders such as schizophrenia.

### 14.3.1 $NK_3$ Receptors

The $NK_3$ receptor is expressed almost exclusively within the mammalian nervous system, irrespective of the species studied. However there are conflicting reports on the neuroanatomical location of $NK_3$ receptors across species ([29, 34, 35]). Generally within the mammalian brain, $NK_3$ receptor mRNA and protein are consistently detected in the frontal, parietal and cingulate cortices, amygdala, hippocampus, substantia nigra (SN), ventral tegmental area (VTA), raphe nucleus, locus ceruleus (LC), and both septal and basal nuclei ([34, 36, 37]. However, interspecies variation in this $NK_3$ receptor localization and function has added to the complexity of unraveling $NK_3$ receptor biology. For example, $NK_3$ receptors are distributed in the medial and deep layer structures of the cortex, hypothalamus, and midbrain dopaminergic structures such as the SN and VTA of the rat. In the guinea pig, distribution in mid- and deep layer cortical structures is largely similar to the rat but differs in the midbrain dopaminergic neurons where $NK_3$ receptor expression has not been detected [38]. However, $NK_3$-mediated functional responses in these nuclei, measured using electrophysiological recordings and subsequent neurochemical output, have been demonstrated [39, 40]. PCR [41] and, more recently, immunocytochemistry techniques [29, 30] have established that $NK_3$ receptors are also expressed, albeit in low abundance, in the primate CNS, and human distribution studies have shown that the deep layer cortical distribution appears to be maintained [37]. However, $NK_3$ receptor expression has not been detected, to date, within human mesencephalic dopaminergic neurons [28, 42]. Thus, in addition to the complications of using preclinical species to evaluate the functional role of the $NK_3$ receptors, there is also some controversy with regard to the specific localization and density of $NK_3$ receptors within the human brain [36]. In this regard, our own studies, using autoradiographic and immunohistochemical techniques, have detected widespread but low level expression of the $NK_3$ receptors within the human brain (unpublished data). A further added complication is the different protein sequence homology between species. The $NK_3$ receptor protein consists of 440–470 amino acids (human = 465 rat = 452, and guinea pig = 440), and although sequence homology across species is generally high (>90%), small differences in amino acid sequence in transmembrane domain II markedly affect the cross-species affinity of ligands for this receptor [43]. Thus, while gerbil and guinea pig $NK_3$ receptor affinities tend to agree well with human, affinity for the rat $NK_3$ receptor is generally at least one order of magnitude lower. This has precluded the evaluation of $NK_3$ receptor ligands in many of the preclinical rodent models of antipsychotic activity (e.g., rat amphetamine-induced locomotor activity) and has necessitated the development of new gerbil and guinea pig based *in vivo* assays (see Section 14.3.1).

Consistent with its general localization pattern, $NK_3$ receptor activation stimulates both the noradrenergic and dopaminergic neurotransmitter systems, augmenting noradrenergic [44] and dopaminergic cell firing [39] in the locus ceruleus and VTAs, respectively. These actions are thought to account, at least in part, for senktide-induced increases in extracellular DA levels in the nucleus accumbens and striatum [40, 45, 46] and increases in noradrenaline levels in the mPFC [44, 47]. Conversely, $NK_3$ receptor antagonists attenuated haloperidol-induced A9/A10 dopaminergic cell firing [48] as well as haloperidol-stimulated DA efflux (arising from dopamine $D_2$ autoreceptor blockade), although they do not affect basal extracellular DA levels or cell firing per se [49, 50]. Furthermore, in freely moving guinea pigs, $NK_3$ receptor antagonism produced similar increases in both DA (PFC) and noradrenaline (PFC and hippocampus) levels to those induced by the atypical antipsychotic drug clozapine [50]. Beyond the monoaminergic system, $NK_3$ receptors have been demonstrated to regulate γ-aminobutyric (GABA)ergic neurotransmission [46] and colocalization studies in the rat indicate that $NK_3$ receptors are expressed on GABAergic interneurons of basal ganglia nuclei including striatum, globus pallidus, ventral pallidum, and substantia inominata [46, 51]. Furthermore, subpopulations of basal ganglia GABAergic neurons appear to send projections to the cerebral cortex [51]. Interestingly, a proportion of these GABAergic neurons are parvalbumin positive, and this subpopulation of interneurons have been implicated in the pathophysiology of schizophrenia (for review see Reference [52]). Functional evaluation of $NK_3$ receptors, using electrophysiological techniques in rat entorhinal cortex [53], gerbil cingulate cortex [54] and guinea pig PFC [55], have all demonstrated that these receptors appear to also play an excitatory role in modulating cortical glutamatergic neurotransmission irrespective of species. Finally, $NK_3$ receptor activation has also been suggested to increase 5-HT tone at 5-$HT_{1A}$ and 5-$HT_{2A}$ receptors through modulation of serotoninergic synaptic transmission and to increase the release/efflux of acetylcholine (ACh) in the hippocampus, striatum, and nucleus accumbens [40, 45].

Clearly $NK_3$ receptors appear to have diverse modulatory roles on a number of key neurotransmitter systems and many if not all of these have been mooted to be involved in the pathophysiology of schizophrenia. The "dopamine hypothesis of schizophrenia" [3] has proposed that a hyperactivity in mesolimbic projection systems underlies the positive symptoms of the disorder, while a hypofunctionality in mesocortical projections may result in negative and cognitive symptoms. Therefore, simplistically, since $NK_3$ receptor antagonists appear to attenuate subcortical while enhancing cortical DA output [50], one may conclude that this would provide therapeutic benefits in the treatment of the positive, negative, and the cognitive symptoms of schizophrenia. Clearly our understanding of the underlying neurochemical framework of this disease has progressed markedly in recent years with the repetition of genetic findings [1] and recent demonstration of clinical efficacy of non-DA-based therapeutics [56, 57]. Accordingly, a circuitry-based "disinhibition theory" has been proposed (recently reviewed in Reference [58]), which focuses on GABAergic interneuron/glutamatergic pyramidal neuronal interfaces and specifically on a dysfunction in the NMDA receptors on these interneurons. These circuits subsequently regulate multiple other neurotransmitter systems including DA. Although it is not entirely clear at present where $NK_3$ receptors specifically lie within these circuits, the information we have to date suggests they may have a modulatory role on at least some of the key facets of this theory (i.e., pyramidal neurons and GABAergic interneuron activity). If the effects seen in preclinical species (highlighted previously) translate into man, it is feasible that $NK_3$ receptor intervention may have therapeutic efficacy against a number of the symptom domains of schizophrenia via modulation of multiple neurotransmitter systems. A discussion of the current clinical findings using $NK_3$ receptor selective ligands will be presented later in this review.

Interestingly the evaluation of $NK_3$ receptor modulation in the "classical antipsychotic" behavioural models has been somewhat limited. The reason for this is probably twofold: first, the distribution of the receptor from rodent to man can be quite different (as highlighted above), and second the affinity of many of the newer small molecule ligands can be much reduced in those rodent species traditionally used for the preclinical evaluation of antipsychotic activity. Thus, the therapeutic predictive validity and translation of these mechanistic signals from rodents to man may be questionable. That said, there are data, if somewhat mixed, on the effects of either $NK_3$ receptor gene deletion or selective ligands in various behavioral paradigms. Data on two independently derived knockout mice have recently been reported. Siuciak and coworkers [59] demonstrated that in several tests, including spontaneous locomotor activity, elevated plus maze, forced swim, and hot plate, wild-type, and knockout mice performed similarly. However, in several cognition tests, including passive avoidance, acquisition of conditioned avoidance responding (CAR), and the Morris water maze (MWM), $NK_3$ receptor knockout mice displayed deficits in both acquisition and retention compared with wild-type mice. In contrast, Nordquist et al. [60] evaluated their mice in delayed matching to position (DMTP), spontaneous alternation, MWM and active avoidance, and demonstrated an improved operant performance (but not working memory per se in the DMTP) and a more rapid response latency. No difference in MWM performance was seen in this study. A follow-on study [61] demonstrated no overt change in behavioral responsiveness to amphetamine and some quite subtle changes in markers of DA function in these mice. As highlighted, the extrapolation of data generated in mice to the human is very difficult. One could argue that the somewhat enhanced cognitive performance seen in the Nordquist study [60] may also have been observed in the clinical studies with talnetant (see Section 14.3.4). However, the question as to why there are two different profiles in two different knockout animals is somewhat perplexing.

The small molecule $NK_3$ receptor antagonist SR142801 [62] has been shown to attenuate cocaine-induced behavioral activation yet, somewhat paradoxically, potentiated its DA-enhancing action in the nucleus accumbens core of the rat [63]. Interestingly, the attenuation of the psychostimulant-induced behaviour was subsequently repeated in a nonhuman primate (*Callithrix penicillata*; the common marmoset [64]) arguably a more suitable species for examining the role of $NK_3$ receptors in relation to man. Taken together, these data support a modulatory role of $NK_3$ receptors on subcortical dopaminergic neurotransmission. Similarly, in preclinical models of psychosis, SR142801 reversed apomorphine-induced deficits in PPI [65] and partially reversed D-amphetamine induced hyperactivity [66], both in gerbils. Interestingly, there are data (again somewhat mixed) demonstrating effects of $NK_3$ receptor ligands in behavioral models of anxiety. In this regard, SR-142801 has been shown to be efficacious in the gerbil social interaction [67] and rat forced swim test [68] but was without effect in the mouse elevated plus maze (while the

$NK_3$ receptor agonist senktide was anxiolytic; [69]), possibly suggesting utility of this target in anxiety disorders, although clinical evaluation of SR142801 has not confirmed this hypothesis (see Clinical Utility section). Taken together, it is fair to say that the behavioral evaluation of this target, although producing some supportive observations for therapeutic potential, has been less than consistent and it is largely our functional understanding of the target that led to its progression into the clinical arena.

### 14.3.2 Ligands for the $NK_3$ Receptor

There is an extensive literature detailing many $NK_3$ receptor ligands including both peptide agonists and nonpeptide antagonists (for further details see Reference [70] and references therein). This section therefore represents a brief overview of the most significant compounds described to date.

*Agonists* A number of naturally occurring nonmammalian tachykinin peptides such as eledoisin (originally isolated from Octopus salivary gland) and kassinin (isolated from the skin of the African frog *Kassina senegalensis*) are potent $NK_3$ receptor agonists and have been used experimentally. However, these generally show limited selectivity across the tachykinin receptor subtypes [70] although overall receptor subtype selectivity is often complicated due to interspecies differences in neurokinin receptor sequence [71, 72]. Systematic modification of several of the endogenous tachykinins has been carried out and the residues critical for subtype selectivity identified. This has led to the development of a number of novel selective agonist peptides. Of relevance here is the work carried out on both NKB and SP to generate selective $NK_3$ receptor agonists (Table 14.2). Replacement of Val-7 in NKB with MePhe increases affinity and selectivity for the $NK_3$ receptor. Several important NKB analogs with this modification (full length or truncated at the N-terminal) have been characterized. In an alternative approach, N-methylation of individual residues in SP C-terminal hexapeptide led to the identification of other $NK_3$ receptor-selective agonists including senktide, the most selective ligand to date. As such, senktide and the NKB analogs described have been extensively used in receptor localization and characterization studies (e.g., [73, 74]).

Solution NMR and modeling studies suggest that the N-methylation of the phenyl alanine residue common to all the selective $NK_3$ receptor agonists has a profound effect in restricting the peptide conformation. This may be responsible for the observed receptor selectivity [75, 76].

*Antagonists*

PEPTIDE AND DIPEPTIDE-DERIVED ANTAGONISTS In addition to the discovery of selective agonists, structural modifications to the tachykinin peptides also led to reports of the identification of selective peptide $NK_3$ receptor antagonists including MEN 10295 (Table 3.5) [77, 78] and GR138676 [79]. However,

**TABLE 14.2 Selective Synthetic NK3 Receptor Agonists**

| Agonist | Structure | Comments | Reference |
|---|---|---|---|
| MePhe7 NKB(4-10) | 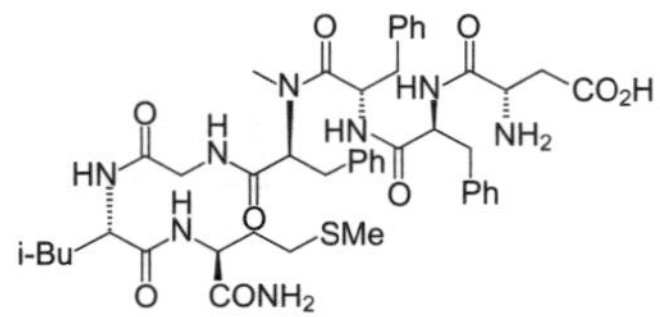 Asp-Phe-Phe-**NMePhe**-Gly-Leu-MetNH$_2$ | Analogs of NKB-(4-10) prepared. Replacement of Val7 with MePhe increased the affinity of NKB-(4-10) for the NKB receptor and conferred marked selectivity. | [179] |
| MePhe7 NKB | Asp-Met-His-Asp-Phe-Phe-**NMePhe**-Gly-Leu-Met-NH$_2$ | Selectivity and affinity for NKB receptors is markedly increased when Val7 is replaced with MePhe in both the fragment NKB (4-10) and NKB. | [180] |
| [$^{125}$I]iodohistidyl, [MePhe7] Neurokinin B | 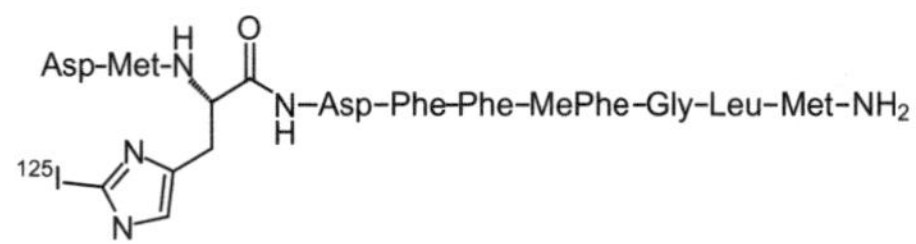 | High-affinity NK$_3$ receptor radioligand | [181] |
| Senktide | 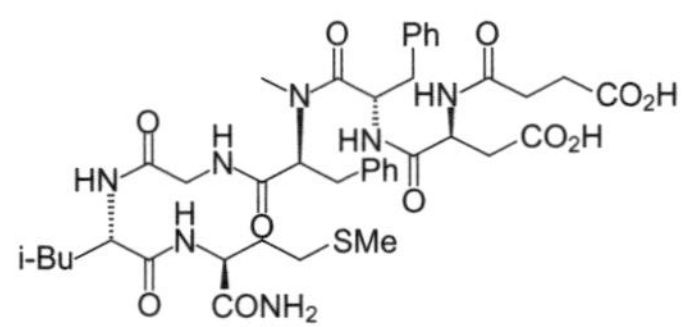 SuccinylAsp-Phe-**NMePh**-Gly-Leu-MetNH$_2$ | Systematic N-methylation of individual peptide bonds in the C-terminal hexapeptide of substance P gave rise to agonists that specifically act on different receptor subtypes. Senktide is the most selective analog of this series. | [77] |
| [pGlu6,N-Me-Phe8, Aib9] substance P (6-11) | 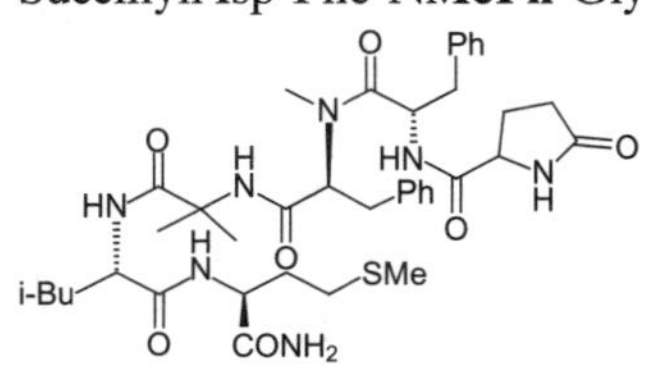 | Exists as a mixture of isomers: *cis* and *trans* Phe-N-MePhe peptide bonds. The main isomer, containing a *cis* Phe-N-MePhe peptide bond, shows a preferred folded conformation characterized by a type VI -turn with Phe and N-MePhe in the i + 1 and i + 2 positions. The turn is followed by a helical segment extending to the C-terminal. | [76] |

work to develop large peptide antagonists was quickly overtaken by rapid progress in the identification of lower molecular weight non-peptide antagonists. In early studies, chemists at ParkeDavis (Pfizer) built and screened a library of dipeptides based on weak $NK_3$ receptor antagonist with Boc-Phe-Phe$NH_2$ being the lead compound. This subsequently led to the identification of a series of low molecular weight, high affinity "peptoid" $NK_3$ receptor antagonists including PD157672 and PD161182 [80–82].

NONPEPTIDE ANTAGONISTS The aryl piperidine benzamide osanetant (SR142801) was the first nonpeptide-derived $NK_3$ receptor antagonist to be reported in the literature (Table 14.3) [62]. This highly potent selective antagonist is structurally related to the earlier reported selective $NK_2$ receptor antagonist, saredutant (formally through introduction of the core piperidine amide as a conformational constraint; [33]). The first publication on a structurally unrelated series of quinoline $NK_3$ receptor antagonists (including talnetant; SB223412) appeared shortly afterward [83]. Many years of subsequent medicinal chemistry have been carried out on both of these templates by several research groups, and there have been many publications and reviews in this area. Remarkably, over 10 years after these original publications, most of the potent nonpeptide $NK_3$ receptor antagonists reported to date can still be broadly assigned into one of these two general classes with only isolated reports of alternative chemotypes showing useful activity

**TABLE 14.3 Selective Peptide- and Dipeptide-Derived $NK_3$ Receptor Antagonists**

| | |
|---|---|
| Asp-Ser-Phe-Trp-β-Ala-Leu-Met$NH_2$ (MEN 10295; R 486; [Trp7,β-Ala8] neurokinin A (4-10)) | 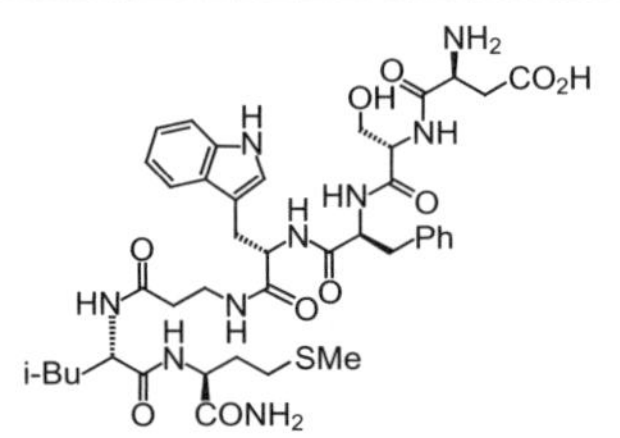 |
| GR138686 | 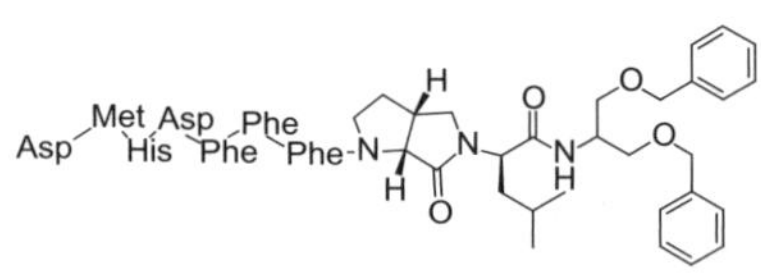 |
| PD157672 | 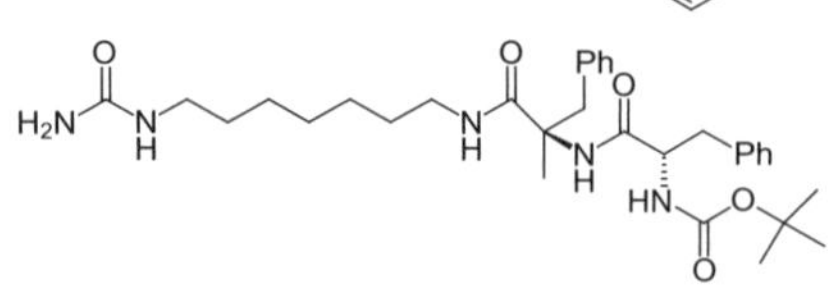 |
| PD161182 | 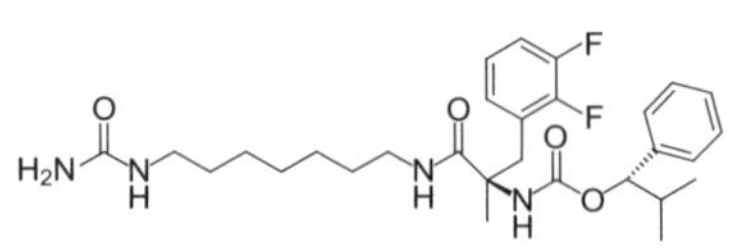 |

(e.g., weak $NK_3$ receptor antagonism seen for some angiotensin II receptor antagonists) [84].

Appropriate modification of the osanetant/saredutant scaffold and pendant substituents has led to the identification of selective antagonists for all of the neurokinin receptor subtypes. Additionally it has also been possible to produce many mixed antagonists ($NK_{1/2}$, $NK_{2/3}$, and $NK_{1/2/3}$; selected examples and associated references in Table 14.4). Using these and related compounds, pharmacophore models for antagonism at the neurokinin receptors have been developed [85, 86]. Despite the discovery of many potent neurokinin receptor antagonists from this class, and the progression of a number of these (in addition to osanetant) into early clinical development, the general physicochemical characteristics particularly for entry into the CNS are not ideal (e.g., high molecular weight, generally greater than 500 D, poor solubility, and high protein binding).

A number of research groups have reported medicinal chemistry studies on the alternative quinoline series of $NK_3$ receptor antagonists (Table 14.5). The prototype compounds from this series were originally designed as $NK_1$ receptor antagonists. However, the first examples synthesized were found to be weak $NK_3$ receptor antagonists devoid of any significant $NK_1$ receptor affinity [83]. Further modification of the substituents on the quinoline ring led to marked increases in $NK_3$ receptor affinity and the identification of talnetant (SB-223412) and a number of other high-affinity $NK_3$ receptor antagonists.

Subsequent work in this chemical class also identified mixed $NK_{2/3}$ and selective $NK_2$ receptor antagonists. Structure–activity relationship (SAR) at the quinoline C2, 3, and 4 position has been extensively investigated and numerous patent applications in the quinoline series were filed during the mid-late 1990s (reviewed in References [87, 88]). Receptor selectivity is controlled by judicious choice of quinoline C3 and C4 substituents. Remarkably, however, all the quinolines reported to date show high selectivity over $NK_1$ receptors.

In addition to modification of the quinoline ring substituents, considerable effort has also been directed to finding alternatives to the quinoline ring. Although early efforts generally produced analogs with weak $NK_3$ receptor affinity [89], some recent patent applications describing imidazole and pyrazole analogues appear to have been more successful [90, 91].

Following the reports from the schizophrenia clinical studies with osanetant and talnetant (detailed below) there has been an increased number of recent quinoline publications (e.g., [92, 93]) and patent applications from other research groups (for recent review see [70]).

### 14.3.3 Emerging Areas

Recently reports of the first mixed dual $NK_{1/3}$ receptor antagonists have emerged in the patent literature (Table 14.6). These compounds are structurally distinct from both the quinoline and osanetant series and are based on a

**TABLE 14.4 Nonpeptide Neurokinin Receptor Antagonists Based on Osanetant and Saredutant**

| Selective $NK_3$ | Selective $NK_2$ | Selective $NK_1$ | Mixed Antagonists |
|---|---|---|---|
| Sanofi Osanetant (SR142801)<br>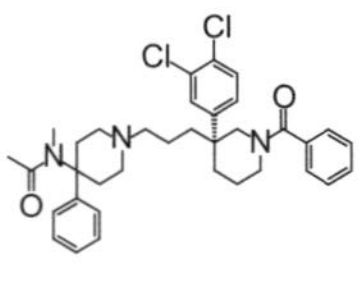<br>[182] [62], | Sanofi Saredutant (SR49868)<br>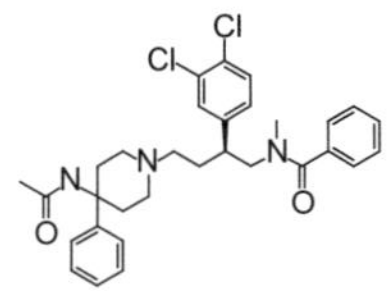<br>[33] [183], | Sanofi Nolpitantium besilate (SR140333)<br>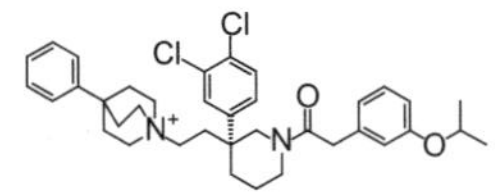<br>[184, 185] | Astra Zeneca $NK_{1/2/3}$<br>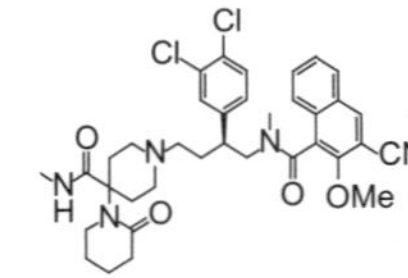<br>[186] |
| Sanofi (SR146977)<br>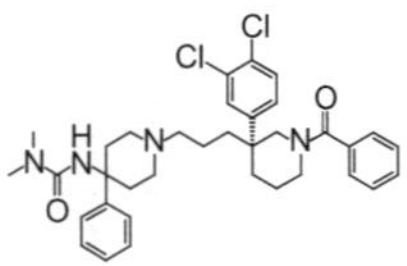<br>[187] | Astra Zeneca (ZD7944)<br>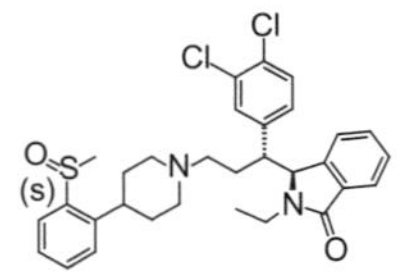<br>[186] | Sanofi (SR240600)<br>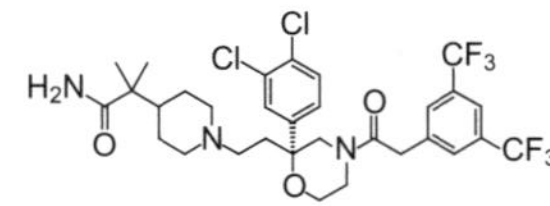<br>[187, 188] | AstraZeneca $NK_{1/2/3}$<br>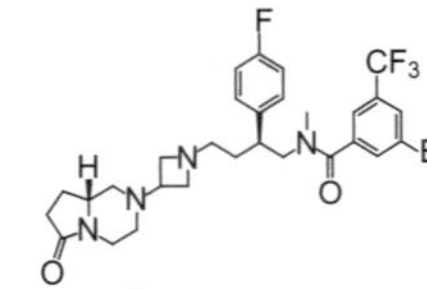<br>[189] |
| Lundbeck<br>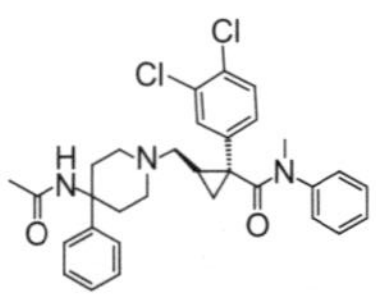<br>[190] | Sanofi (SR144190)<br>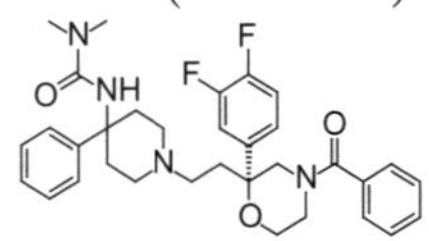<br>[191] | Novartis (NKP-608)<br>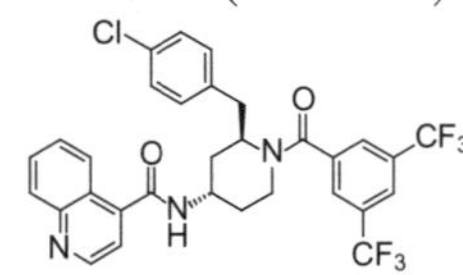<br>[192] (Currently Licensed to Avera) | Sankyo $NK_{1/2/3}$ (CS-003)<br>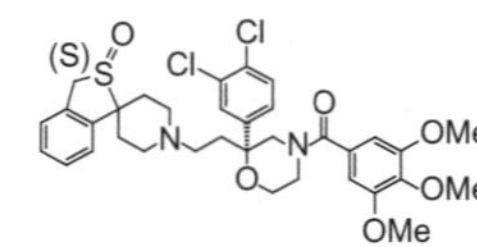<br>[193, 194] |
| Merck<br>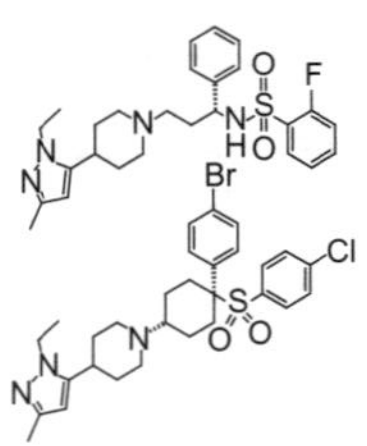 | Yamanouchi (YM38336)<br>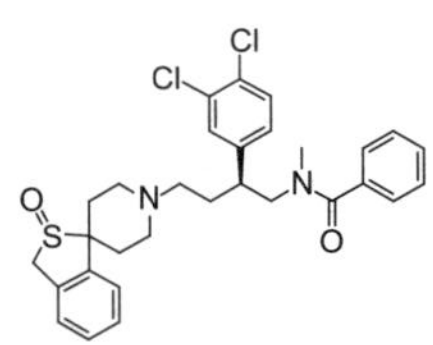 | Janssen<br>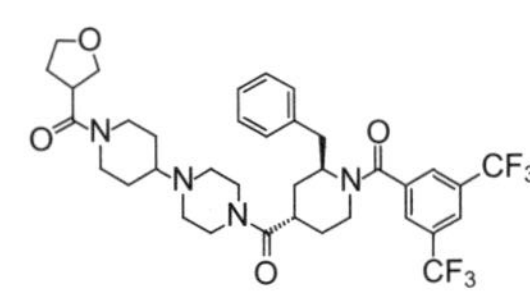<br>$NK_1 > NK_{2,3}$ | Schering $NK_{1/2/3}$ (SCH206272)<br>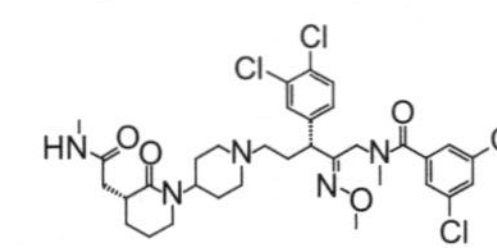 |

| | | | |
|---|---|---|---|
| [195, 196]<br>Merck<br>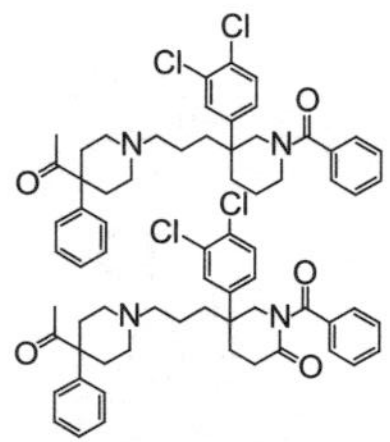<br>$NK_3 > NK_{1/2}$ and $NK_2 > NK_{1/3}$<br>[200] | [197]<br>Solvay (SLV-332)<br>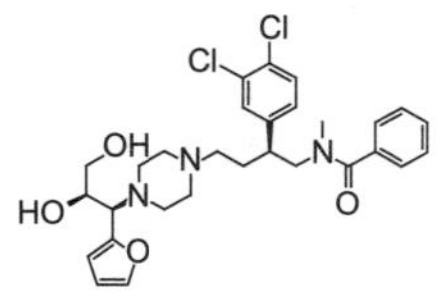<br>[201]<br>Pfizer (UK224671 and UK290795)<br>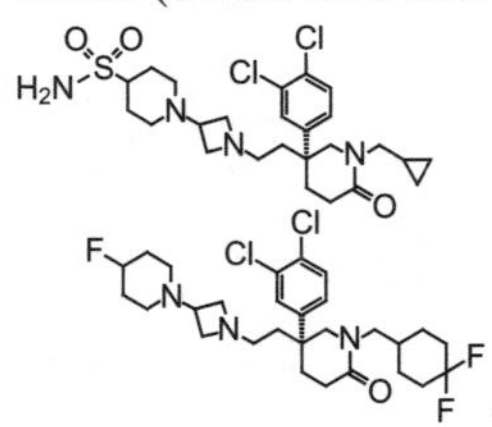<br>$NK_2$ & $NK_{2/3}$<br>[203, 204] | [198] | [199]<br>Rhone Poulenc (MDL105212)<br>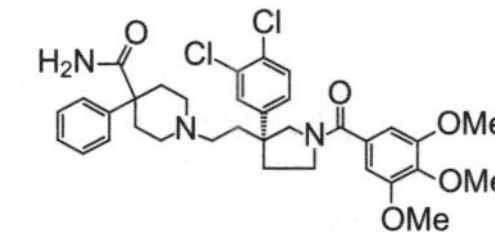<br>$NK_{1/2} > NK_3$<br>[202] |

**TABLE 14.5 Representative Quinoline $NK_3$ Receptor Antagonists**

| Compound | Profile/Comments | Reference | Compound | Profile/Comments | Reference |
|---|---|---|---|---|---|
| 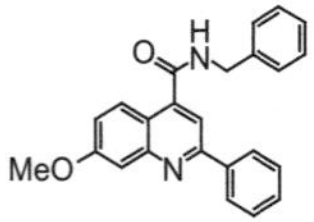 | Prototype quinoline designed as $NK_1$ receptor antagonist. | [83], [205] | 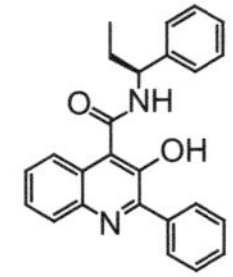 | Talnetant (SB223412) | [49, 50, 205] |
| 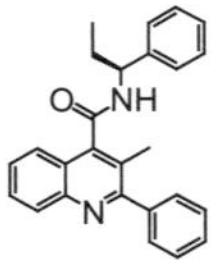 | SB222200 | [206] | 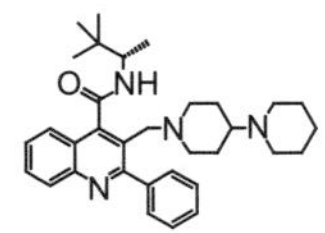 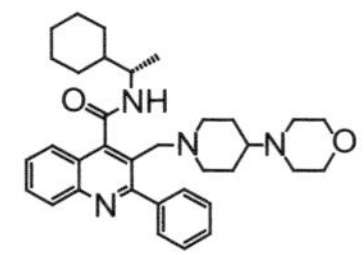 | SB414240 $NK_2$<br>SB400238 $NK_{2/3}$ | [207] |
| 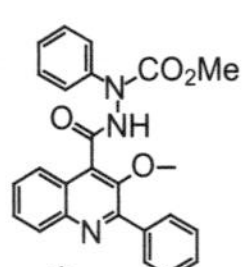 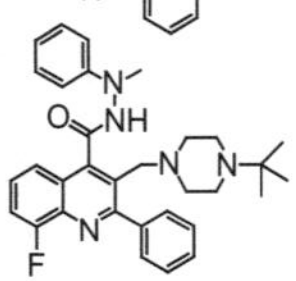 | Occupy $NK_3$ receptors in gerbil brain | [92, 93] | 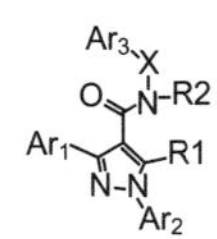 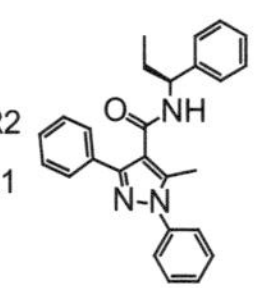 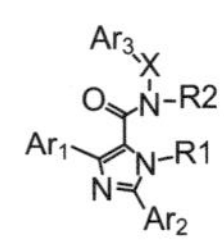 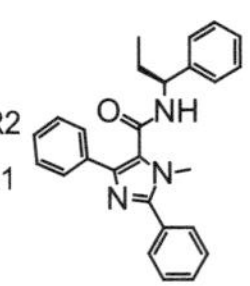 | Alternative replacements of the quinoline ring | [90, 91] |

**TABLE 14.6 Dual $NK_{1/3}$ Receptor Antagonists**

| | |
|---|---|
| 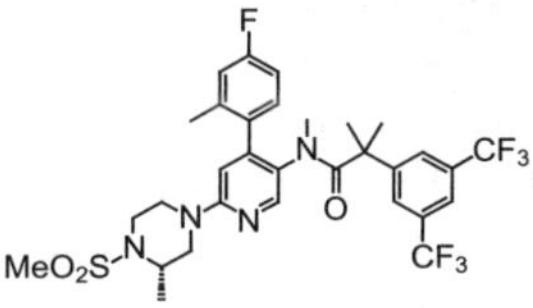 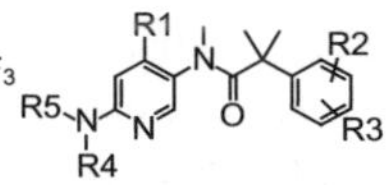 | [208] |
| 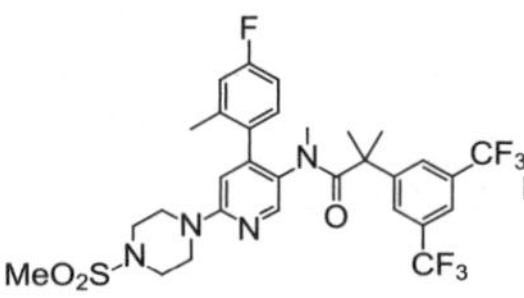 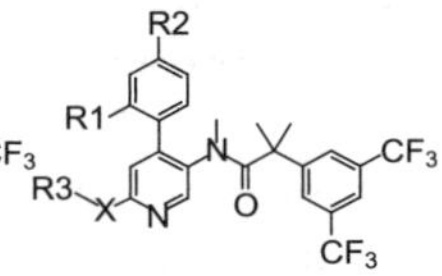 | [209] |
| 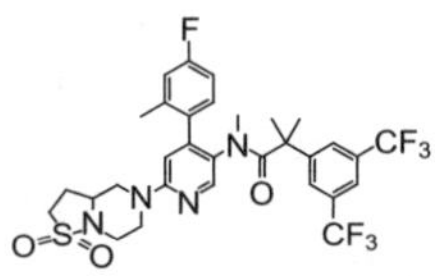 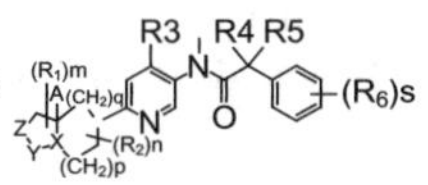 | [210] |

**TABLE 14.7 Additional Neurokinin Receptor Ligands Referred to in Text**

| | |
|---|---|
| $NK_3$ allosteric modulators [94] | 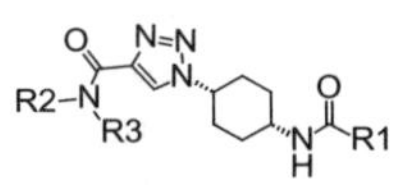 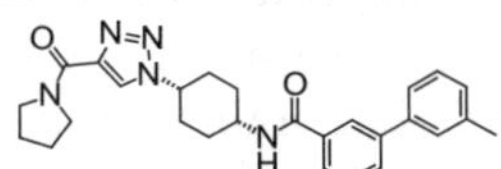 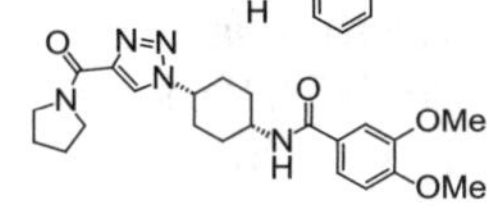 |
| Aprepitant | 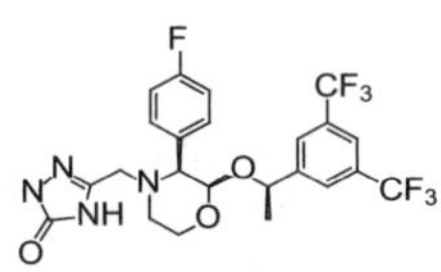 |

pyridine template. A number of examples with very high receptor binding affinities for both $NK_1$ and $NK_3$ have been described.

Finally a recent patent publication has described a new and distinct series of $NK_3$ receptor modulators (Table 14.7). In an *in vitro* functional assay the two examples shown below potentiated the effects of NKB at concentrations in the micromolar range, suggesting that these compounds bind at an allosteric site on the receptor and may act as positive allosteric modulators [94].

### 14.3.4 Clinical Findings with Selective $NK_3$ Receptor Antagonists

Although preclinically $NK_3$ receptor-mediated physiology and pharmacology has been relatively well studied and understood for many years, it is recent clinical observations that have re-ignited interest in this target from a therapeutic stand point. In this regard, the $NK_3$ receptor antagonist SR142801 (osanetant; [24]) was evaluated as one of a number of novel pharmacologies in a 6-week multi-center clinical study in hospitalized schizophrenic and schizoaffective disorder patients ($n = 481$) who were experiencing an acute exacerbation of hallucinatory symptoms. In this trial, SR142801 (200 mg/day; $n = 70$ patients) significantly improved, compared with placebo, four primary efficacy measures, that is, the total score from the Positive and Negative Scale for Schizophrenia (PANSS), the derived score for the Brief Psychiatric Rating Scale (BPRS), the BPRS positive symptom subscale (delusions, hallucinations, conceptual disorganization, and bizarre behavior), and the Clinical Global Impression Scale (CGI-S). Furthermore, the improvement in these patients was not significantly different from that achieved with haloperidol (10 mg/day; $n = 98$) and the magnitude of the haloperidol-induced improvement was typical of that previously observed in other schizophrenia clinical trials. The compound was well tolerated with a low incidence of EPS. Interestingly, the response to osanetant was found to correlate with plasma concentrations of the parent molecule. In this regard, reductions in BPRS total (scores of −7.9 to −9.8) correlated to median plasma concentrations of 20 ng/mL at the 200 mg/day dose [95]. These relatively low exposures suggested that higher doses may produce further improvements, and this was evaluated further by Sanofi. Although no formal details or data have been released from these studies, it has been suggested [96] that these higher doses were ineffectual and the development of this compound for schizophrenia has been stopped (http://ww.Sanofi-aventis.com). Interestingly, osanetant has also been examined in panic disorder [97], Parkinson's disease [98], and depression (http://ww.Sanofi-aventis.com), but without any clear evidence of efficacy.

In a further placebo-controlled trial, schizophrenic individuals (n = 236) received oral talnetant (200 mg) or risperidone (3 to 6 mg) for 6 weeks. The primary endpoint examined was a change in total score on the PANSS positive and negative scales. A 20% reduction in PANSS score was achieved in 40% of patients who received talnetant compared with 48% of those treated with risperidone, and 30% who received placebo [99]. An overview of data from a 20-patient, placebo-controlled Phase II clinical trial of talnetant in schizophrenia using talnetant at "high exposure" is also available (actual dose not disclosed). A reduction of approximately 20% in PANSS score was seen in 25% of patients treated with talnetant compared with 49% and 29% of those receiving risperidone and placebo, respectively. In addition, talnetant treatment significantly increased total scores on the Brief Assessment on Cognition in Schizophrenia Scale (BACS) to +0.3, compared with a score of −0.04 in placebo-treated patients. The drug was well tolerated and patients had no weight gain following high doses of talnetant versus vehicle; in contrast risperidone-treated patientsshowed a weight gain of ~1.9-kg. Talnetant also had a significantly better tolerability profile compared with risperidone, with a lower incidence of prolactin elevations (6% and 69%, respectively; placebo = 12%) and testosterone reduction (28% and 57%, respectively; placebo = 18%; [99]) and a low incidence of EPS.

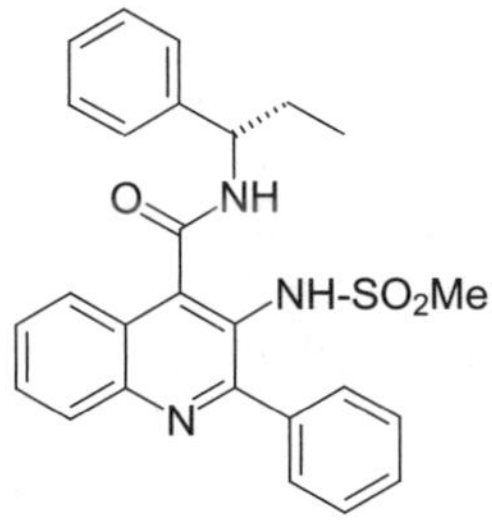

AZD2624

**FIGURE 14.1** Clinical candidate AZD2624.

Interestingly, a recent report has described the psychomotor and cognitive effects of a single 200 mg dose of talnetant in healthy volunteers [100]. Talnetant produced a similar effect to haloperidol (3 mg) in decreasing α—power spectra (as measured using electroencephalography [EEG]) but in all other aspects was dissimilar. In this regard, talnetant improved adaptive tracking and reduced calmness on the VAS (visual analog scale) Bond and Lader assessment, while haloperidol impaired alertness and reduced mood. Furthermore, haloperidol caused elevations in prolactin while talnetant was without effect. All observations correlated with the temporal aspects of the pharmacokinetic profiles of these two compounds. It is obviously difficult to draw too many conclusions from these limited data, but they may be suggestive of CNS penetration without $D_2$-like side effects. One could further speculate that the observed effects (i.e., an increase in attention) may be dopaminergic in nature, perhaps mediated via enhanced cortical DA as seen preclinically [50] and reduced calmness. Generally, the preclinical data do seem to be largely supportive of the clinical observations to date.

Finally, and most recently, AZD2624, a new quinoline derivative developed by AstraZeneca was tested in schizophrenic subjects (see Fig. 14.1). A 4-week Phase II study (following a 2-week washout of previous antipsychotic medication) was performed with 40 mg twice daily dosing of AZD2624 compared with olanzepine (15 mg) as a positive comparator. While olanzepine produced significant efficacy on PANSS positive measures after 3 weeks, AZD2624 showed no efficacy on positive symptoms (despite reaching exposures equivalent to those that had previously been shown to enhance endogenous DA efflux in the striatum of a primate, as measured using $^{11}C$ NMPA PET displacement). Clinical $C_{max}$ was 719 ng/mL with a $t_{1/2}$ of 8 hours. The compound was safe and well tolerated up to 80 mg single dose and 40 mg BID repeat dose with the only reported change being a reduction in serum testosterone levels (personal communication).

### 14.3.5 Clinical Evidence of the Utility of Other NK Receptor Antagonist

It is worth briefly highlighting the potential for the utility of ligands targeted at the other neurokinin receptor family member in schizophrenia. Particularly, some of the synthetic ligands have (by design or otherwise) adopted a polypharmacy approach or "pan" NK intervention strategy. $NK_2$ receptor antagonism has not been tested in patients with schizophrenia per se, so whether this activity will bring anything further in terms of therapeutic efficacy is largely unknown. However, the $NK_1$ receptor antagonist MK-869 (aprepitant; 400 mg, Table 14.7) was evaluated in acutely psychotic patients, but proved to be ineffectual [101]. Both $NK_1$ and $NK_2$ receptor antagonists have proven to be efficacious in depression. MK-869 (aprepitant; [102]) produced an improvement in the total Hamilton Rating Scale for Depression (HAM-D) that was similar to the positive comparator, paroxetine, in a 6-week placebo-controlled major depression outpatient trial. In a separate study [103], the selective $NK_1$ antagonist, L759274 (structure not disclosed) showed a similar profile of improvement in outpatients diagnosed with major depression disorder with melancholia. However, the hypothesis of $NK_1$-mediated antidepressive efficacy has perhaps lost some favor in recent years with the report that MK-869 failed to produce significant improvements in five additional double-blind placebo-controlled trials [104]. Saredutant (SR489686, [33]), a selective $NK_2$ receptor antagonist, has been reported to have shown efficacy in two of four Phase III clinical trials in MDD, although the development of this compound has more recently been reported to have been discontinued. Comorbid depression has a lifetime prevalence in schizophrenics of as high as 80% [105], compared with 8–26% in the general population [106], and comorbid mood disorders have also been linked to an elevated rate of suicide in schizophrenics (for review see Reference [107]); so efficacy against this symptom domain would be of clinical benefit.

In summary, the preclinical data on $NK_3$ receptor antagonists suggest potential efficacy in multiple symptom domains of schizophrenia. All three selective $NK_3$ receptor antagonists were well tolerated clinically and showed no evidence of any of the adverse effects normally associated with conventional antipsychotic therapies. However, although preliminary evidence with both talnetant and osanetant supported the preclinical hypothesis, the subsequent discontinuation of osanetant, due to inability to confirm efficacy, and the recent failure of AZ2624 to show any efficacy have raised questions with regard to the ultimate therapeutic utility of $NK_3$ receptor antagonists as antipsychotics. That said, the development and testing of other, either selective or combined, $NK_{1-3}$ receptor antagonist with improved drug-like characteristics (i.e., with enhanced brain penetration etc) is obviously still ongoing and may yet provide definitive evidence of efficacy. We await the release of these data with interest.

## 14.4 THE NEUROTENSIN SYSTEM

Neurotensin (NT) is a tridecapeptide (pGlu-Leu-Tyr-Glu-Asn-Lys-Pro-Arg-Arg-Pro-Tyr-Ile-Leu-OH) and was first isolated from bovine hypothalamus [108]. It is synthesized from a precursor protein (pro-NT) by pro-hormone convertases. This processing also produces other bioactive peptides including the hexapeptide neuromedin N (Lys-Ile-Pro-Tyr-Ile-Leu-OH), which can also activate NT receptors [109]. Greater than 90% of NT is found in the periphery and largely in the gastrointestinal tract; however, NT is also found in the CNS, where it produces a wide range of physiological and pharmacological effects [110]. In neurons, NT is stored in vesicles and is released in a calcium-dependent manner and inactivated by a range of peptidases [111] or via internalization and subsequent degradation [112]. Three NT receptor subtypes have been identified, cloned, and characterized. $NT_1$ and $NT_2$ are seven transmembrane Gq-protein-coupled receptors, while $NT_3$ is a type 1 receptor with a single transmembrane spanning domain. Although NT is the endogenous ligand for all three receptor subtypes, it has significantly higher affinity for $NT_1$ [113]. A potential fourth NT receptor has been identified as the previously characterized SorLA/LR11 [114]. Despite the wide range of NT-mediated functional and physiological activities and high peripheral expression, there is continued interest in this neuropeptide and its receptors with regard to the pathophysiology and potential treatment of psychiatric and neurological disorders. Indeed a recent review [115] and articles therein, summarize the field and the potential role of NT in the pathophysiology of schizophrenia and as a potential target class for new antipsychotic drugs. The key preclinical findings that support the hypotheses behind NT-targeted therapeutics will be summarized here.

NT and NT receptors colocalize in brain areas generally associated with the pathophysiology of schizophrenia and the proposed sites of action of current antipsychotic medications (i.e., hypothalamus, amygdala, SN, VTA, nucleus accumbens, cortical structures, and hippocampus). Probably not surprisingly given this distribution, NT appears to play roles in regulating dopaminergic, glutamatergic, GABAergic, and serotonergic circuits in these brain structures, again all neurotransmitter systems mooted to be involved in the pathophysiology and treatment of schizophrenia. Specifically, NT appears to be associated with central dopaminergic function, with NT containing neurons showing close neuroanatomical localization with the dopaminergic cell bodies of the VTA and >80% of dopaminergic neurons expressing $NT_1$ receptors [116, 117]. NT receptors have also been demonstrated to be present on cholinergic neurons of the VTA [118]. Functionally, NT selectively attenuates VTA firing and mesolimbic but not nigrostriatal DA output [119], although it should be noted that exogenously administered NT can produce quite different responses depending on the brain region examined and the concentration used. These differences can potentially be explained by heterogenous localization of receptors [111], but also by differing sensitivities to, and concentrations of NT applied. Interestingly, NT also appears to decrease the sensitivity of $D_2$ receptors for endogenous DA and DA receptor agonists [120], potentially via an interaction between the two systems at the level of their signal transduction pathways [121]. Furthermore, NT's role in the modulation of GABA and ACh systems within these dopaminergic brain regions can also complicate the interpretation and isolation of the specific functional role of this neuropeptide on the DA system.

In behavioral models that are thought to be indicative of antipsychotic action, many of the observations have focused on the activity of NT analog agonists such as NT69L. NT69L and NT attenuated apomorphine-induced climbing [122], while NT69L attenuated haloperidol-induced catalepsy without being cataleptogenic in its own right [123]. Both NT69L and a novel peptide agonist, PD149163, attenuated amphetamine, MK801, 5-$HT_{2A}$, and $\alpha 1$ adrenergic receptor agonist-induced PPI deficits [124–128]. Furthermore, PD149163 also reversed a PPI deficit seen in Brattleboro rats that have an endogenous sensory motor function deficit due to a vasopressin mutation [124]. More recently [129], it has been demonstrated that acute administration of PD149163 attenuated fear-potentiated startle in rats, suggesting an anxiolytic-like efficacy. There is also preclinical evidence to suggest that NT receptor agonists may be pro-cognitive [130], and additional data to support this hypothesis in an associative learning paradigm [131]. The authors speculate that the pro-cognitive effect may be a result of modulating the mesocortical DA system, although they do acknowledge that further studies would be required to fully assess this interpretation.

There is a general concern that agonist drug therapies may result in tolerance to therapeutic utility following repeat or chronic administration. This has been investigated to some extent with NT or its analog, but such studies have proven largely inconclusive with regard to the question of tolerance. Hertel et al. [132, 133],demonstrated a tolerance effect, while other groups demonstrated no tolerance [134, 135] or even potentiation [136] of behavioral responses, in paradigms considered indicative of antipsychotic activity. However, differences in the methods and procedures in these studies could have contributed to these apparently discrepant results. In order to investigate this in a more robust manner, Norman et al. [137] have recently determined the effect of continual agonism of NT receptors on amphetamine-induced hyperactivity in rodents. In this study, NT and PD149163 were assessed under the same experimental procedure, with respect to route of administration and dosing period, to better enable a direct comparison. Interestingly, 7-day administration of both agents had no effect on amphetamine-induced hyperactivity, suggesting tolerance, whereas 21 days administration actually potentiated the amphetamine-induced behavior. This finding clearly suggests that the biological actions of NT are more complex than previously thought, and perhaps challenges the concept that chronically stimulating this peptide system will prove efficacious in schizophrenia. Further studies using different agents are required to resolve this controversy. In contrast to the NT receptor agonist approaches, SR142948A has been reported as an $NT_1$ receptor selective antagonist that has been used in several studies to determine the outcome of central $NT_1$ receptor activation. These studies implicated the role of $NT_1$ receptors in the attenuation of mesolimbic dopaminergic activity, and Marie-Claire et al. [138] have recently reported data to further substantiate this hypothesis, in that SR142948A attenuated the hyperactivity induced by the psychoactive compound, MDMA. Interestingly, these studies also suggested that $NT_1$ receptors are involved in the expression, but not acquisition, of conditioned place preference induced by MDMA.

Thus, taken together, these studies suggest that administration of NT, or analogs appear to produce both behavioral and neurochemical effects broadly parallel to those of atypical antipsychotics. In addition, more recent evidence has suggested that NT or its analogs could represent a novel treatment for more than one symptom domain of the disease. Despite the evidence that agonizing NT receptors may prove beneficial in schizophrenia, it cannot be ignored that there are some preclinical data that apparently contradict this approach. In this regard, NT has been shown to increase the firing of dopaminergic neurons and the subsequent release of DA in the Nacc and striatum *in vitro* and *in vivo*. Moreover, local injections of NT into the VTA increased locomotor activity and potentiated the disruption of PPI produced by DA receptor agonists [139]. Very potent and selective nonpeptidic NT receptor antagonists such as SR48692 and SR142948 have been identified [140, 141]. When given chronically, SR48692 decreased the spontaneous electrical activity of dopaminergic neurons in the VTA but not in the SN and selectively decreased basal DA efflux in the Nacc [142, 143]. Moreover, SR48692 antagonized the behavioral effects of psychostimulants [144]. NT receptor antagonists may, thus, represent a new type of antipsychotic drug that acts by preventing excessive dopaminergic neuron activity via a blockade of a pathologically enhanced NT tone on these neurons. The validity of this approach has been clinically assessed and will be discussed.

### 14.4.1 Ligands for Neurotensin Receptors

Numerous reports have been published describing the identification of both neurotensin agonists (truncated peptides/peptide analogs) and antagonists (both peptide and nonpeptide). This research has already been extensively reviewed elsewhere [115]. Herein we summarize some of the key compounds reported in the literature and highlight recent progress.

Interestingly, it is the last six amino acid residues of the NT peptide (residues 8–13) that are thought to mediate the majority of its biological effect. However, the truncated peptide NT(8–13) is rapidly degraded by endogenous peptidases when administered *in vivo* via systemic routes and, thus, must be delivered directly into the brain to exert any observable pharmacological action [145]. Thus, much of the more recent research efforts have focused on NT receptor agonists based on analogs of this truncated peptide but with improved metabolic stability and hence ability to cross the blood–brain barrier when administered *in vivo*. From this research, numerous analogs have been identified that are both CNS penetrant and active *in vivo* following systemic delivery. A selection of some of the NT receptor agonists derived from NT(8-13) are presented in Table 14.8.

**TABLE 14.8 Neurotensin Receptor Agonists**

| Compound | Organisation | Structure | Comments | Reference |
|---|---|---|---|---|
| $NT_1$ | Esai | (Me)Arg-Lys-Pro-Trp-*tert*Leu-Leu | First NT receptor agonist reported to be CNS penetrant<br>Effects on locomotor activity (LMA) measures; none cataleptogenic | [211–213] |
| PD149163 | Parke-Davis (Pfizer) | 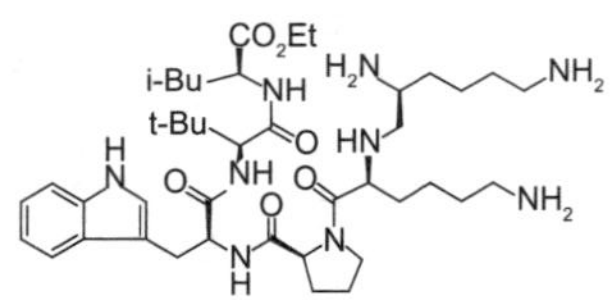<br>(N2-[(2S)-2,6-diaminohexyl]-Lys-Pro-Tryp-3MeVal-LeuOEt) | Reversed amphetamine and dizocilpine (MK-801)-induced PPI deficits in rats | [126] |
| NT69L | Mayo Foundation | 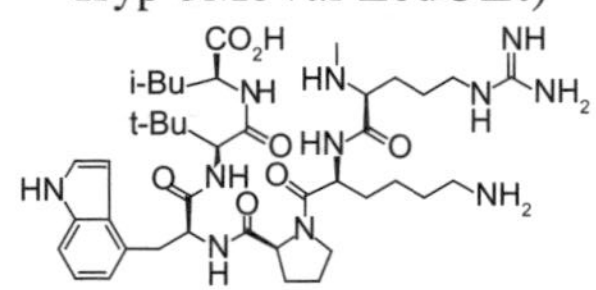<br>($N_2$-MeArg-Lys-Pro-neoTrp-3MeVal-Leu) | Induced hypothermia and was antinociceptive.<br>Increased PPI at baseline and following amphetamine.<br>Attenuated PPI deficits produced by dizocilpine with no effect on startle.<br>Blocked hyperactivity induced by both cocaine and amphetamine. | [128, 158, 214] |
| NT66L<br>NT67L | Mayo Foundation | 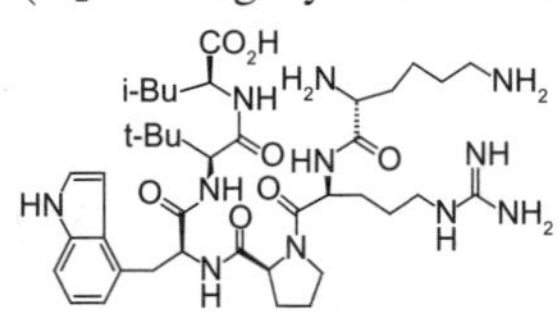<br>(D-lys-Arg-Pro-NeoTrp-3MeVal-Leu)<br>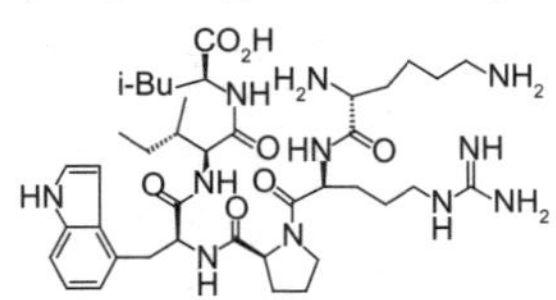<br>(D-Lys-Arg-Pro-NeoTrp-lle-Leu) | Synthesis, stability, *in vitro* activity described.<br>Hypothermic and antinociception. | [215, 216] |

| | | | | |
|---|---|---|---|---|
| JMV-449 | Lundbeck | 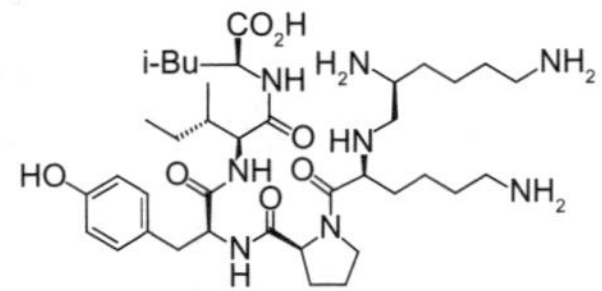 | Induced hypothermia and nociceptive. | [217] |
| ABS-201 | Univ South Carolina | 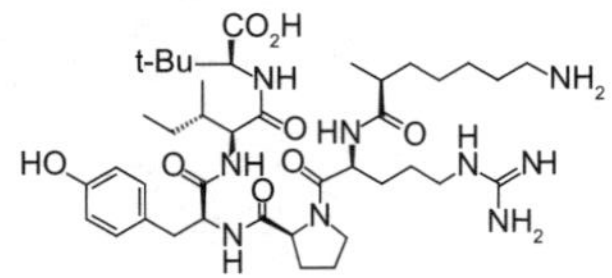 | Induced hypothermia but was not cataleptogenic. | [135, 218, 219] |
| AdaKPYIL | Dupont Merck | 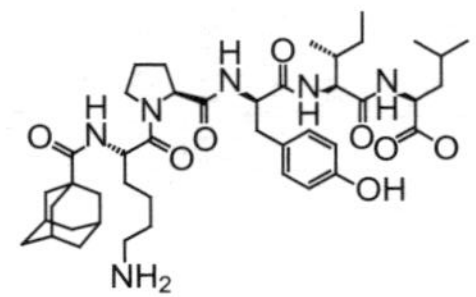 | Orally inactive. | [220] |
| NT34 | Mayo Foundation | 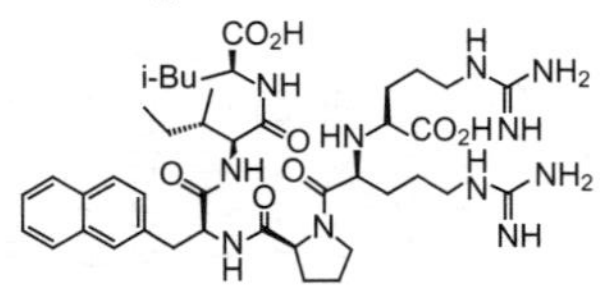 | Higher affinity for rat over human NTS1. | [123] |
| Contulakin G | Cognetix | 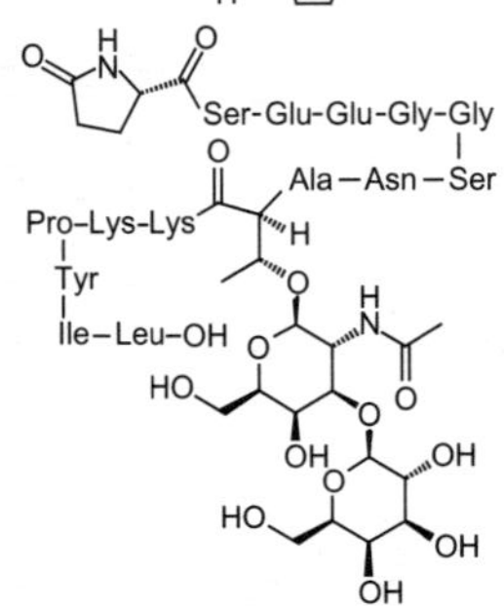 | | [152, 153] |

Several SAR studies have been carried out to investigate the contributions of individual residues in NT(8-13). A diverse selection of unnatural, reduced, and conformationally constrained amino acids have been introduced into the peptide to increase metabolic stability and facilitate the development of pharmacophore models for use in the search for nonpeptide agonists (see, e.g., References [146–151]). Despite this work, nonpeptide NT receptor agonists have not yet been described in the literature.

To date, the only NT receptor agonist that has advanced into clinical trials is Contulakin G (CGX1160). This is an O-glycosylated invertebrate NT isolated from a marine snail venom [152, 153]. Early studies to investigate the potential of this compound as an analgesic were conducted in patients with chronic intractable pain caused by spinal cord injury. Intrathecal administration produced analgesic activity, with no serious adverse events (http://www.Cognetix.com, January 28, 2005). However, the current status is unclear as there have been no recent developments reported.

*Antagonists* With the early advent of nonpeptide antagonist ligands and the inherent difficulties in optimizing peptides, there are few reports describing peptide antagonists. Rhone Poulenc Rorer (now Sanofi-Aventis) reported a weak peptide metabolite RP66453 (Table 14.9) isolated from streptomyces as a potential lead with modest affinity at guinea pig neurotensin receptor ($IC_{50}$ = 30 μg/mL). However, no subsequent publications have appeared in this area [154, 155].

A series of partially nonpeptidic mimetics of NT(8–13) based on an indole core were designed using molecular modeling [156]. Functional evaluation in neuroblastoma N1E-115 cells showed the C-3/C-5 regioisomer to be an NT receptor antagonist, while the C-3/C-7 regioisomer was found to be an NT receptor antagonist at low concentrations and an NT receptor agonist at higher concentrations in the 10–100 $\mu mol/dm^3$ range.

In the early 1990s, screening programs at several pharmaceutical companies led to the the successful identification of nonpeptide NT receptor antagonists. At Pfizer, the lead compound, UK-73,093 [157], was reported to displace [$^3$H]-NT from its bovine brain receptor with modest affinity ($IC_{50}$ = 5.5 μM). A functional assay confirmed it to be a competitive antagonist (Ki = 4.4 μM). UK-73093 also reversed NT-induced behavioral effects in rat after i.p. dosing. Shortly after this publication, scientists at Sanofi described the identification and initial characterization of SR48692 (Meclinertant; [158]). SR48692 was obtained from optimization of a weak screening lead, SR45398. *In vitro*, SR48692 is a potent competitive antagonist at $NT_1$ receptors ($pA_2$ 8.1), and it reverses NT-induced behaviors *in vivo* in mice with similar potency by either i.p. or oral delivery and with a long duration of action (6 hours).

The identification of SR48692 was an important breakthrough which facilitated the identification and characterization of NT receptor subtypes [159] since SR-48692 has significantly lower affinity for the $NT_2$ receptor. A number of analogues of SR48692 have been subsequently reported [160]. SR48527 (S-isomer) is substantially more active than its enantiomer (SR49711) [161].

**TABLE 14.9 Neurotensin Receptor Antagonists**

| | | |
|---|---|---|
| RP66453 | 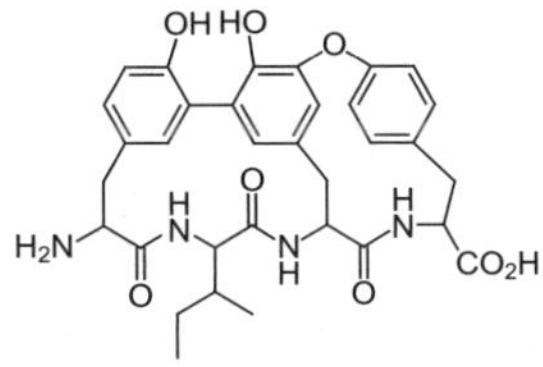 | [154, 155] |
| NT(8-13) mimetics | 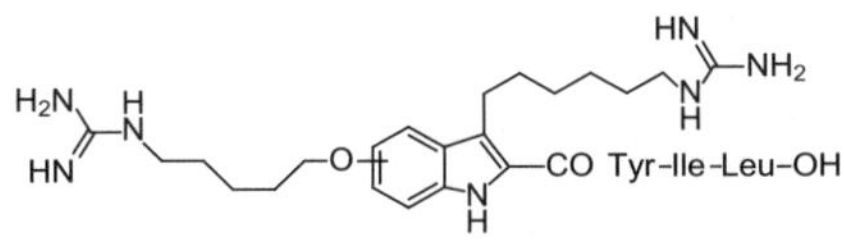 | [156] |
| UK-73,093 | 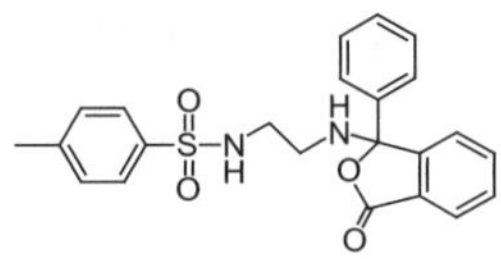 | [157] |
| SR45398, SR48692 | 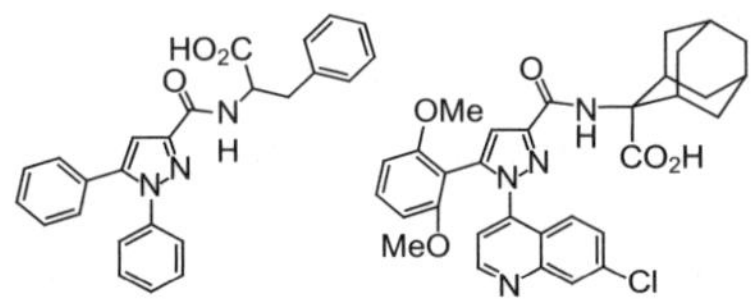 | [158] |
| SR48527, SR142498 | 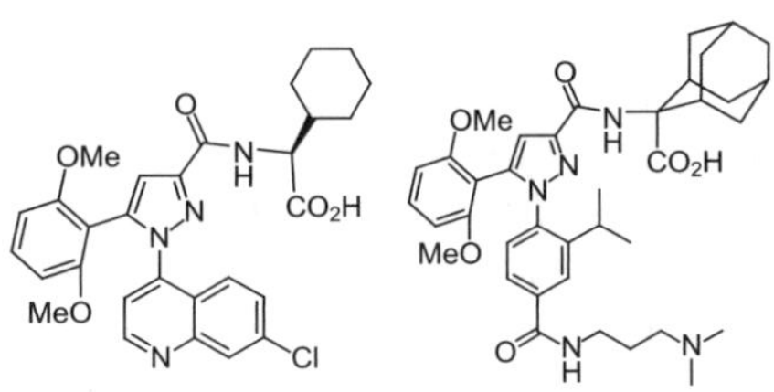 | [140, 144, 164] |
| Parke-Davis | 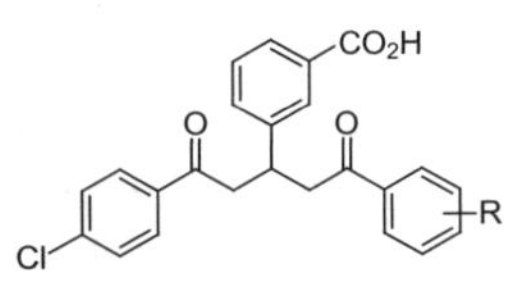<br>R = 4-Cl NT Ki 450 nM,<br>R = 3,4-di-OMe Ki 42 nM | [165] |

Modification of the quinoline substituent resulted in the identification of SR142948 which is 10-fold more potent than SR48692 at $NT_1$ receptors and has similar affinity at both $NT_1$ and $NT_2$ [140, 144]. *In vivo*, SR142948 displays a wider spectrum of activity than SR48692, notably it antagonises NT—induced hypothermia, analgesia and DA efflux. The X-ray structures of SR142948 and SR48692 have been reported and a bioactive conformation proposed [162, 163].

In contrast to their antagonist activity at $NT_1$, both SR48692 and SR142498A were found to be potent agonists of $NT_2$ in a human recombinant *in vitro* CHO cell assay [164].

Screening of the Parke Davis (now Pfizer) compound collection led to the identification of a series of diaryldioxobenzoic acid derivatives. Using an immature mouse brain binding assay SAR was developed which resulted in a 10-fold increase in affinity from the initial lead [165].

Scientists at Merck published a series of patent applications in 1993–1994 highlighting non-peptide NT receptor antagonists [166–173] but no further publications appeared on these compounds and no development was reported.

## 14.5 CLINICAL PERSPECTIVE

The results of studies examining the NT system in schizophrenia have been extensively reviewed [174] In brief, one of the most compelling pieces of evidence comes from the measurement of CSF NT levels in drug-free and treated schizophrenia patients [175]. Low levels of NT have been robustly measured in a subset of drug-free patients whereby clinical improvement was related to a normalization of CSF levels. Low levels of NT also positively correlated with the severity of the psychopathology of the disease [176, 177].In contrast, CSF NT levels were elevated in Parkinsonian patients, thus suggesting an antagonistic relationship between the NT and DA system in the CNS. To date, the only clinical trial that has been performed using an NT ligand is that reported by Meltzer et al. [24]. Here the $NT_1$ receptor antagonist, SR 48692, was assessed in a placebo-controlled study in schizophrenic and schizoaffective patients designed to assess four different investigational drugs, including the previously discussed $NK_3$ receptor antagonist osanetant (SR142801). Patients were randomizely assigned to receive fixed doses of investigational drug, placebo, or haloperidol for 6 weeks. The primary outcome measures were changes from baseline in total score on the PANSS total, severity of illness score on CGI, and total score and psychosis cluster on the BPRS. SR48692 (180 mg/day) was well tolerated but did not differ from placebo on any of the outcome measures, while in contrast the positive control haloperidol showed significant improvement in all primary measures. The preclinical rationale to support an antagonist approach has been described previously. Although alternative reasons for the negative clinical outcome could be poor CNS penetration or insufficient occupancy of $NT_1$ receptors, one could speculate, from the literature to date, that stimulating, rather than blocking, NT receptors could offer therapeutic potential. Although this would appear an obvious conclusion, an agonist approach is not without concerns. For example, preclinical studies to date have suggested that $NT_1$ receptors are implicated but others receptor subtypes cannot be ruled out. In this regard recent studies by Boules et al. [178] have reported on an NT analog (NT79) that is highly selective for $NT_2$ receptors and demonstrates an antipsychotic-like effect preclinically but is devoid of peripherally mediated adverse events. Therefore, aside from the concerns already touched upon for an agonist approach, for example, tolerance to effect and peripherally mediated side effects, there will now be controversy as to which NT subtype to target. These questions will remain unanswered until selective, developable agonists become available in the clinical setting.

## REFERENCES


1. Harrison, P.J., Weinberger, D.R. (2005). Schizophrenia genes, gene expression, and neuropathology: on the matter of their convergence. *Mol Psychiatry*, *10*, 40–68.
2. Kapur, S., Mizrahi, R., Li, M. (2005). From dopamine to salience to psychosis—linking biology, pharmacology and phenomenology of psychosis. *Schizophr Res*, *79*, 59–68.
3. Carlsson, A., Hansson, L.O., Waters, N., Carlsson, M.L. (1997). Neurotransmitter aberrations in schizophrenia: new perspectives and therapeutic implications. *Life Sci*, *61*, 75–79.
4. Lieberman, J.A., Stroup, T.S., McEvoy, J.P., Swartz, M.S., Rosenheck, R.A., Perkins, D.O., Keefe, R.S., Davis, S.M., Davis, C.E., Lebowitz, B.D., Severe, J., Hsiao, J.K., Clinical Antipsychotic Trials of Intervention Effectiveness (CATIE) Investigators (2005). Effectiveness of antipsychotic drugs in patients with chronic schizophrenia. *N Engl J Med*, *353*, 1209–1223.
5. Laruelle, M. (1998). Imaging dopamine transmission in schizophrenia. A review and meta-analysis. *Q J Nucl Med*, *42*, 211–221.
6. Hahn, C.G., Wang, H.Y., Cho, D.S., Talbot, K., Gur, R.E., Berrettini, W.H., Bakshi, K., Kamins, J., Borgmann-Winter, K.E., Siegel, S.J., Gallop, R.J., Arnold, S.E. (2006). Altered neuregulin 1-erbB4 signaling contributes to NMDA receptor hypofunction in schizophrenia. *Nat Med*, *12*, 824–828.
7. Carlsson, A., Waters, N., Holm-Waters, S., Tedroff, J., Nilsson, M., Carlsson, M. (2001). Interactions between monoamines, glutamate and GABA in schizophrenia: new evidence. *Annu Rev Pharmacol Toxicol*, *41*, 237–260.
8. Laruelle, M., Kegeles, L., Abi-Dargham, A. (2003). Glutamate, dopamine and schizophrenia: from pathophysiology to treatment. *Ann N Y Acad Sci*, *1003*, 138–158.
9. Keefe, R.S., Bilder, R.M., Harvey, P.D., Davis, S.M., Palmer, B.W., Gold, J.M., Meltzer, H.Y., Green, M.F., Miller, D.D., Canive, J.M., Adler, L.W., Manschreck, T.C., Swartz, M., Rosenheck, R., Perkins, D.O., Walker, T.M., Stroup, T.S., McEvoy, J.P., Lieberman, J.A. (2006). Baseline neurocognitive deficits in the CATIE schizophrenia trial. *Neuropsychopharmacology*, *31*, 2033–2046.
10. Rosenheck, R., Leslie, D. (2003). Administrative prescription review procedures and use of atypical antipsychotic medications in the Department of Veterans Affairs. *Ment Health Serv Res*, *5*, 149–153.
11. Jones, P.B., Barnes, T.R., Davies, L., Dunn, G., Lloyd, H., Hayhurst, K.P., Murray, R.M., Markwick, A., Lewis, S.W. (2006). Randomized controlled trial of effect on quality of life of second-generation versus first-generation antipsychotic drugs in schizophrenia. *Arch Gen Psychiatry*, *63*, 1079–1087.
12. Davies, L.M., Lewis, S., Jones, P.B., Barnes, T.R., Gaughran, F., Hayhurst, K., Markwick, A., Lloyd, H., CUtLASS team (2007). Cost-effectiveness of first- v. second-generation antipsychotic drugs: results from a randomised controlled trial in schizophrenia responding poorly to previous therapy. *Br J Psychiatry*, *191*, 14–22.

13. Raybould, H.E. (2007). Mechanisms of CCK signaling from gut to brain. *Curr Opin Pharmacol*, *7*, 570–574.
14. Rasmussen, K. (1994). CCK, schizophrenia, and anxiety. CCK-B antagonists inhibit the activity of brain dopamine neurons. *Ann N Y Acad Sci*, *713*, 300–311.
15. Nemeroff, C.B., Bissette, G. (1992). Neuropeptides, dopamine, and schizophrenia. *Ann N Y Acad Sci*, *668*, 273–291.
16. Nair, N.P.V., Lal, S., Bloom, D.M. (1986). Cholecystokinin and schizophrenia. *Prog Brain Res*, *65*, 237–257.
17. Beinfeld, M.D., Garver, D.L. (1991). Concentration of cholecystokinin in cerebrospinal fluid is decreased in psychosis: relationship to symptoms and drug response. *Prog Neuropsychopharmacol Biol Psychiatry*, *15*, 601–609.
18. Schalling, M., Friberg, K., Seroogy, K. (1990). Analysis of expression of cholecystokinin in dopamine cells in the ventral mesencephalon of several species and human with schizophrenia. *Proc Natl Acad Sci U S A*, *87*, 8427–8431.
19. Montgomery, S.A., Green, M.C. (1988). The use of cholecystokinin in schizophrenia: a review. *Psychol Med*, *18*, 593–603.
20. Müller-Vahl, K.R., Emrich, H.M. (2008). Cannabis and schizophrenia: towards a cannabinoid hypothesis of schizophrenia. *Expert Rev Neurother*, *8*, 1037–1048.
21. French, E.D. (1997). delta9-Tetrahydrocannabinol excites rat VTA dopamine neurons through activation of cannabinoid CB1 but not opioid receptors. *Neurosci Lett*, *226*, 159–162.
22. Rinaldi-Carmona, M., Barth, F., Héaulme, M., Alonso, R., Shire, D., Congy, C., Soubrié, P., Brelière, J.C., Le Fur, G. (1995). Biochemical and pharmacological characterisation of SR141716A, the first potent and selective brain cannabinoid receptor antagonist. *Life Sci*, *56*, 1941–1947.
23. Rinaldi-Carmona, M., Barth, F., Héaulme, M., Shire, D., Calandra, B., Congy, C., Martinez, S., Maruani, J., Néliat, G., Caput, D. (1994). SR141716A, a potent and selective antagonist of the brain cannabinoid receptor. *FEBS Lett*, *350*, 240–244.
24. Meltzer, H.Y., Arvanitis, L., Bauer, D., Rein, W. (2004). Placebo-controlled evaluation of four novel compounds for the treatment of schizophrenia and schizoaffective disorder. *Am J Psychiatry*, *161*, 975–984.
25. Deutch, A.Y., Bubser, M. (2007). The orexins/hypocretins and schizophrenia. *Schizophr Bull*, *33*, 1277–1283.
26. Almeida, T.A., Rojo, J., Nieto, P.M., Pinto, F.M., Hernandez, M., Martín, J.D., Candenas, M.L. (2004). Tachykinins and tachykinin receptors: structure and activity relationships. *Curr Med Chem*, *11*, 2045–2081.
27. Saffroy, M., Beaujouan, J.C., Torrens, Y., Besseyre, J., Bergström, L., Glowinski, J. (1988). Localization of tachykinin binding sites ($NK_1$, $NK_2$, $NK_3$ ligands) in the rat brain. *Peptides*, *9*, 227–241.
28. Dietl, M.M., Palacios, J.M. (1991). Phylogeny of tachykinin receptor localization in the vertebrate central nervous system: apparent absence of neurokinin-2 and neurokinin-3 binding sites in the human brain. *Brain Res*, *539*, 211–222.
29. Mileusnic, D., Lee, J.M., Magnuson, D.J., Hejna, M.J., Krause, J.E., Lorens, J.B., Lorens, S.A. (1999). Neurokinin-3 receptor distribution in rat and human brain: an immunohistochemical study. *Neuroscience*, *89*, 1269–1290.

30. Koutcherov, Y., Ashwell, K.W., Paxinos, G. (2000). The distribution of the neurokinin B receptor in the human and rat hypothalamus. *Neuroreport*, *11*, 3127–3131.
31. Alvaro, G., Di Fabio, R. (2007). Neurokinin 1 receptor antagonists—current prospects. *Curr Opin Drug Discov Devel*, *10*, 613–621.
32. Micale, V., Tamburella, A., Leggio, G.M., Mazzola, C., Li Volsi, V., Drago, F. (2008). Behavioral effects of saredutant, a tachykinin $NK_2$ receptor antagonist, in experimental models of mood disorders under basal and stress-related conditions. *Pharmacol Biochem Behav*, *90*, 463–469.
33. Emonds-Alt, X., Vilain, P., Goulaouic, P., Proietto, V., Van Broeck, D., Advenier, C., Naline, E., Neliat, G., Le Fur, G., Breliere, J.C. (1992). A potent and selective non-peptide antagonist of the neurokinin A (NK2) receptor. *Life Sci*, *50*, PL101–PL106.
34. Langlois, X., Wintmolders, C., te Riele, P., Leyson, J.E., Jurzak, M. (2001). Detailed distribution of Neurokinin 3 receptors in the rat, guinea pig and gerbil brain: a comparative autoradiography study. *Neuropharmacology*, *40*, 242–253.
35. Rigby, M., O'Donnell, R., Rupniak, N.M. (2005). Species differences in tachykinin receptor distribution: further evidence that the substance P ($NK_1$) receptor predominates in human brain. *J Comp Neurol*, *490*, 335–353.
36. Mussap, C.J., Geraghty, D.P., Bircher, E. (1993). Tachykinin receptors: a radioligand binding perspective. *J Neurochem*, *69*, 1987–2009.
37. Tooney, P.A., Au, G.G., Chahl, L.A. (2000). Tachykinin $NK_1$ and $NK_3$ receptors in the prefrontal cortex of the human brain. *Clin Exp Pharmacol Physiol*, *27*, 947–949.
38. Yip, J., Chahl, L.A. (2001). Localization of $NK_1$ and $NK_3$ receptors in guinea-pig brain. *Regul Pept*, *98*, 55–62.
39. Nalivaiko, E., Michaud, J.-C., Soubrie, P., Le Fur, G., Feltz, P. (1997). Tachykinin neurokinin1 and neurokinin3 receptor mediated responses in guinea pig substantia nigra: in vitro electrophysiological study. *Neuroscience*, *78*, 745–757.
40. Marco, N., Thirion, A., Mons, G., Bougault, I., Le Fur, G., Soubrie, R., Steinberg, R. (1998). Activation of dopaminergic and cholinergic neurotransmission by tachykinin $NK_3$ receptor stimulation: an in vivo microdialysis approach in guinea pig. *Neuropeptides*, *32*, 481–488.
41. Buell, G., Schulz, M.F., Arkinstall, S.J., Maury, K., Missotten, M., Adami, N., Talabot, F., Kawashima, E. (1992). Molecular characterisation, expression and localisation of human neurokinin-3 receptor. *FEBS Lett*, *299*, 90–95.
42. Whitty, C.J., Paul, M.A., Bannon, M.J. (1997). Neurokinin receptor mRNA localisation in human midbrain dopamine neurons. *J Comp Neurol*, *382*, 394–400.
43. Maggi, C.A. (1995). The mammalian tachykinin receptors. *Gen Pharmacol*, *26*, 911–944.
44. Jung, M., Michaud, J.C., Steinberg, R., Barnouin, M.C., Hayar, A., Mons, G., Souilhac, J., Emonds-Alt, X., Soubrie, P., Le Fur, G. (1996). Electrophysiological, behavioural and biochemical evidence for activation of brain noradrenergic systems following neurokinin $NK_3$ receptor stimulation. *Neuroscience*, *74*, 403–414.
45. Alonso, R., Fournier, M., Carayon, P., Petitpretre, G., Le Fur, G., Soubrie, P. (1996). Evidence for the modulation of dopamine-neuronal function by tachykinin $NK_3$ receptor stimulation in gerbils. *Eur J Neurosci*, *8*, 801–808.

46. Preston, Z., Richardson, P.J., Pinnock, R.D., Lee, K. (2000). $NK_3$ receptors are expressed on mouse striatal gamma-aminobutyric acid-ergic interneurones and evoke [$^3$H] gamma-aminobutyric acid release. *Neurosci Lett*, *284*, 89–92.

47. Bert, L., Rodier, D., Bougault, I., Allouard, N., Le Fur, G., Soubrie, P., Steinberg, R. (2002). Permissive role of Neurokinin $NK_3$ receptors in $NK_1$ receptor-mediated activation of the locus coeruleus revealed by SR142801. *Synapse*, *43*, 62–69.

48. Gueudet, C., Santucci, V., Soubrie, P., Le Fur, G. (1999). Blockade of neurokinin3 receptors antagonizes drug-induced population response and depolarization block of midbrain dopamine neurons in Guinea pigs. *Synapse*, *33*, 71–79.

49. Sarau, H.M., Griswold, D.E., Potts, W., Foley, J.J., Schmidt, D.B., Webb, E.F., Martin, L.D., Brawner, M.E., Elshourbagy, N.A., Medhurst, A.D., Giardina, G.A., Hay, D.W. (1997). Nonpeptide tachykinin receptor antagonists: I. Pharmacological and pharmacokinetic characterization of SB 223412, a novel, potent and selective neurokinin-3 receptor antagonist. *J Pharmacol Exp Ther*, *281*, 1303–1311.

50. Dawson, L.A., Cato, K.J., Scott, C., Watson, J.M., Wood, M.D., Foxton, R., de la Flor, R., Soffin, E., Jones, G.A., Kew, J.N.C., Cluderay, J.E., Southam, E., Gartlon, J., Pemberton, D., Jones, D.N.C., Davies, C.H., Hagan, J.J. (2008). In vitro and in vivo characterisation of the non-peptide $NK_3$ receptor antagonist SB-223412 (talnetant): potential therapeutic utility in the treatment of schizophrenia. *Neuropsychopharmacology*, *33*, 1642–1652.

51. Furuta, T., Koyano, K., Tomioka, R., Yanagawa, Y., Kaneko, T. (2004). GABAergic basal forebrain neurons that express receptor for neurokinin B and send axons to the cerebral cortex. *J Comp Neurol*, *473*, 43–58.

52. Lewis, D.A., Hashimoto, T., Volk, D.W. (2005). Cortical inhibitory neurons and schizophrenia. *Nat Rev Neurosci*, *6*, 312–324.

53. Stacy, A.E., Woodhall, G.L., Jones, R.S. (2002). Neurokinin-receptor-mediated depolarization of cortical neurones elicits increase in glutamate release at excitatory synapses. *Eur J Neurosci*, *16*, 1896–1906.

54. Rekling, J.C. (2004). NK-3 receptor activation depolarizes and induces an after-depolarization in pyramidal neurons in gerbil cingulate cortex. *Brain Res Bull*, *63*, 85–90.

55. Simmons, M.A., Sobotka-Briner, C., Medd, A.M. (2008). Localization and function of NK3 recepotrs of layer V pyramidal neurons of the guinea pig medial prefrontal cortex. *Neurosci*, *156*, 987–994.

56. Coyle, J.T., Tsai, G. (2004). The NMDA receptor glycine modulatory site: a therapeutic target for improving cognition and reducing negative symptoms in schizophrenia. *Psychopharmacology (Berl)*, *174*, 32–38.

57. Patil, S.T., Zhang, L., Martenyi, F., Lowe, S.L., Jackson, K.A., Andreev, B.V., Avedisova, A.S., Bardenstein, L.M., Gurovich, I.Y., Morozova, M.A., Mosolov, S.N., Neznanov, N.G., Reznik, A.M., Smulevich, A.B., Tochilov, V.A., Johnson, B.G., Monn, J.A., Schoepp, D.D. (2007). Activation of mGlu2/3 receptors as a new approach to treat schizophrenia: a randomized Phase 2 clinical trial. *Nat Med*, *13*, 1102–1107.

58. Lisman, J.E., Coyle, J.T., Green, R.W., Javitt, D.C., Benes, F.M., Heckers, S., Grace, A.A. (2008). Circuit-based framework for understanding neurotransmitter and risk gene interactions in schizophrenia. *Trends Neurosci*, *31*, 234–242.

59. Siuciak, J.A., McCarthy, S.A., Martin, A.N., Chapin, D.S., Stock, J., Nadeau, D.M., Kantesaria, S., Bryce-Pritt, D., McLean, S. (2007). Disruption of the neurokinin-3 receptor (NK3) in mice leads to cognitive deficits. *Psychopharmacology (Berl)*, *194*, 185–195.

60. Nordquist, R.E., Delenclos, M., Ballard, T.M., Savignac, H., Pauly-Evers, M., Ozmen, L., Spooren, W. (2008). Cognitive performance in neurokinin 3 receptor knockout mice. *Psychopharmacology (Berl)*, *198*, 211–220.

61. Nordquist, R.E., Savignac, H., Pauly-Evers, M., Walker, G., Knoflach, F., Borroni, E., Glaentzlin, P., Bohrmann, B., Messer, J., Ozmen, L., Albientz, A., Spooren, W. (2008). Characterization of behavioral response to amphetamine, tyrosine hydroxylase levels, and dopamine receptor levels in neurokinin 3 receptor knockout mice. *Behav Pharmacol*, *19*, 518–529.

62. Emonds-Alt, X., Bichon, D., Ducoux, J.P., Heaulme, M., Miloux, B., Poncelet, M., Proietto, V., Van Broeck, D., Vilain, P., Neliat, G., Soubrie, P., Le Fur, G., Breleère, J.C. (1995). SR 142801, the first potent non-peptide antagonist of the tachykinin $NK_3$ receptor. *Life Sci*, *56*, PL27–PL32.

63. Jocham, G., Lezoch, K., Müller, C.P., Kart-Teke, E., Huston, J.P., de Souza Silva, M.A. (2006). Neurokinin receptor antagonism attenuates cocaine's behavioural activating effects yet potentiates its dopamine-enhancing action in the nucleus accumbens core. *Eur J Neurosci*, *24*, 1721–1732.

64. De Souza Silva, M.A., Mello, E.L. Jr, Müller, C.P., Jocham, G., Maior, R.S., Huston, J.P., Tomaz, C., Barros, M. (2006). The tachykinin NK3 receptor antagonist SR142801 blocks the behavioral effects of cocaine in marmoset monkeys. *Eur J Pharmacol*, *536*, 269–278.

65. Man, J., Jurzak, M., Stohr, T. (2000). The $NK_3$ receptor antagonist SR142801 reverses apomorphine-induced deficits on prepulse inhibition in gerbils. *Behav Pharmacol*, *11*, 343.

66. Pouzet, B., Moller Nielson, N.S. (2003). Preclinical investigation of the antipsychotic-like effect of $NK_3$ receptor antagonists versus marketed antipsychotics in gerbils. *J Psychopharmacol*, *17*(S), A46.

67. Salome, N., Stemmelin, J., Cohen, C., Griebel, G. (2006). Selective blockade of $NK_2$ or $NK_3$ receptors produces anxiolytic- and antidepressant-like effects in gerbils. *Pharmacol Biochem Behav*, *83*, 533–539.

68. Dableh, L.J., Yashpal, K., Rochford, J., Henry, J.L. (2005). Antidepressant-like effects of neurokinin receptor antagonists in the forced swim test in the rat. *Eur J Pharmacol*, *507*, 99–105.

69. Ribeiro, S.J., Teixeira, R.M., Calixto, J.B., De Lima, T.C. (2000). Tachykinin NK(3) receptor involvement in anxiety. *Neuropeptides*, *33*, 181–188.

70. Smith, P.W., Dawson, L.A. (2008). Neurokinin 3 ($NK_3$) receptor modulators for the treatment of psychiatric disorders. *Recent Pat CNS Drug Discov*, *3*, 1–15.

71. Regoli, D., Dion, S., Rhaleb, N.E., Rouissi, N., Tousignant, C., Jukic, D., D'Orleans-Juste, P., Drapeau, G. (1989). Selective agonists for receptors of substance P and related neurokinins. *Biopolymers*, *28*, 81–90.

72. Regoli, D., Drapeau, G., Dion, S., Couture, R. (1988). New selective agonists for neurokinin receptors: pharmacological tools for receptor characterization. *Trends Pharmacol Sci*, *9*, 290–295.

73. Dam, T.V., Escher, E., Quirion, R. (1990). Visualization of neurokinin-3 receptor sites in rat brain using the highly selective ligand [$^3$H]senktide. *Brain Res*, *506*, 175–179.
74. Stoessl, A.J., Hill, D.R. (1990). Autoradiographic visualization of $NK_3$ tachykinin binding sites in the rat brain, utilizing [$^3$H] senktide. *Brain Res*, *534*, 1–7.
75. Sumner, S.C., Jiang, S.P., Jernigan, R.L., Ferretti, J.A. (1992). Conformational analysis of receptor selective tachykinin analogs: senktide and septide. *J Biomol Struct Dyn*, *10*, 429–439.
76. Tallon, M., Ron, D., Halle, D., Amodeo, P., Saviano, G., Temussi, P.A., Selinger, Z., Naider, F., Chorev, M. (1993). Synthesis, biological activity, and conformational analysis of [pGlu6,N-MePhe8,Aib9] substance P (6–11): a selective agonist for the NK-3 receptor. *Biopolymers*, *33*, 915–926.
77. Wormser, U., Laufer, R., Hart, Y., Chorev, M., Gilon, C., Selinger, Z. (1986). Highly selective agonists for substance P receptor subtypes. *EMBO J*, *5*, 2805–2808.
78. Regoli, D., Nguyen, Q.T., Jukic, D., Rouissi, N. (1993). Functional characterization of neurokinin receptors with agonists and antagonists. *Regul Pept*, *46*, 287–289.
79. Stables, J.M., Beresford, I.J., Arkinstall, S., Ireland, S.J., Walsh, D.M., Seale, P.W., Ward, P., Hagan, R.M. (1994). GR138676, a novel peptidic tachykinin antagonist which is potent at $NK_3$ receptors. *Neuropeptides*, *27*, 333–341.
80. Boden, P., Eden, J.M., Hodgson, J., Horwell, D.C., Hughes, J., McKnight, A.T., Lewthwaite, R.A., Pritchard, M.C., Raphy, J., Meecham, K., Ratcliffe, G.S., Suman-Chauhan, N., Woodruff, G.N. (1996). Use of a dipeptide chemical library in the development of non-peptide tachykinin NK3 receptor selective antagonists. *J Med Chem*, *39*, 1664–1675.
81. Boden, P., Eden, J.M., Hodgson, J., Horwell, D.C., Pritchard, M.C., Raphy, J., Suman-Chauhan, N. (1995). The development of a novel series of non-peptide tachykinin $NK_3$ receptor selective antagonists. *Bioorg Med Chem Lett*, *5*, 1773–1778.
82. Boden, P., Eden, J.M., Hodgson, J., Horwell, D.C., Howson, W., Hughes, J., McKnight, A.T., Meecham, K., Pritchard, M.C., Raphy, J., Ratcliffe, G.S., Suman-Chauhan, N., Woodruff, G.N. (1994). The rational development of small molecule tachykinin $NK_3$ receptor selective antagonists—the utilization of a dipeptide chemical library in drug design. *Bioorg Med Chem Lett*, *4*, 1679–1684.
83. Giardina, G.A., Sarau, H.M., Farina, C., Medhurst, A.D., Grugni, M., Foley, J.J., Raveglia, L.F., Schmidt, D.B., Rigolio, R., Vassallo, M., Vecchietti, V., Hay, D.W. (1996). 2-Phenyl-4-quinolinecarboxamides: a novel class of potent and selective non-peptide competitive antagonists for the human neurokinin-3 receptor. *J Med Chem*, *39*, 2281–2284.
84. Chretien, L., Guillemette, G., Regoli, D. (1994). Non-peptide angiotensin receptor antagonists bind to tachykinin NK3 receptors of rat and guinea pig brain. *Eur J Pharmacol*, *256*, 73–78.
85. Poulsen, A., Bjornholm, B., Gundertofte, K., Pogozheva, I.D., Liljefors, T. (2003). Pharmacophore and receptor models for neurokinin receptors. *J Comput Aided Mol Des*, *17*, 765–783.
86. Poulsen, A., Liljefors, T., Gundertofte, K., Bjornholm, B. (2002). A pharmacophore model for NK2 antagonist comprising compounds from several structurally diverse classes. *J Comput Aided Mol Des*, *16*, 273–286.

87. Giardina, G., Raveglia, L.F. (1997). Neurokinin-3 receptor antagonists. *Expert Opin Ther Pat*, *7*, 307–323.

88. Giardina, G., Grugni, M., Raveglia, L.F. (2000). Recent advances in neurokinin-3 receptor antagonists. *Expert Opin Ther Pat*, *10*, 939–960.

89. Giardina, G.A., Artico, M., Cavagnera, S., Cerri, A., Consolandi, E., Gagliardi, S., Graziani, D., Grugni, M., Hay, D.W., Luttmann, M.A., Mena, R., Raveglia, L.F., Rigolio, R., Sarau, H.M., Schmidt, D.B., Zanoni, G., Farina, C. (1999). Replacement of the quinoline system in 2-phenyl-4-quinolinecarboxamide NK-3 receptor antagonists. *Farmaco*, *54*, 364–374.

90. Maynard, G.D., Rachwal, S., Pringle, W.C., Yuan, J., Xie, L., Xu, Y., Han, B. (2005). Preparation of diaryl imidazoles as neurokinin-3 receptor modulators. U.S. Pat. Appl. Publ. US 2005148601.

91. Maynard, G.D., Yuan, J., Peterson, J.M. (2005). Preparation of diaryl pyrazoles as neurokinin-3 receptor modulators. PCT Int. Appl. WO 2005061462.

92. Elliott, J.M., Carling, R.W., Chambers, M., Chicchi, G.G., Hutson, P.H., Jones, A.B., MacLeod, A., Marwood, R., Meneses-Lorente, G., Mezzogori, E., Murray, F., Rigby, M., Royo, I., Russell, M.G., Sohal, B., Tsao, K.L., Williams, B. (2006). N′,2-diphenylquinoline-4-carbohydrazide based $NK_3$ receptor antagonists. *Bioorg Med Chem Lett*, *16*, 5748–5751.

93. Elliott, J.M., Carling, R.W., Chicchi, G.G., Crawforth, J., Hutson, P.H., Jones, A.B., Kelly, S., Marwood, R., Meneses-Lorente, G., Mezzogori, E., Murray, F., Rigby, M., Royo, I., Russell, M.G., Shaw, D., Sohal, B., Tsao, K.L., Williams, B. (2006). N′,2-diphenylquinoline-4-carbohydrazide based $NK_3$ receptor antagonists II. *Bioorg Med Chem Lett*, *16*, 5752–5756.

94. Gobbi, L.C., Hoener, M., Riemer, C., Spooren, W. (2007). Substituted triazole derivatives as modulators of NK-3 receptors for treating nervous system disorders. U.S. Pat. Appl. Publ. US 2007021475.

95. Spooren, W., Riemer, C., Meltzer, H. (2005). Opinion: $NK_3$ receptor antagonists: the next generation of antipsychotics? *Nat Rev Drug Discov*, *4*, 967–975.

96. Meltzer, H.Y., Prus, A. (2006). $NK_3$ receptor antagonists for the treatment of schizophrenia. *Drug Discov Today*, *3*, 555–560.

97. Kronenberg, G., Berger, P., Tauber, R.F., Bandelow, B., Henkel, V., Heuser, I. (2005). Randomized, double-blind study of SR142801 (Osanetant). A novel neurokinin-3 ($NK_3$) receptor antagonist in panic disorder with pre- and posttreatment cholecystokinin tetrapeptide (CCK-4) challenges. *Pharmacopsychiatry*, *38*, 24–29.

98. Mesnage, V., Houeto, J.L., Bonnet, A.M., Clavier, I., Arnulf, I., Cattelin, F., Le Fur, G., Damier, P., Welter, M.L., Agid, Y. (2004). Neurokinin B, neurotensin, and cannabinoid receptor antagonists and Parkinson disease. *Clin Neuropharmacol*, *27*, 108–110.

99. Evangelista, S. (2005). Talnetant. *Curr Opin Investig Drugs*, *6*, 717–721.

100. Liem-Moolenaar, M., Gray, F., de Visser, S., Franson, K., Schoemaker, R., Schmitt, J., Cohen, A., van Gerven, J. (2008). Psychomotor and cognitive effects of a single oral dose of talnetant (SB223412) in healthy volunteers compared with placebo or haloperidol. *J Psychopharmacol*, *24*, 73–82.

101. Rupniak, N.M., Kramer, M.S. (1999). Discovery of the antidepressant and anti-emetic efficacy of substance P receptor ($NK_1$) antagonists. *Trends Pharmacol Sci*, *20*, 485–490.

102. Kramer, M.S., Cutler, N., Feighner, J., Shrivastava, R., Carman, J., Sramek, J.J., Reines, S.A., Liu, G., Snavely, D., Wyatt-Knowles, E., Hale, J.J., Mills, S.G., MacCoss, M., Swain, C.J., Harrison, T., Hill, R.G., Hefti, F., Scolnick, E.M., Cascieri, M.A., Chicchi, G.G., Sadowski, S., Williams, A.R., Hewson, L., Smith, D., Carlson, E.J., Hargreaves, R.J., Rupniak, N.M. (1998). Distinct mechanism for antidepressant activity by blockade of central substance P receptors. *Science*, *281*, 1640–1645.

103. Kramer, M.S., Winokur, A., Kelsey, J., Preskorn, S.H., Rothschild, A.J., Snavely, D., Ghosh, K., Ball, W.A., Reines, S.A., Munjack, D., Apter, J.T., Cunningham, L., Kling, M., Bari, M., Getson, A., Lee, Y. (2004). Demonstration of the efficacy and safety of a novel substance P (NK1) receptor antagonist in major depression. *Neuropsychopharmacology*, *29*, 385–392.

104. Keller, M., Montgomery, S., Ball, W., Morrison, M., Snavely, D., Liu, G., Hargreaves, R., Hietala, J., Lines, C., Beebe, K., Reines, S. (2006). Lack of efficacy of the substance P (neurokinin1 receptor) antagonist aprepitant in the treatment of major depressive disorder. *Biol Psychiatry*, *59*, 216–223.

105. Fenton, W.S. (2000). Depression, suicide, and suicide prevention in schizophrenia. *Suicide Life Threat Behav*, *30*, 34–49.

106. Hausmann, A., Fleischhacker, W.W. (2002). Differential diagnosis of depressed mood in patients with schizophrenia: a diagnostic algorithm based on a review. *Acta Psychiatr Scand*, *106*, 83–96.

107. Montross, L.P., Zisook, S., Kasckow, J. (2005). Suicide among patients with schizophrenia: a consideration of risk and protective factors. *Ann Clin Psychiatry*, *17*, 173–182.

108. Carraway, R., Leeman, S.E. (1973). The isolation of a new hypotensive peptide, neurotensin, from bovine hypothalami. *J Biol Chem*, *248*, 6854–6861.

109. Friry, C., Feliciangeli, S., Richard, F., Kitabgi, P., Rovere, C. (2002). Production of recombinant large proneurotensin/neuromedin N-derived peptides and characterization of their binding and biological activity. *Biochem Biophys Res Commun*, *290*, 1161–1168.

110. Kitabgi, P., Rostene, W., Dussaillant, M., Schotte, A., Laduron, P.M., Vincent, J.P. (1987). Two populations of neurotensin binding sites in murine brain: discrimination by the antihistamine levocabastine reveals markedly different radioautographic distribution. *Eur J Pharmacol*, *140*, 285–293.

111. Kinkead, B., Nemeroff, C.B. (2004). Neurotensin, schizophrenia, and antipsychotic drug action. *Int Rev Neurobiol*, *59*, 327–349.

112. Mazella, J. (2001). Sortilin/neurotensin receptor-3: a new tool to investigate neurotensin signalling and cellular trafficking? *Cell Signal*, *13*, 1–6.

113. Vincent, J.P., Mazella, J., Kitabgi, P. (1999). Neurotensin and neurotensin receptors. *Trends Pharmacol Sci*, *20*, 302–309.

114. Jacobsen, L. (2001). Activation and functional characterization of the mosaic receptor SorLA/LR11. *J Biol Chem*, *276*, 22788–22796.

115. Boules, M., Shaw, A., Fredrickson, P., Richelson, E. (2007). Neurotenisn agonists—potential in the treatment of schizophrenia. *CNS Drugs*, *21*, 13–23.

116. Nicot, A., Rostene, W., Berod, A. (1994). Neurotensin receptor expression in the rat forebrain and midbrain: a combined analysis by in situ hybridization and receptor autoradiography. *J Comp Neurol*, *341*, 407–419.

117. Palacios, J.M., Kuhar, M.J. (1981). Neurotensin receptors are located on dopamine containing neurones in rat midbrain. *Nature*, *294*, 587–589.
118. Quirion, R., Rowe, W.B., Lapchak, P.A., Araujo, D.M., Beaudet, A. (1992). Distribution of neurotensin receptors in mammalian brain. What it is telling us about its interactions with other neurotransmitter systems. *Ann N Y Acad Sci*, *668*, 109–119.
119. Grace, A.A., Bunney, B.S., Moore, H., Todd, C.L. (1997). Dopamine-cell depolarization block as a model for the therapeutic actions of antipsychotic drugs. *Trends Neurosci*, *20*, 31–37.
120. Fuxe, K., Von Euler, G., Agnati, L.F., Merlo Pich, E., Tanganelli, S., Li, X.M., Tinner, B., Cintra, A., Carani, C. (1992). Intramembrane interactions between neurotensin receptors and dopamine D2 receptors as a major mechanism for the neuroleptic-like action of neurotensin. *Ann N Y Acad Sci*, *668*, 186–204.
121. Farkas, R.H., Chien, P.Y., Nakajima, S., Nakajima, Y. (1997). Neurotensin and dopamine D2 activation oppositely regulate the same Kþ conductance in rat midbrain dopaminergic neurons. *Neurosci Lett*, *231*, 21–24.
122. Jolicoeur, F.B., Rivest, R., Stpierre, S., Gagne, M.A., Dumais, M. (1985). The effects of neurotensin and [D-Tyr11]-NT on the hyperactivity induced by intraaccumbens administration of a potent dopamine receptor agonist. *Neuropeptides*, *6*, 143–156.
123. Cusack, B., Jansen, K., McCormick, D.J., Chou, T., Pang, Y., Richelson, E. (2000). A single amino acid of the human and rat neurotensin receptors (subtype 1) determining the pharmacological profile of a species-selective neurotensin agonist. *Biochem Pharmacol*, *60*, 793–801.
124. Feifel, D., Melendez, G., Shilling, P.D. (2004). Reversal of sensorimotor gating deficits in Brattleboro rats by acute administration of clozapine and a neurotensin agonist, but not haloperidol: a potential predictive model for novel antipsychotic effects. *Neuropsychopharmacology*, *29*(4), 731–738.
125. Feifel, D., Melendez, G., Shilling, P.D. (2003). A systemically administered neurotensin agonist blocks disruption of prepulse inhibition produced by a serotonin-2A agonist. *Neuropsychopharmacology*, *28*, 651–653.
126. Feifel, D., Reza, T.L., Wustrow, D.J., Davis, M.D. (1999). Novel antipsychotic-like effects on prepulse inhibition of startle produced by a neurotensin agonist. *J Pharmacol Exp Ther*, *288*, 710–713.
127. Feifel, D. Melendez, G., Shilling, P.D., (2003). Neurotensin agonists block the prepulse inhibition deficits produced by a 5-HT(2A) and an α(1) agonist. *Neuropsychopharmacology (Berl)*, *28*, 651–654.
128. Shilling, P.D., Richelson, E., Feifel, D. (2003). The effects of systemic NT69L, a neurotensin agonist, on baseline and drug-disrupted prepulse inhibition. *Behav Brain Res*, *143*, 7–14.
129. Shilling, P.D., Feife, D. (2008). The neurotensin-1 receptor agonist PD149163 blocks fear-potentiated startle. *Pharmacol Biochem Behav*, *90*, 748–752.
130. Azmi, N., Norman, C., Spicer, C.H., Bennett, G.W. (2006). Effects of a neurotensin analogues (PD149163) and antagonist (SR142948A) on the scopolamine-induced deficits in a novel object discrimination task. *Behav Pharmacol*, *17*, 357–362.
131. Grimond-Billa, S.K., Norman, C., Bennett, G.W., Cassaday, H.J. (2008). Selectively increased trace conditioning under the neurotensin agonist PD149163 in an

aversive procedure in which SR142948A was without intrinsic effect. *J Psychopharmacol*, *22*, 290–299.

132. Hertel, P., Byskov, L., Didriksen, M., Arnt, J. (2001). Induction of tolerance to the suppressant effect of NT analog NT69L on amphetamine-induced hyperactivity. *Eur J Pharmacol*, *422*, 77–81.
133. Hertel, P., Olsen, C.K., Didriksen, M., Arnt, J. (2002). Repeated administration of the NT analogue NT69L induces tolerance to its suppressant effect on conditioned avoidance behaviour. *Eur J Pharmacol*, *439*, 107–111.
134. Boules, M., McMahon, B., Wang, R., Warrington, L., Stewart, J., Yerbury, S., Faug, A., McCormack, D., Richelson, E. (2003). Selective tolerance to the hypothermic effects of a NT analog that crosses the blood brain barrier. *Brain Res*, *987*, 39–48.
135. Hadden, M.K., Orwig, K.S., Kokko, K.P., Mazella, J., Dix, T.A. (2005). Design, synthesis and evaluation of the antipsychotic potential of orally bioavailable NT (8-13) analogues containing non-natural arginine and lysine residues. *Neuropharmacology*, *49*, 1149–1159.
136. Rompre, P.P. (1997). Repeated activation of NT receptors sensitises to the stimulant effect of amphetamine. *Eur J Pharmacol*, *328*, 131–134.
137. Norman, C., Beckett, S.R.G., Spicer, C.H., Ashton, D., Langlois, X., Bennett, G.W. (2008). Ffects of chronic infusion of neurotensin and a neurotensin NT1 selective analogue PD149163 on amphetamine-induced hyperlocomotion. *J Psychopharmacol*, *22*, 300–307.
138. Marie-Claire, C., Palminteri, S., Romualdi, P., Noble, F. (2008). Effects of the selective neurotensin antagonist SR 142948A on 3,4-methylenedioxymethamphetamine-induced behaviours in mice. *Neuropharmacology*, *54*, 1107–1111.
139. Feifel, D., Roza, T.L., Robeck, S.L. (1997). Pro-dopamine effects of neurotensin on sensorimotor gating deficits. *Peptides*, *18*, 1457–1460.
140. Gully, D., Labeeuw, B., Boigegrain, R., Oury-Donat, F., Bachy, A., Poncelet, M., Steinberg, R., Suaud-Chagny, M.F., Santucci, V., Vita, N., Pecceu, F., Labbe-Jullie, C., Kitabgi, P., Soubrie, P., Le Fur, G., Maffrand, J.P. (1997). Biochemical and pharmacological activities of SR 142948A, a new potent neurotensin receptor antagonist. *J Pharmacol Exp Ther*, *280*, 802–812.
141. Gully, D., Canton, M., Boigegrain, R., Jeanjean, F., Molimard, J.C., Poncelet, M., Gueudet, C., Heaulme, M., Leyris, R., Brouard, A. (1993). Biochemical and pharmacological profile of a potent and selective nonpeptide antagonist of the neurotensin receptor. *Proc Natl Acad Sci U S A*, *90*, 65–69.
142. Santucci, V., Geuudet, C., Steinberg, R., Le Fur, G., Soubrie, P. (1997). Involvement of cortical neurotensin in the regulation of rat mesocorticolimbic dopamine neurons: evidence from changes in the number of spontaneously active A10 cells after neurotensin receptor blockade. *Synapse*, *28*, 370–380.
143. Azzi, M., Betancur, C., Sillaber, I., Spangel, P., Rostene, W., Berod, A. (1998). Repeated administration of the neurotensin receptor antagonist SR 48692 differentially regulates mesocortical and mesolimbic dopaminergic systems. *J Neurochem*, *71*, 1158–1167.
144. Betancur, C., Cabrera, R., De Kloet, E., Pelaprat, D., Rostene, W. (1998). Role of endogenous neurotensin in the behavioural and neuroendocrine effects of cocaine. *Neuropsychopharmacology*, *19*, 322–332.

145. Clineschmidt, B.V., McGuffin, J.C. (1977). Neurotensin administered intracisternally inhibits responsiveness of mice to noxious stimuli. *Eur J Pharmacol*, *46*, 395–396.

146. Sefler, A.M., He, J.X., Sawyer, T.K., Holub, K.E., Omecinsky, D.O., Reily, M.D., Thanabal, V., Akunne, H.C., Cody, W.L. (1995). Design and structure-activity relationships of C-terminal cyclic neurotensin fragment analogues. *J Med Chem*, *38*, 249–257.

147. Lundquist, J.T. IV, Dix, T.A. (1999). Preparation and receptor binding affinities of cyclic C-terminal neurotensin (8-13) and (9-13) analogues. *Bioorg Med Chem Lett*, *9*, 2579–2582.

148. Lundquist, J.T. IV, Bullesbach, E.E., Dix, T.A. (2000). Synthesis of neurotensin(9–13) analogues exhibiting enhanced human neurotensin receptor binding affinities. *Bioorg Med Chem Lett*, *10*, 453–455.

149. Kokko, K.P., Hadden, M.K., Orwig, K.S., Mazella, J., Dix, T.A. (2003). In vitro analysis of stable, receptor-selective neurotensin [8-13] analogues. *J Med Chem*, *46*, 4141–4148.

150. Nock, B.A., Nikolopoulou, A., Reubi, J., Maes, V., Conrath, P., Tourwe, D., Maina, T. (2006). Toward stable N4-modified Neurotensins for NTS1-receptor-targeted tumor imaging with 99mTc. *J Med Chem*, *49*, 4767–4776.

151. Einsiedel, J., Hubner, H., Hervet, M., Harterich, S., Koschatzky, S., Gmeiner, P. (2008). Peptide backbone modifications on the C-terminal hexapeptide of neurotensin. *Bioorg Med Chem Lett*, *18*, 2013–2018.

152. Craig, A.G., Griffen, D., Olivera, B.M., Watkins, M., Hillyard, D.R., Imperial, J., Cruz, L.J., Wagstaff, J.D., Layer, R.T., Jones, R.M., McIntosh, J.M., McCabe, R.T. (2000). Contulakin-G and analogs for therapeutic use. PCT Int. Appl. WO 2000023092.

153. Craig, A.G., Norberg, T., Griffin, D., Hoeger, C., Akhtar, M., Schmidt, K., Low, W., Dykert, J., Richelson, E., Navarro, V., Mazella, J., Watkins, M., Hillyard, D., Imperial, J., Cruz, L.J., Olivera, B.M. (1999). Contulakin-G, an O-glycosylated invertebrate neurotensin. *J Biol Chem*, *274*, 13752–13759.

154. Clerc, F.-F., Dubroeucq, M.-C., Helynck, G., Leboul, J., Martin, J.-P. (1995). Neurotensin antagonist peptides. PCT Int. Appl WO 9532218.

155. Helynck, G., Dubertret, C., Frechet, D., Leboul, J. (1998). Isolation of RP 66453, a new secondary peptide metabolite from Streptomyces sp. useful as a lead for neurotensin antagonists. *J Antibiot (Tokyo)*, *51*, 512–514.

156. Kozikowski, A.P., Dodd, D.S., Zaidi, J., Pang, Y.-P., Cusack, B., Richelson, E. (1995). Synthesis of partial nonpeptidic peptide mimetics as potential neurotensin agonists and antagonists. *J Chem Soc Perkin Trans 1*, 1615–1621.

157. Snider, R.M., Pereira, D.A., Longo, K.P., Davidson, R.E., Vinick, F.J., Laitinen, K., Genc-Sehitoglu, E., Crawley, J.N. (1992). UK-73,093: a non-peptide neurotensin receptor antagonist. *Bioorg Med Chem Lett*, *2*, 1535–1540.

158. Tyler-McMahon, B.M., Stewart, J.A., Farinas, F., McCormick, D.J., Richelson, E. (2000). Highly potent neurotensin analog that causes hypothermia and antinociception. *Eur J Pharmacol*, *390*, 107–111.

159. Dubuc, I., Costentin, J., Terranova, J.P., Barnouin, M.C., Soubrie, P., Le Fur, G., Rostene, W., Kitabgi, P. (1994). The nonpeptide neurotensin antagonist, SR 48692,

used as a tool to reveal putative neurotensin receptor subtypes. *Br J Pharmacol*, *112*, 352–354.

160. Labeeuw, B., Gully, D., Jeanjean, F., Molimard, J.-C., Boigegrain, R. (1996). 1-Phenylpyrazole-3-carboxamides acting on neurotensin receptors. PCT Int. Appl. WO 9632382.
161. Maffrand, J.-P., Gully, D., Boigegrain, R., Jeanjean, F. (1995). New potent and selective non-peptide antagonists of neurotensin. *Eur J Med Chem*, *30* (Suppl., Proceedings of the 13th International Symposium on Medicinal Chemistry, 1994), 551s–573s.
162. Quere, L., Boigegrain, R., Jeanjean, F., Gully, D., Evrard, G., Durant, F. (1996). Structural requirements of non-peptide neurotensin receptor antagonists. *J Chem Soc Perkin Trans 2*, 2639–2646.
163. Quere, L., Longfils, G., Boigegrain, R., Labeeuw, B., Gully, D., Durant, F. (1998). X-ray structural characterization of SR 142948, a novel potent synthetic neurotensin receptor antagonist. *Bioorg Med Chem Lett*, *8*, 653–658.
164. Vita, N., Oury-Donat, F., Chalon, P., Guillemot, M., Kaghad, M., Bachy, A., Thurneyssen, O., Garcia, S., Poinot-Chazel, C., Casellas, P., Keane, P., Le Fur, G., Maffrand, J.P., Soubrie, P., Caput, D., Ferrara, P. (1998). Neurotensin is an antagonist of the human neurotensin NT2 receptor expressed in Chinese hamster ovary cells. *Eur J Pharmacol*, *360*, 265–272.
165. Johnson, S.J., Akunne, H.C., Heffner, T.G., Kesten, S.R., Pugsley, T.A., Wise, L.D., Wustrow, D.J. (1997). Novel small molecule neurotensin antagonists: 3-(1,5-diaryl-1,5-dioxopentan-3-yl)benzoic acids. *Bioorg Med Chem Lett*, *7*, 561–566.
166. Chakravarty, P.K., Ransom, R.W. (1993). Substituted pyrazoles, isoxazoles and isothiazoles as neurotensin antagonists. Brit. UK Pat. Appl. GB 2263638.
167. Chakravarty, P.K., Ransom, R.W. (1993). Substituted triazoles as neurotensin antagonists. Brit. UK Pat. Appl. GB 2263635.
168. Chakravarty, P.K., Ransom, R.W. (1993). Substituted triazolinones, triazolinethiones, and triazolinimines as neurotensin antagonists. Brit. UK Pat. Appl. GB 2263636.
169. Chakravarty, P.K., Naylor, E.M., Chen, A. (1994). (Biphenylylmethyl)phthalazinones as neurotensin antagonists. PCT Int. Appl. WO 9410151.
170. Chakravarty, P.K., Chen, A., Ransom, R.W. (1993). Substituted imidazo-fused 6-membered carbocycles or heterocycles as neurotensin antagonists. Brit. UK Pat. Appl. GB 2263637.
171. Chakravarty, P.K., Naylor, E.M., Ransom, R.W. (1993). Substituted pyrimidinones as neurotensin antagonists. Brit. UK Pat. Appl. GB 2263639.
172. Chakravarty, P.K., Naylor, E.M., Ransom, R.W. (1993). Substituted quinazolinones as neurotensin antagonists useful in the treatment of CNS disorders. US 5204354.
173. Chakravarty, P.K., Ransom, R.W. (1995). Neurotensin receptor antagonists. *Curr Pharm Des*, *1*, 317–324.
174. Caceda, R., Kinkead, B., Nemeroff, C.B. (2006). Neurotensin: role in psychiatric and neurological diseases. *Peptides*, *27*, 2385–2404.
175. Widerlöv, E., Lindström, L.H., Besev, G., Manberg, P.J., Nemeroff, C.B., Breese, G.R., et al. (1982). Subnormal CSF levels of neurotensin in a subgroup of schizophrenic patients: normalization after neuroleptic treatment. *Am J Psychiatry*, *139*, 1122–1126.

176. Sharma, R.P., Janicak, P.G., Bissette, G., Nemeroff, C.B. (1997). CSF neurotensin concentrations and antipsychotic treatment in schizophrenia and schizoaffective disorders. *Am J Psychiatry*, *154*, 1019–1021.

177. Garver, D.L., Bissette, G., Yao, J.K., Nemeroff, C.B. (1991). Relation of CSF neurotensin concentrations to symptoms and drug response of psychotic patients. *Am J Psychiatry*, *148*, 484–488.

178. Boules, M., Liang, Y., Briody, S., Miura, T., Fauq, I., Oliveros, A., et al. (2010). NT79: a novel neurotensin analog with selective behavioural effects. *Brain Res*, *1308*, 35–46.

179. Drapeau, G., D'Orleans-Juste, P., Dion, S., Rhaleb, N.E., Rouissi, N.E., Regoli, D. (1987). Selective agonists for substance P and neurokinin receptors. *Neuropeptides*, *10*, 43–54.

180. Drapeau, G., d'Orleans-Juste, P., Dion, S., Rhaleb, N.E., Regoli, D. (1987). Specific agonists for neurokinin B receptors. *Eur J Pharmacol*, *136*, 401–403.

181. Sadowski, S., Huang, R.R., Fong, T.M., Marko, O., Cascieri, M.A. (1993). Characterization of the binding of [125I-iodo-histidyl, methyl-Phe7] neurokinin B to the neurokinin-3 receptor. *Neuropeptides*, *24*, 317–319.

182. Kamali, F. (2001). Osanetant (Sanofi-Synthelabo). *Curr Opin Investig Drugs*, *2*, 950–656.

183. Emonds-Alt, X., Goulaouic, P., Proietto, V., Van Broeck, D. (1994). Piperidine- and piperazine-containing arylalkylamines, process for their preparation, and pharmaceutical compositions containing them as neurokinin receptor antagonists. Eur. Pat. Appl. EP 474561.

184. Emonds-Alt, X., Doutremepuich, J.D., Heaulme, M., Neliat, G., Santucci, V., Steinberg, R., Vilain, P., Bichon, D., Ducoux, J.P., Proietto, V., et al. (1993). In vitro and in vivo biological activities of SR140333, a novel potent non-peptide tachykinin $NK_1$ receptor antagonist. *Eur J Pharmacol*, *250*, 403–413.

185. Ahluwalia, A. (1999). SR-140333 Sanofi-Synthelabo. *Curr Opin Anti-Inflam Immunomod Investig Drugs*, *1*, 472–481.

186. Albert, J.S., Aharony, D., Andisik, D., Barthlow, H., Bernstein, P.R., Bialecki, R.A., Dedinas, R., Dembofsky, B.T., Hill, D., Kirkland, K., Koether, G.M., Kosmider, B.J., Ohnmacht, C., Palmer, W., Potts, W., Rumsey, W., Shen, L., Shenvi, A., Sherwood, S., Warwick, P.J., Russell, K. (2002). Design, synthesis, and SAR of tachykinin antagonists: modulation of balance in $NK_1/NK_2$ receptor antagonist activity. *J Med Chem*, *45*, 3972–3983.

187. Emonds-Alt, X., Proietto, V., Steinberg, R., Advenier, C., Daoui, S., Naline, E., Gueudet, C., Michaud, J.C., Oury-Donat, F., Poncelet, M., Vilain, P., Le Fur, G., Maffrand, J.P., Soubrie, P., Pascal, M. (2002). Biochemical and pharmacological activities of SSR 146977, a new potent nonpeptide tachykinin NK3 receptor antagonist. *Can J Physiol Pharmacol*, *80*, 482–488.

188. Steinberg, R., Alonso, R., Rouquier, L., Desvignes, C., Michaud, J.C., Cudennec, A., Jung, M., Simiand, J., Griebel, G., Emonds-Alt, X., Le Fur, G., Soubrie, P. (2002). SSR240600 [(R)-2-(1-[2-[4-[2-[3,5-bis(trifluoromethyl)phenyl]acetyl]-2-(3,4-dichloro phenyl)-2-morpholinyl]ethyl]-4-piperidinyl)-2-methylpropanamide], a centrally active nonpeptide antagonist of the tachykinin neurokinin 1 receptor: II. Neurochemical and behavioral characterization. *J Pharmacol Exp Ther*, *303*, 1180–1188.

189. Bergman, R., Holmqvist, S., Von Unge, S. (2007). Azetidine compounds as neurokinin receptor antagonists, their preparation, pharmaceutical compositions, and use in therapy. PCT Int. Appl. WO 2007037743.

190. Kehler, J., Hansen, T., Poulsen, A., Bjornholm, B., Ruhland, T., Norgaard, M.B., Nielsen, S.M. (2005). Preparation of 1-phenylcyclopropane-1-carboxamide derivatives as tachykinin NK3 receptor antagonists. PCT Int. Appl. WO 2005016884.

191. Emonds-Alt, X., Advenier, C., Cognon, C., Croci, T., Daoui, S., Ducoux, J.P., Landi, M., Naline, E., Neliat, G., Poncelet, M., Proietto, V., Van Broeck, D., Vilain, P., Soubrie, P., Le Fur, G., Maffrand, J.P., Breliere, J.C. (1997). Biochemical and pharmacological activities of SR 144190, a new potent non-peptide tachykinin $NK_2$ receptor antagonist. *Neuropeptides*, *31*, 449–458.

192. File, S.E. (2000). NKP608, an $NK_1$ receptor antagonist, has an anxiolytic action in the social interaction test in rats. *Psychopharmacology (Berl)*, *152*, 105–109.

193. Nishi, T., Ishibashi, K., Takemoto, T., Nakajima, K., Fukazawa, T., Iio, Y., Itoh, K., Mukaiyama, O., Yamaguchi, T. (2000). Combined tachykinin receptor antagonist: synthesis and stereochemical structure-activity relationships of novel morpholine analogues. *Bioorg Med Chem Lett*, *10*, 1665–1668.

194. Tsuchida, H., Takahashi, S., Nosaka, E., Mukaiyama, O., Yamashita, M., Morimoto, K. (2008). Novel triple neurokinin receptor antagonist CS-003 strongly inhibits neurokinin related responses. *Eur J Pharmacol*, *586*, 306–312.

195. Chambers, M.S., Jones, P., Szekeres, H.J. (2004). Preparation of N-(3-(4-substituted-1-piperidinyl)-1-phenylpropyl) substituted sulfonamides as NK-3 receptor antagonists. U.S. Pat. Appl. Publ. US 2004002504.

196. Dirat, O., Elliott, J.M., Owens, A.P., Shaw, D.E., Sternfeld, F., Williams, B.J. (2007). Preparation of substituted cyclohexyl derivatives as NK-3 receptor antagonists. 2007 PCT Int. Appl. WO 2007003965.

197. Kubota, H., Kakefuda, A., Nagaoka, H., Yamamoto, O., Ikeda, K., Takeuchi, M., Shibanuma, T., Isomura, Y. (1998). Spiro-substituted piperidines as neurokinin receptor antagonists. II. Syntheses and $NK_2$ receptor-antagonistic activities of N-[2-aryl-4-(spiro-substituted piperidin-1′-yl)butyl]carboxamides. *Chem Pharm Bull (Tokyo)*, *46*, 242–254.

198. Janssens, F.E., Sommen, F.M., De Boeck, B.C.A.G., Leenaerts, J.E. (2005). Preparation of alkyl- and alkanoyl-piperazine derivatives as neurokinin antagonists. PCT Int. Appl. WO 2005097774.

199. Anthes, J.C., Chapman, R.W., Richard, C., Eckel, S., Corboz, M., Hey, J.A., Fernandez, X., Greenfeder, S., McLeod, R., Sehring, S., Rizzo, C., Crawley, Y., Shih, N.Y., Piwinski, J., Reichard, G., Ting, P., Carruthers, N., Cuss, F.M., Billah, M., Kreutner, W., Egan, R.W. (2002). SCH 206272: a potent, orally active tachykinin NK(1), NK(2), and NK(3) receptor antagonist. *Eur J Pharmacol*, *450*, 191–202.

200. Harrison, T., Korsgaard, M.P., Swain, C.J., Cascieri, M.A., Sadowski, S., Seabrook, G.R. (1998). High affinity, selective neurokinin 2 and neurokinin 3 receptor antagonists from a common structural template. *Bioorg Med Chem Lett*, *8*, 1343–1348.

201. Jasserand, D., Preuschoff, U., Antel, J., David, S., Sann, H., Brueckner, R., Reiche, D., Eeckhout, C. (2003). Preparation of 1-[1-(hetero)aryl-1-hydroxyalkylmethyl] piperazines as NK-2 receptor antagonists. Eur. Pat. Appl EP 1293506.

202. Burkholder, T.P., Kudlacz, E.M., Le, T.-B., Knippenberg, R.W., Shatzer, S.A., Maynard, G.D., Webster, M.E., Horgan, S.W. (1996). Identification and chemical synthesis of MDL 105,212, a non-peptide tachykinin antagonist with high affinity for NK1 and NK2 receptors. *Bioorg Med Chem Lett*, *6*, 951–956.

203. MacKenzie, A.R., Marchington, A.P., Middleton, D.S., Newman, S.D., Jones, B.C. (2002). Structure-activity relationships of 1-alkyl-5-(3,4-dichlorophenyl)-5-[2-[(3-substituted)-1-azetidinyl]ethyl]-2-piperidones. 1. Selective antagonists of the neurokinin-2 receptor. *J Med Chem*, *45*, 5365–5377.

204. Middleton, D.S., MacKenzie, A.R., Newman, S.D., Corless, M., Warren, A., Marchington, A.P., Jones, B. (2005). Structure-activity relationships of 1-alkyl-5-(3,4-dichlorophenyl)-5-{2-[3-(substituted)-1-azetidinyl]-ethyl}-2-piperidones. Part 2: improving oral absorption. *Bioorg Med Chem Lett*, *15*, 3957–3961.

205. Giardina, G.A., Sarau, H.M., Farina, C., Medhurst, A.D., Grugni, M., Raveglia, L.F., Schmidt, D.B., Rigolio, R., Luttmann, M., Vecchietti, V., Hay, D.W. (1997). Discovery of a novel class of selective non-peptide antagonists for the human neurokinin-3 receptor. 1. Identification of the 4-quinolinecarboxamide framework. *J Med Chem*, *40*, 1794–1807.

206. Sarau, H.M., Griswold, D.E., Bush, B., Potts, W., Sandhu, P., Lundberg, D., Foley, J.J., Schmidt, D.B., Webb, E.F., Martin, L.D., Legos, J.J., Whitmore, R.G., Barone, F.C., Medhurst, A.D., Luttmann, M.A., Giardina, G.A., Hay, D.W. (2000). Nonpeptide tachykinin receptor antagonists. II. Pharmacological and pharmacokinetic profile of SB-222200, a central nervous system penetrant, potent and selective $NK_3$ receptor antagonist. *J Pharmacol Exp Ther*, *295*, 373–381.

207. Blaney, F.E., Raveglia, L.F., Artico, M., Cavagnera, S., Dartois, C., Farina, C., Grugni, M., Gagliardi, S., Luttmann, M.A., Martinelli, M., Nadler, G.M., Parini, C., Petrillo, P., Sarau, H.M., Scheideler, M.A., Hay, D.W., Giardina, G.A. (2001). Stepwise modulation of neurokinin-3 and neurokinin-2 receptor affinity and selectivity in quinoline tachykinin receptor antagonists. *J Med Chem*, *44*, 1675–1689.

208. Hoffmann, T., Koblet, A., Peters, J.-U., Schnider, P., Sleight, A., Stadler, H. (2005). Preparation of 2-phenyl-N-(pyridin-3-yl)-N-methylisobutyramide derivatives as dual NK1/NK3 antagonists for treating schizophrenia. PCT Int. Appl. WO 2005002577.

209. Schnider, P. (2006). Preparation of bistrifluoromethylphenylisobutyric acid pyridinylamides as dual tachykinin NK1/NK3 antagonists for treatment of schizophrenia. PCT Int. Appl. WO 2006013050.

210. Alvaro, G., Andreotti, D., Belvedere, S., Di Fabio, R., Falchi, A., Giovannini, R. (2007). Pyridine derivatives as NK receptor inhibitors and their preparation, pharmaceutical compositions, and use in the treatment of psychotic disorders. PCT Int. Appl. WO 2007028654.

211. Tokumura, T., Tanaka, T., Sasaki, A., Tsuchiya, Y., Abe, K., Machida, R. (1990). Stability of a novel hexapeptide, (Me)Arg-Lys-Pro-Trp-tert-Leu-Leu-OEt, with neurotensin activity, in aqueous solution and in the solid state. *Chem Pharm Bull (Tokyo)*, *38*, 3094–3098.

212. Machida, R., Tokumura, T., Tsuchiya, Y., Sasaki, A., Abe, K. (1993). Pharmacokinetics of novel hexapeptides with neurotensin activity in rats. *Biol Pharm Bull*, *16*, 43–47.

213. Sarhan, S., Hitchcock, J.M., Grauffel, C.A., Wettstein, J.G. (1997). Comparative antipsychotic profiles of neurotensin and a related systemically active peptide agonist. *Peptides*, *18*, 1223–1227.

214. Boules, M., Warrington, L., Fauq, A., McCormick, D., Richelson, E. (2001). A novel neurotensin analog blocks cocaine- and D-amphetamine-induced hyperactivity. *Eur J Pharmacol*, *426*, 73–76.

215. Richelson, E., Cusack, B.M., Pang, Y.-P., McCormick, D.J., Fauq, A.T., Marie, B., Boules, M. (1999). Preparation of neo-tryptophan and peptides containing neo-tryptophan as pharmaceuticals. PCT Int. Appl WO 9952539.

216. Tyler, B.M., Douglas, C.L., Fauq, A., Pang, Y.P., Stewart, J.A., Cusack, B., McCormick, D.J., Richelson, E. (1999). In vitro binding and CNS effects of novel neurotensin agonists that cross the blood-brain barrier. *Neuropharmacology*, *38*, 1027–1034.

217. Dubuc, I., Costentin, J., Doulut, S., Rodriguez, M., Martinez, J., Kitabgi, P. (1992). JMV 449: a pseudopeptide analogue of neurotensin-(8-13) with highly potent and long-lasting hypothermic and analgesic effects in the mouse. *Eur J Pharmacol*, *219*, 327–329.

218. Dix, T.A. (2006). Preparation of non-natural amino acids. PCT Int. Appl. WO 2006009902.

219. Brower, J.O., Dix, T.A. (2007). Semisynthetic peptides containing non-natural amino acids with resistance to aminopeptidase degradation as drugs and cosmetics. PCT Int. Appl WO 2007070672.

220. Christos, T.E., Arvanitis, A., Cain, G.A., Johnson, A.L., Potorf, R.S., Tam, S.W., Schmidt, W.K. (1993). Stable isosteres of neurotensin C-terminal pentapeptides derived by modification of the amide function. *Bioorg Med Chem Lett*, *3*, 1035–1040.

# 15

# GABA AND SCHIZOPHRENIA

JOHN H. KEHNE AND GEORGE D. MAYNARD

## 15.1 GABA PATHWAYS AND DRUGS, AND UNMET NEEDS IN SCHIZOPHRENIA

### 15.1.1 GABA and Schizophrenia: A Hypothesis Revisited

> 1983: "A role for GABA in the pathophysiology of schizophrenia was first suggested by Eugene Roberts in 1972. . . . neither biochemical nor pharmacological studies have been able to demonstrate a clear and reproducible GABA disturbance in schizophrenia. . . . Interest in GABA research in schizophrenia appears to have waned . . ." [1]
>
> 2008: "Studies of postmortem brain have provided strong evidence that the GABAergic system is impaired in schizophrenia . . ." [2]; "reduced mRNA for GAD67 is one of the most consistent findings in postmortem studies of individuals with schizophrenia" [3]; ". . . abnormal GABA neurotransmission could form a "final common pathway" to prefrontal dysfunction in schizophrenia . . ." [3]

γ-Aminobutyric acid (GABA) is the major inhibitory amino acid neurotransmitter in the central nervous system (CNS) and is widely distributed at all levels of the neuraxis, from the spinal cord to the neocortex. GABA's effects are mediated through two major subtypes of receptors: $GABA_A$, an ionotropic receptor that controls a chloride ($Cl^-$) channel, and $GABA_B$, a metabotropic

*Targets and Emerging Therapies for Schizophrenia*, First Edition.
Edited by Jeffrey S. Albert and Michael W. Wood.

receptor that controls a potassium channel. Given their prevalence and widespread distribution in the CNS, and importance in shaping spatiotemporal patterns of electrical signaling [4], it is not surprising that GABAergic neurons and their postsynaptic receptors (referred hereafter as "GABA pathways") have been implicated in a variety of neurophysiological and behavioral processes and their dysfunction is thought to contribute a spectrum of CNS disorders including anxiety, depression, epilepsy, insomnia, and motor disorders [5–10]. In recent years, a growing body of evidence indicates that GABA plays an important role in the etiology of schizophrenia and pharmacological agents that target GABA pathways are increasingly being explored for their potential as novel therapeutic approaches. The overall aim of this chapter is to provide a broad overview of the current status of GABAergic approaches in the treatment of schizophrenia. Where appropriate, citations are made for relevant, in-depth reviews.

### 15.1.2 GABA Pharmacology

Table 15.1 summarizes the different classes of pharmacological agents used to modify transmission in GABAergic pathways. These include agents that affect the availability of GABA at the synapse (e.g., GABA transaminase inhibitors, GABA uptake inhibitors) and agents that directly affect $GABA_A$ or $GABA_B$ receptor subtypes.

With regard to agents that affect GABA receptors, the $GABA_A$ receptor complex is a particularly fertile target for pharmacological intervention, based on the presence of a diverse number of receptor subtypes and their heterogeneous distribution throughout the nervous system. Figure 15.1 depicts the physiological $GABA_A$ receptor complex, which is a pentameric protein composed of five subunits forming a $Cl^-$ conducting channel in the center. $GABA_A$ receptors that respond to a structural class of agents referred to as the 1,4-benzodiazepines (BZDs) are comprised of α, β, and γ subunits assembled in a 2:2:1 ratio, respectively. GABA binds to its recognition site, which is located at the interface between α and β subunits, causing $Cl^-$ to enter the cell, which in turn produces hyperpolarization and inhibition of postsynaptic cell firing. Many drugs that are members of the BZD structural class have been shown to act on a distinct allosteric modulatory site (the "BZD recognition-site" or "BZD receptor"), which is located at the interface between α and γ subunits (Fig. 15.1). Binding of a BZD such as diazepam to this site does not cause hyperpolarization by itself but rather enhances the ability of GABA to produce influx of $Cl^-$ into the cell. Agents like diazepam have been generally referred to as "positive allosteric modulators" (PAMs) or "allosteric activators" of GABA transmission. As noted in Table 15.1, they are also referred to as agonists at the BZD recognition site.

As the BZD site is an allosteric modulatory site, under conditions of basal GABA activation, there exists a bidirectional dynamic range of activities that can be produced by different agents. As illustrated in Figure 15.2, this range

**Table 15.1 Representative Pharmacological Agents Used to Manipulate GABA Pathways**

| Targeted Overall Effect | Site of Action | Specific Action | Representative Agents[a] and References | Direction of Effect on GABA Neurotransmission |
|---|---|---|---|---|
| Alter synaptic availability of GABA in all GABA neurons | GABA transporter | Blocker | Tiagabine [179, 180] | ↑ |
| | Glutamatic acid decarboxylase | Inhibitor | Allyglycine [181] | ↑ |
| | GABA transaminase | Inhibitor | $\Gamma$-Vinyl-GABA (Vigabatrin) [182, 183] | ↑ |
| Nonselectively alter activity of all $GABA_A$ receptors | GABA recognition site | Agonist | Muscimol [184] | ↑ |
| | | Antagonist | Bicuculline [185, 186] | ↓ |
| | Picrotoxin recognition site | Antagonist | Picrotoxin [185, 186] | ↓ |
| | Neurosteroid recognition site | Agonist | Allopregnanolone [187, 188] | ↑ |
| | BZD recognition site | Agonist | Chlordiazepoxide, diazepam, lorazepam, triazolam [5, 9, 189, 190] | ↑ |
| | | Partial agonist | Abercarnil [11], | ↑ |
| | | | Bretazenil [11, 192] | ↑ |
| | | | Imidazenil | ↑ |
| | | Partial inverse agonist | FG-7142 [191] | ↓ |
| Selectively alter activity of $GABA_A$ receptor subtypes (BZD sensitive) | α1-$GABA_A$ receptor | Agonist | Zolpidem (Ambien) [193–195] | ↑ |
| | | | (*S*)-Zopiclone (Lunesta) [195, 196] | ↑ |
| | | | Zaleplon [197] | ↑ |
| | | | Indiplon [195] | ↑ |
| | | | Ocinaplon [11, 198] | ↑ |
| | α2-$GABA_A$ receptor | Agonist | SL651498 [199, 200] (also α3 full agonist) | ↑ |
| | Partial agonist at α2-$GABA_A$ receptor | Partial agonist | L-838,417 [11, 193] | ↑ |
| | | | TPA023 [201] | ↑ |
| | α3-$GABA_A$ receptor | Agonist | ELB-139 [142] | ↑ |
| | | | Pagoclone [11]; | ↑ |
| | | | TP003 [11] | ↑ |
| | | Partial agonist | Adipiplon [148, 149, 202] | ↑ |
| | | Partial inverse agonist | α3IA (Merck) [191] | ↓ |

(*Continued*)

**TABLE 15.1 (*Continued*)**

| Targeted Overall Effect | Site of Action | Specific Action | Representative Agents[a] and References | Direction of Effect on GABA Neurotransmission |
|---|---|---|---|---|
| | α5-$GABA_A$ receptor | Agonist | QH-ii-66 [203–205] | ↑ |
| | | Partial inverse agonist | L-655,708 [153] | ↓ |
| | | | α5IA (Merck) [19, 156] | ↓ |
| | | | FG-7142 [21] | ↓ |
| Alter activity of $GABA_B$ receptor | GABA recognition site | Agonist | Baclofen [206] | ↑ |
| | | Antagonist | CGP 35348 [207, 208] | ↓ |
| | | | SGS742 [170] | ↓ |
| | | | SCH50911 [171] | ↓ |

[a]Chemical names: Abecarnil: 4-(methoxymethyl)-6-(phenylmethoxy)-9H-pyrido[3,4-*b*]indole-3-carboxylic acid, 1-methylethyl ester; Adipiplon: 7-[[2-(3-fluoro-2-pyridinyl)-1*H*-imidazol-1-yl]methyl]-2-methyl-8-propyl-[1,2,4]triazolo[1,5-c]pyrimidine (2*E*)-2-butenedioate); Allopregnanolone: 3-hydroxy-(3α,5α)-pregnan-20-one; Allylglycine: 2-amino-4-pentenoic acid; α3IA: 6-(4-pyridyl)-5-(4-methoxyphenyl)-3-carbomethoxy-1-methyl-1*H*-pyridin-2-one; Baclofen: β-(aminomethyl)-4-chloro-benzenepropanoic acid; Bicuculline: 6-[(5*S*)-5,6,7,8-tetrahydro-6-methyl-1,3-dioxolo[4,5-*g*]isoquinolin-5-yl]-(6*R*)- furo[3,4-*e*]-1,3-benzodioxol-8(6*H*)-one; Bretazenil: (13a*S*)-8-bromo-11,12,13,13a-tetrahydro-9-oxo-9*H*-imidazo[1,5-a]pyrrolo[2,1-*c*][1,4]benzodiazepine-1-carboxylic acid 1,1-dimethylethyl ester; CGP 35348: P-(3-aminopropyl)-P-(diethoxymethyl)-phosphinic acid; Chlordiazepoxide: 7-chloro-*N*-methyl-5-phenyl-3*H*-1,4-benzodiazepin-2-amine-4-oxide; Diazepam: 7-chloro-1,3-dihydro-1-methyl-5-phenyl-2*H*-1,4-benzodiazepin-2-one; ELB-139: 1-(4-chlorophenyl)-1,5-dihydro-4-(1-piperidinyl)- 2*H*-Imidazol-2-one; FG-7142: *N*-methyl-β-carboline-3-carboxamide; Gaboxadol: 4,5,6,7-tetrahydro-isoxazolo[5,4-*c*]pyridin-3(2*H*)-one; Vigabatrin: γ-vinyl-GABA; α5IA: 3-(5-methylisoxazol-3-yl)-6-[(1-methyl-1,2,3-triazol-4-yl)methyloxy]-1,2,4-triazolo[3,4-*a*]phthalazine; Imidazenil: 6-(2-bromophenyl)-8-fluoro-4*H*-imidazo[1,5-*a*][1,4]benzodiazepine-3-carboxamide; Indiplon: *N*-methyl-*N*-[3-[3-(2-thienylcarbonyl)pyrazolo[1,5-*a*]pyrimidin-7-yl]phenyl]-acetamide; L-655,708: (ethyl (S)-11,12,13,13a-tetrahydro-7-methoxy-9-oxo-9H-imidazo[1,5-a]pyrrolo[2,1-c][1,4]benzodiazepine-1-carboxylate);L-838,417:3-(2,5-difluorophenyl)-7-(1,1-dimethylethyl)-6-[(1-methyl-1*H*-1,2,4-triazol-5-yl)methoxy]-1,2,4-triazolo[4,3-*b*]pyridazine; Lorazepam: 7-chloro-5-(2-chlorophenyl)-1,3-dihydro-3-hydroxy-2*H*-1,4-benzodiazepin-2-one; Muscimol: 5-(aminomethyl)-3(2*H*)-isoxazolone; Pagoclone: (+)-2-(7-chloro-1,8-naphthyridin-2-yl)-2,3-dihydro-3-(5-methyl-2-oxohexyl)-1*H*-isoindol-1-one; Ocinaplon: 2-pyridinyl[7-(4-pyridinyl)pyrazolo[1,5-*a*]pyrimidin-3-yl]-methanone; QH-ii-066: 7-acetyleno-1,3-dihydro-1-methyl-5-phenyl-2H-1,4-benzodiazepin-2-one; SCH50911: 5,5-dimethyl-2-morpholineacetic acid hydrochloride; SL651498: 6-fluoro-2,9-dihydro-9-methyl-2-phenyl-4-(1-pyrrolidinylcarbonyl)- 1*H*-pyrido[3,4-*b*] indol-1-one; (*S*)-Zopiclone: (5*S*)-6-(5-chloro-2-pyridinyl)-6,7-dihydro-7-oxo-5*H*-pyrrolo[3,4-*b*]pyrazin-5-yl ester 4-methyl-1-piperazinecarboxylic acid; SGS742: P-(3-aminopropyl)-P-butyl-phosphinic acid; Tiagabine: (3*R*)-1-[4,4-bis(3-methyl-2-thienyl)-3-buten-1-yl]-3-piperidinecarboxylic acid; TP003: (4,2′-difluoro-5′-[8-fluoro-7-(1-hydroxy-1-methylethyl)imidazo[1,2-*a*]pyridin-3-yl]biphenyl-2-carbonitrile); TPA023: 7-(1,1-dimethylethyl)-6-(2-ethyl-2*H*-1,2,4-triazol-3-ylmethoxy)-3-(2-fluorophenyl)-1,2,4-triazolo[4,3-*b*]pyridazine; Triazolam: 8-chloro-6-(2-chlorophenyl)-1-methyl-4*H*-[1,2,4]triazolo[4,3-*a*][1,4]benzodiazepine; Zaleplon: *N*-[3-(3-cyanopyrazolo[1,5-*a*]pyrimidin-7-yl)phenyl]-*N*-ethyl-acetamide; Zolpidem: *N,N*,6-trimethyl-2-(4-methylphenyl)-imidazo[1,2-*a*]pyridine-3-acetamide.

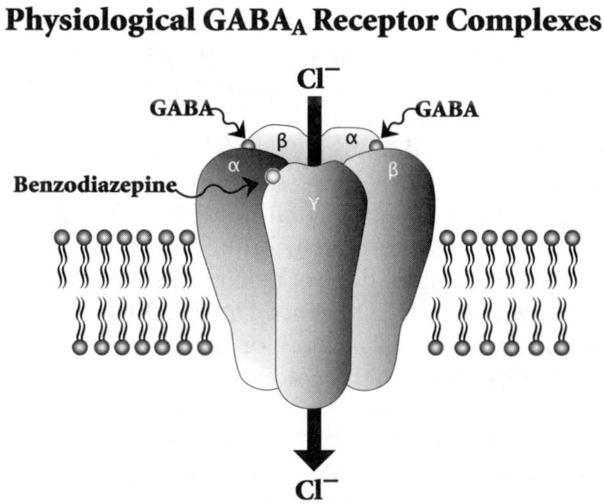


**FIGURE 15.1** Cartoon depicting the $GABA_A$ receptor complex showing the GABA binding site and the benzodiazepine (BZD) binding site. $Cl^-$, chloride ion.

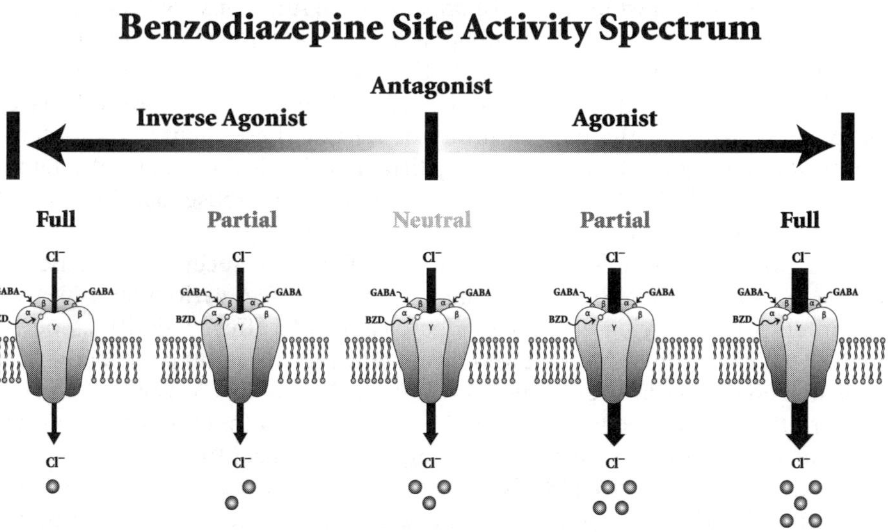


**FIGURE 15.2** Cartoon depicting positive and negative allosteric modulation of the $GABA_A$ receptor complex. BZD, benzodiazepine; $Cl^-$, chloride ion.

of activity spans from positive allosteric modulation represented on the right of the diagram to negative allosteric modulation (also known as "inverse agonism" or "allosteric inhibition") on the left. A drug that is a BZD-site antagonist (e.g., flumazenil) does not have any effect on GABA-induced $Cl^-$ influx but rather prevents the effects of allosteric activators or inhibitors. As most BZD agents are full allosteric activators, one pharmacological strategy for designing new agents that has been pursued by a number of pharmaceutical companies is to "dial in" a level of partial agonism that is sufficient to produce full efficacy while minimizing side effects associated with full agonists. This strategy will be discussed in greater detail below.

The $GABA_A$ receptor story is more complex (for reviews see References [7, 11–15]), as it is currently believed that more than 20 subtypes of $GABA_A$ receptor complexes exist in the human brain. Of these subtypes, which are assembled from various combinations of at least nine distinct subunits, approximately 75% are sensitive to BZD agents. The BZD-sensitive $GABA_A$ receptor subtypes are comprised of $\alpha1$, $\alpha2$, $\alpha3$, or $\alpha5$ subunits co-assembled with $\beta$ (1 or 2) or $\gamma2$ subunits. $GABA_A$ receptors containing the $\alpha1$ subnit are the most prevalent subtype, comprising approximately 60% of the receptors in the CNS, followed by $\alpha2$ (15–20%), $\alpha3$ (10–15%), and $\alpha5$ (<5%) [13]. Other $GABA_A$ receptor subtypes containing $\alpha4$ or $\alpha6$ subunits (each <5%) are insensitive to BZD agents [13]. BZDs have been generally found to be nonselective allosteric agonists as they fully activate all BZD-sensitive $GABA_A$ receptor subtypes [12, 16].

The widespread distribution of $GABA_A$ subtypes in different neuronal circuits subserving a wide variety of physiological functions confers BZDs with diverse therapeutic actions, including anticonvulsant, anxiolytic, muscle relaxant, and sedative–hypnotic activity [5, 17]. However, this nonselective agonist profile at the BZD site is also associated with undesirable side effects and properties that limit the clinical utility of BZDs. These include the potential for producing cognitive and motor impairments, the development of tolerance after chronic administration, and the potential for abuse liability and the development of physical dependence.

The presence of diverse BZD-sensitive $GABA_A$ receptor subtypes has enabled efforts to develop agents that specifically affect various subtypes, with the intent of improving efficacy or decreasing side effect liability associated with the BZD agents. As reviewed elsewhere [12, 16] subtype selectivity can be achieved in two different ways. One approach is to develop agents that have higher affinity for specific subtypes. An example is zolpidem, which has preferential affinity for $\alpha1$ subunit containing $GABA_A$ receptors, where it acts like a full allosteric activator [18]. Notably, as drug concentration increases with dose, zolpidem loses $\alpha1$ selectivity as it will now also activate $\alpha2$ and $\alpha3$ subtypes, whereas it appears to have minimal activity at $\alpha5$ even at very high concentrations. Thus, zolpidem's selectivity as an $\alpha1$-selective allosteric activator is dependent on synaptic concentration of the drug achieved when the drug is taken orally.

A second approach is to develop agents that, while having equal affinity for the different subtypes, have different levels of intrinsic activity at each subtype. Agents can vary considerably in their profiles, having different levels of efficacy ranging from a neutral antagonist to partial agonist to full agonist, and in this way, may confer functional selectivity to certain $GABA_A$ receptor subtypes.

It is important to emphasize that drugs may also be allosteric inhibitors (inverse agonists; negative allosteric modulators) at different subtypes, and this may give rise to some desirable properties as well as side effect liabilities [19, 20]. For example, β-carboline-derived agents such as FG-7142 [21] are known to be negative allosteric modulators at $GABA_A$ receptors containing α5 subunits and have cognition-enhancing effects in animals and in humans. However, there are undesirable side effects associated with inverse agonism at other α-subunits such as the potential for producing anxiety and seizures. In order to minimize these effects, drugs such as α5IA have been developed as selective α5 partial inverse agonists which retain cognition-enhancing efficacy but which have reduced anxiogenic or seizurogenic potential [19].

There are other modulatory sites on the $GABA_A$ receptor complex (not depicted in Fig. 15.1) that are potential targets for drugs, including a neurosteroid binding site (affected by agents such as allopregnanolone, see Table 15.1) and a picrotoxin binding site.

Table 15.1 also lists representative agents that act as agonists or antagonists at the GABA recognition site of the $GABA_B$ receptor. $GABA_B$ agonists such as baclofen are noted for their therapeutic activity in treating spasticity and related dysfunctions [22, 23] and may be novel approaches for treating gastroesophageal reflux disorder [24].

### 15.1.3 Schizophrenia: The Challenge and Unmet Medical Needs

Schizophrenia is a complex and serious neurodevelopmental psychiatric disorder that affects approximately 1% of the world population. It is the most common severe mental illness and usually emerges in the late teens or early twenties, although a rare form, childhood-onset schizophrenia, is expressed at a younger age. Schizophrenia is characterized by three clusters of symptoms that may be present to different degrees in different patients. "Positive symptoms" refer to active hallucinations and delusions; "negative symptoms" refer to anergia, flat affect, apathy, social isolation, and poverty of thought; and "cognitive symptoms" refer to abnormalities in working attention, processing speed, visual and verbal learning and memory, reasoning and problem solving, and social cognition [25]. Cognitive impairments in particular are associated with poor functional outcome in patients with schizophrenia [26, 27].

The origins of schizophrenia are unknown, although numerous environmental and genetic contributions have been proposed. The classic "hyperdopaminergia" hypothesis of schizophrenia implicating hyperactive subcortical (mesostriatal) dopamine (DA) systems has been supported by positron emission tomography (PET) imaging studies in schizophrenics demonstrating hyperresponsive striatal DA pathways [28–32]. Contemporary theories also suggest hypoactivity in the mesocortical DA pathways [33, 34], possibly underlying negative symptoms, although the relative importance of hyper- versus hypodopaminergia to the disease is not certain. Notably, $D_2$ antagonism is the key common feature of all marketed antipsychotics [35] and is associated with the common therapeutic action of these agents to reduce positive symptoms. Agents such as haloperidol, which are most clearly associated with $D_2$ receptor antagonism, are referred to as "typical antipsychotics," or "first-generation antipsychotics," (FGAs), whereas agents such as clozapine, olanzapine, or risperidone, which are associated with other neurochemical activities in addition to $D_2$ antagonism, are referred to as "atypical antipsychotics," or "second-generation antipsychotics" (SGAs). A number of these agents are high-potency antagonists at the 5-$HT_{2A}$ receptor, and the ratio of 5-$HT_{2A}$ to $D_2$ affinity has been proposed as a predictor of "atypicality" [36]. The SGAs clozapine and olanzapine have complex neurochemical profiles, and aripiprazole is the first U.S. Food and Drug Administration (FDA)-approved treatment for schizophrenia that has the profile of a $D_2$ receptor partial agonist.

There are significant unmet needs in treating schizophrenia, from both efficacy and side effect perspectives. While adequately treating positive symptoms, FGAs have limited efficacy (and may even be detrimental) against negative symptoms [37] and cognitive deficits [38]. Relative to FGAs, SGAs have been associated with improvements in efficacy or side effect profiles [39], although recent results in a large clinical trial in the United States (Clinical Antipsychotic Trials of Intervention Effectiveness [CATIE]) failed to demonstrate substantial advantages of these agents relative to first-generation drugs [40]. However, it has been suggested that full analysis of the potential benefits of SGAs agents with regard to long-term safety and prevention of recurrence of schizophrenia may require trials of longer than the 5-year duration of the CATIE trial [41].

As noted previously, cognitive impairment is a core feature of schizophrenia and is particularly resistant to current therapies. As a major unmet medical need, treating cognitive deficits in schizophrenia is a primary focus for new therapeutic approaches [38, 42–46]. Importantly, agents with specific cognition-enhancing actions may be viable for development as adjunctive agents to current antipsychotics, thereby treating the multiple symptom clusters that are present in schizophrenia.

Side effects are a major consideration in antipsychotic treatment. Extrapyramidal side effects (EPS), for example, akathisia, parkinsonism, and dystonia, and tardive dyskinesia have been linked, respectively, to acute and chronic blockade of $D_2$ receptors of the motor areas of the striatum, but are considered to be less of an issue with SGAs relative to FGAs possibly due to ameliorating neurochemical actions such as 5-$HT_{2A}$ receptor antagonism [36] or faster dissociation off-rates at the $D_2$ receptor associated with agents such as the $D_2$ receptor partial agonist aripiprazole [47]. Stimulation of prolactin release [48] is another potential issue associated with $D_2$ receptor blockade, although, again, some second-generation, multimechanistic agents have improved upon this hormonal side effect [48]. A very significant side effect associated with most SGAs is weight gain, glucose dysregulation, and dyslipidemia [49, 50]. Three of the four SGAs tested (ziprasidone being the exception) were shown to have this action in the recent CATIE trial [51]. Another side effect also encountered with many antipsychotics is sedation.

In summary, despite intensive industry efforts, significant unmet medical needs remain with regard to both efficacy and side effects in the treatment of schizophrenia. The remainder of this chapter will focus on GABAergic pathways as targets for improved schizophrenia pharmacotherapies.

## 15.2 GABA: ROLE IN SCHIZOPHRENIA

### 15.2.1 Neural Circuitry and Schizophrenia

Decades of research have yielded important clues for elucidating the complex neuronal circuitries in the brain that are dysfunctional in schizophrenia. Although the focus has traditionally been on DA pathways, GABAergic pathways have come to play an increasingly important core role in a number of these models. The following discussion highlights some key brain circuitries containing GABA components that have been implicated in the etiology of schizophrenia and the action of antipsychotic drugs.

Although ascending dopaminergic pathways have been emphasized, increasing attention has been focused on the critical role of cortical neurons that utilize amino acids as neurotransmitters. Figure 15.3 is a simplified version of circuitry described in several recent reviews [2, 3] that describe the influence of glutamatergic and GABAergic neurons on cortical pyramidal neurons. Pyramidal neurons located in hippocampus and cerebral cortex mediate the outflow of information from these regions, and inhibitory modulation provided by certain GABAergic inputs is thought to be important for filtering and sculpting this flow of information. Importantly, glutamatergic neurons are proposed to provide a key excitatory "drive" on these cortical GABAergic interneurons. Reductions of this excitatory input would therefore decrease GABA inhibition of pyramidal neurons, causing a loss of inhibitory filtering and a subsequent hyperactivation (disinhibition) of pyramidal neurons [52]. Hyperactivation of pyramidal neurons could be a central feature underlying positive symptoms such as hallucinations and disorganized thinking or cognitive deficits.

Notably, other inputs are thought to modulate this pathway, including cholingeric neurons, and evidence has been provided for interactions between nicotinic acetylcholine neurons working through $\alpha$7-nicotinic receptors and GABAergic cortical neurons [53]. Electrophysiological data indicated that GABA release is modulated by $\alpha$7 nicotinic acetylcholine receptors (nAChRs) and that selective allosteric modulators of $\alpha$7 nAChRs could have potential therapeutic utility in schizophrenia [53].

Several important points about this GABA circuit should be emphasized: First, a more complex formulation of this circuitry describes interactions with ascending dopaminergic neurons and may explain their hyperresponsiveness

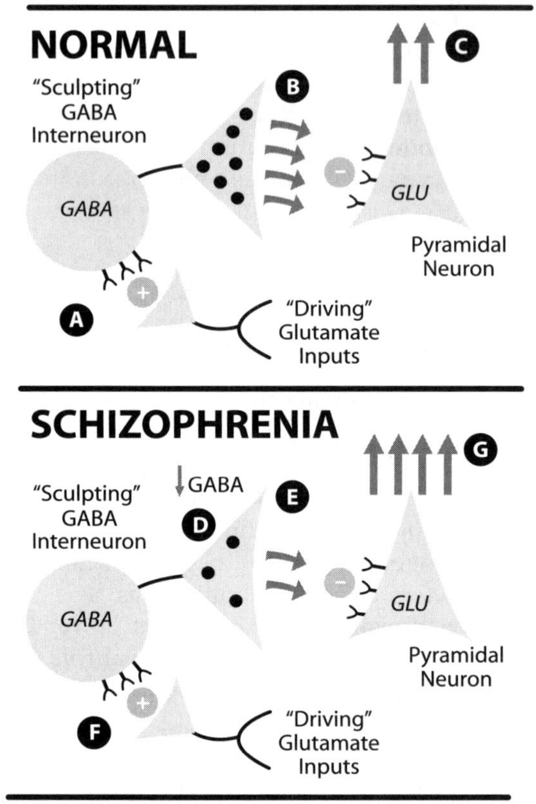


**FIGURE 15.3** Cartoon depicting GABA modulation of pyramidal neurons in the normal (top) and schizophrenic (bottom) brain. In the normal brain (top), a subset of GABA interneurons, driven by excitatory glutamate inputs (A) release GABA onto $GABA_A$ receptors (B) located on pyramidal neurons in the cortex and hippocampus. $GABA_A$ receptor-mediated inhibition "sculpts" the mass activity of pyramidal neurons, allowing optimal neuronal synchrony (e.g., γ-oscillations) needed for performance of certain cognitive tasks. In the schizophrenic brain (bottom), decreased presynaptic GABA availability and release (as evidenced by decreased GABA levels and decreased GAD67), possibly due to a primary GABA deficiency or to a secondary reduction in glumatergic drive, reduces inhibitory modulation of pyramidal neurons, thereby resulting in dysfunctional pyramidal synchrony (e.g., decreased γ-oscillatory activity under cognitive load) and impaired cognitive performance on working memory tasks. According to this conception, the GABA interneuron and its postsynaptic receptors could serve as a "final common pathway" for glutamatergic excitatory inputs (mediated by, e.g., mGlu2/3 receptors, not shown) and for cholinergic inputs (mediated by, e.g., α7-nicotinic receptors, not shown). Novel therapeutic approaches for treating deficits in GABA pathways include agents that increase the availability of GABA in the synapse (to overcome the GABA synaptic deficit) and agents that activate relevant postsynaptic $GABA_A$ receptor subtypes (e.g., α2-$GABA_A$ receptors). The "driving" glutamate inputs may be collaterals from pyramidal neurons mediating recurrent inhibition [2] or from other brain regions [3]. Figure adapted from previously published figures [2, 3].

in schizophrenia [2]. Second, dysfunction of glutamatergic inputs to GABA neurons as described above could explain the well-documented psychotomimetic actions of NMDA receptor antagonists, in that blocking the NMDA receptors on GABA interneurons would diminish GABA-mediated inhibition of cortical neurons. Accordingly, glutamate pathways are highly promising targets for schizophrenia as discussed elsewhere in this book. Third, the "driving" glutamatergic input to GABA neurons may be from other brain regions or from pyramidal neurons themselves (which utilize glutamate as a transmitter). Thus, phasic glutamate-mediated GABA inhibition could serve as a critical "filter" needed to produce synchronous neural activity during conditions of cognitive load that optimize working memory processes, or it could serve as a simple feedback "sensor" for regulating pyramidal activity. Finally, the unique configuraton of these GABAergic neurons places them in a position of being a "final common path" for modulating pyramidal neuron activity. Thus, deficits in other neurotransmitter pathways that are ultimately mediated through these GABAergic neurons may, in theory, be ameliorated by pharmacological treatments that restore normal GABAergic activity. Importantly, as summarized in the next section, there is strong evidence from the schizophrenic postmortem brain that these GABAergic neurons are dysfunctional and exist in a state of hypoactivity.

Although there is currently a major emphasis on GABA circuits modulating pyramidal cells, it is important to note that GABA neurons found in other brain neural circuits may be important for the etiology or treatment of schizophrenia. For example, pallidotegmental GABAergic neurons projecting to $GABA_B$ receptors located on pedunculo-pontine ventral tegmental neurons have been implicated in mediating sensorimotor gating processes that are disrupted in schizophrenia [54]. In humans, there is also a major GABA input to the substantia nigra, the source of nigrostriatal DA neurons. As the nigrostriatal pathway is a key modulator of the extrapyramidal motor system, this GABA modulatory pathway may play an important role in EPS. Immunohistochemical studies of the human substantia nigra have identified specific $GABA_A$ receptor subtypes on DA neurons of the pars compacta (primarily $\alpha 3$, some $\alpha 1$) and on GABAergic parvalbumin-positive projection neurons of the pars reticulata ($\alpha 1$, $\alpha 3$ subunit containing) [55]. This subunit heterogeneity suggests the possibility that subtype-selective $GABA_A$ agents could have different functional effects on substantia nigra-mediated pathways. In the ventral tegmental area, GABAergic neurons project to cortical and subcortical regions, which, based on lesion studies, have an inhibitory influence on behavior [56].

A potential locus of interaction with GABA neurons that may have relevance to negative symptoms and altered emotional responses in schizophrenia is a projection from the basolateral amygdala innervating GABAergic neurons of the medial prefrontal cortex (mPFC). Studies exploring the anatomical development of these connections reported that they were primarily established during adolescence and suggested that they could serve to integrate emotional and attentional or other cognitive processes [57], processes that are dysfunctional in schizophrenia.

Thalamo-cortical GABAergic pathways, which link the thalamus to high-order association cortex, may be potentially important loci for attentional and sensory gating processes in schizophrenia [58]. Two distinct classes of GABA neurons, parvalbumin- or calbindin-containing, project to middle cortical layers or superficial prefrontal layers, respectively, of the PFC, and receive reciprocal glutamatergic inputs.

Interactions between neurotensin and GABA pathways may be important for schizophrenia [59]. Neurotensin regulation of DA release in the nucleus accumbens may be mediated indirectly by glutamate-induced GABA release [59], again placing GABA in the position of the "final common pathway" regulating a key circuit involved in schizophrenia.

In summary, GABAergic neurons are localized in multiple neuronal circuits that may be impacted in schizophrenia or by pharmacological treatments used for the treatment of schizophrenia. The next section will review some key data that support the role of GABA in schizophrenia.

### 15.2.2 GABA Pathway Alterations in Schizophrenia

As is evident from the quote at the beginning of this article, the idea that GABA is involved in schizophrenia is not a new one, having been proposed over 35 years ago, although a 1983 review indicated that over a decade of research had failed to establish a clear link between GABA and schizophrenia and interest in this connection had "waned." However, subsequent technological improvements in methods for quantifying tissue concentrations of messenger RNAs in the postmortem human brain tissue [60], advances in studying brain circuitry, and refinements of pharmacological probes for studying the function of GABA pathways, have all contributed to a revival of interest in GABA as a key player in schizophrenia.

***15.2.2.1 Postmortem Studies*** A key finding that has solidified a central role for GABA is the demonstration of reproducible deficits in cortical GABAergic pathways measured in schizophrenic postmortem brain tissues. As reviewed elsewhere [2, 3, 60–65], these changes include reductions in cortical GABA concentrations and decreases in the activity of the enzyme that synthesizes GABA, glutamic acid decarboxylase (GAD), the predominant form of which is the 67 kD form, GAD67. As there are multiple classes of GABA interneurons, an important finding is that the reported changes are generally only seen in certain subsets of GABA interneurons, that is, those that (1) electrophysiologically are fast-spiking; (2) anatomically are either "basket" type or "chandelier" type; (3) contain the calcium binding protein parvalbumin; and (4) synapse on the periosmatic region of the pyramidal cells.

The prefrontal cortex (PFC) is a brain area of great importance for selecting relevant signals and suppressing distractors [66], for integrating cognitive and motivational context information [67], and for working memory. Loss of PFC neurons leads to lack of flexibility in decision making [68]. Modern theories of schizophrenia have incorporated an important role of the PFC. One of the key regions of interest where reductions of GAD67 have been extensively studied is the dorsolateral region of the PFC, although similar findings have been reported in other cortical areas (anterior cingulate cortex, and primary motor and primary visual cortices) and in limbic system paleocortex, particularly the CA2/3 and stratum oriens regions of the hippocampus [69–71]. These findings are consistent with the hypothesis that reductions in GABA neurotransmission may contribute to the pathophysiology of different clinical aspects of schizophrenia (sensory, affective, cognitive) that are mediated by different brain regions [72, 73].

***15.2.2.2 γ-Oscillatory Activity*** Several lines of evidence have been cited to support the potential link between alterations in cortical GABA activity and functional deficits in schizophrenia, cognition in particular. One line of evidence involves use of an electrophysiological technique referred to as transcranial magnetic stimulation (TMS) to measure cortical inhibitory processes in the brain believed to be mediated by GABA interneurons. Using the TMS technique, deficits in cortical inhibition were measured in schizophrenics, consistent with a presumed deficit in cortical GABAergic transmission [74, 75].

Another line of evidence utilized electrophysiological measurements of synchronized neuronal cortical activity. (For reviews on importance of neural synchrony in schizophrenia see References [76–78].) A number of perceptual and cognitive processes are thought to require synchronization of cortical neuronal activity, expressed as electroencephalogram (EEG) signals at γ-band frequencies (30–50 Hz). Furthermore, it is proposed that activation of GABA interneurons synapsing onto $GABA_A$ receptors on pyramidal neurons is important for induction of γ-band oscillations during certain cognitive tasks. Dysfunctional GABA transmission has been proposed to contribute to the cognitive deficits seen in schizophrenia by interfering with these critical neural synchronization processes. Relative to normal individuals, schizophrenics show a deficit in γ-band activation in the PFC during performance of a working memory task under conditions of demanding cognitive load. Thus, dysfunctional GABA interneurons in a state of hypoactivity are unable to provide adequate phasic synaptic inhibition necessary for synchronized network oscillations that are important for coordinating neural activity at the level of PFC pyramidal neurons.

One of the challenges of interpreting these data is ascertaining what changes are primary and what may be secondary, compensatory changes. Lewis and colleagues suggest that some of the changes that they have measured anatomically in postmortem brain (e.g., increases in the GABA transporter; upregulation of postsynaptic $GABA_A$ receptors—see Section 15.3.2.2. result from compensatory processes that are engaged to counteract the primary deficit (i.e., reduced GABA activation of postsynaptic receptors) which attempt to partially restore inhibitory synaptic efficacy [3, 61–63]. This systems-based scenario is analogous to, for example, the substantial compensatory processes that are engaged in Parkinson's disease as the nigrostriatal DA system undergoes degeneration and postsynaptic receptors are denervated. Lewis argues that for cortical GABA pathways that are impaired in schizophrenia, engagement of compensatory processes is not adequate to restore normal function, resulting in deficient $\gamma$-oscillatory activity and impaired cognitive function, which necessitate pharmacological approaches to restore normal GABA neurotransmission [78].

***15.2.2.3 Computer Modeling*** The dynamics underlying schizophrenia-associated dysfunction of cortical GABA circuits are clearly more complex than the simplified conception presented herein. The reader is referred to recent publications in which computer modeling techniques have been applied to dysfunction of GABAergic cortical circuitry in the dorsolateral PFC (DLPFC) in schizophrenia [65, 79–81]. One study used a computational model to investigate the dynamics of the PFC circuit and showed that abnormal reduction of GABA-mediated cell-inhibition (as thought to exist in schizophrenia) uniquely shifted the PFC toward a "hyperactive mode" with concomitant hyperdopaminergic transmission, a condition that is consistent with increased vulnerability to psychosis [65].

***15.2.2.4 Genetic and Epigenetic Studies*** Currently, the etiology of cortical GABA deficiency and associated cognitive deficits in schizophrenia is not known, although a recent study in humans [82] has strengthened the argument for a genetic basis. A key finding was that impaired cognition and decreased PFC GAD1 mRNA expression in the schizophrenic brain was associated with a single nucleotide polymorphism (SNP) in the 5′ untranslated region for GAD1 (which encodes GAD67). Evidence was also provided for a potential biological synergism between catechol-o-methyltransferase (COMT) and GAD1 SNPs which could lead to increased risk for schizophrenia. Overall, the authors concluded that the results implicate GAD1 and diminished cortical GABA inhibition (with a possible dopaminergic component) in schizophrenia.

Costa and colleagues have proposed potential epigenetic mechanisms, that is, DNA (cytosine-5) methylation, chromatin remodeling, and post-translational covalent modifications of histones, which may contribute to changes in the regulation of GAD1 gene expression and dysfunctional alterations of GAD67 in schizophrenia. As a detailed discussion of these studies is beyond the scope of this chapter, the reader is referred to several recent reviews [83, 84].

### 15.2.3 GABA and Animal Models of Schizophrenia

Animal models are important from two different perspectives: first, for elucidating the anatomical and functional aspects of the complex neural circuitry underlying schizophrenia, and second, for evaluating compounds for therapeutic potential in schizophrenia prior to human testing.

Animal models of schizophrenia with high construct validity strive to successfully reproduce the hypothesized or demonstrated underlying neurochemical imbalance (as well as their neurodevelopmental time course), and replicate the symptom clusters seen in humans as well as their response to pharmacological agents. Identifying animal models that fulfill these criteria is a tremendous challenge in that the underlying neurochemical imbalances in schizophrenia have not been clearly delineated (as they have, for example, in Parkinson's disease) and the symptoms such as hallucinations, delusions, and cognitive impairments are difficult to model. Furthermore, animal models of schizophrenia that have the highest level of validity may be time-consuming and complex, for example, the methylazoxymethanol acetate (MAM) neurodevelopment model in rats [85], and although they may be the most relevant to understanding the underlying circuitry, they are not as amenable to compound screening as simpler, higher-throughput models.

With regard to drug screening, pharmacological challenge models are widely used to evaluate compounds for their antipsychotic potential. For example, locomotor hyperstimulation of DA receptors by agents such as amphetamine or apomorphine is used to model schizophrenic hyperdopaminergia, and therapeutic potential in these models is indicated by a compound's activity in reversing this locomotor stimulation. NMDA glutamate receptor antagonists (phencyclidine [PCP], MK-801, ketamine) model the hypothesized hypoglutamatergia in schizophrenia, and reversal of behavioral social withdrawal and cognitive deficits produced by NMDA antagonists is proposed to predict efficacy in treating negative [86] and cognitive [87, 88] symptoms of schizophrenia, respectively.

A sizeable literature has studied deficits in gating of sensory transmission using electrophysiological models (P50 gating) or behavioral models (prepulse inhibition [PPI]). Deficits in these measures are seen in schizophrenics and can be modeled in animals using various manipulations, including pharmacological stimulation of DA receptors (amphetamine, apomorphine) or blockade of NMDA receptors (PCP, MK-801, ketamine). Recent clinical work demonstrating that PPI in schizophrenics is improved by olanzapine, but not by haloperidol or risperidone, indicates that this deficit is not simply ameliorated by $D_2$ receptor blockade [89].

Other animal models strive to measure side effect liability. These include reversal of amphetamine or apomorphine-induced stereotyped behaviors, indicative of blockade of striatal $D_2$ receptors and therefore EPS liability. Tardive dyskinesia, a movement disorder that occurs as the result of chronic blockade of $D_2$ receptors, has been modeled in both rat and nonhuman primate models [90].

Additional models provide specialized cognitive assessment, that is, using procedures such as set-shifting to measure PFC function that is disrupted in schizophrenia [91, 92]; measures that may be related to negative symptoms, such as amygdala-mediated emotional blunting [93]; and environmental manipulations such as isolation rearing during a critical period of development [94] that produce a schizophrenia-like phenotype. Genetic models under investigation include FEZ1 (fasciculation and elongation protein zeta) knockout (KO) mice, DARPP-32 KO mice [95], and the reeler model of schizophrenia [96].

With this background, the remaining discussion will review preclinical and clinical evidence that drugs that affect GABAergic pathways may be useful in treating schizophrenia.

***15.2.3.1 Animal Models with GABA Dysfunctions*** As mentioned earlier and summarized in Figure 15.3, a current hypothesis posits that glutamatergic neurons "drive" a subset of cortical parvalbumin-containing GABAergic interneurons, which, in turn, through $GABA_A$ receptor activation, "sculpt" or filter the activity of cortical pyramidal neurons. In schizophrenia, it is proposed that there is an abnormal reduction of GABA-mediated inhibition, which results in a loss of filtering of pyramidal neurons and production of schizophrenic symptoms. The reduction in GABA activity could be due to a primary deficit in GABA neurons or it could be secondary to an abnormal reduction in the ability of glutamate to activate GABA interneurons. Given this conception, increasing attention in animal models is being directed toward measuring disruptions or alterations in GABA interneurons produced indirectly by disruption of glutamate excitatory input. Thus, repeated exposure to NMDA antagonists (e.g., ketamine, PCP, MK-801) that produce a schizophrenia-like phenotype in animals is accompanied by a dysfunction of a subset of cortical fast-spiking inhibitory interneurons, as measured by decreased parvalbumin and GAD67 [97]. Rats exposed to subchronic MK-801 also exhibited a decreased density of parvalbumin-positive GABA neurons in the hippocampus [98]. Recent work further extended these findings by describing a model that reproduces the core PFC functional and anatomical deficits of schizophrenia. In this model, subchronic and chronic intermittent PCP produced hypofrontality as measured by reduced glucose utilization in the PFC which was not reversible by haloperidol or clozapine (mimicking clinical data); decreased parvalbumin-containing GABA interneurons; and cognitive deficits in executive function as measured with a set-shifting task [99]. It is important to emphasize that the lack of efficacy of typical or atypical antipsychotics in ameliorating cognitive deficits in this model is consistent with clinical data in humans. The authors suggested that this model should be useful for evaluating novel treatments for potential therapeutic efficacy, particularly in treating cognitive deficits in schizophrenia.

Exposure to an environmental stressor referred to as "isolation rearing" in rodents during a critical period post weaning has been proposed as a nonpharmacological animal model of schizophrenia [94] and has been recently shown to impact GABA pathways in the hippocampus. Isolation rearing produced deficits in sensory gating as measured by PPI (as seen in schizophrenics) and reductions in hippocampal GABAergic cells expressing the calcium-binding proteins parvalbumin and calbindin, but not calretinin, anatomical findings that are consistent with those seen in schizophrenic brain [94]. In addition, the GABA-transporter 1 (GAT-1) in parvalbumin-containing cartridges was reduced in the ventral prelimbic cortex of isolation-reared rats [100], a change that is also analogous to that reported in the PFC of schizophrenic postmortem brain tissues.

A related model of impoverished rearing of Mongolian gerbils combined with dopaminergic stimulation produced by the DA-releasing agent methamphetamine given on postnatal day 14 produced anatomical evidence indicative of altered postnatal maturation of the prefrontal cortical GABAergic neurons, which is possibly associated with a dysfunctional PFC [101].

In the MAM model, a developmental insult (prenatal exposure to the mitogenic agent MAM) produces a schizophrenia-like behavioral phenotype that has been attributed to a pathological enhancement in the output of the hippocampus and resulting hyperactivation of DA neurons located in the ventral tegmental area (VTA) [85, 102]. Recent work has demonstrated that parvalbumin-positive GABA neurons in mPFC and ventral hippocampus were decreased in the MAM animal model [103]. Furthermore, this GABA deficit was expressed electrophysiologically as a decrease in $\gamma$-oscillatory activity measured during performance of a cognitive task (latent inhibition), and functionally as a cognitive impairment in the latent inhibition task. The authors also proposed that a deficit in intrinsic GABAergic signaling may be the origin of the hippocampal hyperactivity purported to underlie the DA dysfunction in psychosis.

Several genetically based animal models relevant to schizophrenia have implicated involvement of GABA pathways. For example, the reeler mouse has been proposed as an animal model of schizophrenia and demonstrates decreases in GAD67 [96]. In addition, FEZ1 has been shown to interact with DISC1 (disrupted in schizophrenia 1), a schizophrenia susceptibility gene product, and polymorphisms of human FEZ1 have been associated with schizophrenia. In mice, FEZ1 is predominantly localized in GABAergic neurons. FEZ1 KO mice showed hyperactivity, enhanced behavioral responses to MK-801 and methamphetamine, and enhanced methamphetamine-induced release of DA in the nucleus accumbens, indicative of an overactive mesolimbic dopaminergic system [104]. Thus, impaired FEZ1 function mediated through GABAergic neurons may be important in the pathogenesis of schizophrenia.

Finally, there is evidence for involvement of ventral tegmental GABA, and $GABA_B$ receptors in particular, in mediating PPI [105]. The disruption of PPI by DA agonists has been attributed to reduced ventral pallidal GABAergic transmission as the DA agonist quinelorane reduced GABA efflux in the ventral pallidum and disrupted PPI [106].

In summary, a variety of animal models of schizophrenia have provided evidence for GABAergic deficits in the brain and functional deficits reminiscent of those seen in schizophrenia. With this background in place, pharmacological studies in animals and humans assessing the potential of various classes of GABAergic agents for utility in schizophrenia will be reviewed.

## 15.3 TARGETING GABAERGIC PATHWAYS FOR SCHIZOPHRENIA

The data thus far indicate that GABA pathways play a potentially important role in schizophrenia and could be a rational target for pharmacological intervention. Postmortem studies indicate consistent deficits in subsets of GABA pathways that interact with cortical pyramidal neurons. Furthermore, the presence of GABA interneurons in multiple points of the complex subcortical and cortical circuitries postulated to be dysfunctional in schizophrenia suggests that GABA neurons could impact positive, negative, and cognitive symptoms of schizophrenia, and could be important for motor side effects associated with neuroleptic administration. This section will review the effects of various GABAergic agents in human trials in schizophrenia or in animal models, and will highlight potential future directions in this area.

### 15.3.1 Global Activation of GABA Pathways

***15.3.1.1 GABA Uptake Inhibitors*** GABA uptake inhibitors nonselectively increase availability of GABA at both $GABA_A$ and $GABA_B$ receptors. Recent work indicates that the GABA uptake inhibitor tiagabine has functional effects relevant to potential utility in schizophrenia in that the drug entrained cortical networks, measured using EEG $\gamma$-band synchrony during cognitive control in healthy human subjects [107]. Notably, tiagabine-enhanced BZD binding as measured with $[^{11}C]$flumazenil positron emission tomography (PET) binding in the major functional domains of the cerebral cortex (association, sensory, and limbic-medial temporal lobe), and this correlated with EEG entrainment. These data were cited as supportive evidence for a relationship between enhanced $GABA_A$ receptor neurotransmission and EEG $\gamma$-band activity, although a potential contribution of $GABA_B$ receptors cannot be ruled out. Based on these findings, it would be of interest to evaluate tiagabine or related compounds for potential efficacy in schizophrenics.

***15.3.1.2 GABA Prodrugs*** Another approach to globally enhancing GABA transmission is to administer a GABA ester prodrug that facilitates entry of GABA into the brain and subsequent availability at the synaptic cleft. BL-1020 (Bioline Rx), an agent described as a "GABA-enhanced antipsychotic," is perphenazine (a $D_2$/5-$HT_2$ antagonist) with an attached GABA moiety that is thought to act like a GABA prodrug. Animal studies [108, 109] demonstrated that BL-1020 binds to $D_2$ (Ki ~ 0.06 nM, $D_2$ short or long) and 5-$HT_{2A}$

($K_i$ = 0.21 nM) receptors, blocked amphetamine-induced locomotion (indicative of antipsychotic efficacy), increased prefrontal and hippocampal DA neurotransmitter release (indicative of the potential to reverse hypodopaminergia), and demonstrated reduced catalepsy and sedation relative to perphenazine (indicative of a reduced side effect profile). In a recent Bioline Rx company press release (http://www.biolinerx.com), reference was made to preclinical data indicating that BL-1020 has the potential to improve cognition. BL-1020 and perphenazine stimulated prolactin secretion equally, suggesting that the additional GABAergic action would not counteract this effect of $D_2$ receptor antagonism [108]. In addition, positive top-line results from a 6-week, open label Phase IIa clinical trial were announced. In this trial, with 36 treatment-resistant schizophrenia patients, BL-1020 significantly improved Positive and Negative Syndrome Scale (PANSS) and Clinical Global Impression of Severity and Improvement (CGI), which are measures of severity and improvement in schizophrenia. This efficacy occurred without significantly affecting weight gain or EPS, although clearly additional trials are needed to fully evaluate this potential advantage. Increased prolactin, typically seen with $D_2$ antagonists, was seen, so it would appear that the additional GABAergic stimulation did not ameliorate this side effect. It was also reported that there was high compliance relative to other antipsychotics as measured by a low withdrawal rate (3/36 patients). Overall, these initial data were interpreted as promising, and additional Phase IIb trials were being pursued.

***15.3.1.3 GABA Transaminase Inhibitors*** A small trial evaluating the effects of the GABA transaminase inhibitor, vigabatrin, on tardive dyskinesia in schizophrenics, demonstrated that the drug increased CSF levels of GABA, which were also depressed in patients with tardive dyskinesia, and reduced symptoms [110]. However, several comprehensive Cochrane summaries [111, 112] reviewing the effects of GABA agonists in tardive dyskinesia concluded that the therapeutic effects are not clear, indicating that further work is needed to fully assess the utility of these agents for this indication.

***15.3.1.4 $GABA_A$ Receptor Agonists*** In general, agents that act at the GABA recognition site on $GABA_A$ receptors as agonists (muscimol) have limited therapeutic utility as they tend to be proconvulsive and therefore are not considered viable therapeutic agents for schizophrenia.

***15.3.1.5 Allosteric Activators of $GABA_A$ Receptors*** BZDs are widely used in treating schizophrenia, although there have been limited controlled clinical studies that have systematically assessed their specific efficacy in treating different aspects of the disease. It is beyond the scope of this chapter to extensively review all of the studies that have been performed to date. However, the reader is referred to two Cochrane reviews of clinical studies exploring the utility of BZDs, either as monotherapy or as adjunctive treatment, in treating psychoses in general [113] or in schizophrenia specifically [114]. Several conclusions from those reviews are worth emphasizing. First, patients receiving BZDs as a monotherapy generally showed a greater clinically significant response, although overall improvement in the Brief Psychiatric Rating Scale (BPRS) mental state was found in only one small study. Second, although effects of BZDs on relapse prevention have been reported, antipsychotics were found to be superior in this regard. Third, when given in combination with an antipsychotic, improvements in global state were seen, although this benefit waned over time and was not measurable at 2 hours or longer. Finally, the co-administration of BZDs also resulted in the less frequent use of anti-parkinson medications to treat EPS.

Despite some positive reports, the overall conclusion was that, based on the results of rigorously designed clinical trials, BZDs could not be strongly recommended as either monotherapy or adjunctive therapy in the treatment of schizophrenia or schizophrenia-like psychoses, although longer-term, more highly powered clinical trials were recommended to evaluate the possible efficacy of combination therapies [114].

BZDs, especially clonazepam [115–117], have been proposed as useful treatments for neuroleptic-induced tardive dyskinesia. This indication has been reviewed extensively in a recent Cochrane report [118] which concluded that there was preliminary evidence in one small study that BZDs had some efficacy in treating tardive dyskinesia; however, routine clinical use was not indicated given inconclusive results seen in other studies.

Given the apparent inconsistent effects in schizophrenia, one conclusion is that BZDs simply have little or no efficacy in schizophrenia. However, there are several alternative explanations for their apparent inconsistent effects. First, tolerance may occur as is well documented for the chronic treatment of seizures in epilepsy [119], and therefore improved $GABA_A$ receptor modulators with reduced tolerance might show increased efficacy in schizophrenia. The topic of subtype-selective agents that may have reduced tolerance is discussed later. Second, as noted previously, schizophrenia is a complex disorder that is comprised of multiple symptom clusters. Thus, it is possible that BZDs may be useful in treating one domain of symptoms but may exacerbate other symptoms, thereby masking the useful actions of the drugs.

As noted previously, cognitive deficits are pervasive in schizophrenia and are particularly resistant to current treatments. An issue not addressed in the Cochrane reviews is the question of the effects of BZDs on cognitive deficits in schizophrenia, which is not surprising since there are very few studies that have explored this question. However, it is well known that BZDs can have cognition-impairing actions, and this is one of the major drawbacks to their therapeutic use, particularly in those conditions that require chronic administration and sustained daytime coverage. If cognitive impairment with BZDs occurs in schizophrenia, this detrimental action could serve to mask other beneficial actions.

A number of experimental clinical studies have explored the effects of BZDs on cognition in normal volunteers [120–125]. These studies have found that BZDs given at sedating doses generally impair learning and memory in an anterograde fashion (i.e., new learning is impaired when it takes place after drug administration, while drug levels are substantial), whereas retrograde memory (memory for events that occurred before drug ingestion) tends to be unaffected.

Studies in healthy volunteers are important, but it is critical to evaluate drug effects in the schizophrenia target population. Menzies and colleagues [126] performed a pharmacological functional magnetic resonance imaging (fMRI) study in 11 chronic schizophrenics. In this study, the BZD lorazepam impaired performance in a working memory task (N-back test) to a greater extent than it did in healthy controls. fMRI measurements made during the cognitive task demonstrated that schizophrenics given placebo had abnormally attenuated activation of fronto-parietal cortex and deactivation of temporo-cingulate cortex. This pattern was induced by lorazepam in healthy controls and exacerbated by lorazepam in schizophrenics. These data thus indicated that lorazepam impaired cognitive performance and attenuated deactivation of task-related brain functional systems. The data also emphasize the importance of evaluating drug effects in the target population, in this case, schizophrenia.

Taken together, these data support the conclusion that BZDs, which nonspecifically activate $GABA_A$ receptors of different subtypes, may exacerbate cognitive deficits in schizophrenia, and this action, along with the possible development of tolerance, may mask any positive effects of BZDs in treating schizophrenia. However, as described later, there is evidence that subtype-selective agents may provide a potentially promising alternative to BZDs.

Two additional actions of BZDs that may be of benefit in schizophrenia are in treating anxiety and catatonia. Anxiety disorders are often comorbid in schizophrenia [127, 128] and anxiety has even been suggested to be a core symptom dimension [128]. Thus, the well-documented anxiolytic actions of BZDs may be beneficial in treating anxiety symptoms in schizophrenia. The neural substrate through which BZD anxiolysis occurs is likely the amygdala complex, a key limbic system structure that mediates fear and anxiety [129]. Extinction of fear responses is a critical active learning process that involves developing new memory traces that inhibit or overcome exising fear memory traces [130]. Recent work in animals indicates that acquisition of fear produces a downregulation of mRNA markers, which is indicative of decreased GABAergic function in the amydala, whereas acquisition of fear extinction produced an upregulation, which is indicative of enhanced GABA transmission [131]. Furthermore, specific subtypes of the $GABA_A$ receptor (i.e., those containing $\alpha 2$ and/or $\alpha 3$ subunits) have been implicated in the anxiolytic actions of BZDs, suggesting the possibility that subtype selective agents would be attractive in schizophrenia [132], an idea that will be revisited later.

Catatonia is a stupor-like state that is sometimes seen in schizophrenics and in other psychiatric states [133–135]. A recent review [134] concludes that catatonia is a syndrome with different subtypes and treatment responses.

Catatonia has been linked to deficits in $GABA_A$ transmission (for discussion see Reference [135]), a conclusion that is supported by the striking efficacy of BZDs in the treatment of catatonia. However, BZDs are less effective when the symptoms are more chronic, which is likely due to the development of tolerance. Thus, development of active agents that have reduced tolerance could provide improved treatment of catatonia in schizophrenia and other disorders.

***15.3.1.6 Partial Allosteric Activators*** The overall lack of compelling findings for nonselective BZD agents in the treatment of schizophrenia may be attributable to the presence of predominant side effects that interfere with, or mask, beneficial actions of the drugs, or to the development of tolerance. As noted earlier, one approach to optimizing efficacy and reducing side effects is to use agents that are partial allosteric activators at the BZD site. In fact, several agents that are partial allosteric activators lacking selectivity for $GABA_A$ receptor subtypes have been evaluated in schizophrenia. In an open label trial in 66 patients with moderate to severe acute schizophrenia, the nonselective BZD site partial allosteric activator bretazenil demonstrated moderate antipsychotic efficacy, good tolerability, and no EPS [136]. Although no further work with this agent has been reported, the results were consistent with the idea that implementing partial allosteric activation may give rise to improved therapeutic agents for treating schizophrenia.

### 15.3.2 $GABA_A$ Subtype Selective Allosteric Modulators

Another approach to improving the therapeutic profile of BZDs is to design agents that achieve selectivity for certain $GABA_A$ receptor subtypes, with or without partial agonism. The following sections will explore the role of different BZD-sensitive $GABA_A$ subtypes in schizophrenia.

***15.3.2.1 $\alpha$1-$GABA_A$ Receptors*** As noted previously, $GABA_A$ receptors containing the $\alpha$1 subunit are the most prevalent BZD-sensitive $GABA_A$ receptor subtype in the brain and only a few regions lack this subunit, that is, the reticular thalamic nucleus, spinal motorneurons, and granule cell layer of the olfactory bulb [10, 13]. To date, the potential utility in schizophrenia has not been reported for agents such as zolpidem that have functional selectivity for the $\alpha$1 subunit and that act as full allosteric activators at this site. However, it is not clear if these agents would be viable given their marked sedative–hypnotic effects.

***15.3.2.2 $\alpha$2-$GABA_A$ Receptors*** Selective allosteric activation at $GABA_A$ receptors that contain $\alpha$2 subunits may be of benefit in schizophrenia for treating anxiety as well as cognitive deficits. With regard to anxiety, as noted previously, activation of the $\alpha$2 subunit has been implicated in the anxiolytic effects of BZDs, and agents that selectively target this subunit may have less sedative liability [16]. As anxiety is prevalent in schizophrenia and anxiety disorders are often comorbid [127, 128], agents that specifically activate α2 subunits may be useful in treating this symptom. To date, this hypothesis has not been tested in formal clinical trials.

As mentioned previously, a major unmet medical need in schizophrenia is cognitive deficits, which include attentional impairments, executive function, visual and verbal learning and memory, working memory, processing speed, and social cognition [27]. Cognitive deficits in schizophrenia may, at least in part, be mediated by a reduction in GABA-mediated inhibition in cortical areas such as the DLPFC. Lewis and colleagues have reported that, in postmortem tissues from schizophrenic brains, postsynaptic $GABA_A$ receptors containing α2 subunits on axon initial segments of pyramidal neurons in the DLPFC were upregulated, indicative of a compensatory upregulation in response to diminished presynaptic GABA input [3, 62, 63, 137]. If these receptors are supersensitive, then allosteric activation at α2-containing $GABA_A$ receptors might restore deficient cortical GABAergic tone and improve cognition. Because these may be supersensitive receptors, compounds that are low efficacy partial agonists may be desirable in restoring cognition without overstimulation, or without adversely affecting GABAergic activity in nonsupersensitive pathways. In contrast, full α2 agonists or full nonselective agonists may be suboptimal and possibly even cognitively impairing.

MK-0777 (Merck), a reported α2 selective partial allosteric activator, has been evaluated in an initial proof-of-concept, double-blind, placebo-controlled clinical trial in 15 male schizophrenics [138]. The results of this trial demonstrated that MK-0777 did not produce changes in the BPRS or in the Repeatable Battery for the Assessment of Neuropsychological Symptoms (RBANS), whereas it did improve performance of three tests of working memory and/or cognitive control (N-back test, AX-continuous performance task [CPT], and Preparing to Ovecome Prepotency [POP] task). In addition, MK-0777 increased prefrontal γ-oscillation power during the POP task. The authors concluded that these data provided preliminary support for the hypothesis that enhanced GABA activity at α2 subunit-containing $GABA_A$ receptors improved behavioral and electrophysiological measures of prefrontal function in schizophrenia. The authors also emphasized the importance of using relevant and sensitive cognitive measures for detecting drug-induced changes in cognition as opposed to standard neuropsychological batteries.

MK-0777 is currently being evaluated in a multicenter, Phase II trial in the TURNS (Treatment Units for Research in Neurocognitive Science) Program for safety and efficacy in improving cognition in schizophrenia (ClinicalTrials.gov identifier: NCT00505076; see http://clinicaltrials.gov/ct/show/NCT00505076?order=1). Two doses of MK-0777, 3 mg BID and 8 mg BID, are being tested. A key primary measure is the MATRICS Consensus Cognitive Battery (MCCB), and a secondary measure is the UCSD Performance-Based Skills Assessment (UPSA), which is designed to assess skills in five areas: household chores, communication, finance, transportation, and planning recreational activities. Another secondary measure is the Schizophrenia Cognition Rating Scale (SCoRS), which is a rating scale designed to elicit information from the subject and informant on the level of cognitive function of the subject. The outcome of this study will be of further importance in assessing the utility of α2-subtype selective partial agonists in treating cognitive deficits in schizophrenia.

***15.3.2.3 α3-GABA$_A$ Receptors*** GABA$_A$ receptors containing α3 subunits are localized in a number of brain regions implicated in the neural circuitry of schizophrenia. One important site of action is in the brainstem, where α3 is the primary subunit that modulates DA neurons [139]. In a study with genetically modified mice [140], the α3 receptor was knocked out without evidence for compensatory upregulation in other subunits. The α3 KO mice demonstrated disrupted PPI (sensorimotor gating), which was reversed by the DA $D_2$ receptor antagonist, haloperidol, providing evidence for an α3–DA interaction that was functionally relevant to schizophrenia. The reduction of PPI was not attributable to a sensory deficit, as KO mice responded equally well to the startle-eliciting stimulus. In electrophysiological studies in brain slices, GABA-induced inhibition of VTA DA neurons was greatly reduced (50%) in α3 KO mice relative to wild-type controls, with the residual response likely attributable to actions on a different subtype. These data indicated that α3-GABA$_A$ neurons contribute to a tonic inhibition of VTA DA neurons and that deficits in their transmission result in hyperactivation of DA pathways and, functionally, in disrupted sensorimotor gating. Also indicative of elevated DA tone was the finding that α3 KO mice showed locomotor hyperactivity. Amphetamine produced a further augmentation of locomotor activity in both wild-type and α3-KO mice, presumably due to amphetamine-induced release of DA from terminals that were "downstream" from the modulatory influence of the α3 receptors. Overall, these findings support a potentially important role of α3-GABA$_A$ receptors in the etiology of hyperdopaminergia in schizophrenia, and furthermore suggest that drugs that have agonist activity at α3 subunits might be useful in treating schizophrenia. In addition, because they would be indirectly modulating VTA DA neurons, such agents could have reduced potential for producing EPS associated with $D_2$ receptor antagonists [141].

Several compounds have been reported to have profiles as α3-preferring allosteric activators. ELB139 is described as an α3 subunit-selective partial agonist for the BZD binding site of GABA$_A$ receptors, which has anxiolytic, antidepressant, and anticonvulsant activity that has reduced side effect liability [142–146]. ELB139 has highest potency at α3-containing receptors but highest efficacy on α1- or α2-containing receptors, respectively. ELB139 binds with an $IC_{50}$ = 1390 nM to the flunitrazepam binding site in rat forebrain cortical membranes and in rat hippocampal neurons and was a partial agonist with 40–50% of the efficacy of diazepam in potentiating GABA-induced currents [145]. Antipsychotic-like activity was reported in ELB139's ability to reduce amphetamine- or MK-801-induced hyperactivity, and these effects were reversed by the BZD receptor antagonist flumazenil [143]. In the same assays, the nonselective BZD agonist diazepam did not have an antipsychotic profile at a dose that was nonsedating, suggesting that the α3 selectivity conferred ELB139 with a unique functional profile.

A microdialysis study demonstrated that ELB139 increased extracellular 5-HT (with no effect on DA) in the striatum and the mPFC of rats [144]. The BZD antagonist flumazenil administered systemically or locally into the dorsal raphe nucleus, an α3 receptor-rich monoamine nucleus, reversed the ELB139-induced 5-HT increase in the striatum. These results suggested that at least some of the effects of ELB139 might be mediated indirectly through 5-HT neurons. ELB139's unique profile as an antipsychotic was emphasized in that an antidepressant-like profile may be useful for treating negative symptoms [144].

Notably, ELB139 was also shown to have less anxiolytic tolerance following chronic administration relative to the BZD diazepam [142]. As noted previously, reduced tolerance could be important for a drug that is administered chronically, as is the case for antipsychotics. It has not been reported whether tolerance to the antipsychotic effects of ELB139 is seen.

TP003 is another selective α3 agonist that has the preclinical profile of a nonsedating anxiolytic agent [147]. No information is available on the activity of this compound in animal models of schizophrenia, including measures of psychosis or cognition. Regarding side effect profile, Dias et al [147] noted that TP-003 is nonsedating at low doses.

Adipiplon is a partial allosteric activator of $GABA_A$ receptors with preferential activity on $GABA_A$ receptors containing α3 subunits [148]. Stated differently, adipiplon is a partial agonist at α1, α2, α3, and α5 subunit-containing $GABA_A$ receptors, while having greatest efficacy (intrinsic activity) at α3 subunits. As expected for an α3 partial agonist, adipiplon is anxiolytic in rats [149]. A closely related analog, NG2-83, shows robust anxiolysis with a substantially greater therapeutic index compared with the BZD triazolam in rhesus monkeys [150]. Adipiplon has weak partial agonist activity on α2 subunits (approximately half of its efficacy on α3) [148], although given the upregulation of α2 subunits reported in the DLPFC of schizophrenics, this activity may be sufficient to produce cognition-enhancing effects. Thus, based on its partial agonist activity at α3- and, to a lesser degree, α2-$GABA_A$ receptors, adipiplon may be effective in restoring tone to deficient cortical and subcortical $GABA_A$ receptors in schizophrenia. Additional work is required to test this hypothesis.

***15.3.2.4 α5-Selective Agents*** As cognitive deficits are pervasive in schizophrenia, receptor targets that are implicated in cognition are of potential therapeutic interest. Several lines of evidence indicate that activation of $GABA_A$ receptors containing α5 subunits impairs cognition and that inverse agonists at this site have the potential to be cognition enhancing [20, 151–153].

$GABA_A$ α5 receptors are considered extrasynaptic and mediate a tonic conductance [154], with low concentrations of transmitter required to produce continuous inhibition. Intravenous or volatile anesthetics that have marked amnestic effects in humans potentiated this slow inhibition, supportive of a cognition-impairing action of allosteric activation at the α5 site. Studies utilizing α5-KO mice also demonstrate a critical role of the α5 subtype. Early proof of concept was provided by the finding that intravenous ZK-93,426, a weak partial inverse agonist at the α5 subtype, improved memory in animal models and in a double-blind, placebo-controlled Phase I trial in healthy volunteers. However, this compound was not further developed because of pharmacokinetic issues.

Merck has described an agent, "α5IA," as a partial inverse agonist selective for α5-$GABA_A$ receptors [19]. In human studies, alcohol-induced cognitive deficits were reversed by α5IA, with a partial reversal of sedation, and no effect on intoxication, alcohol liking or slowing of eye movements [155]. Unfortunately, α5IA cannot be used for chronic dosing studies [156], however, given the link between α5 subunits and cognition, it would be of interest to evaluate a mechanistically-similar agent in schizophrenics for possible utility in reversing cognitive deficits.

A study by Menzies and colleagues in which lorazepam was reported to produce a greater disruptive effect on working memory in schizophrenics relative to normal controls also reported that the BZD antagonist flumazenil significantly improved cognition in schizophrenics [126] wheras it tended to decrease cognition in healthy volunteers. The authors also reported that the cognitive changes correlated with expected changes in regional brain activity as measured by fMRI.

In the Menzies study, flumazenil was cited as a "partial inverse agonist" that would inhibit $GABA_A$ receptor-mediated transmission. However, other data suggest that flumazenil may behave like a partial agonist. For example, flumazenil is anxiolytic (reflecting an agonist action) in some mouse strains [157], although inconsistent anxiolysis relative to full agonists is more consistent with a weak partial agonist profile. Flumazenil enhanced the hypnotic properties of propofol [158], also consistent with an agonist action. Thus, the precise mechanism underlying the reported cognitive benefit in schizophrenia is not clear.

Although the primary focus of discussion of α5 has been on cognition, there is recent evidence that this subunit may be relevant to negative symptoms. In a PET imaging study in 11 schizophrenics (six drug-naïve and six drug-free) performed using the α5-preferring ligand [$^{11}$C]Ro 15-4513, a negative correlation was seen between binding potential in the hippocampus and PFC and negative symptoms as measured using PANSS [159].

Imidazenil, a full allosteric modulator of $GABA_A$ receptors expressing α5 subunits, was reported to reduce psychotic symptomatology without producing sedation [84]. However, as discussed previously, imidazenil may have actions at subunits other than α5, limiting conclusions regarding the precise mechanism of action.

### 15.3.3 Treatments That Affect $GABA_B$ Receptors

$GABA_B$ agonists and antagonists have potential in a variety of CNS disorders (for review see References [160, 161]), although the primary current use of agonists (e.g., baclofen) is in the treatment of spasticity in spinal cord injury and other motor disorders.

***15.3.3.1 $GABA_B$ Agonists*** Several animal studies suggest the potential of baclofen in treating sensorimotor processing deficits in schizophrenia [54, 162] Studies in mice indicate that pallidotegmental GABAergic neurons projecting to $GABA_B$ receptors on pedunculo-pontine ventral tegmental neurons modulate sensorimotor gating as measured with PPI [54]. Baclofen attenuated disrupted PPI produced by methamphetamine or by MK-801, suggesting that $GABA_B$ agonism might be therapeutically useful in disorders with sensorimotor gating deficits, including schizophrenia [54].

In a second study [162], baclofen, like the atypical antipsychotic clozapine, improved spontaneous sensorimotor gating deficits seen in DBA/2J mice, and this effect was reversed by the $GABA_B$ antagonist SCH50211. Notably, baclofen did not alter PPI in C57BL/6J mice, a finding possibly related to reported strain differences in $GABA_B$ receptor expression in PFC and hippocampus in DBA/2J versus C57BL/6J mice.

Microdialysis studies in the rat mPFC indicated that $GABA_B$ receptors tonically inhibit pyramidal neurons that project to the VTA [163], where they synapse on mesocorticolimbic DA cell bodies and GABA interneurons. Thus, the $GABA_B$ receptor antagonist CGP35348 but not the $GABA_A$ receptor antagonist bicuculline reversed stimulation of glutamate release in the VTA produced by activation of mPFC pyramidal neurons. This effect was reversed by baclofen. These results suggest a role for the PFC in the regulation of glutamate release in the VTA and a critical modulatory role for cortical $GABA_B$ receptors.

A number of older clinical studies provided mixed results with baclofen in schizophrenia, with both positive [164, 165] and negative [166–168] outcomes reported. Furthermore, based on limited clinical evaluation of baclofen, it has been suggested that GABA agonist drugs may exacerbate psychotic symptoms [111].

Another suggested therapeutic use for $GABA_B$ agonists is in the treatment of tardive dyskinesia in schizophrenia, although a Cochrane review concluded that evidence for utility of baclofen in tardive dyskinesia was "inconclusive and unconvincing" and that "any possible benefits are likely to be outweighed by the adverse effects associated with their use." An earlier Cochrane study [112] reported a tendency for "some degree of improvement," but these were accompanied by "confusion and sedation and a deterioration of the person's mental state."

***15.3.3.2 $GABA_B$ Antagonists*** Studies in animals and in humans have indicated that $GABA_B$ receptor antagonists have cognition-enhancing properties and therefore may be of potential interest for treating cognitive deficits in schizophrenia. Thus, SGS742 demonstrated precognitive effects in a spatial memory task in rats [169] and in several tasks in different strains of mice [170]. Another $GABA_B$ antagonist, SCH50911, increased $\gamma$-oscillatory activity in DBA/2J mice [171]. Positive Phase II clinical trial results for SGS742 were reported in mild cognitive impairment [172, 173] and plans to further test the compound in Alzheimer's disease were reported. Currently, however, no data are available with regard to treating cognitive deficits in schizophrenia.

## 15.4 SUMMARY AND FUTURE DIRECTIONS

There has been a long-standing interest in the potential of GABA pathways in the brain for their potential role in schizophrenia and as a possible target for therapeutic intervention, although interest has been rekindled in the last decade based on converging studies from a variety of disciplines. The demonstration that GABA deficits are reliably detected in certain subsets of cortical GABA interneurons that play an important role in modulating pyramidal neuron activity has been a key stimulus in this reawakening of interest in GABA. In addition, strides made in understanding the potential role of glutamate pathways, and the evidence suggesting important functional interactions with cortical GABA neurons, have once again placed GABA on the radar as a potential key mediator in schizophrenia. Although there is considerable evidence in support of a role for GABA, identifying suitable GABAergic agents that will provide effective, safe, and improved therapies in schizophrenia is in its early stages. The heterogeneous symptom clusters seen in schizophrenia suggest the possibility of multiple impairments at different sites in the complex circuitries that are dysfunctional in this complex disease. However, given the presence of GABA components in those circuits, it is not unreasonable to expect that a fairly discrete impairment in GABAergic function, expressed in multiple pathways, could give rise to a diversity of symptoms. One major challenge will be to identify pharmacological agents that act selectively on pathways uniquely disrupted in schizophrenia, thereby avoiding the undesirable side effects that are associated with agents that nonselectively affect GABA pathways. The $GABA_A$ receptor complex, with its BZD allosteric site and the spectrum of possibilities afforded by a diversity of subtypes, is a particularly promising target for new therapeutic agents. Preliminary efficacy in treating cognitive deficits in schizophrenia has been shown for MK-0777, an allosteric activator at $\alpha 2$-$GABA_A$ receptor subtypes, and preclinical studies suggest a potentially important role of $\alpha 3$-$GABA_A$ receptor activation in the control of hyperdopaminergic states in schizophrenia. The $GABA_B$ receptor also has potential, particularly with regard to treatment of cognitive deficits based on the known therapeutic profiles of $GABA_B$ receptor antagonists. Furthermore, progress is even reported for agents that globally affect GABA transmission, in that their administration as adjunctive agents to established antipsychotics has promise for improving their efficacy or decreasing their side effect profiles. Finally, although the discussion herein has been exclusively focused on schizophrenia, it should be emphasized that GABA deficits may be important in other disorders, such as autism [174], bipolar disorder [175, 176], and depression [177, 178]. Given the ever-growing evidence implicating the importance of GABA in schizophrenia and more broadly, in a range of CNS disorders, and the potential of GABA pathways as a target for novel therapeutic drugs, these are indeed exciting times, although clearly much work remains to be done.

## ACKNOWLEDGMENT

The authors thank Elizabeth Kehne for expert graphics assistance in figure preparation.

## REFERENCES

1. Garbutt, J.C., van Kammen, D.P. (1983). The interaction between GABA and dopamine: implications for schizophrenia. *Schizophrenia Bulletin*, *9*, 336–353.
2. Lisman, J.E., Coyle, J.T., Green, R.W., Javitt, D.C., Benes, F.M., Heckers, S., Grace, A.A. (2008). Circuit-based framework for understanding neurotransmitter and risk gene interactions in schizophrenia. *Trends in Neurosciences*, *31*, 234–242.
3. Lewis, D.A., Moghaddam, B. (2006). Cognitive dysfunction in schizophrenia: convergence of gamma-aminobutyric acid and glutamate alterations. *Archives of Neurology*, *63*, 1372–1376.
4. Huang, Z.J., Di Cristo, G., Ango, F. (2007). Development of GABA innervation in the cerebral and cerebellar cortices. *Nature Reviews. Neuroscience*, *8*, 673–686.
5. Tallman, J.F., Paul, S.M., Skolnick, P., Gallager, D.W. (1980). Receptors for the age of anxiety: pharmacology of the benzodiazepines. *Science*, *207*, 274–281.
6. Mendelson, W.B. (1992). Neuropharmacology of sleep induction by benzodiazepines. *Critical Reviews in Neurobiology*, *6*, 221–232.
7. Rudolph, U., Mohler, H. (2004). Analysis of GABAA receptor function and dissection of the pharmacology of benzodiazepines and general anesthetics through mouse genetics. *Annual Review of Pharmacology and Toxicology*, *44*, 475–498.
8. Haefely, W., Martin, J.R., Schoch, P. (1990). Novel anxiolytics that act as partial agonists at benzodiazepine receptors. *Trends in Pharmacological Sciences*, *11*, 452–456.

9. Costa, E. (1998). From GABAA receptor diversity emerges a unified vision of GABAergic inhibition. *Annual Review of Pharmacology and Toxicology*, *38*, 321–350.
10. Mohler, H. (2006). GABAA receptors in central nervous system disease: anxiety, epilepsy, and insomnia. *Journal of Receptor and Signal Transduction Research*, *26*, 731–740.
11. Whiting, P.J. (2006). GABA-A receptors: a viable target for novel anxiolytics? *Current Opinion in Pharmacology*, *6*, 24–29.
12. Whiting, P.J. (2003). The GABAA receptor gene family: new opportunities for drug development. *Current Opinion in Drug Discovery & Development*, *6*, 648–657.
13. Mohler, H. (2006). GABA(A) receptor diversity and pharmacology. *Cell and Tissue Research*, *326*, 505–516.
14. Mohler, H., Rudolph, U. (2004). Selective GABAA circuits for novel GABAA CNS drugs. *Drug Discovery Today*, *1*, 117–123.
15. Rudolph, U., Mohler, H. (2006). GABA-based therapeutic approaches: GABAA receptor subtype functions. *Current Opinion in Pharmacology*, *6*, 18–23.
16. Atack, J.R. (2005). The benzodiazepine binding site of GABA(A) receptors as a target for the development of novel anxiolytics. *Expert Opinion on Investigational Drugs*, *14*, 601–618.
17. Tallman, J.F., Gallager, D.W. (1985). The GABA-ergic system: a locus of benzodiazepine action. *Annual Review of Neuroscience*, *8*, 21–44.
18. Sanger, D.J. (2004). The pharmacology and mechanisms of action of new generation, non-benzodiazepine hypnotic agents. *CNS Drugs*, *18*(Suppl 1), 9–15, discussion 41, 43–15.
19. Dawson, G.R., Maubach, K.A., Collinson, N., Cobain, M., Everitt, B.J., MacLeod, A.M., Choudhury, H.I., McDonald, L.M., Pillai, G., Rycroft, W., Smith, A.J., Sternfeld, F., Tattersall, F.D., Wafford, K.A., Reynolds, D.S., Seabrook, G.R., Atack, J.R. (2006). An inverse agonist selective for alpha5 subunit-containing GABAA receptors enhances cognition. *The Journal of Pharmacology and Experimental Therapeutics*, *316*, 1335–1345.
20. Maubach, K. (2003). GABA(A) receptor subtype selective cognition enhancers. *Current Drug Targets. CNS and Neurological Disorders*, *2*, 233–239.
21. Evans, A.K., Lowry, C.A. (2007). Pharmacology of the beta-carboline FG-7,142, a partial inverse agonist at the benzodiazepine allosteric site of the GABA A receptor: neurochemical, neurophysiological, and behavioral effects. *CNS Drug Reviews*, *13*, 475–501.
22. Brennan, P.M., Whittle, I.R. (2008). Intrathecal baclofen therapy for neurological disorders: a sound knowledge base but many challenges remain. *British Journal of Neurosurgery*, *22*, 508–519.
23. McClelland, S. 3rd, Bethoux, F.A., Boulis, N.M., Sutliff, M.H., Stough, D.K., Schwetz, K.M., Gogol, D.M., Harrison, M., Pioro, E.P. (2008). Intrathecal baclofen for spasticity-related pain in amyotrophic lateral sclerosis: efficacy and factors associated with pain relief. *Muscle & Nerve*, *37*, 396–398.
24. Blackshaw, L.A. (2008). New insights in the neural regulation of the lower oesophageal sphincter. *European Review for Medical and Pharmacological Sciences*, *12*(Suppl 1), 33–39.

25. Nuechterlein, K.H., Barch, D.M., Gold, J.M., Goldberg, T.E., Green, M.F., Heaton, R.K. (2004). Identification of separable cognitive factors in schizophrenia. *Schizophrenia Research*, *72*, 29–39.

26. Green, M.F. (1996). What are the functional consequences of neurocognitive deficits in schizophrenia? *The American Journal of Psychiatry 153*, 321–330.

27. Green, M.F., Kern, R.S., Heaton, R.K. (2004). Longitudinal studies of cognition and functional outcome in schizophrenia: implications for MATRICS. *Schizophrenia Research 72*, 41–51.

28. Laruelle, M. (1998). Imaging dopamine transmission in schizophrenia. A review and meta-analysis. *The Quarterly Journal of Nuclear Medicine*, *42*, 211–221.

29. Laruelle, M., Abi-Dargham, A. (1999). Dopamine as the wind of the psychotic fire: new evidence from brain imaging studies. *Journal of Psychopharmacology (Oxford, England)*, *13*, 358–371.

30. Laruelle, M., Abi-Dargham, A., Gil, R., Kegeles, L., Innis, R. (1999). Increased dopamine transmission in schizophrenia: relationship to illness phases. *Biological Psychiatry*, *46*, 56–72.

31. Laruelle, M., Abi-Dargham, A., van Dyck, C., Gil, R., D'Souza, D.C., Krystal, J., Seibyl, J., Baldwin, R., Innis, R. (2000). Dopamine and serotonin transporters in patients with schizophrenia: an imaging study with [(123)I]beta-CIT. *Biological Psychiatry*, *47*, 371–379.

32. Laruelle, M., Abi-Dargham, A., van Dyck, C.H., Gil, R., D'Souza, C.D., Erdos, J., McCance, E., Rosenblatt, W., Fingado, C., Zoghbi, S.S., Baldwin, R.M., Seibyl, J.P., Krystal, J.H., Charney, D.S., Innis, R.B. (1996). Single photon emission computerized tomography imaging of amphetamine-induced dopamine release in drug-free schizophrenic subjects. *Proceedings of the National Academy of Sciences of the United States of America*, *93*, 9235–9240.

33. Doran, A.R., Boronow, J., Weinberger, D.R., Wolkowitz, O.M., Breier, A., Pickar, D. (1987). Structural brain pathology in schizophrenia revisited. Prefrontal cortex pathology is inversely correlated with cerebrospinal fluid levels of homovanillic acid. *Neuropsychopharmacology*, *1*, 25–32.

34. Guillin, O., Abi-Dargham, A., Laruelle, M. (2007). Neurobiology of dopamine in schizophrenia. *International Review of Neurobiology*, *78*, 1–39.

35. Seeman, P. (2002). Targeting the dopamine D2 receptor in schizophrenia. *Expert Opinion on Therapeutic Targets*, *10*, 515–531.

36. Meltzer, H.Y., Matsubara, S., Lee, J.C. (1989). The ratios of serotonin2 and dopamine2 affinities differentiate atypical and typical antipsychotic drugs. *Psychopharmacology Bulletin*, *25*, 390–392.

37. Schlagenhauf, F., Juckel, G., Koslowski, M., Kahnt, T., Knutson, B., Dembler, T., Kienast, T., Gallinat, J., Wrase, J., Heinz, A. (2008). Reward system activation in schizophrenic patients switched from typical neuroleptics to olanzapine. *Psychopharmacology*, *196*, 673–684.

38. Green, M.F. (2007). Stimulating the development of drug treatments to improve cognition in schizophrenia. *Annual Review of Clinical Psychology*, *3*, 159–180.

39. Breier, A. (1999). Cognitive deficit in schizophrenia and its neurochemical basis. *The British Journal of Psychiatry. Supplement*, *37*, 16–18.

40. Lieberman, J.A. (2007). Effectiveness of antipsychotic drugs in patients with chronic schizophrenia: efficacy, safety and cost outcomes of CATIE and other trials. *The Journal of Clinical Psychiatry*, *68*, e04.
41. Meyer, J.M. (2007). Antipsychotic safety and efficacy concerns. *The Journal of Clinical Psychiatry*, *68*(Suppl 14), 20–26.
42. Kerns, J.G., Nuechterlein, K.H., Braver, T.S., Barch, D.M. (2008). Executive functioning component mechanisms and schizophrenia. *Biological Psychiatry*, *64*, 26–33.
43. Dickinson, D., Harvey, P.D. (2009). Systemic hypotheses for generalized cognitive deficits in schizophrenia: a new take on an old problem. *Schizophrenia Bulletin*, *35*, 403–414.
44. Buchanan, R.W., Freedman, R., Javitt, D.C., Abi-Dargham, A., Lieberman, J.A. (2007). Recent advances in the development of novel pharmacological agents for the treatment of cognitive impairments in schizophrenia. *Schizophrenia Bulletin*, *33*, 1120–1130.
45. Meltzer, H.Y. (1997). Treatment-resistant schizophrenia—the role of clozapine. *Current Medical Research and Opinion*, *14*, 1–20.
46. Keefe, R.S., Bilder, R.M., Davis, S.M., Harvey, P.D., Palmer, B.W., Gold, J.M., Meltzer, H.Y., Green, M.F., Capuano, G., Stroup, T.S., McEvoy, J.P., Swartz, M.S., Rosenheck, R.A., Perkins, D.O., Davis, C.E., Hsiao, J.K. Lieberman, J.A. (2007). Neurocognitive effects of antipsychotic medications in patients with chronic schizophrenia in the CATIE Trial. *Archives of General Psychiatry*, *64*, 633–647.
47. Kapur, S., Seeman, P. (2001). Does fast dissociation from the dopamine d(2) receptor explain the action of atypical antipsychotics?: a new hypothesis. *The American Journal of Psychiatry*, *158*, 360–369.
48. Dickson, R.A., Glazer, W.M. (1999). Neuroleptic-induced hyperprolactinemia. *Schizophrenia Research*, *35*(Suppl), S75–S86.
49. Henderson, D.C. (2007). Weight gain with atypical antipsychotics: evidence and insights. *The Journal of Clinical Psychiatry*, *68*(Suppl 12), 18–26.
50. Nasrallah, H.A. (2008). Atypical antipsychotic-induced metabolic side effects: insights from receptor-binding profiles. *Molecular Psychiatry*, *13*, 27–35.
51. Meyer, J.M., Davis, V.G., Goff, D.C., McEvoy, J.P., Nasrallah, H.A., Davis, S.M., Rosenheck, R.A., Daumit, G.L., Hsiao, J., Swartz, M.S., Stroup, T.S., Lieberman, J.A. (2008). Change in metabolic syndrome parameters with antipsychotic treatment in the CATIE Schizophrenia Trial: prospective data from phase 1. *Schizophrenia Research*, *101*(1–3), 273–286.
52. Homayoun, H., Moghaddam, B. (2007). NMDA receptor hypofunction produces opposite effects on prefrontal cortex interneurons and pyramidal neurons. *The Journal of Neuroscience*, *27*, 11496–11500.
53. Arnaiz-Cot, J.J., Gonzalez, J.C., Sobrado, M., Baldelli, P., Carbone, E., Gandia, L., Garcia, A.G., Hernandez-Guijo, J.M. (2008). Allosteric modulation of alpha 7 nicotinic receptors selectively depolarizes hippocampal interneurons, enhancing spontaneous GABAergic transmission. *The European Journal of Neuroscience*, *27*, 1097–1110.
54. Arai, S., Takuma, K., Mizoguchi, H., Ibi, D., Nagai, T., Takahashi, K., Kamei, H., Nabeshima, T., Yamada, K. (2008). Involvement of pallidotegmental neurons in

methamphetamine- and MK-801-induced impairment of prepulse inhibition of the acoustic startle reflex in mice: reversal by GABA(B) receptor agonist baclofen. *Neuropsychopharmacology*, *33*(13), 3164–3175.

55. Waldvogel, H.J., Baer, K., Gai, W.P., Gilbert, R.T., Rees, M.I., Mohler, H., Faull, R.L. (2008). Differential localization of GABA(A) receptor subunits within the substantia nigra of the human brain: an immunohistochemical study. *The Journal of Comparative Neurology*, *506*, 912–929.
56. Shank, E.J., Seitz, P.K., Bubar, M.J., Stutz, S.J., Cunningham, K.A. (2007). Selective ablation of GABA neurons in the ventral tegmental area increases spontaneous locomotor activity. *Behavioral Neuroscience*, *121*, 1224–1233.
57. Cunningham, M.G., Bhattacharyya, S., Benes, F.M. (2008). Increasing interaction of amygdalar afferents with GABAergic interneurons between birth and adulthood. *Cerebral Cortex*, *18*, 1529–1535.
58. Zikopoulos, B., Barbas, H. (2007). Parallel driving and modulatory pathways link the prefrontal cortex and thalamus. *PLoS ONE*, *2*, e848.
59. Ferraro, L., Tomasini, M.C., Fuxe, K., Agnati, L.F., Mazza, R., Tanganelli, S., Antonelli, T. (2007). Mesolimbic dopamine and cortico-accumbens glutamate afferents as major targets for the regulation of the ventral striato-pallidal GABA pathways by neurotensin peptides. *Brain Research Reviews*, *55*, 144–154.
60. Lewis, D.A., Mirnics, K. (2006). Transcriptome alterations in schizophrenia: disturbing the functional architecture of the dorsolateral prefrontal cortex. *Progress in Brain Research*, *158*, 141–152.
61. Lewis, D.A., Gonzalez-Burgos, G. (2008). Neuroplasticity of neocortical circuits in schizophrenia. *Neuropsychopharmacology*, *33*, 141–165.
62. Lewis, D.A., Hashimoto, T. (2007). Deciphering the disease process of schizophrenia: the contribution of cortical GABA neurons. *International Review of Neurobiology*, *78*, 109–131.
63. Lewis, D.A., Gonzalez-Burgos, G. (2006). Pathophysiologically based treatment interventions in schizophrenia. *Nature Medicine*, *12*, 1016–1022.
64. Sakai, T., Oshima, A., Nozaki, Y., Ida, I., Haga, C., Akiyama, H., Nakazato, Y., Mikuni, M. (2008). Changes in density of calcium-binding-protein-immunoreactive GABAergic neurons in prefrontal cortex in schizophrenia and bipolar disorder. *Neuropathology*, *28*, 143–150.
65. Tanaka, S. (2008). Dysfunctional GABAergic inhibition in the prefrontal cortex leading to "psychotic" hyperactivation. *BMC Neuroscience*, *9*, 41.
66. Barbas, H., Zikopoulos, B. (2007). The prefrontal cortex and flexible behavior. *The Neuroscientist*, *13*, 532–545.
67. Watanabe, M., Sakagami, M. (2007). Integration of cognitive and motivational context information in the primate prefrontal cortex. *Cerebral Cortex*, *17*(Suppl 1), i101–i109.
68. Sakagami, M., Watanabe, M. (2007). Integration of cognitive and motivational information in the primate lateral prefrontal cortex. *Annals of the New York Academy of Sciences*, *1104*, 89–107.
69. Benes, F.M. (2007). Searching for unique endophenotypes for schizophrenia and bipolar disorder within neural circuits and their molecular regulatory mechanisms. *Schizophrenia Bulletin*, *33*, 932–936.

70. Benes, F.M., Lim, B., Matzilevich, D., Walsh, J.P., Subburaju, S., Minns, M. (2007). Regulation of the GABA cell phenotype in hippocampus of schizophrenics and bipolars. *Proceedings of the National Academy of Sciences of the United States of America*, *104*, 10164–10169.

71. Benes, F.M., Gisabella, B. (2006). Rat modeling for GABA defects in schizophrenia. *Advances in Pharmacology (San Diego, Calif.)*, *54*, 73–93.

72. Hashimoto, T., Bazmi, H.H., Mirnics, K., Wu, Q., Sampson, A.R., Lewis, D.A. (2008). Conserved regional patterns of GABA-related transcript expression in the neocortex of subjects with schizophrenia. *The American Journal of Psychiatry*, *165*, 479–489.

73. Woo, T.U., Shrestha, K., Lamb, D., Minns, M.M., Benes, F.M. (2008). N-Methyl-D-Aspartate receptor and calbindin-containing neurons in the anterior cingulate cortex in schizophrenia and bipolar disorder. *Biological Psychiatry*, *64*(9), 803–809.

74. Daskalakis, Z.J., Christensen, B.K., Chen, R., Fitzgerald, P.B., Zipursky, R.B., Kapur, S. (2002). Evidence for impaired cortical inhibition in schizophrenia using transcranial magnetic stimulation. *Archives of General Psychiatry*, *59*, 347–354.

75. Daskalakis, Z.J., Fitzgerald, P.B., Christensen, B.K. (2007). The role of cortical inhibition in the pathophysiology and treatment of schizophrenia. *Brain Research Reviews*, *56*(2), 427–442.

76. Ford, J.M., Krystal, J.H., Mathalon, D.H. (2007). Neural synchrony in schizophrenia: from networks to new treatments. *Schizophrenia Bulletin*, *33*, 848–852.

77. Ford, J.M., Mathalon, D.H. (2008). Neural synchrony in schizophrenia. *Schizophrenia Bulletin*, *34*, 904–906.

78. Gonzalez-Burgos, G., Lewis, D.A. (2008). GABA neurons and the mechanisms of network oscillations: implications for understanding cortical dysfunction in schizophrenia. *Schizophrenia Bulletin*, *34*, 944–961.

79. Rolls, E.T., Loh, M., Deco, G., Winterer, G. (2008). Computational models of schizophrenia and dopamine modulation in the prefrontal cortex. *Nature Reviews. Neuroscience*, *9*, 696–709.

80. Santana, N., Mengod, G., Artigas, F. (2008). Quantitative analysis of the expression of dopamine D1 and D2 receptors in pyramidal and GABAergic neurons of the rat prefrontal cortex. *Cerebral Cortex*, *19*(4), 849–860.

81. Loh, M., Rolls, E.T., Deco, G. (2007). A dynamical systems hypothesis of schizophrenia. *PLoS Computational Biology*, *3*, e228.

82. Straub, R.E., Lipska, B.K., Egan, M.F., Goldberg, T.E., Callicott, J.H., Mayhew, M.B., Vakkalanka, R.K., Kolachana, B.S., Kleinman, J.E., Weinberger, D.R. (2007). Allelic variation in GAD1 (GAD67) is associated with schizophrenia and influences cortical function and gene expression. *Molecular Psychiatry*, *12*, 854–869.

83. Costa, E., Dong, E., Grayson, D.R., Guidotti, A., Ruzicka, W., Veldic, M. (2007). Reviewing the role of DNA (cytosine-5) methyltransferase overexpression in the cortical GABAergic dysfunction associated with psychosis vulnerability. *Epigenetics*, *2*, 29–36.

84. Costa, E., Davis, J.M., Dong, E., Grayson, D.R., Guidotti, A., Tremolizzo, L., Veldic, M. (2004). A GABAergic cortical deficit dominates schizophrenia pathophysiology. *Critical Reviews in Neurobiology*, *16*, 1–23.

85. Moore, H., Jentsch, J.D., Ghajarnia, M., Geyer, M.A., Grace, A.A. (2006). A neurobehavioral systems analysis of adult rats exposed to methylazoxymethanol

acetate on E17: implications for the neuropathology of schizophrenia. *Biological Psychiatry*, *60*, 253–264.

86. Snigdha, S., Neill, J.C. (2008). Efficacy of antipsychotics to reverse phencyclidine-induced social interaction deficits in female rats—a preliminary investigation. *Behavioural Brain Research*, *187*, 489–494.
87. Grayson, B., Idris, N.F., Neill, J.C. (2007). Atypical antipsychotics attenuate a sub-chronic PCP-induced cognitive deficit in the novel object recognition task in the rat. *Behavioural Brain Research*, *184*, 31–38.
88. Abdul-Monim, Z., Reynolds, G.P., Neill, J.C. (2006). The effect of atypical and classical antipsychotics on sub-chronic PCP-induced cognitive deficits in a reversal-learning paradigm. *Behavioural Brain Research*, *169*, 263–273.
89. Wynn, J.K., Green, M.F., Sprock, J., Light, G.A., Widmark, C., Reist, C., Erhart, S., Marder, S.R., Mintz, J., Braff, D.L. (2007). Effects of olanzapine, risperidone and haloperidol on prepulse inhibition in schizophrenia patients: a double-blind, randomized controlled trial. *Schizophrenia Research*, *95*, 134–142.
90. Casey, D.E. (2000). Tardive dyskinesia: pathophysiology and animal models. *The Journal of Clinical Psychiatry*, *61*(Suppl 4), 5–9.
91. Robbins, T.W., Roberts, A.C. (2007). Differential regulation of fronto-executive function by the monoamines and acetylcholine. *Cerebral Cortex*, *17*(Suppl 1), i151–i160.
92. Robbins, T.W. (2007). Shifting and stopping: fronto-striatal substrates, neurochemical modulation and clinical implications. *Philosophical Transactions of the Royal Society of London. Series B, Biological Sciences*, *362*, 917–932.
93. Pietersen, C.Y., Bosker, F.J., Doorduin, J., Jongsma, M.E., Postema, F., Haas, J.V., Johnson, M.P., Koch, T., Vladusich, T., den Boer, J.A. (2007). An animal model of emotional blunting in schizophrenia. *PLoS ONE*, *2*, e1360.
94. Harte, M.K., Powell, S.B., Swerdlow, N.R., Geyer, M.A., Reynolds, G.P. (2007). Deficits in parvalbumin and calbindin immunoreactive cells in the hippocampus of isolation reared rats. *Journal of Neural Transmission*, *114*, 893–898.
95. Trantham-Davidson, H., Kroner, S., Seamans, J.K. (2008). Dopamine modulation of prefrontal cortex interneurons occurs independently of DARPP-32. *Cerebral Cortex*, *18*, 951–958.
96. Pillai, A., Mahadik, S.P. (2008). Increased truncated TrkB receptor expression and decreased BDNF/TrkB signaling in the frontal cortex of reeler mouse model of schizophrenia. *Schizophrenia Research*, *100*, 325–333.
97. Behrens, M.M., Ali, S.S., Dao, D.N., Lucero, J., Shekhtman, G., Quick, K.L., Dugan, L.L. (2007). Ketamine-induced loss of phenotype of fast-spiking interneurons is mediated by NADPH-oxidase. *Science*, *318*, 1645–1647.
98. Braun, I., Genius, J., Grunze, H., Bender, A., Moller, H.J., Rujescu, D. (2007). Alterations of hippocampal and prefrontal GABAergic interneurons in an animal model of psychosis induced by NMDA receptor antagonism. *Schizophrenia Research*, *97*, 254–263.
99. Pratt, J.A., Winchester, C., Egerton, A., Cochran, S.M., Morris, B.J. (2008). Modelling prefrontal cortex deficits in schizophrenia: implications for treatment. *British Journal of Pharmacology*, *153*(Suppl 1), S465–S470.
100. Bloomfield, C., French, S.J., Jones, D.N., Reavill, C., Southam, E., Cilia, J., Totterdell, S. (2008). Chandelier cartridges in the prefrontal cortex are reduced in isolation reared rats. *Synapse (New York, N.Y.)*, *62*, 628–631.

101. Brummelte, S., Neddens, J., Teuchert-Noodt, G. (2007). Alteration in the GABAergic network of the prefrontal cortex in a potential animal model of psychosis. *Journal of Neural Transmission*, *114*, 539–547.
102. Lodge, D.J., Grace, A.A. (2007). Aberrant hippocampal activity underlies the dopamine dysregulation in an animal model of schizophrenia. *The Journal of Neuroscience*, *27*, 11424–11430.
103. Lodge, D., Behrens, M., Grace, A. (2008). A loss of parvalbumin containing interneurons is associated with diminished gamma oscillatory activity in an animal model of schizophrenia. *Schizophrenia Research*, *102*, 112.
104. Sakae, N., Yamasaki, N., Kitaichi, K., Fukuda, T., Yamada, M., Yoshikawa, H., Hiranita, T., Tatsumi, Y., Kira, J.I., Yamamoto, T., Miyakawa, T. Nakayama, K.I. (2008). Mice lacking the schizophrenia-associated protein FEZ1 manifest hyperactivity and enhanced responsiveness to psychostimulants. *Human Molecular Genetics*, *17*(20), 3191–3203.
105. Kodsi, M.H., Swerdlow, N.R. (1995). Ventral pallidal GABA-A receptors regulate prepulse inhibition of acoustic startle. *Brain Research*, *684*, 26–35.
106. Qu, Y., Swerdlow, N.R., Weber, M., Stouffer, D., Parsons, L.H. (2008). Quinelorane, a dopamine D3/D2 receptor agonist, reduces prepulse inhibition of startle and ventral pallidal GABA efflux: time course studies. *Pharmacology, Biochemistry, and Behavior*, *90*(4), 686–690.
107. Frankle, W.G., Cho, R.Y., Narendran, R., Mason, N.S., Vora, S., Litschge, M., Price, J.C., Lewis, D.A., Mathis, C.A. (2008). Tiagabine increases [(11)C]flumazenil binding in cortical brain regions in healthy control subjects. *Neuropsychopharmacology*, *34*(3), 624–633.
108. Geffen, Y., Nudelman, A., Gil-Ad, I., Rephaeli, A., Huang, M., Savitsky, K., Klapper, L., Winkler, I., Meltzer, H.Y., Weizman, A. (2008). BL-1020: a novel antipsychotic drug with GABAergic activity and low catalepsy, is efficacious in a rat model of schizophrenia. *European Neuropsychopharmacology*, *19*(1), 1–13.
109. Nudelman, A., Gil-Ad, I., Shpaisman, N., Terasenko, I., Ron, H., Savitsky, K., Geffen, Y., Weizman, A., Rephaeli, A. (2008). A mutual prodrug ester of GABA and perphenazine exhibits antischizophrenic efficacy with diminished extrapyramidal effects. *Journal of Medicinal Chemistry*, *51*, 2858–2862.
110. Thaker, G.K., Tamminga, C.A., Alphs, L.D., Lafferman, J., Ferraro, T.N., Hare, T.A. (1987). Brain gamma-aminobutyric acid abnormality in tardive dyskinesia. Reduction in cerebrospinal fluid GABA levels and therapeutic response to GABA agonist treatment. *Archives of General Psychiatry*, *44*, 522–529.
111. Soares, K., Rathbone, J., Deeks, J. (2004). Gamma-aminobutyric acid agonists for neuroleptic-induced tardive dyskinesia. *Cochrane Database of Systematic Reviews*, (4), CD000203.
112. Soares, K.V., McGrath, J.J., Deeks, J.J. (2000). Gamma-aminobutyric acid agonists for neuroleptic-induced tardive dyskinesia. *Cochrane Database of Systematic Reviews*, (2), CD000203.
113. Gillies, D., Beck, A., McCloud, A., Rathbone, J., Gillies, D. (2005). Benzodiazepines alone or in combination with antipsychotic drugs for acute psychosis. *Cochrane Database of Systematic Reviews*, (4), CD003079.
114. Volz, A., Khorsand, V., Gillies, D., Leucht, S. (2007). Benzodiazepines for schizophrenia. *Cochrane Database of Systematic Reviews*, (1), CD006391.

115. Tarsy, D. (2000). Tardive dyskinesia. *Current Treatment Options in Neurology*, *2*, 205–214.
116. Marsalek, M. (2000). Tardive drug-induced extrapyramidal syndromes. *Pharmacopsychiatry*, *33*(Suppl 1), 14–33.
117. Thaker, G.K., Nguyen, J.A., Strauss, M.E., Jacobson, R., Kaup, B.A., Tamminga, C.A. (1990). Clonazepam treatment of tardive dyskinesia: a practical GABAmimetic strategy. *The American Journal of Psychiatry*, *147*, 445–451.
118. Bhoopathi, P.S., Soares-Weiser, K. (2006). Benzodiazepines for neuroleptic-induced tardive dyskinesia. *Cochrane Database of Systematic Reviews*, (3), CD000205.
119. Loscher, W., Schmidt, D. (2006). Experimental and clinical evidence for loss of effect (tolerance) during prolonged treatment with antiepileptic drugs. *Epilepsia*, *47*, 1253–1284.
120. Mintzer, M.Z., Frey, J.M., Griffiths, R.R. (1998). Zolpidem is differentiated from triazolam in humans using a three-response drug discrimination procedure. *Behavioural Pharmacology*, *9*, 545–559.
121. Mintzer, M.Z., Frey, J.M., Yingling, J.E., Griffiths, R.R. (1997). Triazolam and zolpidem: a comparison of their psychomotor, cognitive, and subjective effects in healthy volunteers. *Behavioural Pharmacology*, *8*, 561–574.
122. Mintzer, M.Z., Griffiths, R.R. (1999). Triazolam and zolpidem: effects on human memory and attentional processes. *Psychopharmacology*, *144*, 8–19.
123. Mintzer, M.Z., Griffiths, R.R. (1999). Selective effects of zolpidem on human memory functions. *Journal of Psychopharmacology (Oxford, England)*, *13*, 18–31.
124. Mintzer, M.Z., Griffiths, R.R., Contoreggi, C., Kimes, A.S., London, E.D., Ernst, M. (2001). Effects of triazolam on brain activity during episodic memory encoding: a PET study. *Neuropsychopharmacology*, *25*, 744–756.
125. Mintzer, M.Z., Kuwabara, H., Alexander, M., Brasic, J.R., Ye, W., Ernst, M., Griffiths, R.R., Wong, D.F. (2006). Dose effects of triazolam on brain activity during episodic memory encoding: a PET study. *Psychopharmacology*, *188*(4), 445–461.
126. Menzies, L., Ooi, C., Kamath, S., Suckling, J., McKenna, P., Fletcher, P., Bullmore, E., Stephenson, C. (2007). Effects of gamma-aminobutyric acid-modulating drugs on working memory and brain function in patients with schizophrenia. *Archives of General Psychiatry*, *64*, 156–167.
127. Braga, R.J., Petrides, G., Figueira, I. (2004). Anxiety disorders in schizophrenia. *Comprehensive Psychiatry*, *45*, 460–468.
128. Muller, J.E., Koen, L., Soraya, S., Emsley, R.A., Stein, D.J. (2004). Anxiety disorders and schizophrenia. *Current Psychiatry Reports*, *6*, 255–261.
129. Davis, M. (2006). Neural systems involved in fear and anxiety measured with fear-potentiated startle. *The American Psychologist*, *61*, 741–756.
130. Davis, M., Myers, K.M., Chhatwal, J., Ressler, K.J. (2007). Pharmacological treatments that facilitate extinction of fear: relevance to psychotherapy. *NeuroRx*, *3*, 82–96.
131. Heldt, S.A., Ressler, K.J. (2007). Training-induced changes in the expression of GABAA-associated genes in the amygdala after the acquisition and extinction of Pavlovian fear. *The European Journal of Neuroscience*, *26*, 3631–3644.

132. Atack, J.R. (2003). Anxioselective compounds acting at the GABA(A) receptor benzodiazepine binding site. *Current Drug Targets. CNS and Neurological Disorders*, *2*, 213–232.

133. Seethalakshmi, R., Dhavale, S., Suggu, K., Dewan, M. (2008). Catatonic syndrome: importance of detection and treatment with lorazepam. *Annals of Clinical Psychiatry*, *20*, 5–8.

134. Weder, N.D., Muralee, S., Penland, H., Tampi, R.R. (2008). Catatonia: a review. *Annals of Clinical Psychiatry*, *20*, 97–107.

135. Carroll, B.T., Goforth, H.W., Thomas, C., Ahuja, N., McDaniel, W.W., Kraus, M.F., Spiegel, D.R., Franco, K.N., Pozuelo, L., Munoz, C. (2007). Review of adjunctive glutamate antagonist therapy in the treatment of catatonic syndromes. *The Journal of Neuropsychiatry and Clinical Neurosciences*, *19*, 406–412.

136. Delini-Stula, A., Berdah-Tordjman, D. (1996). Antipsychotic effects of bretazenil, a partial benzodiazepine agonist in acute schizophrenia—a study group report. *Journal of Psychiatric Research*, *30*, 239–250.

137. Volk, D.W., Lewis, D.A. (2002). Impaired prefrontal inhibition in schizophrenia: relevance for cognitive dysfunction. *Physiology & Behavior*, *77*, 501–505.

138. Lewis, D.A., Cho, R.Y., Carter, C.S., Eklund, K., Forster, S., Kelly, M.A., Montrose, D. (2008). Subunit-selective modulation of GABA type a receptor neurotransmission and cognition in schizophrenia. *The American Journal of Psychiatry*, *165*, 1585–1593.

139. Fritschy, J.M., Mohler, H. (1995). GABAA-receptor heterogeneity in the adult rat brain: differential regional and cellular distribution of seven major subunits. *The Journal of Comparative Neurology*, *359*, 154–194.

140. Yee, B.K., Keist, R., von Boehmer, L., Studer, R., Benke, D., Hagenbuch, N., Dong, Y., Malenka, R.C., Fritschy, J.M., Bluethmann, H., et al. (2005). A schizophrenia-related sensorimotor deficit links alpha 3-containing GABAA receptors to a dopamine hyperfunction. *Proceedings of the National Academy of Sciences of the United States of America*, *102*, 17154–17159.

141. Yee, B.K., Hauser, J., Dolgov, V.V., Keist, R., Mohler, H., Rudolph, U., Feldon, J. (2004). GABA receptors containing the alpha5 subunit mediate the trace effect in aversive and appetitive conditioning and extinction of conditioned fear. *The European Journal of Neuroscience*, *20*, 1928–1936.

142. Langen, B., Egerland, U., Bernoster, K., Dost, R., Unverferth, K., Rundfeldt, C. (2005). Characterization in rats of the anxiolytic potential of ELB139 [1-(4-chlorophenyl)-4-piperidin-1-yl-1,5-dihydro-imidazol-2-on], a new agonist at the benzodiazepine binding site of the GABAA receptor. *The Journal of Pharmacology and Experimental Therapeutics*, *314*, 717–724.

143. Langen, B. (2005). Antipsychotic and antidepressive activity of the alpha-3 subunit selective benzodiazepine agonist ELB139 in rats. *Abstracts of the 11th Biennial EBPS Meeting* 11, S47.

144. Langen, B., Rundfeldt, C. (2007). ELB139 an agonist at the benzodiazepine binding site increases 5-HT in the striatum and prefrontal cortex of rats: a microdialysis study. *Pharmacology, Biochemistry, and Behavior*, *86*, 79–85.

145. Rabe, H., Kronbach, C., Rundfeldt, C., Luddens, H. (2007). The novel anxiolytic ELB139 displays selectivity to recombinant GABA(A) receptors different from diazepam. *Neuropharmacology*, *52*, 796–801.

146. Grunwald, C., Rundfeldt, C., Lankau, H.J., Arnold, T., Hofgen, N., Dost, R., Egerland, U., Hofmann, H.J., Unverferth, K. (2006). Synthesis, pharmacology, and structure-activity relationships of novel imidazolones and pyrrolones as modulators of GABAA receptors. *Journal of Medicinal Chemistry*, *49*, 1855–1866.

147. Dias, R., Sheppard, W.F., Fradley, R.L., Garrett, E.M., Stanley, J.L., Tye, S.J., Goodacre, S., Lincoln, R.J., Cook, S.M., Conley, R., Conley, R. Hallett, D., Humphries, A.C., Thompson, S.A., Wafford, K.A., Street, L.J., Castro, J.L., Whiting, P.J., Rosahl, T.W., Atack, J.R., McKernan, R.M., Dawson, G.R., Reynolds, D.S. (2005). Evidence for a significant role of alpha 3-containing GABAA receptors in mediating the anxiolytic effects of benzodiazepines. *The Journal of Neuroscience*, *25*, 10682–10688.

148. Krause, J.E., Matchett, M., Crandall, M., Yu, J., Baltazar, C., Brodbeck, R.M., Kehne, J.H., Maynard, G.D., Shaw, K.R., Chenard, B.L., Hutchison, A.J., Xie, L., Yu, W. (2007). I. Preclinical characterization in vitro of NG2-73 as a potent and selective partial allosteric activator at the benzodiazepine site of GABAA receptors with predominant efficacy at the $\alpha 3$ subunit, in *Society for Neuroscience Annual Meeting* (San Diego, CA).

149. Rajachandran, L., McCloskey, T.C., Chock, M., Gambini-Elwood, D., Xie, L., Kehne, J.H. (2007). III. Preclinical characterization in vivo of NG2-73, an alpha3-subunit preferring GABAA receptor partial allosteric activator, as a sedative-hypnotic agent with an improved side effect profile relative to zolpidem, in *Society for Neuroscience Abstract* (San Diego, CA).

150. Rowlett, J.K., Bano, K.M., Sprenger, K., Liu, Y., Kehne, J.H. (2008). Anxiolytic-like effects of NG2-83, a novel compound with selectivity for alpha3 subunit-containing GABA(A) receptors, in a monkey conflict model, in *American Psychiatric Association Annual Meeting* (Washington, D.C.).

151. Collinson, N., Kuenzi, F.M., Jarolimek, W., Maubach, K.A., Cothliff, R., Sur, C., Smith, A., Otu, F.M., Howell, O., Atack, J.R., McKernan, R.M., Seabrook, G.R., Dawson, G.R., Whiting, P.J., Rosahl, T.W. (2002). Enhanced learning and memory and altered GABAergic synaptic transmission in mice lacking the alpha 5 subunit of the GABAA receptor. *The Journal of Neuroscience*, *22*, 5572–5580.

152. Collinson, N., Atack, J.R., Laughton, P., Dawson, G.R., Stephens, D.N. (2006). An inverse agonist selective for alpha5 subunit-containing GABA(A) receptors improves encoding and recall but not consolidation in the Morris water maze. *Psychopharmacology*, *188*(4), 619–628.

153. Atack, J.R., Bayley, P.J., Seabrook, G.R., Wafford, K.A., McKernan, R.M., Dawson, G.R. (2006). L-655,708 enhances cognition in rats but is not proconvulsant at a dose selective for alpha5-containing GABAA receptors. *Neuropharmacology*, *51*, 1023–1029.

154. Glykys, J., Mody, I. (2007). Activation of GABAA receptors: views from outside the synaptic cleft. *Neuron*, *56*, 763–770.

155. Nutt, D.J., Besson, M., Wilson, S.J., Dawson, G.R., Lingford-Hughes, A.R. (2007). Blockade of alcohol's amnestic activity in humans by an alpha5 subtype benzodiazepine receptor inverse agonist. *Neuropharmacology*, *53*, 810–820.

156. Atack, J.R. (2008). GABA(A) receptor subtype-selective efficacy: TPA023, an alpha2/alpha3 selective non-sedating anxiolytic and alpha5IA, an alpha5 selective cognition enhancer. *CNS Neuroscience & Therapeutics*, *14*, 25–35.

157. Belzung, C., Le Guisquet, A.M., Crestani, F. (2000). Flumazenil induces benzodiazepine partial agonist-like effects in BALB/c but not C57BL/6 mice. *Psychopharmacology*, *148*, 24–32.

158. Adachi, Y.U., Watanabe, K., Higuchi, H., Satoh, T. (2002). Flumazenil reduces the hypnotic dose of propofol in male patients under spinal anesthesia. *Journal of Anesthesia*, *16*, 9–12.

159. Asai, Y., Takano, A., Ito, H., Okubo, Y., Matsuura, M., Otsuka, A., Takahashi, H., Ando, T., Ito, S., Arakawa, R., Asai, K., Suhara, T. (2008). GABAA/Benzodiazepine receptor binding in patients with schizophrenia using [11C]Ro15-4513, a radioligand with relatively high affinity for alpha5 subunit. *Schizophrenia Research*, *99*, 333–340.

160. Bowery, N.G. (2006). GABAB receptor: a site of therapeutic benefit. *Current Opinion in Pharmacology*, *6*, 37–43.

161. Marshall, F.H. (2005). Is the GABA B heterodimer a good drug target? *Journal of Molecular Neuroscience: MN*, *26*, 169–176.

162. Bortolato, M., Frau, R., Orru, M., Piras, A.P., Fa, M., Tuveri, A., Puligheddu, M., Gessa, G.L., Castelli, M.P., Mereu, G., Marrosu, F. (2007). Activation of GABA(B) receptors reverses spontaneous gating deficits in juvenile DBA/2J mice. *Psychopharmacology*, *194*, 361–369.

163. Harte, M., O'Connor, W.T. (2005). Evidence for a selective prefrontal cortical GABA(B) receptor-mediated inhibition of glutamate release in the ventral tegmental area: a dual probe microdialysis study in the awake rat. *Neuroscience*, *130*, 215–222.

164. Kuhn, R. (1976). [Neuroleptic effect of baclofen in chronic schizophrenia (author's transl)]. *Arzneimittel-Forschung*, *26*, 1187.

165. Gulmann, N.C., Bahr, B., Andersen, B., Eliassen, H.M. (1976). A double-blind trial of baclofen against placebo in the treatment of schizophrenia. *Acta Psychiatrica Scandinavica*, *54*, 287–293.

166. Beckmann, H., Frische, M., Ruther, E., Zimmer, R. (1977). Baclofen (parachlorphenyl-GABA) in schizophrenia. *Pharmakopsychiatrie, Neuro-Psychopharmakologie*, *10*, 26–31.

167. Wolf, M.E., Keener, S., Mathis, P., Mosnaim, A.D. (1983). Phenylethylamine-like properties of baclofen. *Neuropsychobiology*, *9*, 219–222.

168. Schopf, J., Hucker, H. (1977). Baclofen in the treatment of schizophrenia: a pilot study. *Pharmakopsychiatrie, Neuro-Psychopharmakologie*, *10*, 89–91.

169. Helm, K.A., Haberman, R.P., Dean, S.L., Hoyt, E.C., Melcher, T., Lund, P.K., Gallagher, M. (2005). GABAB receptor antagonist SGS742 improves spatial memory and reduces protein binding to the cAMP response element (CRE) in the hippocampus. *Neuropharmacology*, *48*, 956–964.

170. Sunyer, B., Patil, S., Frischer, C., Hoger, H., Selcher, J., Brannath, W., Lubec, G. (2007). Strain-dependent effects of SGS742 in the mouse. *Behavioural Brain Research*, *181*, 64–75.

171. Marrosu, F., Santoni, F., Fa, M., Puligheddu, M., Barberini, L., Genugu, F., Frau, R., Manunta, M., Mereu, G. (2006). Beta and gamma range EEG power-spectrum correlation with spiking discharges in DBA/2J mice absence model: role of GABA receptors. *Epilepsia*, *47*, 489–494.

172. Bullock, R. (2005). SGS-742 Novartis. *Current Opinion in Investigational Drugs*, *6*, 108–113.

173. Froestl, W., Gallagher, M., Jenkins, H., Madrid, A., Melcher, T., Teichman, S., Mondadori, C.G., Pearlman, R. (2004). SGS742: the first GABA(B) receptor antagonist in clinical trials. *Biochemical Pharmacology*, *68*, 1479–1487.

174. Yip, J., Soghomonian, J.J., Blatt, G.J. (2007). Decreased GAD67 mRNA levels in cerebellar Purkinje cells in autism: pathophysiological implications. *Acta Neuropathologica*, *113*, 559–568.

175. Benes, F.M., Berretta, S. (2001). GABAergic interneurons: implications for understanding schizophrenia and bipolar disorder. *Neuropsychopharmacology*, *25*, 1–27.

176. Heckers, S., Stone, D., Walsh, J., Shick, J., Koul, P., Benes, F.M. (2002). Differential hippocampal expression of glutamic acid decarboxylase 65 and 67 messenger RNA in bipolar disorder and schizophrenia. *Archives of General Psychiatry*, *59*, 521–529.

177. Rajkowska, G., Miguel-Hidalgo, J.J. (2007). Gliogenesis and glial pathology in depression. *CNS & Neurological Disorders Drug Targets*, *6*, 219–233.

178. Rajkowska, G., O'Dwyer, G., Teleki, Z., Stockmeier, C.A., Miguel-Hidalgo, J.J. (2007). GABAergic neurons immunoreactive for calcium binding proteins are reduced in the prefrontal cortex in major depression. *Neuropsychopharmacology*, *32*, 471–482.

179. Brodie, M.J. (1995). Tiagabine pharmacology in profile. *Epilepsia*, *36*(Suppl 6), S7–S9.

180. Suzdak, P.D., Jansen, J.A. (1995). A review of the preclinical pharmacology of tiagabine: a potent and selective anticonvulsant GABA uptake inhibitor. *Epilepsia*, *36*, 612–626.

181. Alberici, M., Rodriguez De Lores, A., De Robertis, E. (1969). Glutamic acid decarboxylase inhibition and ultrastructural changes by the convulsant drug allylglycine. *Biochemical Pharmacology*, *18*, 137–143.

182. Richens, A. (1991). Pharmacology and clinical pharmacology of vigabatrin. *Journal of Child Neurology*, *2*(Suppl 2), S7–S10.

183. French, J.A. (1999). Vigabatrin. *Epilepsia*, *40*(Suppl 5), S11–S16.

184. DeFeudis, F.V. (1982). Muscimol and GABA-receptors: basic studies and therapeutic implications. *Reviews in Pure & Applied Pharmacological Sciences*, *3*, 319–379.

185. Olsen, R.W. (1981). The GABA postsynaptic membrane receptor-ionophore complex. Site of action of convulsant and anticonvulsant drugs. *Molecular and Cellular Biochemistry*, *39*, 261–279.

186. Olsen, R.W., Leeb-Lundberg, F. (1981). Convulsant and anticonvulsant drug binding sites related to GABA-regulated chloride ion channels. *Advances in Biochemical Psychopharmacology*, *26*, 93–102.

187. Guidotti, A., Dong, E., Matsumoto, K., Pinna, G., Rasmusson, A.M., Costa, E. (2001). The socially-isolated mouse: a model to study the putative role of allopregnanolone and 5alpha-dihydroprogesterone in psychiatric disorders. *Brain Research. Brain Research Reviews*, *37*, 110–115.

188. Concas, A., Mostallino, M.C., Porcu, P., Follesa, P., Barbaccia, M.L., Trabucchi, M., Purdy, R.H., Grisenti, P., Biggio, G. (1998). Role of brain allopregnanolone in the plasticity of gamma-aminobutyric acid type A receptor in rat brain during pregnancy and after delivery. *Proceedings of the National Academy of Sciences of the United States of America*, *95*, 13284–13289.

189. Pakes, G.E., Brogden, R.N., Heel, R.C., Speight, T.M., Avery, G.S. (1981). Triazolam: a review of its pharmacological properties and therapeutic efficacy in patients with insomnia. *Drugs*, *22*, 81–110.

190. Greenblatt, D.J., Shader, R.I. (1978). Prazepam and lorazepam, two new benzodiazepines. *The New England Journal of Medicine*, *299*, 1342–1344.

191. Atack, J.R., Hutson, P.H., Collinson, N., Marshall, G., Bentley, G., Moyes, C., Cook, S.M., Collins, I., Wafford, K., McKernan, R.M., Dawson, G.R. (2005). Anxiogenic properties of an inverse agonist selective for alpha3 subunit-containing GABA A receptors. *British Journal of Pharmacology*, *144*, 357–366.

192. Mirza, N.R., Nielsen, E.O. (2006). Do subtype-selective gamma-aminobutyric acid A receptor modulators have a reduced propensity to induce physical dependence in mice? *The Journal of Pharmacology and Experimental Therapeutics*, *316*, 1378–1385.

193. Mirza, N.R., Rodgers, R.J., Mathiasen, L.S. (2006). Comparative cue generalization profiles of L-838, 417, SL651498, zolpidem, CL218,872, ocinaplon, bretazenil, zopiclone, and various benzodiazepines in chlordiazepoxide and zolpidem drug discrimination. *The Journal of Pharmacology and Experimental Therapeutics*, *316*, 1291–1299.

194. Doble, A. (1999). New insights into the mechanism of action of hypnotics. *Journal of Psychopharmacology (Oxford, England)*, *13*, S11–S20.

195. Petroski, R.E., Pomeroy, J.E., Das, R., Bowman, H., Yang, W., Chen, A.P., Foster, A.C. (2006). Indiplon is a high-affinity positive allosteric modulator with selectivity for {alpha}1 subunit-containing GABAA receptors. *The Journal of Pharmacology and Experimental Therapeutics*, *317*, 369–377.

196. Najib, J. (2006). Eszopiclone, a nonbenzodiazepine sedative-hypnotic agent for the treatment of transient and chronic insomnia. *Clinical Therapeutics*, *28*, 491–516.

197. Petroski, R.E., Pomeroy, J.E., Das, R., Bowman, H., Yang, W., Chen, A.P., Foster, A.C. (2006). Indiplon is a high-affinity positive allosteric modulator with selectivity for alpha1 subunit-containing GABAA receptors. *The Journal of Pharmacology and Experimental Therapeutics*, *317*, 369–377.

198. Lippa, A., Czobor, P., Stark, J., Beer, B., Kostakis, E., Gravielle, M., Bandyopadhyay, S., Russek, S.J., Gibbs, T.T., Farb, D.H., Skolnick, P. (2005). Selective anxiolysis produced by ocinaplon, a GABA(A) receptor modulator. *Proceedings of the National Academy of Sciences of the United States of America*, *102*, 7380–7385.

199. Griebel, G., Perrault, G., Simiand, J., Cohen, C., Granger, P., Decobert, M., Francon, D., Avenet, P., Depoortere, H., Tan, S., Oblin, A. Schoemaker, H., Evanno, Y., Sevrin, M., George, P., Scatton, B. (2001). SL651498: an anxioselective compound with functional selectivity for alpha2- and alpha3-containing gamma-aminobutyric acid(A) (GABA(A)) receptors. *The Journal of Pharmacology and Experimental Therapeutics*, *298*, 753–768.

200. Griebel, G., Perrault, G., Simiand, J., Cohen, C., Granger, P., Depoortere, H., Francon, D., Avenet, P., Schoemaker, H., Evanno, Y., Sevrin, M., George, P., Scatton,

B. (2003). SL651498, a GABAA receptor agonist with subtype-selective efficacy, as a potential treatment for generalized anxiety disorder and muscle spasms. *CNS Drug Reviews*, *9*, 3–20.

201. Atack, J.R., Wafford, K.A., Tye, S.J., Cook, S.M., Sohal, B., Pike, A., Sur, C., Melillo, D., Bristow, L., Bromidge, F., Ragan, I., Kerby, J., Street, L., Carling, R., Castro, J.L., Whiting, P., Dawson, G.R., McKernan, R.M. (2006). TPA023 [7-(1,1-dimethylethyl)-6-(2-ethyl-2H-1,2,4-triazol-3-ylmethoxy)-3-(2-fluor ophenyl)-1,2,4-triazolo[4,3-b]pyridazine], an agonist selective for alpha2- and alpha3-containing GABAA receptors, is a nonsedating anxiolytic in rodents and primates. *The Journal of Pharmacology and Experimental Therapeutics*, *316*, 410–422.

202. Sprenger, K.J., Aneiro, L., Fung, L., Changchit, A., Rajachandran, L., Kehne, J.H., Xie, L. (2007). III. Clinical trial data demonstrating sedative-hypnotic efficacy of the α3-subunit preferring GABAA receptor partial allosteric activator, NG2-73: Translational validity of pharmacokinetic/pharmacodynamic (PK/PD) relationships derived from preclinical studies, in *Society for Neuroscience Annual Meeting* (San Diego, CA).

203. Lelas, S., Rowlett, J.K., Spealman, R.D., Cook, J.M., Ma, C., Li, X., Yin, W. (2002). Role of GABAA/benzodiazepine receptors containing alpha 1 and alpha 5 subunits in the discriminative stimulus effects of triazolam in squirrel monkeys. *Psychopharmacology*, *161*, 180–188.

204. Skolnick, P., Hu, R.J., Cook, C.M., Hurt, S.D., Trometer, J.D., Liu, R., Huang, Q., Cook, J.M. (1997). [3H]RY 80: a high-affinity, selective ligand for gamma-aminobutyric acidA receptors containing alpha-5 subunits. *The Journal of Pharmacology and Experimental Therapeutics*, *283*, 488–493.

205. Huang, Q., He, X., Ma, C., Liu, R., Yu, S., Dayer, C.A., Wenger, G.R., McKernan, R., Cook, J.M. (2000). Pharmacophore/receptor models for GABA(A)/BzR subtypes (alpha1beta3gamma2, alpha5beta3gamma2, and alpha6beta3gamma2) via a comprehensive ligand-mapping approach. *Journal of Medicinal Chemistry*, *43*, 71–95.

206. Bartholini, G. (1985). GABA receptor agonists: pharmacological spectrum and therapeutic actions. *Medicinal Research Reviews*, *5*, 55–75.

207. Blake, J.F., Cao, C.Q., Headley, P.M., Collingridge, G.L., Brugger, F., Evans, R.H. (1993). Antagonism of baclofen-induced depression of whole-cell synaptic currents in spinal dorsal horn neurones by the potent GABAB antagonist CGP55845. *Neuropharmacology*, *32*, 1437–1440.

208. Tian, N., Slaughter, M.M. (1994). Pharmacology of the GABAB receptor in amphibian retina. *Brain Research*, *660*, 267–274.

# INDEX



*Targets and Emerging Therapies for Schizophrenia*, First Edition.
Edited by Jeffrey S. Albert and Michael W. Wood.